GASTROINTESTINAL ENDOSCOPY IN PRACTICE

Commissioning Editor: *Michael Houston*
Development Editor: *Joanne Scott*
Editorial Assistant: *Poppy Garraway*
Project Manager: *Beula Christopher*
Design: *Charles Gray*
Illustration Manager: *Gillian Richards*
Illustrators: *Michel Politur/Richard Tibbitts*
Marketing Manager(s) (UK/USA): *Gaynor Jones/Abigail Swartz*

GASTROINTESTINAL ENDOSCOPY IN PRACTICE

Jean Marc Canard MD

Gastroenterologist, GI Endoscopist
Past President of the French Society of Gastrointestinal Endoscopy (SFED)
Trocadéro Clinic
Paris, France

Jean-Christophe Létard MD

Gastroenterologist, GI endoscopist
Past Vice President of the French Society of Gastrointestinal Endoscopy (SFED)
General Secretary of the French Association of Private Gastroenterology (CREGG)
Department of Gastroenterology and Hepatology
Polyclinique de Poitiers
Poitiers, France

Laurent Palazzo MD

Gastroenterologist, GI Endoscopist
Past President of the French Society of Gastroenterology (SNFGE)
Past President of the French Society of Gastrointestinal Endoscopy (SFED)
Medical Surgical Federation of Hepato-gastroenterology
Beaujon Hospital, University of Paris, Clichy, France;
Trocadero Clinic, Paris, France

Ian Penman BSc, MD, FRCP Edin

Consultant Gastroenterologist
Centre for Liver and Digestive Disorders
Royal Infirmary of Edinburgh
Edinburgh, UK

Anne Marie Lennon MD, MRCPI, PhD

Assistant Professor of Medicine
Director of the Pancreatic Cyst Clinic
Johns Hopkins Medical Institutions
Baltimore, MD, USA

For additional online content visit expertconsult.com

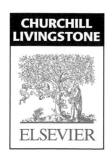

CHURCHILL LIVINGSTONE

ELSEVIER

Edinburgh   London   New York   Oxford   Philadelphia   St Louis   Sydney   Toronto   2011

An imprint of Elsevier Limited

Churchill Livingstone

British Library Cataloguing in Publication Data

Gastrointestinal Endoscopy in Practice.
1. Gastrointestinal system – Diseases – Diagnosis.
2. Gastrointestinal system – Endoscopic surgery.
3. Endoscopy.
I. Canard, Jean.
616.3'307545–dc22

9780702031281

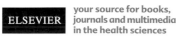
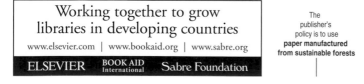
Printed in China
Last digit is the print number: 9   8   7   6   5   4   3   2   1

Contents

Jean Marc Canard MD

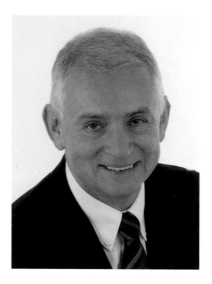

Jean-Christophe Létard MD

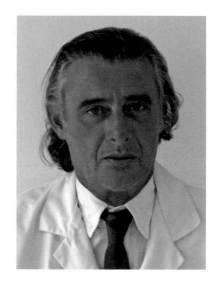

Laurent Palazzo MD

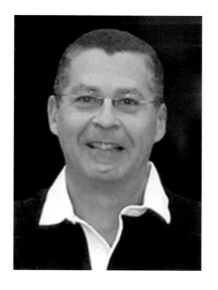

Ian Penman BSc, MD, FRCP Edin

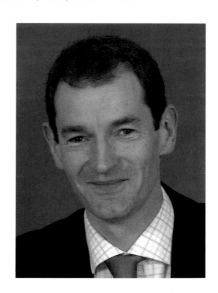

Anne Marie Lennon MD, MRCPI, PhD

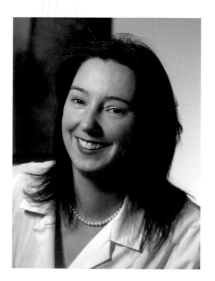

Preface

The first edition of *Gastrointestinal Endoscopy in Practice* was written by leading French endoscopists and published in 1994. Its aim was to provide an easy to read, comprehensive guide to endoscopy. This, the third edition, is the first English language edition of the book. The authorship is truly international and we believe it provides a comprehensive guide to diagnostic and interventional endoscopy. The book adopts a practical approach, with step by step guides to performing procedures, the inclusion of clear algorithms which summarize clinical decision making and approx 1260 high quality endoscopic images and illustrations. Throughout the book, clinical tips are given to aid the endoscopist and potential 'danger' areas to be aware of are highlighted.

This new edition is organised into ten different sections. The first and second sections cover the essential prerequisites for undertaking endoscopic procedures as well as safety and quality issues relating to endoscopy. The third, fourth, fifth and sixth sections provide a step by step guide on performing diagnostic upper endoscopy and colonoscopy as well as imaging the small bowel and advanced imaging techniques: these include confocal endomicroscopy, autofluorescence, narrow band imaging and magnification endoscopy. Section seven covers the most commonly performed interventional techniques including recent developments such as radiofrequency ablation for early Barrett's neoplasia and mucosal resection techniques. The final sections have detailed chapters on two specific procedures: endosonography (EUS) and ERCP. These chapters have been completely rewritten and illustrated. As elsewhere in the book, the emphasis is on practicality and clear instruction on performing these complex procedures to the highest possible standard.

This first English edition strives to uphold the tradition of excellence established in the original French editions. We believe that the third edition of *Gastrointestinal Endoscopy in Practice* remains an ideal resource for everyone involved in endoscopy, from endoscopy trainees and nurse endoscopists to established endoscopists, nursing and technical staff. We hope you agree.

Jean Marc Canard
Jean-Christophe Létard
Laurent Palazzo
Ian Penman
Anne Marie Lennon
2011

List of Contributors

Jean Marc Canard MD
Gastroenterologist, CI Endoscopist
Past President of the French Society of Gastrointestinal
    Endoscopy (SFED)
Trocadéro Clinic
Paris, France

Christophe Cellier MD
Professor of Gastroenterology
President of the French Society of
    Gastrointestinal Endoscopy (SFED)
Department of Endoscopy
Georges Pompidou University Hospital
Paris, France

François Cessot MD
Consultant Gastroenterologist
Department of Gastroenterology and Endoscopy
Centre Hospitalier d Aix en Provence
Aix-en-Provence, France

Nicholas I. Church MD, MRCP
Centre for Liver and Digestive Diseases
Royal Infirmary of Edinburgh
Edinburgh, UK

Pierre-Adrien Dalbies MD
Gastroenterologist
Saint Privat Clinic
Béziers, France

Michel Delvaux MD
Consultant Gastroenterologist
Department of Internal Medicine and Digestive Pathology
University Hospital of Nancy
Hospital de Brabois
Vandoeuvre-les-Nancy, France

Kerry B. Dunbar MD
Assistant Professor of Medicine
Division of Gastroenterology and Hepatology
VA North Texas Heathcare System
University of Texas Southwestern Medical Center at Dallas
Dallas, Texas, USA

Jacques Etienne MD
Specialist PDT in digestive Cancerology
President PDT and Photodiagnostic Commission at CREGG
Trocadero Clinic
Paris, France

Isaac Fassler MD
Consultant Gastroenterologist
Department of Internal Medicine and Digestive Pathology
University Hospital of Nancy
Brabois Hospital
Vandoeuvre les Nancy, France

Muriel Frédéric MD
Consultant Gastroenterologist
Department of Internal Medicine and Digestive
    Pathology
University Hospital of Nancy
Brabois Hospital
Vandoeuvre les Nancy, France

Gérard Gay MD
Professor of Medicine
Department of Internal Medicine and Digestive
    Pathology
Brabois Hospital
Vandoeuvre-les-Nancy, France

Denis Heresbach MD, PhD
Professor of Gastroenterology
Endoscopic Unit
Department of Hepato-gatroenterology
Hospital of Cannes
Cannes, France

Sanjay Jagannath MD, FASGE, AGAF
Director
Center for Comprehenive Pancreatic Care
Mercy Medical Center
Baltimore, MD, USA

Anthony N. Kalloo MD
Moses and Helen Golden Paulson Professor of
    Gastroenterology
Director, Division of Gastroenterology and Hepatology
Johns Hopkins Hospital
Baltimore, MD, USA

Mouen Khashab MD
Assistant Professor of Medicine
Director of Therapeutic Endoscopy
Division of Gastroenterology and Hepatology
Department of Medicine
Johns Hopkins School of Medicine
Baltimore, MD, USA

Jean Lapuelle MD
Gastroenterologist
Saint Jean du Languedoc Clinic
Toulouse, France

Anne Marie Lennon MD, MRCPI, PhD
Assistant Professor of Medicine
Director of the Pancreatic Cyst Clinic
Johns Hopkins Medical Institutions
Baltimore, MD, USA

Anne Le Sidaner MD
Consultant Gastroenterologist
Department of Hepato-Gastroenterology
Limoges University Hospital
Limoges, France

Jean-Christophe Létard MD
Gastroenterologist, GI Endoscopist
Past Vice President of the French Society of
 Gastrointestinal Endoscopy (SFED)
General Secretary of the French Association of Private
 Gastroenterology (CREGG)
Department of Gastroenterology and Hepatology
Polyclinique de Poitiers
Poitiers, France

Bernard Marchetti MD
Gastroenterologist
Biotech-Germande laboratory
Parc scientifique de Luminy
Marseille, France

Bertrand Napoleon MD
Gastroenterologist, GI Endoscopist
Past President of the French Society of Gastrointestinal
 Endoscopy (SFED)
Hôpital Privé Jean Mermoz
Lyon, France

Marcel Happi Nono MD
Gastroenterologist
Private Practice
Tours, France

Geneviève Obel
Chief of the Staff Nurses
Trocadéro Clinic
Paris, France

Patrick Okolo III MBBS, MPH,FASGE
Chief of Endoscopy
Johns Hopkins Hospital
Baltimore, MD, USA

Laurent Palazzo MD
Gastroenterologist, GI Endoscopist
Past President of the French Society of Gastroenterology
 (SNFGE)
Past President of the French Society of Gastrointestinal
 Endoscopy (SFED)
Medical Surgical Federation of Hepato-gastroenterology
Beaujon Hospital, University of Paris, Clichy, France;
Trocadero Clinic, Paris, France

Ian Penman BSc, MD, FRCP Edin
Consultant Gastroenterologist
Centre for Liver and Digestive Disorders
Royal Infirmary of Edinburgh
Edinburgh, UK

Denis Sautereau MD
Professor of Gastroenterology
Past president of the French Society of Gastrointestinal
 Endoscopy (SFED)
Department of Hepato-gastroenterology
Limoges University Hospital
Limoges, France

Vikesh K. Singh MD, MSc
Assistant Professor of Medicine;
Director, Pancreatitis Center;
Medical Director, Pancreatic Islet Cell Autotransplantation
 Program
Division of Gastroenterology
Johns Hopkins Hospital
Baltimore, MD, USA

Pascale Stelian
Consultant
Private Practice
Paris, France

Rémi Systchenko MD
Gastroenterologist
Department of Hepato-gastroenterology
Centre for Liver and Digestive Diseases of South West Lyon
Irigny, France

Dedications

To my wife Marie-Christine, without whom nothing would be possible. To my parents, especially my mother Amélie, my children Jean-Denis, Juliette, Axelle, Lucille and Valentin and Titouan, my grandsons. To my brother Francis, his wife Caroline, to Julien and Charlotte, and all my family and friends, present through the good and bad times.

To my colleagues who have supported me in every sense of the word.

Jean Marc Canard MD

To my wife Mette Galatius Jensen and children Nikita, Louis, Mia Rindra, Marie Fétroline and to my endoscopy mentor Professor Denis Sautereau who is renowned in France for the teaching of digestive endoscopy during the last ten years.

Jean-Christophe Létard MD

To my wife Elisabeth, whom I love, without whom I could never have got involved in the teaching of endoscopy. For my two boys, Maxime and Alexis, who bring me so much kindness and for their love of family and their unwavering support.

Laurent Palazzo MD

To my wife Jacqueline and children Heather and Harris, who put up with so much and are a constant source of support and encouragement to me.

To my endoscopy mentors for their skilful teaching, wisdom and patience – Kelvin Palmer, Robert Hawes and Peter Cotton. Also to John Dagg and Kenneth McColl, who tried to teach me to think like a physician and scientist.

Ian Penman BSc, MD, FRCP Edin

To Robert, for his constant support and encouragement.

Anne Marie Lennon MD, MRCPI, PhD

Acknowledgments

The editors wish to thank all of the book's co-authors, who receive a token of our profound admiration for their qualities as endoscopists and equally for their kindness and friendship which they have shown us by agreeing to take part in writing this book. Dr Zenobia Casey, Johns Hopkins Hospital for her advice on sedation during endoscopic procedures and Ronald J Wroblewski RN, Johns Hopkins Hospital, for his assistance and input with the preendoscopy checklist and Dr Siobhan Mc Grane, for her assistance with the imaging and anatomy sections in chapter 10. We would also like to thank the administrative council of SFED. The editors wish to give their profound thanks to Joanne Scott, Michael Houston and Gavin Smith at Elsevier for their tireless support during preparation of this book.

CHAPTER 1

Introduction to endoscopy

1.1 Anatomy of an endoscope

Jean Marc Canard

Summary

Key Points

- Modern endoscopes are complex and expensive instruments and, for optimum performance and safe use, all endoscopists should be familiar with their design and construction.
- Endoscopists should be able to set up and connect an endoscope for a procedure correctly, and safely disconnect it afterwards.
- Understanding this allows endoscopists to troubleshoot common problems that may occur with e.g. lighting, suction, valves, etc.

Introduction

Although endoscope performance and reliability have vastly improved since they were first introduced in the 1960s, they are still tricky to handle and knowledge of their various components and features will enable their optimum and efficient use.

An endoscope is composed of the following elements: a control handle, the insertion tube and the connecting cable to the processor/generator.

1. The control handle

The control handle (Fig. 1) combines the following elements:

- The main insertion tube, which terminates at the bending section
- The generator connecting cable, which has a connector at the end of it.

The control handle is intended for use with the left hand only, and combines all the necessary controls, which are ergonomically positioned. They consist of the following:

- Suction valve
- Air insufflation and lens cleaning valve

- Bending section and the control wheels
- Instrument elevator lever (depending on model)
- Proximal opening of the operating channel, which combines a watertight seal
- Buttons to freeze or capture an image or start video recording
- Buttons to activate the electronic zoom mechanism or switch imaging modes (e.g. FICE or NBI; see Ch. 6.2).

1.1. Suction and insufflation/cleaning valves

These contain joints that create a watertight seal and operate in cylinders. Suction and insufflation/cleaning occurs continuously so as to minimize delays on activation. The buttons also contain an air vent stack and, when released, return to their resting position by means of retraction springs.

1.1.1. Suction

The cylinder (Fig. 2), which is attached to the aspirator at its base, communicates with the operating channel, to which it is joined by a circular channel.

The plunger houses a vent, which is uppermost when the plunger is in its resting position. The vent points upwards relative to the cylinder lumen, and air enters the cylinder via the plunger's air vent stack.

When the plunger moves downward with its air vent stack occluded, the narrow portion of the vent appears opposite the lumen, followed by the wider portion of the vent, thus ensuring that there is sufficient suction force.

1.1.2. Insufflation–cleaning

The cylinder (Fig. 2) integrates separate inlets and outlets for air and water. The inlet–outlet group that is closest to the base is the insufflation channel. The second group, which is higher up, is the lens cleaning channel.

DOI: 10.1016/B978-0-7020-3128-1.00001-8

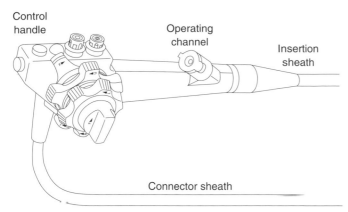

Figure 1 Control handle.

A large water reservoir integrated into the middle section of the button separates the air and water.

The insufflation channel is open while in the resting position, but air escapes from the stack, which is larger than the insufflation tube and combines a one-way anti-insufflation valve.

When the plunger moves downwards, its base closes off the insufflation channel, and the water reservoir is moved into a position facing the cleaning channel. Inasmuch as the air pulsed by the insufflation pump cannot escape, it provides the pressure in the cleaning flask necessary to propel the water into the line.

This mechanism is either fully activated or deactivated, i.e. there is no intermediate position.

 Clinical Tips

- To activate suction, block the orifice of the air vent stack with your left index finger and press down on the button. The amount of suction force is determined by how far the button travels into its cylinder.
- To activate air insufflation, block the orifice of the air vent stack with your left middle finger, but without pressing down on the button. As air can no longer exit the stack, it is forced into the insufflation channel valve.
- To clean the lens, press down on the air button as far as it will go.

1.2. Bending section controls

The two flexing controls (Fig. 3) (large wheel for up/down, small wheel for left/right) are coaxial and each has a separate brake.

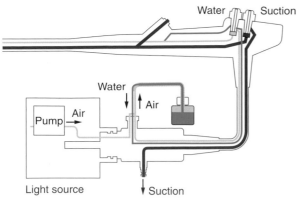

Figure 2 Aspiration and insufflation–cleaning pistons.

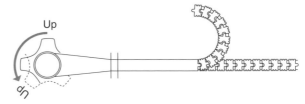

Figure 3 Bending section controls.

The most reliable system currently available comprises a cable wound onto a drum. The control cable is attached to the middle of the drum. Each free element makes a dead turn on the drum before being attached to the bending section cable.

When the drum is rotated using the control wheel, it rolls up the cable, which is attached to the tip of a series of articulated steel rings that are attached to each other (like vertebrae) and can bunch up in such way as to provoke the deformation shown in Figure 3.

There are generally either four or six control buttons housed on top of the control handle.

1.3. Elevator control

The cable's relatively short path enables a bar to be activated by a lever, which in turn mobilizes the elevator.

1.4. Operating channel

This channel has two functions: it allows instruments to be passed to the endoscope's distal tip, and it is also used for suction. The channel is metal from its proximal opening to a point beyond the suction/insufflation buttons but from here distally is made of plastic. The two materials are joined at a cone (via a female element) that occludes the tube's plastic walls.

2. Main insertion tube

The insertion sheath, which is mounted on the handle, combines the following elements:

- The fiberoptic image conductor
- One or more illumination bundles
- The operating channel
- The cleaning, and air/water insufflation channels
- The four bending section cables, which are in a separate sheath
- The elevator control cables.

The sheath, which terminates at the bending section, contains the lens at its distal tip and is used to explore the various parts of the gastrointestinal tract. It is fairly supple for the esophagus and stomach, but far more so in the duodenum. Hence, duodenoscope sheaths exhibit differential flexibility in their distal third segments. The segment of the sheath that is in the stomach is stiff enough to prevent it from forming loops as it passes along the greater curve.

Internally, the sheath (Fig. 4) contains a spiral metal element covered with a metal plait that provides the external synthetic resin coating with support. The characteristics of the spiral determine the texture of the sheath, depending on

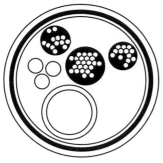

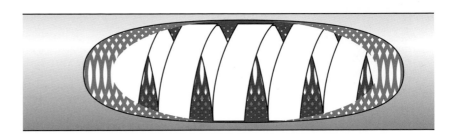

Figure 4 Sheath structure.

the thickness of the metal element, and the extent to which the wound elements tend to form joints with each other. The type of metal used is also a key factor. Stainless steel is used for the upper segment, whereas bronze is used for longer colonoscopes. Alternatively, to obtain better rotational torque, two parallel coaxial spiral elements are integrated and move in opposite directions in such a way that they oppose each other.

3. Bending section

The bending section (Fig. 3), which is the continuation of the main sheath, bears a strong resemblance to an alligator's spine. The bending section is composed of a series of circular rings that are reciprocally articulated at a 90° angle. Each ring combines hinge plates that guide the bending section cables and keep them in place. The cables, which are soldered to the distal chain, pass over the hinge plates, and when they reach the main sheath, they enter the insertion tube. The rings must be non-contiguous, so that when a cable is pulled, causing the rings to bunch up toward the sheath, they cannot pivot on their axes and abut each other. When two cables are pulled concurrently, the flexing occurs at the bisector of the angle formed by the cables. Multidirectionality is obtained by the force of these crossed impulses.

Inasmuch as the rings are non-contiguous, they are covered with a plate that prevents them from pinching the external rubber coating, which is usually glued and stitched to either end of the bending section.

This method, although more rudimentary than vulcanization, is highly advantageous, in that it allows for rapid replacement of the cladding if it shows any signs of weakness.

4. The optical head

The optical head (Fig. 5), which is an endoscope's most distal component, provides either forward or side-viewing optics, depending on its intended destination and use.

The optical head is mounted on the distal end of the bending section, where all of the elements that are accommodated by the main sheath are attached in a watertight manner.

4.1. Forward-viewing optics

The light bundles are sealed in a watertight casing. The lens casing is rendered watertight by a parallel or prismatic porthole that accommodates the lens in its enclosure with or without a focusing element, and then the image conductor, which is wedged into the lens chamber. The air insufflation channel and the cleaning channel are bundled on a sprayer that moves toward the lens porthole to allow it to be washed.

The operating channel terminates at the lens, the head of which accommodates a protective rubber sleeve that prevents contact with the mucosa.

4.2. Side-viewing optics

The elements of this head are connected as described in the previous section.

The light source is bent at an angle and ends at the lens, which is mounted on the axis of the head and shines through a rectifier prism. The operating channel terminates next to the lens and is fitted with an elevator tab, the rest position of which is at a 45° angle relative to the conduit axis.

5. Generator connecting cable

This cable, which is attached to the control lever, accommodates the endoscope's electrical and mechanical

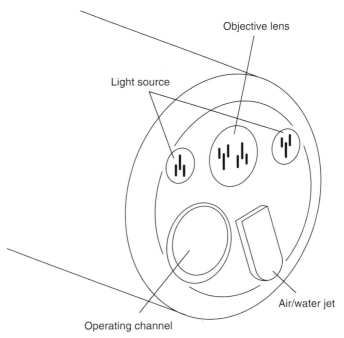

Objective lens

Light source

Air/water jet

Operating channel

Figure 5 Optical head.

connections (tubes that bring fluids and also current from the generator to which the cable is connected via a port).

The sheath is structured in exactly the same way as the main sheath. The connector combines lateral elements that accommodate the suction tube and the water bottle tubing.

Conclusion

Videoendoscopes have supplanted fiberscopes. Fiberoptic image conductors have been replaced by miniature charge coupled devices (CCDs) that are increasingly sophisticated and that allow the operator to see far more detail than would be possible with the naked eye, while still employing the same types of operator controls and channels without compromising robustness or reliability (Fig. 6).

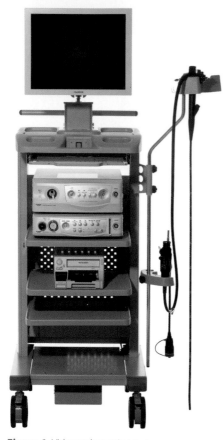

Figure 6 Videoendoscopic tower.

1.2 Electronic videoendoscopy

Jean Lapuelle

Summary

Introduction 5	2. Electronics and the endoscope 7
1. Electronic videoendoscopes 5	Conclusion 8

Key Points

- Videoendoscopes have replaced fiberoptic instruments for almost all indications.
- Endoscopists should have a basic understanding of the principles of light transmission and how electronic video imaging works.
- Coupled charge device (CCD)s are improving all the time with greater numbers of pixels and miniaturization allowing better quality imaging by smaller diameter endoscopes.
- Optical and electronic magnification systems allow greater resolution of surface detail.
- Recent advances in technology allow endoscopists to see more mucosal detail and thus a greater understanding of mucosal anatomy and pathology will be required of endoscopists.

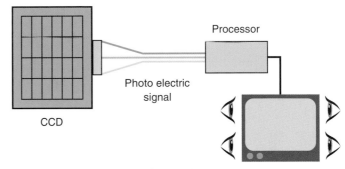

Figure 2 Operating principle of videoendoscope.

Introduction

The endoscope has changed greatly since the Bozzini endoscope was introduced in 1795 as the first instrument that allowed for rectal examinations. In the intervening two centuries, numerous advances have been made, notably the development of the rigid gastroscope, in 1868. The era of modern endoscopy was ushered in when the flexible endoscope came on the market in 1958.

In a fiberoptic endoscope, image resolution is determined by the number of optical fibers in the image bundle. Hence, image resolution is limited by the size of each fiber. This technology gradually improved to the point where, by the mid-1980s, each colonoscope contained 35 000 fibers.

Fiberoptic endoscopes have a number of serious drawbacks:

- Only one lens is available, which makes training in diagnosis and therapy difficult (Fig. 1).
- Endoscope fibers tend to break, such that:
  - Increasing numbers of black dots appear, which greatly reduce image quality
  - Bundle frame changes and color distortion occurs, particularly in terms of red light.

In 1983, Welch Allyn introduced the first electronic endoscope on whose distal end a miniature camera was mounted, thus replacing the fiberoptic bundle.

The first electronic videoendoscope came on the market around 1986 (Fig. 2).

1. Electronic videoendoscopes

The electronic videoendoscope works like a digital camera. Its distal end combines a coupled charge device (CCD; Fig. 3). This technology allows better image transmission and storage, leading to improved diagnosis and therapy. It has a coupled charge device and a color system.

1.1. Coupled charge device (CCD)

A CCD is composed of a silicon semiconductor with an insulating oxide coating to which aluminum electrodes known as MOS (metal oxide semiconductors) are attached. MOS are photosensitive, and convert light to electricity in accordance with the brightness of the light. The atoms of the MOS photosensitive surface store an electric charge when exposed to light. The accumulated electrical charge is proportional to the intensity of the incident light.

The photosensitive surface of a CCD is divided into a large number of photodiodes. This image element is often incorrectly referred to as a pixel. However, the photodiode that captures the light is actually part of the pixel, which is also

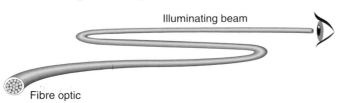

Figure 1 Operating principle of a fiberoptic endoscope.

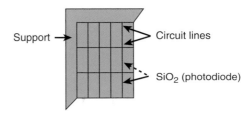

Figure 3 Coupled charge device (CCD) elements.

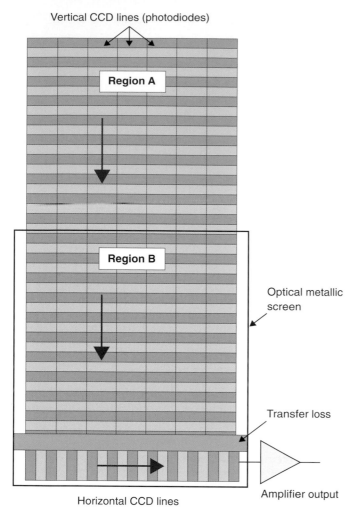

Vertical CCD lines (photodiodes)

Region A

Region B

Optical metallic screen

Transfer loss

Amplifier output

Horizontal CCD lines

Figure 4 Frame transfer.

This transfer process, which occurs extremely rapidly, occurs in various ways depending on the type of CCD used.

1.2. CCD frame transfer (Fig. 4)

CCD frame transfer provides optimal resolution and sensitivity. The image zone that gathers the electrons is transferred to a memory zone of the same size that is shielded from the light source. This separation increases sensitivity, thus providing maximum image-surface efficiency. The drawback of this solution is that it involves the use of a relatively large CCD.

1.3. CCD interline transfer (Fig. 5)

This configuration contains, alternatively, an image element area, as well as an electron transfer area that is shielded from the light source. These frames thus integrate a memory adjacent to each sensitive line and engender substantial dead areas in the final images. This is why relatively small CCDs exhibit limited sensitivity, despite their good resolution.

1.4. Full frame read-out CCD (Fig. 6)

This technology is identical to frame transfer CCD, but lacks a storage area that is shielded from the light source. Hence, these CCDs are small. Their drawback is that the lighting is not available throughout the reading process, as it is desirable to alternate between luminance at the charge creation locus and dark periods during which these charges are transferred.

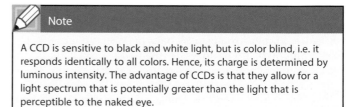

> **Note**
>
> A CCD is sensitive to black and white light, but is color blind, i.e. it responds identically to all colors. Hence, its charge is determined by luminous intensity. The advantage of CCDs is that they allow for a light spectrum that is potentially greater than the light that is perceptible to the naked eye.

the charge transmission channel. Thus a pixel actually refers to a device's resolution, not the number of photosensitive cells (photodiodes) it combines.

If a digital camera is said to have a resolution amounting to 6.2 million pixels, this means that the CCD comprises 3.3 photodiodes. However, this artificially widens the scope of the definition, since additional pixels are produced by means of a software process known as interpolation. Interpolation involves inserting a new pixel into an image via a calculation between a number of existing pixels. It degrades the quality of the original image, which is why it is necessary to speak in terms of photodiodes rather than pixels.

Division of the target allows each photodiode to respond independently to the amount of light reflected by the tissue.

Photodiodes are discharged during the reading process before a new charge acquisition cycle begins. The reading process is extremely rapid, but during it, the electrical charges continue to accumulate on the image that is being transmitted. These additional (thermal) charges accumulate even in the absence of light. This signal is stronger for lines that are read last, i.e. the lines at the top of the image. This results in a problem known as image smearing, which can be resolved by transferring the useful portion of the frame to an area that is shielded from the light source.

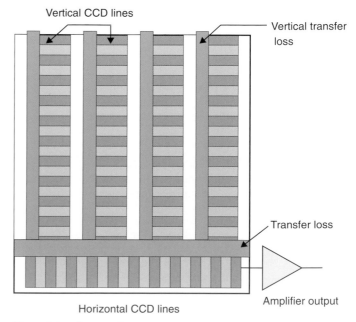

Vertical CCD lines

Vertical transfer loss

Transfer loss

Amplifier output

Horizontal CCD lines

Figure 5 Interline transfer.

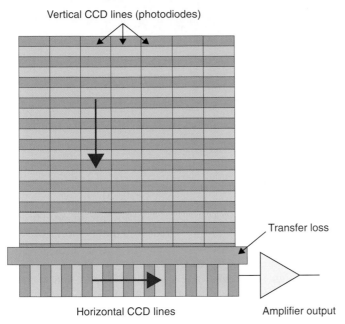

Vertical CCD lines (photodiodes)

Transfer loss

Horizontal CCD lines   Amplifier output

Figure 6 Full-frame read-out.

Color is not a physical reality. It is an impression generated in our brain, via our eyes, by luminous radiation from objects. In 1676, Isaac Newton showed that sunlight can be broken down into the colors of the spectrum by passing light through a prism (Fig. 7).

Light is composed of electromagnetic waves. Visible light comprises a continuous spectrum, the wavelengths of which range from 380 to 780 nanometers (nm). Each element of white light has a refraction coefficient that varies according to the element's wavelength.

1.5. Color system selection

1.5.1. Sequential system: black and white CCD

This system successively analyzes the light reflected by an illuminated object based on the three primary colors: red, green, and blue. Inasmuch as all colors of the rainbow can be created using these primary colors, a color can be reconstituted via color superimposition using a black and white sensor.

Sequential lighting is obtained via a filter wheel that rotates at a rate of 30–50 times per second in front of the light source, while electric signals are emitted sequentially rather than concurrently. Hence, the information must be stored and projected concurrently 25 times per second via a video monitor. The video processor converts the analog information into a digital code, whereupon the inverse operation

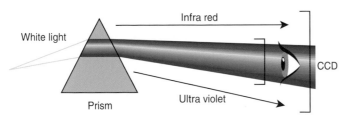

Infra red

White light

CCD

Prism   Ultra violet

Figure 7 White-light decomposition through a prism.

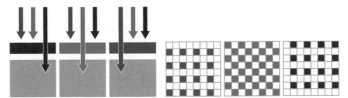

Figure 8 CCD colors.

generates a television image. This system enables the processing and analysis of increasingly sophisticated CCD images, thus in turn giving an improvement in diagnostic capability.

1.5.2. CCD colors: a mosaic system

A CCD combines a mosaic filter that is transparent to one of the primary colors (red, green, or blue) or their complements (cyan, magenta, or yellow). Each photodiode captures a color and then reconstitutes a pixel using four photodiodes. Inasmuch as cyan is composed of blue and green, and yellow is composed of red and green, the color green has more potential luminance, i.e. red and blue have only 25% as much luminance as green (Fig. 8).

2. Electronics and the endoscope

A video processor combines and processes information transmitted by a CCD in order to translate this information into a television image. This image is transmitted in two steps, or rather in two half-images using lines, i.e. odd-numbered lines followed by even-numbered lines. These are called interlaced images. In endoscopy, a CCD image must comprise a certain minimum number of vertical and horizontal pixels, which determine the image's definition. Image resolution is determined by the number of pixels per image unit. Hence, image quality is determined by image definition and resolution. If the image does not contain enough pixels, it will not fill the screen. Latest generation CCDs allow for full-screen images.

2.1. Blooming

The capacity of each CCD pixel to store electrons is limited. If there is too much light, the electrons jump to the adjacent pixels, resulting in image distortion, as well as a phenomenon known as blooming (color dissociation at the edge of the object). Integration of an anti-blooming system changes the sensitivity via a loss of some of the photosensitive surface of a pixel.

2.1. Resolution

A light sensor comprises a fixed number of pixels. A lens's resolution allows it to separate the image details. Resolution patterns make it possible to take real-time measurements in practice. The theoretical limit is reached when a pair of black and white lines is projected onto a pair of pixels.

The best videoendoscope is one whose CCD contains the most pixels, depending on the type of transfer system used. Some CCDs only use a portion of the image elements, while reserving the others for the transfer process.

Box 1 Advantages of electronic videoendoscopes

- Image resolution superior to that obtained with fibroscopes.
- The image can be viewed by a number of people at the same time in the examination room and remotely.
- Electronic videoendoscopes make the endoscopist more efficient by optimizing the intervention procedure and reducing the risk of complications associated with information transfer.
- Allows the operator to freeze images and archive the examination.
- Electronic videoendoscope hardware has a longer service life than that of videoscopes, with no image deterioration over time (black spots).

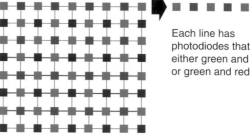

Each line has photodiodes that are either green and blue or green and red

Figure 9 Classic CCDs.

Today, owing to improvements in image stability, color CCDs are gaining ground on their black and white counterparts and manufacturers are currently focusing on the following developments:

- CCD miniaturization, such that the 1/2″ pixel will be replaced by a 1/10″ pixel, which will allow extremely small devices such as transnasal videogastroscopes that are 5–6 mm in diameter, and twin-channel instruments that expand the range of therapeutic options
- High definition CCDs with very high numbers of pixels that allow for full screen images, i.e. very high definition CCDs (≥850 000 pixels).

Completely digital electronic videoendoscope systems (i.e. from the endoscope to the screen) open up (a) a major field of investigation by virtue of the wealth of information that is captured by the CCD; and (b) new image processing options.

Endoscopic imaging is making major advances thanks to the migration to digital technology.

Once the pixel count, lens, and field of exploration have been improved, the range of structures amenable to examination can be expanded by greatly improving the peripheral contrast of a lesion and enhancing its relief.

Addition of a zoom function may represent a major advance, but must nonetheless be validated scientifically. The following types of zooms are currently in use:

- An optical zoom function that allows for 100–150 times magnification of the image of the previously viewed lesion. When combined with chromoendoscopy or narrow band imaging (NBI, FICE, iSCAN), these zoom functions enable the detection and assessment of subtle, superficial lesions in the upper GI tract and colon (see Ch. 6.2).
- An electronic zoom allows artificial magnification of pixels.

Conclusion

Electronic videoendoscopes still await further technological improvements in terms of CCDs and pixel counts.

New high resolution CCDs are 45% smaller than classic CCDs and integrate octagonal photodiodes that theoretically allow storage of more information in the same surface area. With this type of CCD, 1.7 times more photodiodes can be obtained relative to the previous generation of CCDs (Figs 9, 10).

These super-CCDs and their zoom functions facilitate detection and diagnosis of early neoplasia of pit patterns and by characterization of capillary vascular patterns. Other technologies are in the pipeline that are based on certain characteristics of silicon and that will allow a single photodiode to capture three colors. This will obviate the need for colored filters, greatly reduce the scope of color reconstitution calculations and algorithms, increase image processing, and heighten sensitivity.

Thus, in the foreseeable future, we may have videoendoscopes that contain more than 5 million photodiodes.

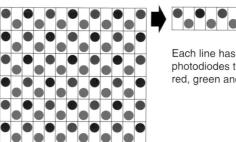

Each line has photodiodes that are red, green and blue

Figure 10 Super CCDs.

Further Reading

Houcke P, Canard J-M, Chirol P-L, et al: Evaluation technique des vidéo-endoscopes couramment utilisés en gastro-entérologie [Technical evaluation of gastroenterological videoendoscopes], *Hépatogastroenterology* 6:495–504, 1997.

Machida H, Sano Y, Hamamoto Y, et al: Narrow-band imaging in the diagnosis of colorectal mucosal lesions: a pilot study, *Endoscopy* 36(12):1094–1098, 2004.

Pelletier M: La technique du zoom ou magnification. [Zoom/magnification techniques] CREGG, Paris, 27 September 2003, *Acta Endoscop* 33(Suppl 3):446, 2003.

Endoscopic accessories

Jean-Christophe Létard, Jean Marc Canard

Summary

Key Points

- A vast array of endoscopic accessories is available and new ones are being developed as novel interventional endoscopic procedures are described.
- Endoscopy units should stock an adequate range and supply of commonly used accessories at all times.
- Endoscopists should be familiar with the appropriate and safe use of all endoscopic accessories.
- All staff should be trained in the safe use of endoscopic accessories.
- In many countries, legislation mandates single-use, disposable accessories to comply with infection control policies.

Introduction

Millions of endoscopic procedures are performed each year around the world and interventions ranging from biopsy to complex therapeutic procedures are increasingly undertaken. At upper endoscopy, biopsies are the most common intervention, while therapeutic procedures, e.g. PEG insertion or variceal therapy, occur in 7–10% of cases. Other procedures such as dilatation, esophageal stenting, argon plasma coagulation (APC), endoscopic mucosal resection (EMR) and polypectomy are increasingly undertaken. Polypectomy is the main therapeutic procedure performed at colonoscopy (10–25%), other interventions being performed in 2.5% of cases (argon plasma coagulation (APC), EMR, dilatation, and stenting).

Medical supplies needed for endoscopic procedures relate to both patients and caregivers: disposable paper hospital gowns, absorbent pads, paper gowns for staff, non-sterile gloves and gauze swabs or compresses. Oxygen masks and tubing, lubricant gel and Xylocaine spray are also necessary. Small transparent caps to facilitate magnifying endoscopy and disposable brushes are also indispensable. Endoscopic accessories must be available that allow for grasping and biopsy, injection, hemostasis, mechanical suture, dilatation, sectioning, and prosthetic re-establishment of gastrointestinal lumens.

1. Tissue grasping and acquisition

Gastrointestinal biopsies pose a major challenge for the endoscopist. They are undertaken using 5 mm-long forceps with spoon-shaped jaws (Fig. 1), which employ one of the following mechanical principles:

- *Pantograph*, whose jaws close via a cable controlled mechanism
- *Passive sheath*, where the jaws scissor and enter via traction provided by a sheathed cable
- *Ball and socket*, which combines the two aforementioned principles, whereby the articulating ball greatly reduces the amount of effort needed to operate the forceps
- *Forceps with a multiple aspiration chamber* and guillotine sectioning, which allow a number of specimens to be taken simultaneously.

Forceps are available in different lengths and external diameters to be compatible with gastroscopes, (including pediatric instruments), colonoscopes, and enteroscopes. Biopsy specimen size appears to correlate with the forceps jaw size. A central metal spike is not mandatory and can in fact damage the endoscope operating channel.

The removal of foreign bodies requires longer, and in some cases rubberized, crocodile or rat-tooth forceps. Dormia baskets, polyp traps and 'Roth' nets can be used for batteries and components. It is useful to have an overtube for the extraction of foreign bodies >6 cm in length, to prevent them being dropped and inhaled on removal, and protective sheaths for the removal of sharp objects.

2. Injection

Injections are performed: (a) with the aid of a basic catheter for fluoroscopic opacification (prior to insertion of a gastrointestinal stent); (b) with the aid of a spray catheter for chromoendoscopy, or (c) via disposable needles for tattooing, hemostasis, variceal sclerotherapy, chromoendoscopy (see Ch. 2.4), EMR, submucosal dissection, and antireflux treatment (Fig. 2).

Injection hemostasis is performed using adrenaline diluted to 1/10 000 for gastroduodenal ulcers, Mallory–Weiss tears, acute Dieulafoy lesions polyps and bleeding diverticula. Polidocanol (1%), or 5% ethanolamine is used for esophageal variceal sclerotherapy. Injection catheters are being improved constantly, with needles ranging from 18 to 23 gauge that slide very easily in 7–8 French catheters, some of which contain a cleaning system. Biological tissue

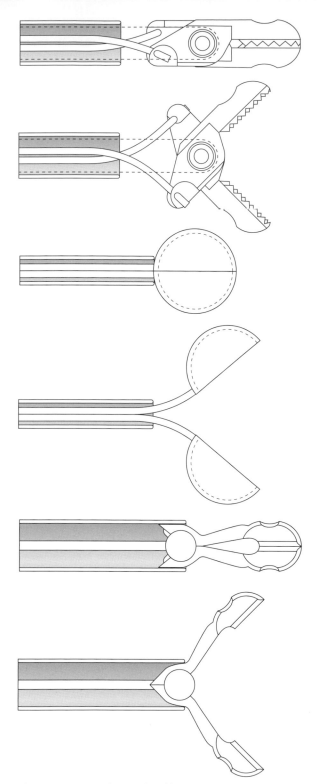

Figure 1 Mechanical principles of biopsy forceps: pantograph, passive sheath, and ball and socket.

adhesives can be used with dual-chamber needles. Precision relies on the length and diameter of the chosen needle (narrow for injection of fluid, larger diameter for injection of carbon for tattooing; short bevelled needle for the colon, longer for the upper GI tract).

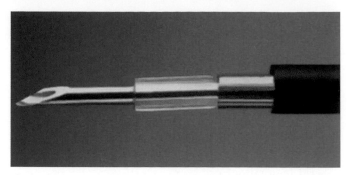

Figure 2 Injection needle with cleaning channel.

3. Clips and ligation devices

Hemostasis can be performed using clips and ligation systems. Reusable and disposable clipping systems are available and their use is described in Chapter 7.8. Clips can also be used for marking the site of a lesion or for closing small perforations that occur during polypectomy, EMR or ESD. Disposable ligation systems are available with 6–10 elastic bands for esophageal variceal ligation and to assist EMR (Ch. 7.8). They are also used for hemostasis of bleeding Dieulafoy lesions, and for Mallory–Weiss tears (Fig. 3).

Disposable *miniloops* that work like clips can also be used, particularly in the gastric cardia. Detachable snares ('endoloops') are very useful for preventing post-polypectomy bleeding. However, they are contraindicated for polyps with thin or short stalks, as premature transection of the stalk and bleeding can occur.

4. Dilatation

Dilatation (see Ch. 7.1) is performed using progressively larger bougie dilators over a rigid or semi-rigid metal guidewire or else using disposable balloons (Fig. 4A). Balloon diameters and length vary. The balloons are passed through the operating channel and dilatation is performed hydrostatically (except in cases of achalasia) under visual and/or fluoroscopic control.

5. Coagulation

Coagulation (see Ch. 1.4) can be monopolar, bipolar (Fig. 4B), or multipolar, and can be performed using dedicated probes. Coagulation is useful for tumor debulking and for hemostasis. In monopolar coagulation, a high-frequency

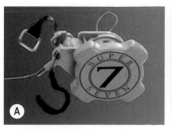
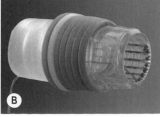

Figure 3 (A) Rotating handle that is attached to the operating channel at the height of endoscope handle. (B) Ring with elastic bands, attached to the distal end of the endoscope.

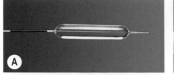 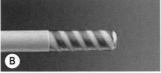

Figure 4 (A) Dilatation balloon. (B) Bipolar coagulation probe.

electric current is applied to the tissue, requiring a patient grounding pad (25–40 watt (W) pulses for 7–10 s). This method is risky as the muscle layer may be coagulated and delayed perforation may occur. Argon plasma coagulation (APC) is less risky, and is also more appealing by virtue of its cost-effectiveness and multifunctionality (60 W, 0.8–1.5 l/mn). The advantage of bipolar coagulation, which uses three electrodes, is that the electric current is conducted back to the electrosurgical generator (useful in the presence of a pacemaker).

Bipolar probes contain a lateral spiral filament at their distal end (10–20 W, 3–4 pulses lasting 10–14 s each). The contact must be tangential as the distal tip of the probe is perforated and has no conductor, thus allowing for cleaning. Some probes are equipped with a distal injection needle. Diathermic heater probes (Fig. 5A), which are used in some countries, comprise an internal thermocouple that generates a constant temperature of 250°C at the distal end (which has an anti-adhesive coating). This system also houses three 1-cm cleaning channels above the active distal portion (8-s 20–30 joule pulses).

6. Tissue resection

Sectioning (see Ch. 7.11) occurs using 200–500 volts HF current that generates an electric arc between the diathermy snare and the tissue. The latest generation of electrosurgical generators allows automatic stabilization of fluctuations in potential and intensity. The heat generated at the points where the electric arc comes into contact with the tissue is so high that the tissue is immediately vaporized. Following this, as the snare moves across the tissue, electric arcs are generated continuously wherever the gap between the tissue and snare is small enough, thus producing the resection.

It is useful to have a range of snares (Figs. 5B,C,D): monofilament; braided; small size (10 mm); large size (20–30 mm); asymmetric for esophageal EMR; and barbed for large colonic EMRs. Transparent caps with an edge groove (into which the loop inserts) are also essential.

7. Gastrointestinal stents

A range of self-expanding metal stents (SEMS) (see Ch. 7.2) are available for use in the esophagus, stomach, duodenum, biliary tree, and colon. Most of today's gastrointestinal prostheses are made of hardened steel (articulated components that are 2.5 cm in diameter and that do not become shorter on expansion), nitinol or Elgiloy (mesh or webbing composed of one or more wires, the length of which decreases by 30% as the prosthesis expands). The stents are straight, and may or may not have funnel-shaped or 'dog-bone' tips. Anchorage, extraction and antireflux valve systems are also available for these devices and some may be completely or partially membrane-covered to minimize tumor ingrowth.

Conclusion

Modern endoscopists must be familiar not only with an increasing range of endoscopes and techniques, but also a growing array of endoscopic accessories with which to undertake interventions. Sophisticated accessories and knowledge of how to use them properly underpin the success of complex therapeutic endoscopy.

> **Note**
>
> The American Society for Gastrointestinal Endoscopy (ASGE) website (www.asge.org) contains technology evaluation reports and guidance covering the majority of accessories used in endoscopic practice and is a valuable resource.

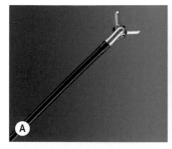 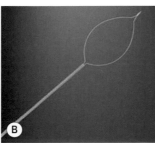 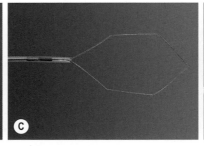 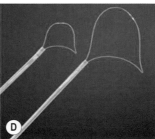

Figure 5 (A) Diathermic forceps. (B) Toothed (polypectomy) loop. (C) Hexagonal (polypectomy) loop. (D) Asymmetrical (mucosectomy) loops.

Further Reading

American Society for Gastrointestinal Endoscopy Committee: Technology Status Evaluation Report. Endoscopic hemostatic devices, *Gastrointest Endosc* 69(6): 987–996, 2009.

American Society for Gastrointestinal Endoscopy Committee: Technology Status Evaluation Report. Guidewires for use in GI endoscopy, *Gastrointest Endosc* 65(4):571–576, 2007.

American Society for Gastrointestinal Endoscopy Committee: Technology Status Evaluation Report, *Gastrointest Endosc* 65:741–749, 2007.

1.4   Electrosurgical generators: procedures and precautions

Jean Marc Canard, Ian Penman

Summary

Introduction   12

1. Electrophysical basis of electrosurgery   12

2. Problems associated with older electrosurgical generators   13

3. Principles of endoscopic diathermy (electrosurgery)   14

4. Coagulation   15

5. Monopolar and bipolar current   15

6. Alarm systems   16

7. Statutory requirements of endoscopy rooms   16

8. Precautions for cleaning and disinfection of equipment   16

9. Practical tips for endoscopic electrosurgery   16

Conclusion   17

Key Points

- Electrosurgical diathermy is an important component of daily endoscopy practice.
- A thorough understanding of the correct use of different types of electrosurgical current is essential.
- Newer generators provide automatic regulation of output power; they integrate an endoscopic diathermy ('endo-cut') mode (fractionated sectioning alternates automatically with low-intensity coagulation).
- Bipolar current does not produce effective tissue sectioning.
- Complications with electrosurgery result from the effects of the electric current. Perforations are almost always attributable to excessive coagulation of the gut wall and bleeding almost always results from unduly rapid cutting.
- Argon plasma electrocoagulation paved the way for the development of interventional endoscopy and has replaced laser methods for most of the latter's indications.

Introduction

To achieve satisfactory results when using electric current for polypectomy, EMR or sphincterotomy, tissue sectioning and hemostasis must be effective, and the following must be avoided:

- Immediate bleeding caused by unduly rapid sectioning or not enough coagulation
- Delayed perforation resulting from unduly slow sectioning or excessive coagulation.

Moreover, sectioning must begin carefully to avoid causing changes in tissues that are being coagulated. Advances in electrosurgical generator techniques help achieve these goals and this chapter describes their safe use.

1.   Electrophysical basis of electrosurgery

In-vivo application of electric current to biological tissues creates an *electrolytic effect, neuromuscular excitation,* and a *thermal effect.*

In endoscopy, only the thermal effect is used. It is obtained via high frequency AC current exceeding 300 kHz which, unlike low frequency current (e.g. household appliances), does not cause neuromuscular excitation or cardiac rhythm disturbances.

The heat provided and the tissue effects engendered by this are determined by *current intensity, specific tissue impedance* and *current-application time.*

- *Tissue resection* is obtained using intense heat. When intense heat is applied to tissues, water rushes out of the cells, which explode, thus triggering the resection. It can only occur in the presence of an electric arc and >200 V of electricity between the tissue and electrode (Fig. 1).
- *Low-intensity coagulation/desiccation* without an electric arc is performed using lesser intensities and engenders less heat. The water flows out of the cells and extracellular space slowly, and the tissues contract. Less than 190 V should be used to ensure that no electric arc forms (Fig. 2).
- *Forced coagulation* involves desiccation but uses higher voltage as for cutting, as well as an electric arc, which carbonizes the tissue.

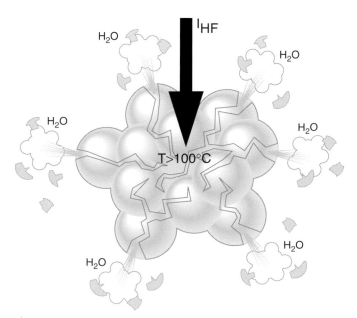

Figure 1 During sectioning, which is performed at temperatures exceeding 100°C, water comes rushing out of the cells and the cells explode.

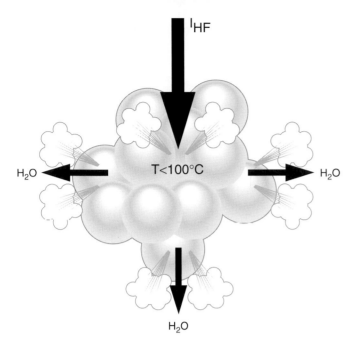

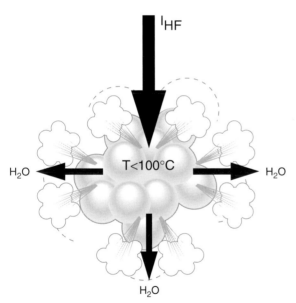

Figure 2 In coagulation, which is realized at temperatures of <100°C, the water emerges slowly from the cells, which retract.

- *Spray or fulguration coagulation* involves surface desiccation of the tissue, which is induced by ultra-high voltage (>4000 V) that produces a very large electric arc. However, the electrode does not come into contact with the tissue.
- *Argon plasma coagulation (APC)* uses very high voltage via a spray. The effect of the electric arc is mitigated by ionized gas, which distributes the energy evenly across the tissue without carbonizing it.

Sectioning, as well as the aforementioned monopolar coagulation methods, necessitates a second pole in the form of a neutral electrode, to recover the energy generated by the activated electrode or probe.

2. Problems associated with older electrosurgical generators

The power created by older electrosurgical generators is constant and does not vary with tissue and cutting surface impedance. Cutting speed and electric arc intensity are the only variable parameters with these devices. In today's generators, electric-arc intensity is constant and controlled. Cutting speed is preadjusted in endoscopic diathermy mode without the need for any action on the part of the operator. The electrosurgical generator's output power is regulated automatically in accordance with the contact surface. The most common unit is the ERBE ICC 200 (Fig. 3), recently replaced by the VIO 200 or 300 series.

2.1. The role of automatic regulation of the electric current

When, for example, 100 W of current pass through the tungsten filament of an electric light bulb, there is a substantial thermal effect that turns the filament white, thus generating light, which is in fact a secondary effect. In the copper wire that provides the electricity for the light bulb, this same electric current engenders little or no heat. Hence, various types of biological tissue exhibit differing levels of current impedance (resistance). In order to obtain a stable effect in tissue, the level of electric current administered to the tissue must be commensurate with the tissue's impedance, which, if elevated, requires relatively little voltage. Conversely, low-impedance tissue needs considerable voltage to achieve the same effect.

2.2. Sectioning may inadvertently result in tissue coagulation

This can occur if too little current is applied to the target contact surface (Fig. 4). Sectioning a 1 mm^2 contact surface requires a high level of current density. This same current applied to a 1 cm^2 surface will be unduly low and will induce coagulation. New electrosurgical generators avoid this problem by automatically adjusting the instrument's output current to the characteristics of the tissue being sectioned, within the limits of the maximum-current setting, which must be high enough to allow sectioning, as otherwise the tissue will be coagulated.

2.3. Consequences of using unsuitable settings for electrosurgical generators

The device settings must be defined in such a way as to (a) prevent the generator from peaking out; and (b) ensure that the device's power is sufficient to perform the section and does not induce coagulation and accidents.

 Clinical Tip

Complications result from the effects of the electric current. Delayed perforations are almost always attributable to excessive gastrointestinal wall coagulation, and bleeding usually results from unduly rapid cutting.

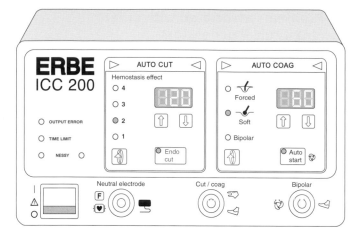

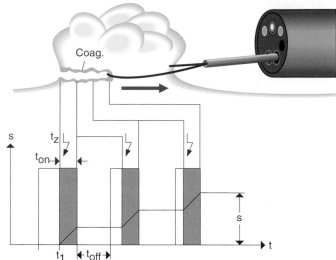

Figure 5 Endocut occurs by automatic alternation between sectioning and coagulation.

arc's voltage and intensity between the tissue and cutting wire are measured, analyzed and stabilized by an onboard microprocessor. Endoscopic diathermy is a fractionated process that is carried out via the following stages:

- The initial incision (variable duration) via the 'Power Peak System' (ERBE) or equivalent facility in other generators
- Sectioning when the electric arc first appears (roughly 50 ms)
- Low intensity (0 to 60 W) coagulation (roughly 750 ms).

All of these parameters are regulated automatically via the device's power.

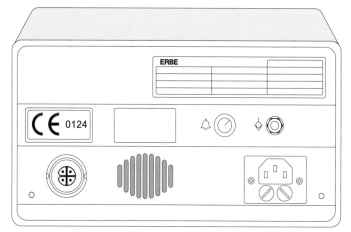

Figure 3 ICC 200 electrosurgical generator with endo-cut mode.

3. Principles of endoscopic diathermy (electrosurgery)

In endoscopic diathermy, all of the electrical settings that are applied to the section and its characteristics are automatically controlled and adjusted so as to achieve optimal cutting performance throughout the process (Fig. 5). The electrical

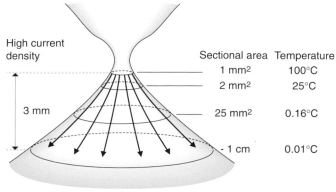

Figure 4 The heat generated increases exponentially as tissue surface area decreases.

3.1. The Power Peak System and Endocut

At the beginning of the process, the Power Peak System (PPS) delivers power exceeding the configured threshold for a few milliseconds (ms) so as to allow rapid initiation of resection.

Following this, in endocut mode, sectioning occurs for 50 ms, followed by low-intensity coagulation for 750 ms. Sectioning and coagulation alternate automatically until the tissue has been completely resected. When using 'endo-cut' mode, the operator should avoid pulling too hard on the snare, or closing it too tightly; it should be in gentle contact with the tissue at all times. This results in a slow cutting process that alternates with coagulation. The risk of hemorrhaging is greatly reduced if the operator does not section mechanically by pulling hard on the snare. By the same token, the risk of secondary perforation and excessive coagulation is reduced if the resection begins immediately on application of current.

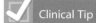 Clinical Tip

During polypectomy, do not pull hard on the snare or close it too tight as this will result in mechanical transection of the stalk and bleeding – let the endo-cut function of the generator section the stalk in a controlled manner.

3.2. What to do if the resection does not start immediately

There are two possible scenarios in this case:

- If you pull too hard on the snare or close too tightly, it will be 'buried' in the tissue and prevent the electric arc from firing.
- The contact surface between the snare and tissue may be unduly large. The larger this surface, the weaker the impedance and the more power needed to start the incision. If the incision fails to start, coagulation will occur instead of cutting (because current is nonetheless administered to the tissue). If this occurs, replace the snare and start again with more power (160–200 W).

The high power generated by an automatically regulated electrosurgical generator poses no risk for the operator for the simple reason that the device only generates the amount of power that is needed for sectioning.

3.3. Endocut for sphincterotomies

Endocut is used frequently for sphincterotomies with lower settings in some cases and identical settings in others, and using less coagulation than for polypectomies (endo-cut I mode in ERBE VIO). The use of an electrosurgical generator for sphincterotomies gives the operator better control over the sectioning process, without provoking bleeding, and this in turn avoids abrupt sectioning, perforations and secondary hemorrhaging. A randomized study comparing an Erbotom T175 (classic electrosurgical generator) with an ERBE ICC 200 (which has an endoscopic diathermy or 'endo-cut' function) revealed a significant difference in terms of reducing secondary bleeding.

3.4. Starting endocut

To start ('endo-cut') mode, press the yellow foot pedal, whereupon the cutting/coagulation cycle will take place automatically. All you need to define is the sectioning power threshold, in accordance with the diameter of the polyp that is being resected (if in doubt, use the 120 W default setting with effect level 3 or 2 hemostasis) and set the coagulation (blue pedal) to 'low' (60 W) to avoid an undesired result in the event of accidentally pressing the wrong pedal.

The low-coagulation power in endo-cut mode is set by default to from 0 to 60 W, which automatically overrides any manual setting on the electrosurgical generator.

4. Coagulation

4.1. Low-intensity coagulation

The low-intensity coagulation provided by using the blue pedal occurs without an electric arc or tissue coagulation. This type of coagulation is slow, penetrating, and provokes no bleeding.

4.2. Forced coagulation

Forced coagulation is obtained using 1300 V resulting in an electric arc and tissue carbonization. This type of coagulation

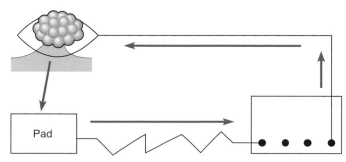

Figure 6 Monopolar current.

is quicker and less penetrating than low-intensity coagulation.

4.3. Spray-mode coagulation

Spray-mode coagulation is only used in gastrointestinal endoscopy in conjunction with an argon plasma coagulator and requires >4000 V of electricity. In this process, ionized argon gas is applied via flexible probes that do not come into contact with the tissue. The gas acts as an electrical conductor between the probe and tissue. Argon plasma distributes heat evenly across a very large surface. The coagulation is very rapid and does not penetrate nearly as deeply as with laser coagulation. However, the coagulation depth is determined by the preset power and particularly by the target-surface application time (there is no automatic regulation in Argon spray mode). For endoscopic procedures, APC is superior to laser coagulation for all indications other than destruction of bulky tumors, where laser still has a role.

5. Monopolar and bipolar current

5.1. Monopolar current (Fig. 6)

Monopolar current circulates between the active electrode (diathermy snare, hot biopsy forceps, sphincterotome), and the patient grounding pad.

5.2. Bipolar current (Fig. 7)

Here, the second electrical pole is located in very close proximity to the active element, and the current circulates between the two ends. If a bipolar snare was used with an electrosurgical generator for a bipolar section, the electric arc (and hence the resection) would occur on one side of the

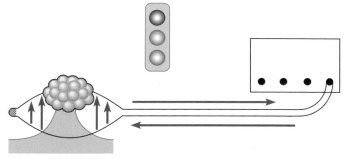

Figure 7 Bipolar current (returns to the electrosurgical generator).

snare only, where there is less contact with the tissue. The other side would assume the function of a neutral electrode and would coagulate rather than section. No bipolar instrument is available for endoscopic sphincterotomy and for polypectomy. Bipolar current is used *solely* for coagulation with specific *bipolar probes*. The coagulation depth obtained with bipolar current is less than with monopolar current owing to the fact that the current is recovered immediately.

> **! Warning!**
>
> Bipolar devices should not be used for gastrointestinal procedures as they do not provide suitable tissue resection. Bipolar current should only be used for coagulation procedures in patients with cardiac pacemakers.

6. Alarm systems

These alarm systems allow for detection of:

- A defective or improperly connected patient grounding pad
- Incorrect voltage
- Improper pedal activation.

They ensure that endoscopic electrosurgery is safe for the patient and operator. The grounding pad monitoring system (NESSY) guarantees that no skin burn will occur under the neutral pad, providing that double-face pads are used (Fig. 8).

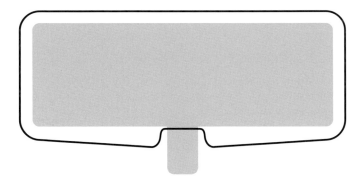

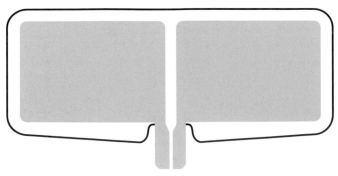

Figure 8 Single-side (A) and two-sided (B) pad. The latter is preferable.

7. Statutory requirements of endoscopy rooms

The endoscopy room must meet the following statutory requirements:

- It must have an antistatic floor
- It must have safe electrical sockets
- It must be devoid of any power strips, extension cords, loose wires or cables
- The electrical mains must be isolated by circuit breakers with a nominal current of 10 A.
- The electrosurgical generator must be set up in a location that is well ventilated to allow proper cooling.

8. Precautions for cleaning and disinfection of equipment

Clean the generator with products that are non-inflammable and non-explosive in a dry atmosphere. Do not clean the front panel of the device using alcohol or any hard or sharp equipment and do not allow any dampness to enter the generator. Argon plasma coagulation probes are single use and disposable in most countries, as are polypectomy snares and sphincterotomes.

9. Practical tips for endoscopic electrosurgery

9.1. General tips

- Only use double-face patient grounding pads
- Press the yellow pedal to cut and the blue pedal to coagulate
- When performing a polypectomy, bear in mind that the larger the contact surface between the snare and polyp, the lower the impedance in the tissue, which means that more power is needed to start sectioning
- An unduly tight snare will make it more difficult to start cutting
- If cutting does not begin immediately, withdraw the device at once, because current is still being administered and will coagulate the tissue instead of sectioning it. In such a case, replace the snare and start again
- If the polyp has a stalk, resect the polyp at the stalk's narrowest point.

9.2. Standard settings for an ERBE ICC 200 electrosurgical generator

The endoscopic diathermy ('endo-cut') function can only be obtained using the yellow pedal, in which case cutting and coagulation will alternate automatically (Fig. 9).

9.3. Polypectomy

- For polyps with a contact surface measuring <1 cm: endo-cut: hemostasis 3; 120 W; low-intensity coagulation: 60 W.
- For polyps with a contact surface measuring >1 cm: endo-cut: hemostasis 3; 160–200 W; low-intensity coagulation: 60 W.

9.4. Sphincterotomy

To avoid the problems caused by excessive contact surface between the sphincterotome and tissue, insert only the distal third of the cutting wire into the papilla. The endoscopic diathermy (endo-cut) function is adjusted for hemostasis and using the same amount of power as for a polypectomy (120 W). Low-intensity coagulation is performed using 60 W.

9.5. Endoscopic mucosal resection (EMR)

- For EMR without a submucosal injection: deactivate the endo-cut function by pressing the endo-cut button on the front of the generator and use hemostasis level 2 and 120 W. For continuous sectioning, press the yellow pedal.
- For EMR with a submucosal injection: endo-cut mode can be used with hemostasis set at 2 and 120 W.

There are small but significant differences with the newest range of ERBE electrosurgical generators (VIO 200 or 300) (Fig. 10). Two different endo-cut functions (Q and I) exist: 'endo-cut Q' is designed for polypectomy and functions much as described above with slow cutting and more coagulation. The standard setting for a polypectomy is 120 W, effect level 3 (the effect level can be reduced to 2 if less coagulation is desired). There are, however, many adjustable settings and general recommendations are outlined in Tables 1 and 2. 'Endo-cut I' is designed for sphincterotomy with a different cutting-coagulation cycle, designed for quick cutting and less coagulation, although it can be adjusted.

9.6. Argon plasma coagulation (APC)

Equipment settings and the use of APC is discussed in detail in Chapter 7.4.

Conclusion

Previous generation HF generators have the following drawbacks relative to the latest-generation devices: less regular cutting speed; sectioning is more difficult to initiate; less regular electrical arc intensity; greater risk of secondary perforation and/or hemorrhaging. New devices are superior in terms of: allowing automatic regulation of output power (regulated electrical arc); they integrate an endoscopic

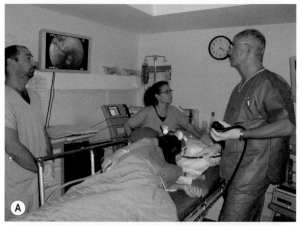

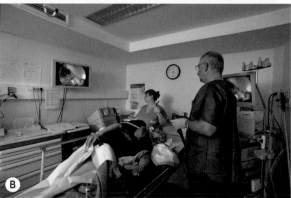

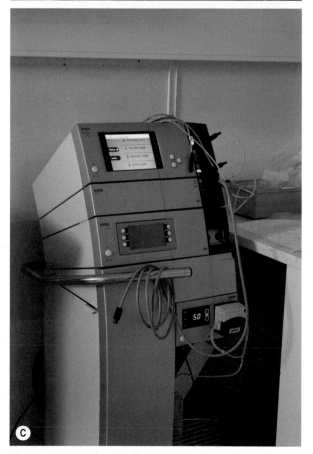

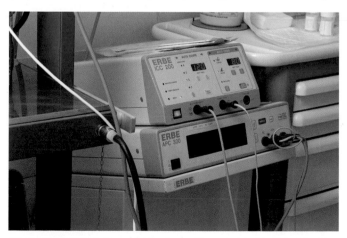

Figure 9 ICC 200 electrosurgical scalpel with a regulated endo-cut function for polypectomies.

Figure 10 (A) ESD for superficial gastric cancer. (B) Argon plasma coagulation for recurrence of esophageal cancer. (C) VIO ERBE 300 D with ERBE JET.

Table 1 Manufacturer's recommended settings for ERBE VIO series electrosurgical generators

Polypectomy

Pre-coagulation	Forced coagulation	Effect 1 – 50 W	Pre-coagulation for stalked polyps and those ≥2 cm
Duodenum-caecum-right colon	Endo-cut Q	Effect 1	Small polyps – no coagulation
		Effect 2	Larger polyps – with coagulation
Left colon-rectum	Endo-cut Q	Effect 2	Average polyp – normal coagulation
		Effect 3	Large polyp – more coagulation

Endoscopic mucosal resection

Marking	Soft coagulation or	Effect 5	Power – 80 W
	Forced coagulation	Effect 1	Power = 20 W
Resection	Endo-cut Q	Effect 2	

Sphincterotomy

Sphincterotomy	Endo-cut I	Effect 1	No coagulation
		Effect 2	With coagulation

Hot biopsy

Hot biopsy	Soft coagulation	Effect 5	Power = 80 W

diathermy ('endo-cut') mode (fractionated sectioning alternates automatically with low-intensity coagulation) and a Power Peak System. The latter system provides a burst of power (above the configured level) for a fraction of a second, thus allowing for a rapid start and avoiding gastrointestinal wall coagulation. These developments have improved the effectiveness and safety of many interventional therapeutic procedures.

Table 2 Manufacturer's recommended settings for ERBE VIO series electrosurgical generators when performing endoscopic submucosal dissection (ESD)

ESD

ERBEJet injection	Esophagus		Pressure 20–30
	Stomach		Pressure 20–40
	Duodenum-caecum-right colon		Pressure 20–30
	Left colon-rectum		Pressure 20–30
Marking	Soft coagulation or	Effect 5	Power 80 W
	Forced coagulation	Effect 1	Power 20 W
Incision	Endo-cut Q	Effect 2	
Dissection	Endo-cut Q	Effect 2	
	Swift coagulation	Effect 4	Power 40 W
Hemostasis	Soft coagulation	Effect 5	Power 80 W

Further Reading

ASGE Technology Committee: Technology status evaluation report. Electrosurgical generators, *Gastrointest Endosc* 58:656–660, 2003.

ASGE Technology Committee: Technology status evaluation report. The argon plasma coagulator, *Gastrointest Endosc* 55:807–810, 2002.

Canard JM, Ponchon T, Napoléon B, et al: Bistouris électriques: principes et précautions d'utilisation [Electrosurgical generators: usage principles and precautions] SFED, September 2003. www.sfed.org.

Canard JM, Védrenne B: Clinical application of argon plasma coagulation in gastrointestinal endoscopy: has the time come to replace the laser? *Endoscopy* 33(4):353–357, 2001.

Farin G, Grund KE: Technology of argon plasma coagulation with particular regard to endoscopic applications, *End Surg* 2:71–77, 1994.

Maier M, Kohler B, Benz C, et al: A new HF current electrosurgical generator with integrated self modifying system (endo-cut mode) for endoscopic sphincterotomy: a prospective randomized trial, *Gastrointest Endosc* 41:308, 1995.

Rey JF, Beilenhoff U, Neumann CS, Dumonceau JM: European Society of Gastrointestinal Endoscopy (ESGE) guideline: the use of electrosurgical units, *Endoscopy* 42(9):764–771, 2010.

1.5 Organizational structure of an endoscopy unit

Jean Marc Canard, Rémi Systchenko

Summary

Introduction 19	4. Information management system 24
1. Rooms 19	5. Quality assurance of endoscopy 24
2. Equipment 23	Conclusion 25
3. Medical and paramedical personnel 23	

Key Points

- Endoscopic procedures should ideally be carried out at dedicated endoscopy centers.
- Endoscopic centers should be equipped with facilities for the whole range of diagnostic and therapeutic endoscopy for the upper and lower GI tract.
- Careful planning is necessary when designing a new endoscopy center with due consideration of: design and layout; endoscopic equipment; infection control measures and disinfection facilities; patient flow and safety, and staffing requirements and needs.
- A quality assurance framework should be developed to cover all aspects of the center's activities and should be part of the endoscopy team's ethos and daily activities.

Introduction

Ever since its advent in the 1970s, gastrointestinal endoscopy has taken place at various types of medical facility.

Ideally, these procedures should be carried out at dedicated, autonomous centers, i.e. facilities that are specifically configured for endoscopy, preferably in an endoscopy room rather than an operating room (OR); or, failing that, in the OR of a dedicated ambulatory endoscopy and day surgery unit, rather than office-based endoscopy.

Endoscopic centers (Fig. 1) should be equipped with facilities for the whole gamut of diagnostic and therapeutic endoscopy for the lower and upper GI tract, and should also be equipped so that non-GI tract endoscopy can also be performed – particularly bronchoscopy, ENT, and urological endoscopy.

In view of the sizeable capital investments that are needed to provide high quality endoscopy, and particularly the safety-related expenditures entailed by modern endoscopy, small private practices may find it increasingly difficult to continue providing all of these services in the future. Modern endoscopy needs to occur in an autonomous endoscopy unit within a private or public hospital. An endoscopy unit is composed of rooms, equipment, and staff.

1. Rooms

An endoscopy unit contains the following types of rooms: endoscopy rooms; disinfection rooms; storage areas for equipment and supplies; waiting areas; office areas; changing rooms; a recovery room for patients who receive general anesthesia; a recovery room for patients who receive IV sedation; and a post-intervention monitoring area. Consultation rooms and offices for the unit's administrator and clerical staff are also indispensable. A radiology room should be provided at centers that undertake complex interventional procedures.

1.1. Endoscopy rooms

The number of endoscopy rooms should be appropriate for the number of procedures that are performed annually. These rooms should be equipped for upper and low GI tract procedures, as well as for endoscopic ultrasound.

1.1.1. Characteristics of an endoscopy room

- Floor dimensions: 20–30 sq meters
- Ceiling height: 2.7 meters
- Floors and walls that are conducive to washing
- Acoustic insulation
- Antistatic floor covering
- Air conditioning
- Automatic sliding doors so that trolleys and beds can be moved in and out
- Technical windows that communicate with the supply and disinfection areas so as to allow separate one-way flow of contaminated and clean equipment. Inasmuch as it is not possible for all endoscopy rooms to be adjacent to the disinfection rooms, trolleys should be available for the transport of endoscopes that are to be disinfected. The endoscopes should be transported in covered containers, with the devices submerged in an appropriate fluid. It is essential that there is a one-way flow of equipment from clean-to-dirty so that there is no chance of cross-contamination of clean equipment.
- Cabling for the following in the walls and ceilings: electricity; vacuum suction; oxygen; nitrogen; audio, video, and data cables.
- Fluid circulation, the number and location of electrical outlets, and emergency circuits must satisfy local health and safety laws and should be bundled on one or two distribution pendants.

1.1.2. Endoscopy room equipment

- The center of the room (Fig. 2) should contain a 60 cm wide trolley that can be oriented in any direction necessary and that has removable side-restraints. This trolley should be placed at a distance from the

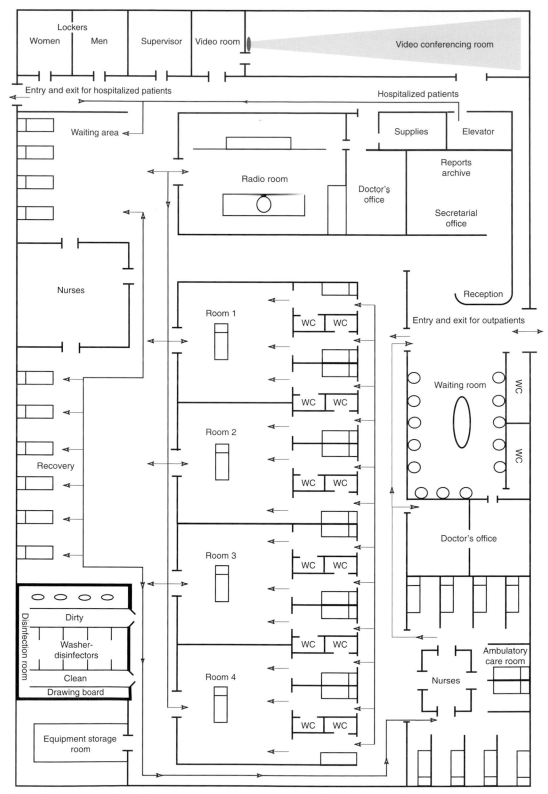

Figure 1 Endoscopic unit with five rooms, as well as separate pathways for outpatients and inpatients.

examination table so as to prevent patients from tampering with it.

- The endoscopy stack accommodates the screen, light source, video processor, electrosurgical generator, DVD/VCR, and photo printer.

- An instrument table containing the equipment that the nurses will need to have at their disposal, including the following: gloves; local anesthesia; lubricant; biopsy fixative jars; forceps; polypectomy snares; sterile brushes in individual pouches (for a multilevel table). The table

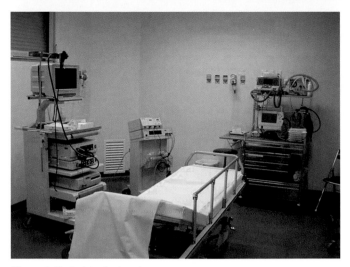

Figure 2 Gastrointestinal endoscopy room.

should also have dedicated spot lighting that is trained directly at it.

- Distribution arm for fluids, electricity, and video/data cabling, located above the video console.
- X-ray film viewer; work surface for patient records.
- A trolley or distribution arm for anesthesia/emergency procedures, equipped and meeting agreed resuscitation standards.
- Under the technical window, on the side containing the cleaning and disinfection surface, a work surface covered with a material that is atraumatic for endoscopes. Trolleys containing the endoscopes and their clean field (outbound) and the endoscope submersion container (inbound) are used in settings where the disinfecting room does not adjoin the endoscopy rooms.
- A washbasin with an automatic control that allows staff members to wash and disinfect their hands.
- A cabinet that is large enough to store all necessary supplies.
- The electrical equipment must comply with all applicable standards and regulations, and must be compatible with the room's specific equipment. Having numerous power cords on the floor of the room should be avoided, and towards this end, the distributing arm should house a sufficient number of outlets (five at a minimum).
- Wall-mounted vacuum suction: two separate connections are needed: one for the endoscope and the other for upper GI tract aspiration.
- Oxygen, supplied under constant pressure, should be available via the distributing arm if any examinations are to be undertaken under sedation or anesthesia.
- Audio/video and data line: the distribution arm should contain at least one audio and video input and output port, and two data ports.
- An endoscopist's desk for computer and dictation equipment.

1.1.3. Anesthesia equipment

Either the trolley containing the endoscopy accessories or a dedicated console must contain the equipment needed for sedation or anesthesia and to monitor patients until they

wake up. Endoscopic procedures that are performed without anesthesia or sedation, however, may also rarely be accompanied by cardiovascular and respiratory complications, particularly in patients at risk – which means that every endoscopy unit must be equipped for the diagnosis and management of such complications. Each endoscopy room must have equipment for monitoring of blood pressure, oxygen saturation, and heart rate. A trolley containing items that may be needed in an emergency should be kept close at hand and it should be checked daily.

1.2. Postoperative monitoring room and recovery room

All endoscopy units that administer general anesthesia or IV sedation should have a postoperative monitoring room where each patient's vital signs are monitored by a nurse (cardiac activity, pulse, blood pressure, and oxygen saturation). When the patient fully awakens they should be taken to the recovery room, where they remain until the doctor in charge authorizes their discharge. In some countries, nurse-led discharge policies exist, allowing them to discharge patients who meet key safety criteria, e.g. mobile, pain-free, normal observations. The postoperative monitoring room must comply with national safety standards (Fig. 3).

1.3. Cleaning room

The disinfecting room (Fig. 4) should be a separate, self-enclosed space that communicates with each endoscopy room via a technical window, or preferably a door that opens automatically. This room is used to clean and disinfect endoscopes. Medical supplies should not be sterilized in the disinfecting room. This should be done in a central sterilization facility that is used for the operating rooms, if the endoscopy unit is part of a hospital. Cleaning and disinfecting rooms for medical equipment must comply with legal regulations pertaining to design, methodology, and personnel training.

There should be one or more work surfaces for non-sterile items. Each surface should be cushioned and covered with a material that is not traumatic for endoscopes. There should

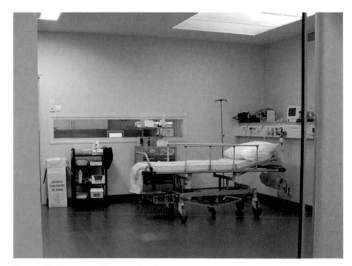

Figure 3 Postoperative monitoring room.

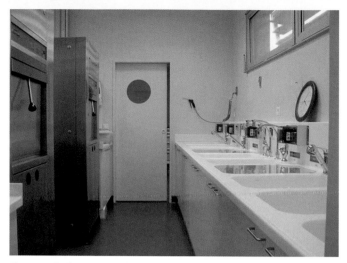

Figure 4 Endoscope disinfecting room.

be 4–6 cleaning sinks of adjustable height in which the endoscopes can be immersed in water. Each basin must have its own tap and drain.

The use of gluteraldehyde is illegal in many countries, as are other aldehyde disinfectants. In some countries it is mandatory to establish a wastewater disposal contract with the municipal authorities in charge of sewage treatment. A separate circuit can be established that allows wastewater to be channeled into a tank if necessary.

In most countries, manual disinfection has been replaced by the use of automated endoscope reprocessors (AERs), but the steps of manual cleaning are described here. There must be separate washing and rinsing basins for each stage of the washing process. A hot and cold water mixer tap must be available for one or two of the basins. In some countries, it is law that the basins used for disinfectant and for the final rinse should contain a 0.22 µm microbiological filter that is autoclaved daily and changed regularly in accordance with the manufacturer's instructions (after every 40–60 autoclave cycles). Basins used for detergent and disinfectant should be equipped with lids.

The microbiological and physical quality of the tap water used must meet the criteria of local health and safety regulations or infection control policies. However, in both treatment and disinfection rooms, so-called 'water for standard medical treatment' is sufficient if the quality of the water used by the unit is under active management. If not, so-called 'bacteriologically managed' water is to be used for the final rinse, as is done in washer-disinfectors.

Basins used for detergent and disinfectant should have a suction connection at the height of the basin and an extraction hood with an absorbent filter. The air recirculation system must have *separate* extraction and fresh air pipes. The fresh-air intake element should be located more than 8 meters away from the air extraction outlet element, and the air in the room should be exchanged at a rate of more than 10 volumes per hour. The room must be depressurized at all times. Endoscopes must be transported in covered plastic containers that are color coded: one color for contaminated endoscopes (e.g. red) and a second color for clean ones (e.g. green). These containers must be disinfected in a basin that is used for this purpose only.

1.3.1. Additional work surfaces should be provided

- A work surface for small components. After the endoscopes have been disinfected, the components are placed in an ultrasonic cleaning unit and are then dried using compressed air and put in pouches prior to being sterilized. In many countries, cleaning of small components by ultrasound is no longer recommended: buttons, valves etc are kept as a unique set with each endoscope and cleaned with the endoscope in the AER. This improves traceability should it be required.
- A 'clean' work surface for compressed air drying of endoscopes prior to storage.

The number of dedicated work surfaces for manual disinfection must be appropriate for the number of endoscopy rooms in the unit. These surfaces may be replaced by washer-disinfectors that do not dispense with the initial manual washing and rinsing phase and for which two dedicated basins are provided, i.e. one for washing and one for rinsing. If the endoscopy unit has only one washer-disinfector, it is essential to provide a work surface with four to six basins as back-up, in case the machine breaks down.

If washing and disinfecting are automated, at least one washer-disinfector should be provided for each endoscopy room. The type of machine should be specified for each room (i.e. synchronous or asynchronous machine; a washer-disinfector that can process one endoscope at a time, or two endoscopes at a time, in accordance with the type of activity in the room). Latest generation machines are 'pass-though', i.e. endoscopes that are contaminated are placed in the washers in one room and are removed from the opposite side in an adjacent clean room.

1.4. Endoscope storage room

The endoscope storage room (Fig. 5) must be separate from the disinfecting room and should contain vented cabinets to store endoscopes, endoscope accessories, and small implements. Endoscopes should be stored vertically. The utility of cabinets with high efficiency particulate air filtration (HEPA) systems, and their location, have yet to be clearly

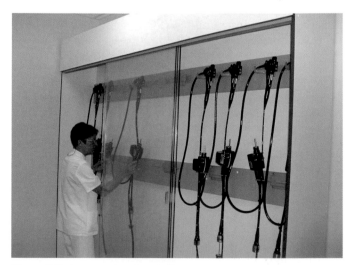

Figure 5 Endoscopes stored vertically.

established but they may allow clean endoscopes to be stored for up to 72 hours without the need for reprocessing prior to use.

1.5. Spaces for patients

An endoscopy unit must contain the following dedicated spaces for patients:

- A waiting room
- Several pre-procedure changing rooms, each containing a trolley and preferably a bathroom
- A recovery area, under a nurse's supervision, containing beds, trolleys, refreshments, and a TV.

1.6. Waiting area and reception desk

This area must be located at the entrance of the endoscopy unit and should be the place where patient records are stored. At endoscopy units that have a large number of patients, there should be one reception desk for appointments and preparing patient records and taking information confidentially from patients, and a second desk where reports are prepared and records are archived.

1.7. Consultation rooms

A consultation room allows a doctor to provide patients with the relevant information prior to and following an endoscopy examination. In endoscopy units that administer general anesthesia and handle large numbers of patients, there should also be an anesthesia-team station that adjoins the recovery area.

1.8. Office for the chief endoscopy nurse

This office allows management of the staff (nurses and doctors) and equipment in an endoscopy unit that handles a large number of patients.

2. Equipment

2.1. Endoscopes

Ideally, each endoscopy room should be equipped with at least four gastroscopes and four colonoscopes so that sufficient time is available for cleaning/disinfection and upkeep without the need to borrow instruments or reduce the unit's activities.

2.2. Medical instruments

This includes all items that are needed for endoscopy and that enhance its diagnostic and therapeutic efficacy. All of the following must be available at all times: biopsy forceps; washing or spray catheters; injection sclerotherapy needles; variceal ligation devices; thermal hemostasis probes; diathermy snares; hemostatic or perforation closure clips; and all necessary pancreaticobiliary endotherapy accessories, if the center performs ERCP. Centers performing EUS must keep a supply of different caliber needles for EUS-guided fine-needle aspiration (19–25 gauge).

3. Medical and paramedical personnel

3.1. Endoscopists

Gastrointestinal endoscopy involves diagnostic and therapeutic procedures for which the operator must possess an extremely high skill level and must be thoroughly conversant with gastrointestinal pathologies. Quality can only be maintained if the operators and their teams are highly experienced and competent. Operators must receive thorough endoscopy training from both a theoretical and a practical standpoint, based on structured training programs. It should begin during the initial months of a gastroenterology training program. The endoscopy trainee's competence should be objectively assessed before certification of competence can be issued.

3.2. Endoscopy nurse assistants

The training program for an endoscopy assistant is demanding and needs to include the following diverse topics:

- Preparing the patient for the procedure from a physical and psychological standpoint
- Technical assistance with endoscopic procedures, particularly for therapeutic endoscopy
- Familiarity with the risks associated with procedures and equipment
- Endoscope cleaning and disinfection
- Accessory sterilization
- Equipment maintenance
- Ordering and managing supplies
- Equipment storage.

It is essential for endoscopy assistants to continue with their training throughout their careers to keep abreast of new equipment and techniques. In many countries endoscopy nurses have their own societies or are officially part of the national society representing endoscopists and membership of such a body should be encouraged.

3.3. Medical secretaries

Endoscopy unit medical secretaries need specific training. Their main tasks involve scheduling appointments and providing operators with information regarding procedures and anesthesiology protocols. Medical secretaries must be sufficiently familiar with endoscopic procedures to provide patients with support in the form of information and encouragement. Endoscopy unit medical secretaries also type up medical reports and manage medical records.

All secretaries should have the same credentials and skill sets and should be interchangeable.

3.4. Endoscopy center administrator

An endoscopy unit requires a dedicated administrator who is in charge of ensuring that the unit functions smoothly. This should not be left to the general administrative department of the hospital. They should be conversant with all diagnostic and therapeutic procedures and the equipment used; and also the applicable regulations and policies regarding endoscope and accessory disinfection. They should also have basic knowledge of equipment management, as well as medical and paramedical personnel management.

4. Information management system

This system comprises the following:

- Medical records
- Patient pathways
- Equipment protocols
- An information network that can be queried remotely at external sites
- Shared medical records.

5. Quality assurance of endoscopy

This mechanism applies in France to institutions that are recognized as health centers within the framework of the institution's accreditation procedures. In other countries, quality metrics are employed for continuous service improvement. The database maintained by the French health public health organization known as Haute Autorité de Santé (HAS), now allows for hospital department self-assessment, which promotes the following: improvements

---

Box 1 The main requirements for the organizational structure of an endoscopy unit

The following requirements must be met in order for a gastrointestinal endoscopy unit to function properly.

- The unit's endoscopists must receive specific initial and continued training in gastrointestinal endoscopy, and this training must be quantifiable.
- The unit's endoscopy assistants, secretaries, and administrator must receive specific initial and continued training.
- The unit must have the capacity to provide all patients who undergo endoscopic procedures with safe and comfortable IV sedation or general anesthesia, subject to the patient's informed consent.
- Optimally safe conditions in all endoscopy rooms, even in the absence of general anesthesia or IV sedation.
- Rigorous and monitored cleaning and disinfection procedures for all equipment used.

- Use of automated washer-disinfectors with a view to improving standardization, tracing, and disinfection procedure monitoring, and in order to minimize factors that have a negative impact on staff performance.
- Use of videoendoscopy and keeping abreast of advances in this field.
- Having a sufficient number of endoscopes available to ensure that procedures can be carried out in light of the following: the time constraints associated with cleaning and disinfection (45–60 min); possible equipment malfunctions, and the need for maintenance and repair. A 'sufficient number' means four gastroscopes and four colonoscopes per endoscopy room.
- Sufficient equipment at all times to handle any complications that may arise without putting the patient at risk.
- Photographic, video and/or digital documentation should be available for each medical report.

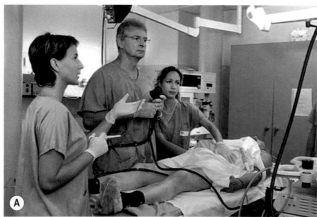

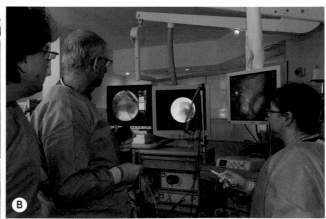

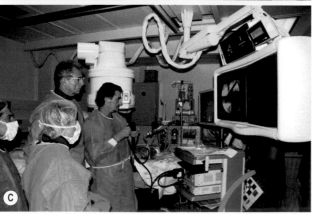

Figures 6 (A–C) Endoscopic praxis in endoscopic units that are part of public or private sector hospitals.

in patient management; reduced risk of nosocomial infection, optimization of department management practices (in terms of human resources, finances, logistics, and information systems); evaluation of professional practices. In the UK, all endoscopy units complete an online self-assessment tool every 6 months called the Global Rating Scale (www.grs.nhs.uk). This assesses multiple aspects of quality, including procedural quality indicators, patient experience, the endoscopy workforce and the quality of training. It provides a benchmark for endoscopy services and highlights areas for improvement.

Conclusion

The manner in which new endoscopy units should be organized is anything but a futuristic vision. It is in fact highly pragmatic, and is based on the principle of unit autonomy (dedicated sites that are configured for the performance of gastrointestinal endoscopy, via resource sharing in settings where other types of endoscopy are carried out), so as to ensure that the unit is able to manage, follow-up and monitor patients in connection with all diagnostic and therapeutic gastrointestinal endoscopy procedures, and in such a way that patients receive competent, safe and comfortable care.

Further Reading

American Society for Gastrointestinal Endoscopy: *Ambulatory Endoscopy Centers. A primer*. Oak Brook, IL, 2009, ASGE.

Global Rating Scale: www.grs.nhs.uk.

1.6 **Gastrointestinal endoscopy training**

Denis Sautereau, François Cessot, Pascale Stelian

Key Points

- Formal training and assessment in all aspects of endoscopy is essential.
- Revalidation of training is recommended to ensure that physicians maintain adequate skills.
- Training can be performed by observation, use of models (animals) and direct training.
- Competence is not solely based on completing a minimum number of procedures, but should also involve direct observation and successful completion of objective criteria.
- Competence will be acknowledged by official certification.

Box 1   American Society for Gastrointestinal Endoscopy (ASGE) guidelines for certification or re-certification

The endoscopist must:
- Understand the indications, contraindications, and alternatives of the procedure.
- Interpret findings correctly.
- Perform the procedure proficiently and safely.
- Integrate findings into therapy or management plans.
- Avoid, recognize, and manage complications.
- Assess pre-procedural and plan post-procedural follow-up care.
- Credentials and privileges should be determined for each procedure.
- Perform continuous quality improvement.
- Obtain training, ideally through a formal training program.

Introduction

Gastrointestinal endoscopy involves diagnostic and therapeutic procedures where the operator must possess an extremely high skill level and be thoroughly acquainted with gastrointestinal pathologies and the devices used to investigate and treat them.

Training in gastrointestinal endoscopy is essential, given the rapid advances in the field in terms of both techniques and devices. This in turn means that gastroenterologists need to update their competencies on an ongoing basis.

Training can be obtained by observation of experts at specialized centers and use of models; however, these cannot replace hands-on training.

1. Principles of certification and re-certification

General principles have been developed by societies which document the minimum requirements for certification or re-certification of an individual. These are listed in Box 1. A minimum number of procedures are still required for general endoscopy (Table 1). A key change in assessing the adequacy of an individual's training is that competence is not solely based on completing a minimum number of procedures, but should also involve direct observation and successful completion of objective criteria. Several societies now require a formal summative assessment prior to certification. Guidelines have also been developed to certify non-physicians performing endoscopy in countries where there are too few endoscopists.

Advanced endoscopic training is usually obtained and additional training and competence assessed and credentialed separately (Box 2). Ideally, a formal training program should be completed. Animal models and short courses are useful adjuncts but cannot replace formal training.

For re-certification, physicians must document evidence of ongoing training and an adequate case load to maintain endoscopic skills. In addition to adequate numbers of procedures, the success, ability to perform therapeutic interventions and complication rate should be assessed (Table 2). Continuing medical education and continuous quality improvement are also key components of re-certification.

Box 2   ASGE guidelines for EUS certification

The endoscopist should demonstrate the following:
- A thorough understanding of the indications, contraindications, individual risk factors, and benefit-risk considerations for the individual patient.
- Clearly describe the endoscopic, not EUS alone, procedure and obtain informed consent.
- Have a sound understanding of gastrointestinal anatomy, and EUS equipment and accessories.
- Be able to safely intubate the esophagus, pylorus, and duodenum, and obtain imaging of the desired organ or lesion.
- Be able to accurately identify and interpret EUS images and recognize normal and abnormal findings.
- Be able to perform imaging, such as tumor staging, in agreement with surgical findings or findings of an EUS trainer.
- Be able to document EUS findings and communicate with referring physicians.

The above requirements are in addition to competence in general endoscopy and the general certification requirements detailed in Box 1.

Table 1 Guidelines for minimum numbers of general endoscopy procedures required for certification

Procedure	Number of supervised procedures	
	USA	France
EGD	130	300
Flexible sigmoidoscopy/ proctoscopy	30	100
Colonoscopy	140	100
Esophageal dilation	20	10
PEG	15	Not stated
Esophageal stent placement	10	10
Pneumatic dilation for achalasia	5	Not Stated
Tumor ablation	20	10
Advanced endoscopy	Not applicable	100[a]
Non-variceal hemostasis	25 (including 10 active bleeders)	30
Variceal hemostasis	20 (including 5 active bleeders)	
Polypectomy	30	50
Abdominal ultrasound	Not applicable	300
pH and manometry	See Box 3	50

[a]This includes laser, APC, dilation, and stent insertion.

the pigs must be sacrificed after two or three procedures due to the fragility of their bile ducts.

2.3. Digital simulators

The Simbionix GI Mentor robot is a computer simulator which consists of an endoscope with sensors at its distal end. Moving the endoscope in a cylinder generates a virtual image. Software applications that integrate diagnostic and therapeutic cases have been developed for the robot, and the graphics are of high quality. Programs available include: investigation of upper and lower GI tract; hemorrhage; polypectomy; EUS and ERCP. However, the mechanical constraints in terms of loops and instruments are not very realistic.

2.4. Erlangen active simulator for interventional endoscopy (EASIE)

EASIE uses resected stomachs of adult pigs which have been washed, and frozen (Figs 1–4). The stomachs are fastened to

2. Endoscopic training using models

Several models exist which allow trainees to improve their manual skills and dexterity. In addition, it allows a trainee to practice invasive procedures such as polypectomy, hemostasis and endoscopic mucosal resection. It is important to understand that although models allow a trainee to hone their skills in a safe environment, they do not replace formal training.

2.1. Plastic models

The Tübingen model is a plastic dummy which allows a number of different pathologies to be assessed. However, the model is not ideal, as it conducts electricity poorly, which affects the ability to perform hemostasis techniques.

2.2. Animal models

Pigs have been used as models, as the digestive system of pigs is similar to that of humans. However, this type of model has a number of drawbacks, including high cost, and

Table 2 Recommended numbers of interventional procedures

Procedure	Number of supervised procedures	
	USA	France
EUS		
Mucosal Lesions	75	150
Submucosal abnormalities	40	
Pancreaticobiliary	75	
EUS-guided FNA: Nonpancreatic Pancreatic	25 25	
ERCP	200 With at least an 80% cannulation rate	150
Laparoscopy	25	50

The ASGE recommend a minimum of 125 supervised cases for competence of mucosal and submucosal abnormalities, with a minimum of 150 supervised cases, of which 75 are pancreaticobiliary and 50 EUS-FNA for comprehensive competence.

a board at six points, with the distal end of the esophagus attached to a tube that simulates the gastrointestinal tract. ERCP training can also be performed, in which case the stomach-duodenum-liver is preserved to allow for access to

the bile ducts via the papilla. Current EASIE models include: hemostasis; polypectomy; APC; dilation; stent placement and ERCP. Endotrainer uses the same models, with some improvements.

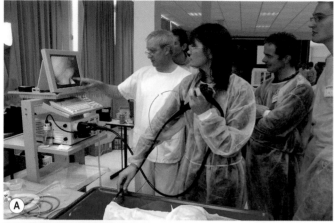

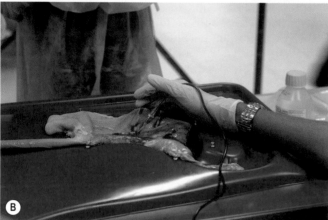

Figure 1 Hemostasis model. (A) A trainee is taught how to perform hemostasis by injection. (B) Hemostasis model with clips placed.

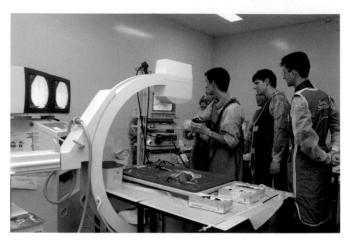

Figure 3 EASIE training model. This model uses pig organs. A trainee is learning how to place esophageal stents.

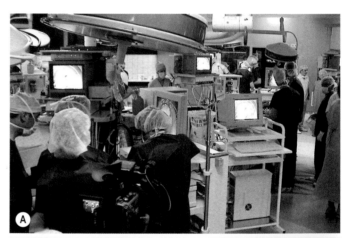

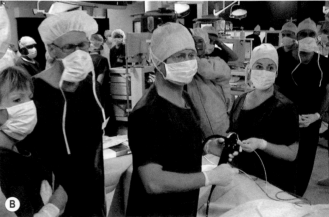

Figure 4 (A) Room at IRCAD in Strasbourg, containing various stations to allow for *in-vivo* work on an animal model. (B) Expert practitioners at a training session.

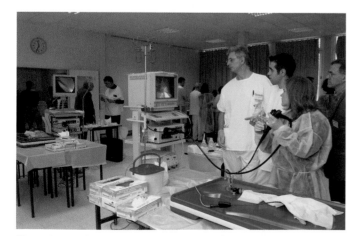

Figure 2 A student is being taught how to perform endoscopic mucosal resection on a model.

Further Reading

Aabakken L, Adamsen S, Kruse A, et al: Performance of colonoscopy simulator: experience from a hands-on endoscopy course, *Endoscopy* 32:911–913, 2000.

American Association for the Study of Liver Diseases, the American College of Gastroenterology, American Gastroenterological Association Institute, American Society for Gastrointestinal Endoscopy: The gastroenterology core curriculum. Third edition, *Gastroenterology* 132:2012–2018, 2007.

ASGE: Guidelines for certification and granting privileges for endoscopic ultrasound, *Gastrointest Endosc* 54:811–814, 2001.

ASGE: Guidelines for certification and granting privileges for gastrointestinal endoscopy, *Gastrointest Endosc* 48:679–682, 1998.

ASGE: Guidelines for training in endoscopic ultrasound, *Gastrointest Endosc* 49:829–833, 1999.

Bar-Meir S: A new endoscopic simulator, *Endoscopy* 32:898–900, 2000.

British Society of Gastroenterology: Non-medical endoscopist. A report of the working party of the British Society of Gastroenterology. www.bsg.org.uk.

Eisen GM, Baron TH, Dominitz JA, et al: Methods of granting hospital privileges to perform gastrointestinal endoscopy, *Gastrointest Endosc* 55:780–783, 2002.

Faigel DO, Baron TH, Adler DG, et al: ASGE. Guidelines for certification and granting privileges for capsule endoscopy, *Gastrointest Endosc* 61:503–505, 2005.

Greff M, Mignon M: Europe and initial and continuing medical education in hepato-gastroenterology, *Gastroenterol Clin Biol* 20(2):13–15, 1996.

Hochberger J, Maiss J, Hahn EG: The use of simulators for training in GI endoscopy, *Endoscopy* 34:727–729, 2002.

Hochberger J, Maiss J, Magdeburg B, et al: Training simulators and education in gastrointestinal endoscopy: current status and perspectives in 2001, *Endoscopy* 33:541–549, 2001.

Ikenberry SO, Anderson MA, Banerjee S, et al: ASGE. Endoscopy by nonphysicians, *Gastrointest Endosc* 69(4):767–770, 2009.

JAG: Guidelines for the training, appraisal and assessment of trainees in gastrointestinal endoscopy. 2004. www.thejag.org.uk.

Neumann M, Hochberger J, Felzmann T, et al: Part 1. The Erlanger endotrainer, *Endoscopy* 33:887–890, 2001.

Jean-Christophe Létard, Jean Marc Canard

Summary

1. Sphere of responsibility 30

Key Points

- Endoscopy nurses have a specialized and important role in the provision of endoscopy services.
- Roles and responsibilities are wide-ranging, from technical expertise in complex and diverse procedures, disinfection, management of the unit activities, budgeting, stock requisition, staffing, training, audit and research.
- Formal training programs and regular update sessions are essential for endoscopy nurses.
- Endoscopy nurses should be members of their national professional society.

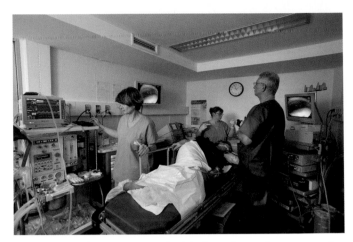

Figure 1 An endoscopist, an anesthesiologist, and an endoscopy nurse for a therapeutic endoscopic upper GI tract procedure.

1. Sphere of responsibility

Endoscopy nurses play a critical role in the provision of safe, high quality endoscopy. They provide nursing care in accordance with doctors' instructions, which includes supporting disease prevention, health education, training, and management.

As much of what endoscopy nurses do centers around the technical aspects of endoscopy, they must have the ability to:

- Take care of all patients who undergo endoscopic examinations (Fig. 1)
- Assist the operator during procedures (Fig. 2)
- Perform endoscopy-related management tasks in connection with scheduling, room availability, endoscopes and equipment, operators, and the various types of procedures that are carried out
- Take the lead in disinfection and infection control
- Undertake training of new staff.

1.1. Dealing with patient needs

An endoscopy nurse must have the ability to admit and prepare patients, provide the patient with the information needed for their examination, ensure their comfort and safety, and give the patient instructions regarding post-procedural aftercare. An endoscopy nurse must also act competently and professionally during emergencies, to ensure that care is given properly and that important tasks are prioritized. To this end, the endoscopy unit should be part of a healthcare system to ensure that these objectives are fulfilled. Endoscopy nurses ensure that patients are properly settled in, that the relevant equipment is available, and conduct pre-procedure instrument checks. They also counsel the patient regarding the endoscopy procedure and the period thereafter.

1.2. Technical knowledge

An endoscopy nurse must have the following technical attributes:

- A thorough understanding of the following techniques: upper GI endoscopy; colonoscopy, enteroscopy, endoscopic ultrasound; ERCP; video capsule endoscopy; laser and argon plasma coagulation techniques; taking biopsies; foreign-body extraction; hemostasis; polypectomy; stricture dilatation; injection sclerotherapy; clipping; mucosal resection; stent placement; hemorrhoid management; intragastric

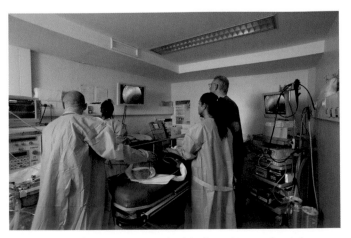

Figure 2 An endoscopist, an anaesthesiologist and two endoscopic nurses during a therapeutic colonoscopy.

Table 1 Endoscopy nurses – societies and training links

Country/Region	Society	Website
USA	Society of Gastrointestinal Nurses and Associates (SGNA)	www.sgna.org
Europe	European Society of Gastroenterology and Endoscopy Nurses and Associates (ESGENA)	www.esgena.org
UK	British Society of Gastroenterology Endoscopy Associates Committee (BSG-EAG)	www.bsg.org.uk; www.jets.nhs.uk/GIN
FRANCE	Groupement des infirmier(e)s pour la formation en endoscopie (GIFE)	www.gife.fr

balloons; pH-metry and manometry, and ablative therapies, e.g. radiofrequency ablation or photodynamic therapy
- A thorough understanding of all endoscopes and accessories that are used
- Good manual dexterity and a good sense of anticipation
- The ability to learn and evolve professionally and personally.

1.3. Management of endoscopes and endoscopic accessories

Management of endoscopy equipment is a highly responsible role, in light of the capital costs involved. These management processes are the responsibility of the endoscopy nurses, in collaboration with decontamination staff, infection control teams and the hospital's technical or medical physics department (a unit's endoscope inventory may cost $500 000–$1.5 m, or even more). Endoscopy nurses are also in charge of ensuring the traceability of endoscopic devices and disinfection processes. An endoscopy nurse is also in charge of inventory management and stock requisition, sterilization of reusable medical devices, and sterilization of linens, biomedical and maintenance equipment.

1.4. Infection control

Endoscopy nurses are also in charge of unit environmental hygiene and endoscopy disinfection processes (see Ch. 1.10).

1.5. Training

Endoscopy nurses play a number of key training roles in terms of induction and knowledge transfer for new staff members and trainees. They are also involved in appraisal, staff development and clinical research. In the UK, the national 'GIN' training program has been developed to train endoscopy nurses to be local facilitators who run regular nurse training courses. In the USA, the Society of Gastrointestinal Nurses and Associates (SGNA) is an important forum for nurse training in endoscopy and gastroenterology. The European Society of Gastroenterology and Endoscopy Nurses and Associates (ESGENA) is similar, and runs regular training and update courses (Table 1).

Further Reading

European Society of Gastroenterology and Endoscopy Nurses and Associates: ESGENA Core curriculum for endoscopy nursing, 2008. www.esgena.org.

European Society of Gastroenterology and Endoscopy Nurses and Associates: European job profile for endoscopy nurses, *Endoscopy* 2004;36(11):1025–1030.

Society of Gastroenterology Nurses and Associates: Standards of clinical nursing practice and role delineations, 2010. www.sgna.org.

1.8 Patient information

Ian Penman

Summary

Patient information   32

Key Points

- Patient information is a key component of high quality endoscopy services, and particularly the process for obtaining consent.
- Written leaflets should be clear, balanced, and written in language that is easy to understand.
- The nature of the procedure, alternatives, and risks should be explained.
- Information provided should be locally adapted, e.g. to include specific contact telephone numbers for queries before procedures and potential problems which may arise afterwards.
- The needs of patients from ethnic minorities and those with disabilities must be taken into account when developing patient information leaflets.

Patient information

Provision of high quality patient information is a key element of successful endoscopic practice. Written patient information leaflets (PIL) help patients recall information discussed during a clinic consultation, allow them to understand their intended procedure, and to contemplate any questions requiring clarification before the procedure is performed.

Endoscopy centers should have printed leaflets available for all major diagnostic and therapeutic procedures that they undertake. While many useful generic PILs are available from national and international endoscopy societies, patient support groups and websites, these should be considered a starting point for development of locally adapted leaflets that relate specifically to the endoscopy center's activities.

PILs should be procedure-specific, developed by the endoscopy team, agreed by the hospital and preferably, should involve patient groups in their development. They should be clear and easy to read, avoiding technical jargon, and seeking the views of patient representative groups can be helpful in this regard. Leaflets should include a section on frequently asked questions (FAQs), deal with common issues (e.g. diabetes, anticoagulation, and the possible need for antibiotics). If appropriate, PILs should be available in locally prevalent, community languages for those from ethnic minorities. If this is not possible, a reliable and readily available language interpretation service is essential for these patients. The needs of disabled patients (e.g. visually impaired) should also be considered and leaflets should be available in large type or Braille.

PILs should be structured and the broad headings listed in Box 1 provide a useful framework for their development.

Most national endoscopy societies have downloadable PILs for common procedures on their websites and some of these are listed below. Boxes 2 and 3 give examples of patient leaflets for colonoscopy and ERCP, which may serve as a useful guide.

Box 1   Key points to consider in developing patient information for endoscopic procedures

- Description of procedure.
- Indications.
- Alternative procedures.
- Any preparation necessary.
- Regular medications (e.g. warfarin, iron, insulin, etc.).
- Need for sedation or anesthesia.
- What happens during the procedure.
- Possible abnormal findings (e.g. polyps, cancer, ulcer).
- Possible interventions (e.g. biopsy, dilatation, polypectomy).
- Risks and complications (e.g. bleeding, perforation, pancreatitis).
- Post-procedure recovery.
- Follow-up plans.
- Contact numbers pre- *and* post-procedure.
- Directions to endoscopy center and map.

Box 2   Colonoscopy Information

Your appointment details, information and consent form

Please bring this booklet with you.

An appointment for your **Colonoscopy** has been arranged at:

Hospital name: _____

Date: _____

Telephone number: _____

Endoscopist/Consultant: _____

Please telephone the Endoscopy Department on the above number. If this is not convenient, or you would like to discuss any aspect of the procedure before your appointment.

Introduction

You have been advised by your GP or hospital doctor to have an investigation known as a colonoscopy. *This procedure requires your formal consent.* If you are unable to keep your appointment, please notify the department as soon as possible. This will enable the staff to give your appointment to someone else and they will be able to arrange another date and time for you. Please bring this booklet with you when you attend. This booklet has been written to enable you to make an informed decision in relation to agreeing to the investigation. At the back of the booklet is the consent form.

The procedure you will be having is called a colonoscopy. This is an examination of your large bowel (colon). It will be performed by or under the supervision of a trained doctor and we will make the investigation as comfortable as possible for you. When you are having a colonoscopy procedure you will usually be given sedation and analgesia.

Why do I need to have a colonoscopy?

You may have been advised to undergo this investigation of your large bowel to try and find the cause for your symptoms, help with treatment, and if necessary, to decide on further investigation. It is sometimes undertaken to follow-up previous disease or abnormalities or to assess the clinical importance of an abnormality seen on an X-ray.

A barium enema examination is an alternative investigation to colonoscopy. It has the disadvantage that samples of the bowel cannot be taken if an abnormality is found. If this is the case, a subsequent endoscopic examination may be required. CT colonography ('virtual colonoscopy') provides high quality CT X-ray pictures of the bowel but, again, if biopsies are required you may subsequently need to have a colonoscopy.

What is a colonoscopy?

This test is a very accurate way of looking at the lining of your large bowel (colon), to establish whether there is any disease present. This test also allows us to take tissue samples (biopsy) for analysis by the pathology department if necessary. The instrument used in this investigation is called a colonoscope (scope), and is flexible. This enables the endoscopist to have a clear view and to check whether or not disease or inflammation is present. During the investigation, the endoscopist may need to take some samples from the lining of your colon for analysis: this is painless. The samples will be retained. A video recording and/or photographs may be taken for your records.

Preparing for the investigation

Eating and drinking

It is necessary to have clear views of the lower bowel. Instructions on what you can and cannot eat, as well as advice on how to take the bowel preparation for your procedure are enclosed separately with this leaflet.

What about my medication?

Your routine medication should be taken. If you are taking iron tablets you must stop these one week prior to your appointment. If you are

taking stool bulking agents (e.g. ispaghula (Fybogel), Loperamide, Co-phenoxylate or Codeine phosphate you must stop these *3 days prior* to your appointment.

Diabetics

If you are diabetic controlled on insulin or medication, please ensure the Endoscopy department is aware so that the appointment can be made at the beginning of the list. Please see advice supplied with your bowel preparation regarding what you can and cannot eat and how to monitor your blood sugar levels.

Anticoagulants/Allergies

Please telephone the Unit if you are taking anticoagulants such as warfarin or antiplatelet drugs such as clopidogrel. Phone for information if you think you have a latex allergy.

How long will I be in the endoscopy department?

This largely depends on how quickly you recover from the sedation and how busy the department is. You should expect to be in the department for approximately 3 hours.

What happens when I arrive?

When you arrive in the department, you will be met by a qualified nurse or healthcare assistant who will ask you a few questions, one of which concerns your arrangements for getting home. You will also be able to ask further questions about the investigation. The nurse will ensure you understand the procedure and discuss any outstanding concerns or questions you may have. As you will be having sedation, she may insert a small cannula (plastic tube) in the back of your hand through which sedation will be administered later.

As you will have sedation you will not be permitted to drive or use public transport so you must arrange for a family member or friend to collect you. The nurse will need to be given their telephone number so that she can contact them when you are ready for discharge.

You will have a brief medical assessment when a qualified endoscopy nurse who will ask you some questions regarding your medical condition and any surgery or illnesses you have had to confirm that you are fit to undergo the investigation. If you have not already done so, and you are happy to proceed, you will be asked to sign your consent form at this point.

Intravenous sedation

The sedation and a painkiller will be administered into a vein in your hand or arm which will make you drowsy and relaxed but not unconscious. You will be in a state called cooperative sedation. This means that, although drowsy, you will still hear what is said to you and therefore will be able to follow simple instructions during the investigation. Sedation makes it unlikely that you will remember anything about the examination. While you are sedated, we will monitor your breathing and heart rate so changes will be noted and dealt with accordingly. Please note as you have had sedation you must not drive, take alcohol, operate heavy machinery or sign any legally binding documents for 24 hours following the procedure and you will need someone to accompany you home.

The colonoscopy investigation

The nurse looking after you will ask you to lie on your left side. The sedative drugs will be administered into a cannula (tube) in your vein. The colonoscopy involves maneuvering the colonoscope around the entire length of your large bowel. There are some bends that naturally occur in the bowel and negotiating these may be uncomfortable for a short period of time but the sedation and analgesia will minimize any discomfort. Air is gently passed into the bowel during the investigation to facilitate the passage of the colonoscope. During the procedure, samples may be taken from the lining of your bowel for analysis in our laboratories. These will be retained.

Box 2 Continued

Risks of the procedure

Lower gastrointestinal endoscopy is classified as an invasive investigation and because of that it has the possibility of associated complications. These occur extremely infrequently; we would wish to draw your attention to them and so with this information you can make your decision. The doctor who has requested the test will have considered this. The risks must be compared to the benefit of having the procedure carried out. The risks can be associated with the procedure itself and with administration of the sedation.

The endoscopic procedure

The main risks are of mechanical damage:

- Perforation (risk approximately 1 for every 1000 examinations) or tear of the lining of the bowel. An operation is nearly always required to repair the hole. The risk of perforation is higher with polyp removal.
- Bleeding may occur at the site of biopsy or polyp removal (risk approximately 1 for every 100–200 examinations where this is performed). Typically minor in degree, such bleeding may either stop on its own or can be controlled by cauterization or injection treatment.

Sedation

Sedation can occasionally cause problems with breathing, heart rate, and blood pressure. If any of these problems do occur, they are normally short lived. Careful monitoring ensures that any potential problems can be identified and treated rapidly.

What is a polyp?

A polyp is a protrusion from the lining of the bowel. Some polyps are attached to the intestinal wall by a stalk, and look like a mushroom, whereas others are flat without a stalk. Polyps when found are generally removed or sampled by the endoscopist as they may grow and later cause problems. Flat polyps are generally a little more difficult to remove.

Polypectomy

A polyp may be removed in one of two ways both using an electrical current known as diathermy. For large polyps a snare (wire loop) is placed around the polyp, a high frequency current is then applied and the polyp is removed. Flat polyps (without any stalk) can be removed by a procedure called EMR (Endoscopic Mucosal Resection). This involves injecting the lining of the bowel that surrounds the flat polyp. This raises the area and allows the wire loop snare to capture the polyp. For smaller polyps, special biopsy forceps are used. These hold the polyp while the diathermy is applied, therefore destroying the polyp.

After the procedure

You will be allowed to rest for as long as is necessary. Your blood pressure and heart rate will be recorded and if you are diabetic, your blood glucose will be monitored. Should you have underlying breathing difficulties or if your oxygen levels were low during the procedure, we will continue to monitor your breathing. Once you have recovered from the initial effects of the sedation (which normally takes 30–60 minutes), you will be moved to a comfortable chair and offered a hot drink and something to eat. Before you leave the department, the nurse or endoscopist will discuss the findings and any medication or further investigations required. She or he will also inform you if you require further appointments.

The sedation may temporarily affect your memory, so it is a good idea to have a member of your family or friend with you when you are given this information although there will be a short written report given to you. Because you have had sedation, the drug remains in your blood system for about 24 hours and you may feel drowsy later on, with intermittent lapses of memory. If you live alone, try and arrange for someone to stay with you or, if possible, arrange to stay with your family or a friend for at least 4 hours.

General points to remember

- If you are unable to keep your appointment please notify the endoscopy department as soon as possible.
- Because you are having sedation, please arrange for someone to collect you.
- If you have any problems with persistent abdominal pain or bleeding please contact your GP immediately informing them that you have had an endoscopy. If you are unable to contact or speak to your doctor, you must go immediately to the Accident and Emergency department.

Box 3 ERCP Information[a]

Your appointment details, information and consent form

Please bring this booklet with you.

An appointment for your **ERCP** has been arranged at:

Hospital name: _____

Date: _____

Telephone number: _____

Endoscopist/Consultant: _____

Please telephone the Endoscopy Department on the above number if this is not convenient or you would like to discuss any aspect of the procedure before your appointment.

What is an ERCP?

An ERCP (Endoscopic Retrograde Cholangio Pancreatography) is a test to examine the tubes that drain bile from your liver (the bile duct and gallbladder), and digestive juices from the pancreas (pancreatic duct). The doctor who is to perform the test will explain what will happen and you will both sign the consent form. You will be required to lie on an X-ray table and you will be given an injection which will make you very sleepy (sedation). Once you are sleepy, an endoscope (a long, thin flexible tube with a bright light at one end) will be passed through your mouth, down into your stomach and the upper part of the small intestine (the duodenum). A small plastic mouth guard will be used to protect your teeth and the endoscope, and you will be given a little oxygen to breathe during the test. X-ray dye will be injected down the endoscope so that the pancreas and bile ducts may be seen on X-ray films. If everything is normal, the endoscope is then removed and the test is complete. The dye is passed out of your body harmlessly.

If the X-rays show a gallstone, the doctor may enlarge the opening of the bile duct (sphincterotomy) to allow the stones to pass into the intestine. If a narrowing is found, bile can be drained by leaving a short plastic or metallic tube (stent) in the bile duct. You will not be aware of the presence of the tube, which may remain in place permanently.

Preparing for the procedure

Prior to the procedure you must have a blood test (unless this test is done, the doctor cannot carry out the ERCP). You will need to telephone the department 2–3 days before your test to arrange to collect a blood test form to take to the Hematology Department

Box 3 Continued

within the hospital. You may go home as soon as the blood has been taken. To allow a clear view, the stomach and duodenum must be empty. *It is essential that you have nothing to eat for at least SIX hours before your procedure and on the day of your procedure to only drink clear fluids, stopping TWO hours prior to your test.*

The day of the procedure

You will be asked to undress and wear a hospital gown. It will also be necessary for you to remove any false teeth.

Sedation

You will be given sedation, which is a medicine to help you to relax. This is given by injection. While this will make you drowsy it does not 'put you to sleep' like a general anesthetic.

Please be aware you cannot have sedation unless you bring someone with you to your appointment. Your escort must stay in the department so they can be with you when the endoscopist discusses the outcome of your procedure – sedation will make you sleepy and therefore you may not remember what is being said. They will also need to escort you home. Someone must then stay with you for 24 hours following your procedure to look out for any complications. During this time, you are advised against doing any of the following:

- Drive a motor vehicle
- Drink alcohol
- Operate machinery
- Sign legal documents

If you have any queries you can phone the Unit on _____ for advice. *We are unable to perform your procedure if you require sedation and do not have an escort.*

Privacy and dignity

Please be aware that in order to protect the privacy and dignity of all patients, some of whom may be undressed for procedures, relatives/carers will NOT be allowed to stay with the patient for the whole time. They are welcome to accompany the patient during the initial admission process but will then be required to leave the admission/recovery area once the patient has been made ready for the procedure. Relatives/carers will be invited back once the patient is recovered and ready for discharge.

Medicines and medical conditions

It is important you bring a list of your current medication with you so that you can give it to the nurse on arrival. If you have a latex allergy, please telephone the Unit for medical advice.

Warfarin/Phenindione /Clopidogrel (Plavix), or any other blood thinning agent (anticoagulant)

If you are taking any of the above, please inform the Endoscopy Unit on _____ as soon as possible, as our doctors may decide that it is necessary for you to stop taking your tablets for a limited time before the procedure.

Diabetes

If you suffer from diabetes, please inform the Gastroenterology Unit as soon as possible, as it may be necessary to change the time of your appointment or be admitted to hospital a day before your procedure for treatment. If your diabetes is managed by your GP please contact the surgery for advice. Otherwise, please contact your Diabetes specialist nurse on _____.

Pregnancy

If you are pregnant or breast-feeding please contact the Endoscopy Unit for advice.

Antimotility drugs (used to treat diarrhea)

If you regularly take Loperamide, Lomita or another medicine to control diarrhea, you are advised to stop taking it one week prior to your procedure. If you are concerned or have any problems, please contact us for advice.

What are the risks and complications?

Sometimes patients may experience discomfort and/or a sore throat for a few days. This can be relieved by normal painkillers such as paracetamol. Although this procedure is very safe, very occasionally, severe complications can occur, the two most common are pancreatitis and bleeding:

- *Acute pancreatitis* This is inflammation of the pancreas and can cause abdominal pain often going into the back and associated with vomiting. This is a severe complication and requires immediate attention.
- *Bleeding* This can occur if a cut has been made to remove stones. Bleeding can cause vomiting of blood which may be black, or the passing of dark black stools.

The incidence of these complications are small, but if you have any problems after ERCP which you feel could be a result of the test please inform your GP who will refer you back to the department if necessary.

Consent

Enclosed is a consent form for you to read before you come for your appointment. This is to ensure that you understand the test and its implications/risks. Please bring it with you to your appointment but DO NOT sign it until AFTER you have had a discussion with the doctor in the Unit. If you have any queries, you can telephone the Unit before your procedure or ask the staff when you have your discussion.

After the procedure

The endoscopist will talk to you at the end of the procedure, explaining what has been found and any treatment given. Once you have returned home, or back to your ward you may begin to eat and drink normally and resume your normal medication, unless instructed otherwise by the Doctor. You will be given an advice sheet on aftercare and any problems to watch for when you have had your procedure.

Useful sources of information

Additional information can be found at these websites:
- National Library of Medicine. www.nlm.nih.gov/portals/public.html
- The American Society of Gastrointestinal Endoscopy. www.askasge.org
- CORE. www.corecharity.org.uk

^aReproduced with permission, courtesy of Dr Richard Tighe, Norfolk and Norwich Hospital, UK.

Further Reading

American Society for Gastrointestinal Endoscopy: www.asge.org/PatientInfoIndex.aspx?id=1022.

British Society of Gastroenterology: www.bsg.org.uk/sections/bsg-endoscopy-general/related-documents.html.

Gastroenterological Society of Australia: www.gesa.org.au/leaflets.cfm.

Societe Francaise d'Endoscopie Digestive: www.sfed.org/Generalites/Fiches-info-patients.html.

1.9 Medicolegal aspects of endoscopy

Ian Penman

Summary

Introduction 36

1. Specific medicolegal aspects of endoscopy practice 36

2. Complications 37

3. Consent for endoscopic procedures 37

Key Points

- Following the principles of good medical practice will help to minimize the medicolegal risks associated with endoscopic practice.
- Direct procedure-related complications and/or failure to recognize and treat them are the commonest causes of endoscopy-related litigation.
- Consent and medication-related issues are less common reasons.
- Measures aimed at prevention of and early recognition of complications are important in reducing patient harm and medicolegal risks; the whole endoscopy team has a role to play in this.

Introduction

Gastrointestinal endoscopy has become increasingly complex and interventional in recent years, and as a procedural specialty, is inherently associated with an element of risk. While the vast majority of endoscopic procedures are undertaken safely and successfully, there is always the potential for harm, and endoscopists may face medicolegal consequences as a result. Much of this risk, however, relates not to specific aspects of endoscopy but to good medical practice and while it is beyond the scope of this brief chapter to discuss good medical practice in depth, it is worth emphasizing some key elements:

- *Good doctors* are competent, up-to-date and always prioritize patient care on the basis of clinical need. They are honest, trustworthy and always act with integrity and have good relations with both patients and colleagues alike.
- *Good care* is essential at all stages of a patient's journey, not just around endoscopy. This includes good history taking, examination, investigations, and treatment. Doctors need to work within the limit of their competence, provide effective evidence-based treatment, respect the rights and wishes of their patients, and keep clear written records and documentation at all times.
- *Maintaining knowledge* Doctors should remain up-to-date with continuing professional development, membership of professional societies, attendance at local and national conferences and regularly read relevant journals and guidelines. They should strive to maintain and continually improve their skills, while promoting a safety culture. Doctors must participate in local and national licensing and revalidation procedures, participate in regular appraisals and play a role in clinical audit and quality improvement projects, and be willing to act on the outcomes of these, in the best interests of their patients.
- *Good relationships with patients* Openness, trust and good communication skills are essential, and doctors must strive to respect patients' views at all times, and maintain their dignity, privacy, and confidentiality. The needs of children, patients from minority backgrounds and those with disabilities must be respected and catered for. Doctors must be open and honest if things go wrong, offer a clear explanation of events, give an apology when appropriate, and continue to provide patient care after a complication occurs.
- *Medicolegal indemnity insurance* cover is essential and must be up to date.
- *Consent* Doctors should have a thorough knowledge of, and follow, local and national policies relating to consent for endoscopic procedures (see below).

1. Specific medicolegal aspects of endoscopy practice

Studies in the USA have found that medicolegal issues relate mainly to iatrogenic harm, i.e. direct procedure-related complications, delay in diagnosis (especially gastric or colonic malignancy), but also delayed diagnosis of other pathology (e.g. lung or ovarian cancer, presenting to gastroenterologists). Drug-prescribing errors (especially anticoagulation) are also a regularly occurring, but uncommon theme. A recent UK analysis of medicolegal claims involving endoscopy-related deaths that proceeded to a court of law found that issues relating to inappropriate treatment or direct complications of procedures accounted for one-half of all claims and a delay in recognizing and/or treating complications accounted for another 40%. Consent issues only accounted for 1 in 20 cases, and the remainder were medication-related. The clear lesson from this study was that the majority of claims relating to cases of death involved the delay in recognizing and dealing with procedure-related complications.

 Clinical Tip

The majority of medicolegal claims relating to endoscopy involve direct procedure–related complications and/or a delay in recognizing and treating these.

2. Complications

Many years ago, the commonest complications arising from endoscopy were sedation-related events, but better sedation practice has made these uncommon nowadays. Large audits suggest that both immediate and delayed complications are perhaps more common than realized, but have also highlighted the fact that many complications are preventable and that delayed recognition is associated with worse patient outcomes and a greater likelihood of litigation. Specific procedure-related complications will, however, inevitably occur from time to time, when undertaking invasive procedures, and these are discussed in detail in Chapter 8.

The best strategy for dealing with endoscopy-related complications is therefore to prevent them, and the following measures may assist this:

- *Promoting a culture of quality and safety* Putting patient safety at the heart of the activities of an endoscopy center is essential. Mapping a patient's complete journey, from initial consultation to final discharge, can highlight areas where safety can be improved at every step. Continuous audit of the performance of endoscopy and quality assurance of the unit's activities with benchmarking against national standards is an important means of measuring and monitoring quality.
- *Fully trained endoscopists* working within their competence limits
- *Adequate supervision of trainee endoscopists* at all times. It is inappropriate to leave trainees to perform procedures unsupervised. This compromises patient care and also the quality of training for trainees.
- *Appropriate endoscopy setting* High quality endoscopy can only occur in adequate facilities with good quality equipment and adequate numbers of fully trained and competent staff (medical, nursing, technical, and clerical).
- *Promoting a culture of team working*
- *Clear local policies* for consent, sedation, use of antibiotics, patients taking antithrombotic therapy, and risk stratification of patients, etc. These need to be understood and followed by all staff.
- *Systematic and regular audit* of performance with regular team meetings to analyse and act on results. This should include near-miss incidents so that lessons can be learned for the future. In the UK, for example, all endoscopy units participate in a rolling audit and quality assurance program, called the Global Rating Scale (GRS, www.grs.nhs.uk), every 6 months. This forms the cornerstone of a national system of accreditation of endoscopy units, and similar systems exist in other countries.
- *Clinical governance* The endoscopy unit and its activities should feed into a larger hospital clinical governance structure, with clear escalation policies for performance related issues.

3. Consent for endoscopic procedures

Personal autonomy is a fundamental human right and failure to obtain informed, valid consent breaches this, and may lead to litigation for assault or battery. Consent is a patient's agreement to treatment and is a process that begins during the initial consultation with the patient, and ends with the completion of treatment. In order for consent to be 'valid', patients must be adequately informed (i.e. have been given sufficient information about the procedure, its benefits, risks, and alternatives). Patients must be mentally competent to decide, must give their consent freely and without duress, and retain the right to refuse or withdraw consent at any time. In some countries, it is a legal requirement that all endoscopic procedures require written consent, but this is not universal; but note that a patient simply attending for a procedure does not imply that consent has been given.

3.1. Patient information

This is discussed in Chapter 1.8 and should include as much information as is reasonable to allow patients to make an informed decision. It must be easy to understand, and patients must have adequate time to read and contemplate the information before making their decision. It is generally not acceptable for patients to be presented with information and/or a consent form for signature immediately prior to the proposed procedure. Knowing how much information to provide to patients without causing undue concern is not easy, but a description of the procedure, alternatives, the need for sedation and potential risks is essential. All common complications (occurring with a frequency of 1% or more) should be discussed, as should rare complications, if they are potentially serious or fatal, or may lead to long-term disability (e.g. perforation, pancreatitis). The principle is that serious complications, no matter how rare, might influence a patient's decision to proceed, and therefore needs to be discussed beforehand.

 Clinical Tip

A signature on a consent form is necessary but not enough. There must be evidence that the patient was given adequate information in a form that is easy to understand, and sufficient time to make an informed decision, without duress.

3.2. Refusal of treatment and withdrawal of consent

Competent adults may refuse treatment or withdraw consent at any time, and no matter how much the endoscopist may disagree with this, the patient's autonomy must be respected. If an unsedated patient withdraws consent during a procedure, the procedure should stop immediately. If a sedated patient indicates that they are in distress or wishes the procedure to stop, the endoscopist must act in the patient's best interests. Sometimes, discussion with the patient and the offer of additional sedation may allow the procedure to proceed and be completed successfully, but if the patient is clear that they wish the procedure to stop, or the patient is combative and safety is jeopardized, the procedure should stop.

3.3. Adults lacking capacity to give consent

The legal situation varies from country to country, but, in general, no one else can give consent on behalf of an incompetent adult, unless they have been appointed by a court of law as a legal guardian or 'power of attorney'. If an endoscopist is in doubt about how to proceed, the hospital's legal department should be consulted for advice beforehand. This may also pertain to patients with 'advanced directives' about life-sustaining treatment.

3.4. Retention and storage of tissue

Specific consent should be obtained for the retention of tissue samples including biopsies. Tissues are useful in teaching and research but patients must be given the opportunity to refuse permission for the use of their tissues for such purposes. If additional tissue samples are to be taken for research purposes, this can only be done with explicit approval from the local Ethics Committee and the patient's written consent.

3.5. Photography and/or videorecording

These may be made for clinical management as part of the patient's medical record but use of imaging for teaching, publication or research requires the patient's formal consent and they must understand that the material may appear in the public domain.

3.6. Patients lacking capacity to give consent

When patients lack capacity to give consent, endoscopists must ensure that they have made every effort to discuss treatment in a way that the patient is best able to understand. Patients should be offered the option of having a relative or carer present to help them make an informed decision. Providing them with a written record of the conversation is sometimes helpful. These situations may arise with patients with mental health problems, brain injury, learning disabilities or dementia, and in those with alcohol or drug misuse. At all times, the endoscopist must act with the patient's best interests at heart and their dignity must be respected. Endoscopists must remain objective and not allow their personal feelings or views to influence them. All available options for treatment should be carefully considered, and the one that is least restrictive to the patient considered. Any previously expressed preferences by the patient must be considered, as should the views of their relatives or partners, etc. Wherever possible, the aim should be to reach a consensus about patient management, but in complex cases, it may be helpful to hold a multidisciplinary meeting to review the clinical and ethical aspects of the patient's case. Only in rare cases is it necessary to seek a formal judicial review. Finally, it is wise to remember always to act in a patient's 'best interests', and to avoid making assumptions or being judgmental.

Further Reading

ASGE Standards of Practice Committee: Informed consent for GI endoscopy, *Gastrointest Endosc* 66(2):213–218, 2007.

British Society of Gastroenterology: Guidance for obtaining a valid consent for elective endoscopic procedures. A Report of the Working Party of the British Society of Gastroenterology. April 2008. www.bsg.org.uk.

Stanciu C, Novis B, Ladas S, et al: Recommendations of the ESGE workshop on Informed Consent for Digestive Endoscopy. First European Symposium on Ethics in Gastroenterology and Digestive Endoscopy, Kos, Greece, June 2003, *Endoscopy* 35(9):772–774, 2003.

1.10 Cleaning, disinfection, sterilization, and storage of endoscopy equipment

Bernard Marchetti, Ian Penman

Summary

Key Points

- Flexible endoscopes cannot be autoclaved for sterilization and have complex requirements for effective disinfection.
- Standard operating procedures for disinfection should be developed and rigorously followed.
- Disinfection should be undertaken by fully trained staff in dedicated cleaning rooms that comply with local health and safety and building regulations.
- Aldehyde and alcohol-based disinfectants may fix prions and proteins inside endoscopes and should be replaced by other agents, e.g. peracetic acid or superoxidized water.
- Special precautions are necessary to identify patients at risk of variant CJD and to minimize risk of transmission.
- The use of automated endoscope reprocessors (AERs) should replace manual cleaning processes.
- The final rinse water from the AER should be regularly tested for microbiological quality.
- There should be systems for tracking all endoscopes, valves, and devices used so that contact tracing can occur in the event of the possibility of transmission of infection.

Introduction

In the course of an endoscopic procedure, the endoscope passes through cavities containing bacteria, some of which may be pathogenic, and the endoscope is contaminated after every examination. Lack of efficient disinfection may result in the transmission of bacteria, viruses, fungi, spores, parasites or prions. Numerous recommendations have been put forward in recent years regarding disinfection procedures for non-autoclavable medical devices and these vary from country to country. The recommendations are broadly similar and all staff working in endoscopy must have a thorough understanding of and be up-to-date with cleaning processes in their country. Links to recommendations from France, the UK and the USA are listed at the end of this chapter.

1. Definitions of terms

1.1. Cleaning

Refers to the removal of biological, organic and liquid particles and other debris using a procedure that is compatible with the characteristics of the surface being treated, and using the following factors in combination with each other: a combination of chemical action, mechanical action and heat, all for an adequate duration.

According to ISO 15883-1, the term 'cleaning' means removing contamination from an object up to the level necessary for the use for which the object is intended. This cleaning phase may include two or more washing phases. Contamination here means debris.

1.2. Disinfection

Disinfection is defined as a procedure, the result of which is transient and that eliminates or kills microorganisms and/or deactivates undesirable viruses that are carried by inert contaminated environments. Such operations, which are carried out in accordance with defined objectives, relate solely to the microorganisms that are present at the time the procedure is carried out.

Disinfection is a generic term that refers to any antimicrobial measure (regardless of the level of the outcome attained), using a product that exhibits *in-vitro* properties that meet the criteria of a disinfectant or antiseptic agent. The name of each disinfection procedure should indicate its application domain, for example, medical device disinfection, floor disinfection, and hand disinfection.

1.3. Disinfectant

A product that is used for disinfecting under defined conditions. If the procedure is selective, this must be specified. A disinfectant is a product that contains one or more active ingredients that exhibit antimicrobial properties and the activity of which is determined by a recognized standard system.

1.4. Sterilization

A thermal operation, the purpose of which is to eliminate all living microorganisms of any kind whatsoever. Items that undergo sterilization are disinfected beforehand and remain so as long as their protective packaging remains intact. Sterilization is used for autoclavable instruments and not for flexible endoscopes.

1.5. Traceability

The purpose of medical device traceability is to enable the relevant agencies to determine how and where a specific medical device was used, based on a registered ID number in accordance with ISO 9000: 2000.

The traceability of disinfection and sterilization procedures is part of the quality control process. In the present context, traceability refers to documentation of all stages of the processing undergone by a medical device so as to allow for certification that the relevant steps were carried out properly. Such documentation, either paper or electronic, relates to all human, technical, and material resources deployed, as well as all procedures used.

1.6. Medical device

A medical device is any instrument, apparatus, material, or product of non-human origin, or any item used alone or in association with such items, including accessories and software, that is intended by the vendor for human medical applications and whose primary effect is not obtained by pharmacological, immunological or metabolic means.

Endoscopes, endoscopic accessories and supplies, disinfectants, and reprocessing machines all count as medical devices and are subject to the CE mark or equivalent.

2. Disinfection phases for immersible flexible endoscopes

In view of the current (but unquantified and non-confirmed) risk of variant Creutzfeldt Jacob Disease (vCJD) transmission during an endoscopic procedure, in France it is recommended that endoscopes be cleaned twice. This is not mandated in all countries. At all times, every step of the cleaning process must be monitored.

2.1. Preliminary cleaning

The purpose of this phase is to remove visible debris. Preliminary cleaning, which is performed immediately following the procedure, comprises the following:

- Wiping down the endoscope using a disposable wipe or cloth
- Aspiration and insufflation of all endoscope channels using water, even if not used during the procedure.

Box 1   Minimizing the risk of transmission of variant CJD

- All patients attending for endoscopy should be assessed by questionnaire for their risk of vCJD:
  - 'Have you a history of CJD or other prion disease in your family?'
  - 'Have you ever received growth hormone or gonadotropin treatment?'
  - 'Have you ever had surgery on your brain or spinal cord?'
  - 'Since 1980, have you had any transfusions of blood or blood components (red cells, plasma, cryoprecipitate or platelets)?'
- Centers serving populations at high risk, e.g. hemophilia centers, should use single use disinfectants.
- All endoscope channels should be brushed with a dedicated single-use brush appropriate for the instrument channel length and diameter.
- 'Invasive' procedures are those that breach gut mucosa and where an unsheathed accessory is then withdrawn up through the scope. Diathermy, APC and laser therapy are also invasive and if such a procedure occurs in an 'at risk' patient, the endoscope must then be quarantined.

The device is then taken to the disinfection room where subsequent steps are carried out. In the interest of preventing the endoscope from drying out if it is not disinfected immediately or if the disinfection room is far from the endoscopy room, the endoscope should be immersed in a cleaning and decontaminating fluid.

However, before an endoscope is immersed, it must undergo a leakage test.

2.2. Initial cleaning (basin 1)

An adequate number of basins must be available for manual cleaning steps. The purpose of this phase is to reduce the endoscope's contamination level and remove any debris by physicochemical means, as well as a mechanical process during which force is applied.

Manual cleaning is undertaken by completely immersing the endoscope in a basin containing an enzymatic detergent solution.

The initial cleaning phase must include the following actions and a minimum of 10 min should be spent on this phase:

- Clean the endoscope insertion tube
- Remove and clean valves, buttons and other moving parts, keeping them with the endoscope for traceability purposes
- Brush down all of the endoscope channels that are accessible. (Note: the length and diameter of cleaning brushes must be suitable for each endoscope.) Single use brushes are recommended.
- Irrigate all of the endoscope's flushable channels.
- Brush out the endoscope's tips and crevices
- Swab the endoscope again if the irrigation fluid is not perfectly clear
- Purge the channels.

 Note

If, in lieu of irrigators or connections provided by the manufacturer, pumps are used, it is absolutely essential to verify that the pumps are at least as efficient as the irrigators or connectors in terms of fluid circulation in the various channels.

2.3. First rinsing (basin 2)

- After immersing the endoscope in the basin, rinse and irrigate it with tap water to remove debris and any traces of detergent. Use a pump or syringe to ensure that the water enters the endoscope's channels
- Then purge the channels
- Change the rinsing water after each use.

2.4. Second cleaning (basin 1)

- Immerse the endoscope and its (dismantled) accessories in a basin containing a fresh detergent solution
- Irrigate all of the endoscope's channels
- Purge the channels.

A minimum of 5 min should be spent on this phase.

2.5. Intermediate rinsing (basin 2)

- After immersing the endoscope in the basin, rinse and irrigate the endoscope with tap water to remove all debris and traces of detergent. Use a pump or syringe to ensure that the water enters the endoscope's channels
- Purge the channels
- Change the rinsing water after each use.

2.6. Disinfection (basin 3)

This phase is efficient only if the cleaning before is well done.

In most countries, manual disinfection is now unacceptable and the use of automated endoscope reprocessing machines (AER) is required. For countries where AERs are not mandatory or widely available, the process for manual cleaning is described below but this practice will have the desired effect *only* if the previous two phases were carried out properly, and is strongly discouraged.

This operation is composed of the following steps:

- Irrigate the endoscope in a basin containing a suitable disinfectant
- Irrigate the channels
- Leave the product on the endoscope for the length of time recommended by the manufacture
- Irrigate and purge the channels.

Disinfectant selection

Use a product that is solely a disinfectant, and not a disinfecting detergent. In selecting a disinfectant, the required level of disinfection must be taken into account: bactericidal, virucidal, fungicidal, etc.

Glutaraldehyde and other aldehydes as well as alcohol-based disinfectants are no longer recommended, as their fixative properties may bind prions and other proteins within the endoscope channels. Products containing group II active agents such as chlorine dioxide or superoxidized water are recommended.

Peracetic acid may also be used. Disinfectants must be prepared and used in accordance with the manufacturer's specifications at all times, especially with reference to duration of use, as some group II agents are unstable. Units undertaking procedures on populations of patients at risk of vCJD should consider using single-use disinfectants.

2.7. Final rinse (basin 4)

The purpose of the final rinse is to reduce toxic risk by eliminating all traces of disinfectant on the device without changing the level of cleanliness and antisepsis that was attained in the previous phases.

- Immerse the endoscope in the basin
- Use a pump or syringe to ensure that the water enters the endoscope's channels
- Rinse thoroughly using abundant water.

The quality of the final rinsing water will be determined by the level of disinfection obtained previously. Bacterial sampling of the final rinse water must be undertaken regularly.

The water quality for gastrointestinal endoscopy must meet either of the following criteria:

- The water must meet bacteriological criteria for potability and must be devoid of *Pseudomonas aeruginosa*, for which the water must be tested at regular intervals.
- The bacteriological content of the water must be controlled; this is generally done via filtration.

Purge the channels, which is the final step in this phase.

Change the final rinsing water after each endoscopy procedure.

 Clinical Tip

Each endoscopy centre should have a regular planned maintenance of their AERs with written records.

2.8. Drying

- Wipe the outside of the endoscope and the endoscope accessories using a suitable element.
- Dry the inside of the channels using filtered medical air. Isopropyl alcohol is no longer recommended because of its fixative properties.

2.9. Storage

Store endoscopes in a clean and dry place, protected from any source of microbial contamination, and preferably in an enclosure whose efficacy has been evaluated. Purpose-built storage cabinets using filtered air have been shown to prevent colonization for up to 72 h and may obviate the need for endoscope reprocessing before every list.

Do not store endoscopes in cases.

2.10. Post-storage disinfection

If an endoscope has been stored for >3 h, it must be disinfected via a procedure comprising, at a minimum, a disinfection and final rinsing phase, in such a way that: (a) the manufacturer's recommended time for soaking the endoscope in disinfectant is observed; and (b) water is circulated in the endoscope's channels.

3. Endoscope disinfection using AERs

Two types of AER are available:

- Those which carry out all of the aforementioned manual phases except for preliminary cleaning. If your AER only performs one cleaning phase, before putting the endoscope into it, it is advisable to use a manual procedure comprising the following phases: preliminary cleaning, leakage test, cleaning, and rinsing.
- Those that only perform disinfection, rinsing and drying phases. All mechanical pre-disinfecting phases should be performed as described above for the manual procedure.

The manufacture and use of AERs must comply with ISO 15883. The use of 'pass-through' machines is recommended in several countries (see Ch. 1.5) but this has major implications for the design and layout of endoscopy units.

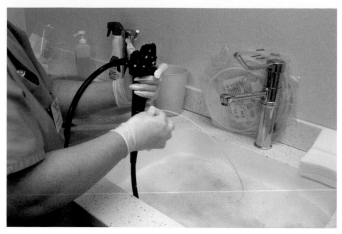

Figure 1 Swabbing an endoscope operating channel.

Today's AERs perform cycles composed of two cleaning phases.

The use of such machines requires a preliminary phase that must be performed immediately following the use of the endoscope and that comprises the following steps:

- Pre-immersion leakage test
- Cleaning the insertion tube
- Air purging
- Aspiration
- Channel swabbing (Fig. 1)
- A rinsing phase if the detergent used could potentially alter the manner in which the AER operates (Fig. 1).

This phase is carried out in water with an enzymatic detergent but containing no disinfectant. The endoscope should be soaked for as long as necessary for swabbing. Place the endoscope in the AER ensuring that all connectors are correctly secured. Start the machine immediately after you place the endoscope in it.

> **Clinical Tip**
>
> It is essential that all endoscopes used in your endoscopy unit, the chosen disinfectant, and the AER and all its connectors are all compatible with each other. This needs to be carefully checked with each manufacturer before purchase.

4. Cleaning procedure for accessories

4.1. Steam-sterilizable instruments

This type of procedure is used less frequently nowadays, as single use disposable accessories are widely used in many countries. Reusable instruments should only be used where no equivalent disposable device exists and in these situations, full traceability is essential. In some countries, economic considerations mean that reusable accessories are still used, in which case, the following procedures should be followed:

- Dismantle the instruments
- Clean and brush them in a cleaning/decontamination solution
- Place instruments in an ultrasonic cleaning basin

- Rinse and dry very carefully, if possible using medically filtered air
- Place the instruments in sealable packets
- Steam-sterilize at 134°C for 18 min
- Store prior to use.

4.2. Non-steam-sterilizable instruments

These types of instruments are rarely used nowadays.

The cleaning procedure is the same as for flexible endoscopes, and should be carried out in such a way that all five phases are followed. It is particularly important that the procedure be carried out immediately following use of the instruments, and that a preliminary cleaning phase occurs.

The instruments must be stored in specialized disposable packaging, the appearance of which is noticeably different from that of sterilization packaging. Stored instruments must undergo a disinfection and rinsing phase prior to use.

4.3. Basin maintenance

The following must be performed after each use:

- Rinse out the basins
- Clean and disinfect them by wiping them down using a soft wipe impregnated with a detergent disinfectant product.

5. The ideal endoscopy unit

5.1. Endoscope cleaning room equipment and layout

The equipment and layout of this room (see also Ch. 1.5) must be specifically intended for the cleaning and maintenance of medical devices. It should designed in accordance with the 'forward movement' principle, i.e. equipment flow is one-way from dirty to clean.

The room must meet the following criteria:

- Good aeration – ventilation suitable for the products being used
- A work surface, plus one or more benches that integrate 4–6 basins
- Pumps that allow solutions to be circulated in endoscope channels. These pumps should be designed in such a way that the tubes connected to the endoscopes can readily undergo all of the various disinfection phases with a minimum of manual intervention
- A filtered medical-air connection for drying the devices
- If AERs are used, a sufficient number of machines must be available to allow all endoscopes that are used to be cleaned concurrently. Manual disinfection should be used in an emergency only, if washer-disinfectors are normally used. It is important, however, that all staff are trained in manual cleaning and understand how to undertake this if necessary. In such a case, it is essential to ensure that the manual procedure does not result in a reduction in disinfection quality
- One or more cabinets for vertical or horizontal endoscope storage

- A hand-washing station for personnel that is separate from the basins used for endoscopes
- Separate containers for biological and non-biological waste.

5.2. Personnel

Each patient is a potential source of infection and endoscopy unit staff should take the following precautions:

- They should be vaccinated against hepatitis A and B and typhoid
- They should wash their hands before and after treating a patient
- They should wear an operating gown during the endoscopy procedure, as well as gloves, operating room shoes, a mask, and protective eyewear
- They should wear single use gloves while cleaning and disinfecting devices. This measure also helps

Box 2	Protection of staff working in decontamination

- Long-sleeved waterproof gowns – change between patients.
- Single-use gloves that cover the forearms.
- Protective goggles or glasses.
- Charcoal-containing facemasks to reduce inhalation of vapors.
- An approved respirator in case of spillages.

protect against any skin irritation caused by the products used

- Disinfection personnel should receive specific training in disinfection processes. This training should be updated at regular intervals, particularly when new endoscopes, reprocessors or cleaning/disinfecting products are developed
- Each endoscopy room should have two endoscopy assistants (one for the patient, the other for the equipment), as well as a trained medical technician.

Box 3	Good practice for endoscope disinfection – 16 key elements

1. Create and follow a written policy for endoscope cleaning that is approved by the hospital's Infection Control and Governance Committees. This policy must be valid for all endoscopic examination settings, e.g. in the operating rooms and in emergency situations.
2. Carry out the cleaning process twice for each cleaning cycle and use a group II procedure in conjunction with a suitable antimicrobial product.
3. When using choledoscopes, repeat the high-level disinfection procedure, regardless of how long the device has been stored.
4. Begin the endoscope cleaning process immediately following the procedure.
5. Carry out disinfection procedures in a dedicated room.
6. Before immersing a videoendoscope, put its sealing cap on.
7. Perform a leakage test before immersing an endoscope. If the test reveals any leaks, send the endoscope for repair in packaging that protects personnel and the environment, and in so doing indicate that the endoscope has *not* been disinfected in accordance with the required procedure.
8. Irrigate all endoscope channels, including the auxiliary (elevator and water jet) channels that some endoscopes have. In most cases, such channels can only be accessed using a special connector. Brush or swab all accessible channels.
9. Change cleaning and rinsing solutions after each use.

10. Do not keep disinfectant solutions for longer than the manufacturer's recommendations, as some, e.g. superoxidized water, are unstable.
11. Perform a final rinsing of the endoscope in a basin containing water whose quality is compatible with the disinfecting level attained, as follows: for choledoscopes, use sterilized bottled water in accordance with the EU pharmacopeia for choledoscopes; for semi-critical endoscopes, use bacteriologically controlled water.
12. The microbiological quality of the final-rinse basin must be at least of the same quality as the water in the basin. This means that the basin must be sterile if sterile bottled water is used.
13. Purge the channels so that all remaining fluid is removed from the channels. Prior to use, choledoscopes may only be purged using sterile physiological saline.
14. Implement a tracking and tracing system for all disinfection procedures. Caps and buttons should be cleaned with the same endoscope that they were used with and be part of the traceability process.
15. Make sure that endoscopes are dried thoroughly, particularly their channels. Store endoscopes in a clean and dry place, in such a way that they are protected against environmental contamination.
16. Any incidents relating to problems with disinfection processes or equipment must be recorded and notified to the local hospital infection control team so that they can be investigated, lessons learnt, and processes modified if necessary.

Further Reading

ASGE Standards of Practice Committee: Infection control during GI endoscopy, *Gastrointest Endosc* 67:781–790, 2008.

Beilenhoff U, Neumann CS, Rey JF, et al: ESGE-ESGENA guideline: Cleaning and disinfection in gastrointestinal endoscopy. Update 2008, *Endoscopy* 40:939–957, 2008.

BSG Guidelines for Decontamination of Equipment for Gastrointestinal Endoscopy: The Report of a working party of the British Society of Gastroenterology

Endoscopy Committee 2008. www.bsg.org.uk/clinical-guidelines/endoscopy

Endoscopy and individuals at risk of vCJD for public health purposes. A consensus statement from the British Society of Gastroenterology Decontamination working group and the ACDP TSE working group; Endoscopy and vCJD sub-group. http://www.dh.gov.uk/ab/ACDP/TSEguidance/index.htm (see Annex F-Endoscopy, updated January 2011).

ISO 15883-15881 Washer-disinfectors. Part 1: General requirements, terms and definitions and tests. www.iso.org

Marchetti B, Boustière C, Chapuis C, et al: La désinfection du matériel en endoscopie digestive, *Acta Endosc* 37:699–704, 2007.

Patient safety and reduction of risk of transmission of Creutzfeldt–Jakob disease (CJD) via interventional procedures, National Institute for Health and Clinical Excellence, 2006. www.nice.org.uk/guidance/IPG196

Jean-Christophe Létard, François Cessot

Key Point

- Close collaboration between gastroenterologists and pathologists is essential.

Box 1   Breached muscularis mucosa

Patients with early cancer in whom the muscularis mucosae has been breached do not require surgery if they have the following four criteria:
- Absence of a mucin or poorly-differentiated focus for colonic polyps
- Absence of lymphatic involvement
- No evidence of venous infiltration
- The resection margin is >1 mm from the tumor.

Introduction

Endoscopic biopsies are an indispensable diagnostic tool, allowing histological, immunological and microbiological studies, as well as tissue culture. Biopsy specimens should include the full depth of the mucosa and if possible the submucosa, particularly in settings involving screening for inflammatory disease (granulomas) or vascular disease (amyloid deposits, vasculitis, lymphangiectasia). Several high quality biopsies should be taken to avoid the creation of artifacts due to erosion, epithelial hemorrhaging, and cytoplasmic vacuolization.

Low-grade dysplasia involves the following cellular changes:

- Preservation of crypt architecture, with mild distortion if present
- Stratified nuclei, especially near the base of the crypts. This stratification typically does not reach the crypt lumen
- Hyperchromatic nuclei; mitoses may be present in the upper portion of the crypt.

High-grade dysplasia demonstrates the following changes:

- High-grade dysplasia includes carcinoma *in situ*
- Stratification of nuclei extends to into the superficial parts of the cells
- Prominent hyperchromatism, large pleomorphic nuclei, numerous mitoses, and substantial structural changes (disorganized glands and crypts; pseudovilli).

A microinvasive malignancy exists if the lesion breaches the muscularis mucosae. When an endoscopic mucosal resection has been performed, the submucosa should be examined to ensure that it has not been infiltrated. Box 1 documents the criteria for careful monitoring versus surgical referral in patients in whom the muscularis mucosa has been breached.

1. Sample collection in endoscopy

Biopsy specimens must be placed in fixative immediately or mounted on slides. The specimens are numbered and patient identification details added. Formaldehyde can be used to stain any specimen, particularly those containing mucin, fat or endocrine cells. Formaldehyde does not alter cellular structures, particularly DNA, so that molecular biology techniques can be performed on the tissue if required. Box 2 shows what to document on a pathology form. Samples that are obtained following endoscopic mucosal resection or dissection should be pinned (Box 3).

2. Processing of biopsy samples

2.1. Biopsies

After being labeled, biopsy specimens are checked against the bottles, as well as the specified biopsy sites, and are then desiccated, incorporated into paraffin, cut into 2 μm slices, and stained using hematoxylin and eosin (H&E). Specific stains can be used if required. Those most frequently requested are: Masson trichrome (stains connective tissue, vascular walls, basal membrane); Perl's (excess iron); PAS (Whipple's disease); Congo red for amyloidosis (homogenous appearance, with green birefringence under polarized light); and Alcian blue for mucin. The lamina propria is seen with silver impregnation (for reticulin) or Giemsa (for lympho-plasmocytotic cells).

Box 2   What to note when taking biopsies

- Location – if necessary by labeling the reference points on a diagram, particularly for Barrett's esophagus
- Relevant aspects of the patient's medical history
- Endoscopic findings.

The editors would like to acknowledge Brigitte Marchetti.

Immunohistochemistry can be performed using specific antibodies which can be used to assess undifferentiated tumors. Markers which can be assessed include:

- Epithelial marker expression (cytokeratin, EMA) for carcinomas
- KIT (CD117), CD34, DOG1 and PDGFRA for gastrointestinal stromal tumors (GIST)
- NSE and chromogranin markers for carcinoids
- Leukocyte antigen and B and T markers for lymphoid tissue markers
- Connective tissue markers (vimentin) in sarcomas
- Flow cytometry or imaging analyses can be performed to determine the aneuploid nature of a tumor (which indicates a poor prognosis)
- PCR studies can also be performed.

2.2. Cytological smears

The endoscopist performs the smear, following aspiration, or brushing. However, a biopsy is always preferable to a cytology smear, regardless of the quality of the specimen or the pathologist's competence. Cytology smear results are only conclusive in the presence of a previously diagnosed tumor.

2.3. Bile or pancreatic juice

This is performed using a dry tube containing at least one drop of formaldehyde. If the specimen is not analyzed immediately, it should be refrigerated at 4°C. The analysis can be performed using the classic method or the so-called monolayer technique, depending on the equipment available. Any contrast material can be used, with Papanicolaou and May-Grünwald-Giemsa (MGG) the most frequently used.

Biliary or pancreatic brush specimens are spread on glass slides, air dried, and then sent to the pathologist for MGG staining. The monolayer technique allows for dilution of the material collected on the brush in a specific liquid, whereupon the cells are spread more evenly so that they form a 'single' layer. This technique allows for better cell visualization as it eliminates cell clumping and superimposition.

3. Histology of the GI tract

3.1. The esophagus

The esophagus consists of the mucosa, submucosa, and muscularis propria (Fig. 1). The mucosa contains non-keratinized stratified squamous epithelium, lamina propria, and muscularis mucosae. The submucosa contains small aciniform cells that secret mucins and connective fibers (papillas), which extend far into the mucosa. The muscularis propria consists of striated muscle in the upper third, both striated and smooth muscle in the middle, and smooth muscle in the lower third. The esophagus contains no serous membrane.

3.1.1. Squamous cell cancer of the esophagus

In microinvasive squamous cell cancer of the esophagus, the tumor extends through the basal membrane up to, but not invading, the muscularis mucosae (PT1m) or submucosa (PT1sm). Lugol's iodine solution is used to identify and determine the extent of squamous cell cancer, as lesions with low levels of glycogen (i.e. tumor cells) do not absorb the contrast material. Other stains which are used include methylene blue, acetic acid, and indigo carmine (see Ch. 2.4).

3.1.2. Barrett's esophagus

Four quadrant biopsies should be taken every 2 cm from the Barrett's mucosa. Advanced imaging techniques (Figs 2, 3) can be used to screen for Barrett's esophagus (see Chs 6.1

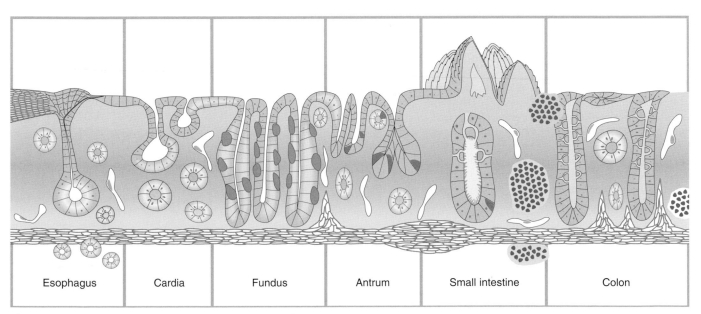

| Esophagus | Cardia | Fundus | Antrum | Small intestine | Colon |

Figure 1 Structure of the GI tract, from the esophagus to the colon.

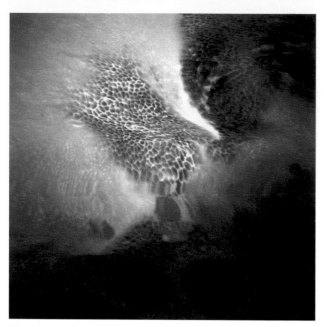

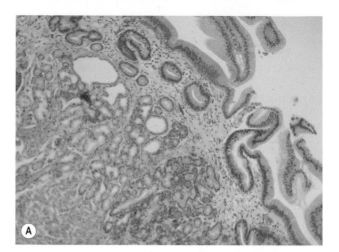

Figure 2 Gastroesophageal junction seen with confocal endomicroscopy.

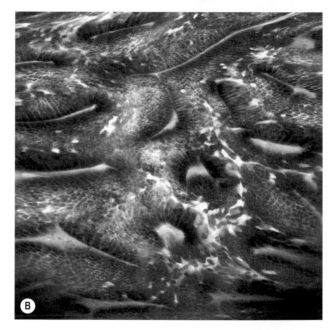

and 6.2). The gastroesophageal junction can be visualized using confocal endomicroscopy (Fig. 2), as can Barrett's esophagus (Fig. 3B) and dysplasia (Fig. 3C), which correlate with the pathological findings (Fig. 3A). Biopsies should be submitted to pathology in separate containers to permit focusing of subsequent biopsies, should dysplasia be detected. Depending on whether high-grade, low-grade or no dysplasia is found, this determines management and endoscopic screening intervals (for screening intervals for Barrett's esophagus, see Ch. 3).

3.2. The stomach

The cardia is a 5–30 mm area composed of individual or interlinked cardiac glands, which contain identical mucus secreting cells. The fundus (Fig. 4A,B) contains two regions. The first is delineated by furrows containing vessels with thick mucosa. Its crypts are round and regular and are surrounded by a vascular web (Fig. 4D), with numerous narrow, rectangular glands, which are perpendicular to the surface. The second region is composed of mucus and parietal cells. The body of the fundic gland is mainly composed of parietal cells, but also contains larger cells that are rich in pepsin or zymogens. The antrum (Fig. 4C) contains a thinner mucosa that is 200–1000 μm thick. Its epithelium is more irregular than the fundus. The antrum's crypts are elongated and contain smaller glands that are mainly composed of mucus cells that occur around primary or secondary crypts. Cells producing gastrin and serotonin are also found here.

3.2.1. *Helicobacter pylori* infection

This initially provokes acute gastritis, accompanied by a polynuclear infiltration, followed by chronic gastritis accompanied by a lympho-plasmocyte infiltration (Fig. 5), which provokes lymphoid follicles. The latter occurs mainly in the antrum, but also extends to the fundus. An endoscopic

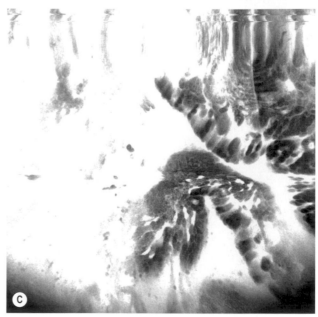

Figure 3 Barrett's esophagus. Seen on (A) histology and (B) endomicroscopy. (C) Dysplasia in Barrett's esophagus on endomicroscopy.

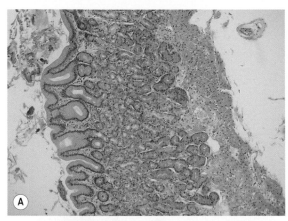

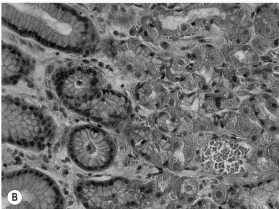

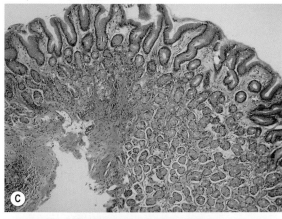

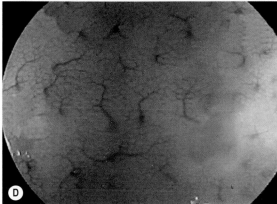

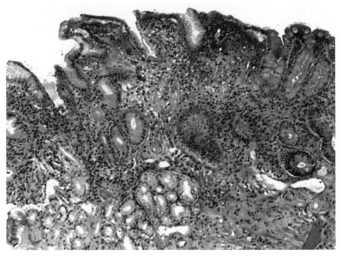

Figure 5 Chronic gastritis with lymphocyte infiltrations on histology.

examination may reveal mini- or macro-nodules that constitute submucosal lymphoid nodules. Micro-ulceration can be seen with zoom magnification (Fig. 6). *Helicobacter pylori* infection is initially accompanied by elevated acid secretion, which induces chronic duodenitis, which in turn is associated with gastric metaplasia and colonization by bacteria. Chronic *Helicobacter pylori* infection is associated with atrophy, which can be associated with reduced acid secretion and should be investigated during screening for intestinal metaplasia (Fig. 7).

Helicobacter pylori is detected via direct examination, culture, or a urease test (CLO test). Culture is considered the gold standard, and allows assessment of antibiotic sensitivity. CAG A+ strains tend to activate inflammatory cells. Specimens should be collected from the antrum (2 cm around the pylorus) and fundus, in accordance with the Sydney classification system (two antral and two fundic specimens). *Helicobacter pylori* distribution is heterogeneous in the stomach, but predominates in the antrum.

Figure 4 Gastric histology. (A,B) Histology of the fundus. (C) Gastric antrum. (D) Vascular network of the fundus (×60).

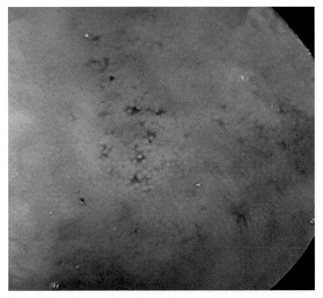

Figure 6 Antral micro-ulcerations (×60).

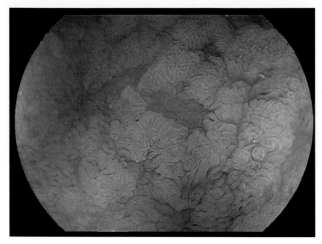

Figure 7 Atrophic gastritis with intestinal metaplasia (×50).

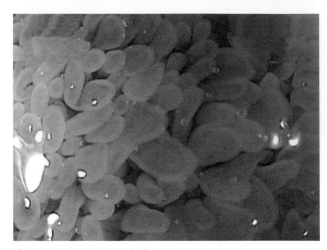

Figure 9 Normal duodenal villi (×120).

3.2.2. Linitis plastica

In cases of gastric linitis plastica (Fig. 8), where there is invasion of the gastric wall by small signet-ring cells, biopsies sometimes yield false negative results and have to be repeated. Endoscopic ultrasound should be used where doubt exists.

3.3. Duodenum and jejunum

The duodenum and jejunum contain villi, which are covered with absorbent cells (enterocytes with microvillous, brush border) as well as a very small number of goblet cells, with crypts of Lieberkühn between the villi.

 Clinical Tip

Duodenal biopsies should be taken in the distal duodenum below the ampulla of Vater, as the villi in the first part of the duodenum are only three-quarters of the height of the villi below the papilla (Fig. 9).

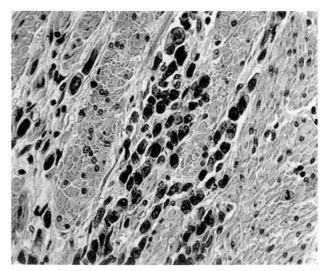

Figure 8 Linitis plastica. Note the submucosal infiltration accompanied by small, signet-ring cells.

Duodenal biopsies should be performed in cases of anemia secondary to iron or folic acid deficiency (or any other nutritional deficiency), chronic diarrhea accompanied by exudative enteropathy or malabsorption, particularly for the diagnosis or monitoring of celiac disease. Duodenal biopsies are also recommended in cases of suspected amebiasis, strongyloidoses, or bacterial overgrowth. Immunohistochemical staining should be performed on biopsies in patients in whom lymphoma is suspected.

3.3.1. Celiac disease

Celiac disease is associated with the following:

- Partial villous atrophy if the villi become short but are still higher than the crypt villi
- Subtotal atrophy if the crypts are higher than the villi
- Total atrophy if there are no villi in the presence of glandular hyperplasia
- An increased number of goblet and intraepithelial lymphocyte cells (>20% of epithelial cells)
- An increase in the number of lympho-plasmocytes in the lamina propria.

Celiac disease is associated with an increased risk of gastrointestinal lymphoma.

3.4. Rectum, colon, and ileum

The ileal mucosa is composed of long villi that are identical to those in the jejunum; goblet cells outnumber absorbent cells by a ratio of 5:1 (Fig. 10).

The colonic mucosa, which is mainly composed of goblet, absorbant and endocrine cells, and varies in thickness from 500–1000 μm (owing to the absence of Paneth cells) (Figs 11–13). Small numbers of intraepithelial lymphocytes (<5% of the epithelial cells) are observed in normal colic mucosa. The basal membrane is <5 μm thick, and the crypts (1700/cm^2), are rectangular, and terminate with parallel intestinal glands. The goblet cells are more numerous in the upper part of the gland. Endocrine cells occur in the lower segment. The lamina propria is composed of fibroblasts, smooth mucosal fibers, macrophages, capillaries and

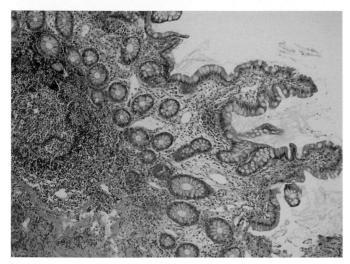

Figure 10 Ileal lymphoid follicle.

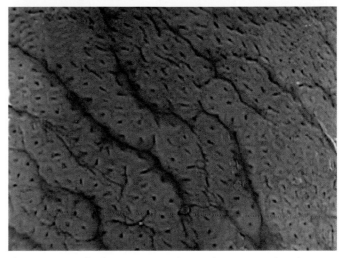

Figure 12 Normal colonic mucosa with a regular pit pattern (×120).

small lymphocytes containing a few lymphoid follicles. The muscularis mucosae is 20–40 µm thick, and the submucosa is composed of loose connective tissue that is rich in arterioles and mini-veins and contains the Meissner plexus. The terminal vascularization is web-like and contains glandular crypts. Peri-cryptic micro-arches are more numerous in the caecum than in the sigmoid colon, whereas colonic mucosa thickness varies inversely.

3.4.1. Benign polyps

Benign polyps include hyperplasic, inflammatory, and juvenile hamartomatous polyps.

- Hyperplastic polyps exhibit a saw-tooth appearance. The epithelium is characterized by elongation of the glandular crypts; the muscularis mucosa is thickened. Hyperplastic polyps are typically located in the recto-sigmoid and are <5 mm in diameter. If multiple, they can be associated with hyperplastic polyposis syndrome (Box 4)
- Inflammatory polyp containing numerous inflammatory cells and a regenerative basal membrane
- Juvenile hamartomatous polyps occur where the epithelium is replaced by tissue composed of pseudocystic crypts, with central thickened fibromuscular stroma and eosinophilic infiltration. If multiple, they can be associated with familial juvenile polyposis syndrome (Box 4).

3.4.2. Neoplastic polyps

There are several types of adenoma:

- *Tubular adenomas* (87%) consist of glandular tubes of irregular size with abundant lamina propria. At least 75% must have a tubular component.
- *Villous adenomas* (5%) are characterized by long, straight glands, which extend from the center of the polyp. At least 75% of the polyp should have a villous component.
- *Tubulovillous adenomas* (8–25%), contain histological features of both tubular and villous adenoma.
- *Serrated adenomas* contain mixed histological features of both hyperplastic and adenomatous polyps. There is

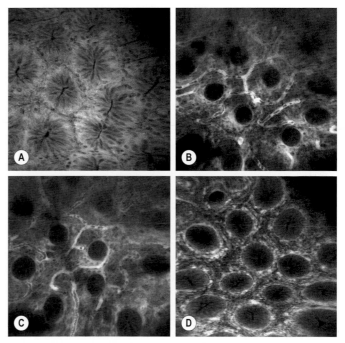

Figure 13 Endomicroscopy (×1000). (A) Sunflower-like colonic mucosa with mucin-rich cells. (B,C) Vascular arches. (D) 150 µm deep.

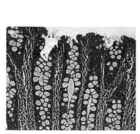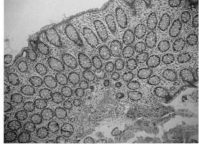

Figure 11 Normal colonic mucosa with regular glands rich in goblet cells. Two axes with perpendicular slices.

Box 4   Hereditary polyposis syndromes

- Hyperplastic polyposis syndrome (HPS).
  This is characterized by multiple, large/proximal hyperplastic polyps and occasionally a smaller number of serrated adenomas. Unlike sporadic hyperplastic polyps, HPS is associated with an increased risk of colorectal cancer. The diagnosis of HPS requires:
  - At least five hyperplastic polyps proximal to the sigmoid colon, with two >1 cm in size *or*
  - Any number of hyperplastic polyps proximal to the sigmoid colon in a person with a 1st-degree relative with HPS *or*
  - >30 hyperplastic polyps throughout the colon.
- Familial adenomatous polyposis (FAP),
  FAP is an autosomal dominant disease involving >100 polyps in the colorectal region with chromosomal mutation 5q21. In addition to developing colorectal cancer at an early age, FAP is associated with duodenal ampullary cancers, gastric cancer, follicular or papillary thyroid cancer, hepatoblastoma and medulloblastomas.
- Familial juvenile polyposis syndrome (FJP).
  Associated with multiple juvenile polyps and inherited in an autosomal dominant fashion. It is associated with an increased risk of developing colorectal cancer, and in some families, gastric cancer.
- Hereditary non-polyposis colorectal cancer (HNPCC).
  HNPCC is due to a mutation in mismatch repair genes, and is associated with gastrointestinal and extraintestinal cancer. HNPCC is associated with the development of colorectal cancer occurring at a younger age (mean 45), which classically occurs in the right colon. The diagnosis can be made using the Amsterdam II criteria (below) or the Bethesda guidelines. FAP must be excluded. The Amsterdam II criteria are:
  - Three members of the same family present with a malignancy associated with HNPCC (colorectal cancer, endometrial cancer, small intestine cancer, transitional cell carcinoma of the ureter or renal pelvis)
  - One individual is a 1st-degree relative of the other two (parent, sibling or child)
  - Two or more successive generations are affected
  - One person developed cancer before the age of 50.
- Peutz–Jeghers syndrome.
  Hamartomatous polyps are found in the colon and small intestine. These consist of a proliferation of smooth muscle extending into the lamina propria with normal overlying epithelium. Associated with an increased risk of gastric, small bowel, colon and pancreatic cancer, as well as non-gastrointestinal cancers.
- Cowden's disease.
  This is associated with multiple hamartomas is accompanied by multiple hamartomas.
- Cronkhite–Canada syndrome.
  This is a non-familal disorder associated with multiple hamartomatous polyps. In addition, patients exhibit alopecia, cutaneous hyperpigmentation, onychodystrophy. Patients present with diarrhea, bleeding, and sepsis.

---

growing evidence that these polyps may be precursor lesions of sporadic microsatellite unstable colon cancers. They should be managed like adenomatous polyps.

- *Microtubular adenomas* with microtubular rings that extend to just below the surface epithelium.
- *Benign adenomas* are polyps that do not exhibit high-grade dysplasia or a malignant focus.

DALM (dysplasia associated lesion or mass), has a different genetic basis from adenomatous polyps. DALM occur in patients with inflammatory bowel disease (ulcerative colitis/Crohn's disease) and are associated with a high risk of colorectal cancer.

Guidelines on who to screen are available in Chapter 4.

3.4.3. Microscopic colitis

There are two types of microscopic colitis: lymphocytic and collagenous. Both are associated with a loss of epithelium surface integrity, a large number of intraepithelial lymphocytes (>20% of all epithelial cells) and lamina propria infiltration by mononuclear cells. Collagenous colitis is associated with an increase in basal membrane thickness to >10 μm. Various areas are affected, although the right colon is more commonly affected. Duodenal biopsies are also useful, as there is an association between lymphocytic gastritis and celiac disease.

3.4.4. Inflammatory bowel disease (IBD)

Patients with IBD should have serial colonic biopsies taken to identify histological signs of the disease. It is important to document carefully the location of these biopsies. In ulcerative colitis, the surface of the glandular epithelium is ulcerated, flat, and associated with regenerative pseudopolyps. In Crohn's disease, there is focal ulceration with acute and chronic inflammation. The focality of the inflammation differs from the diffuse pattern typically seen in ulcerative colitis. Non-caseating granulomata are present in up to 30% of patients.

Patients with long-standing IBD should undergo screening for dysplasia with biopsies taken every 10 cm in addition to targeted biopsies of any focal visible abnormalities (see Ch. 2.4 for details on chromoendoscopy; Ch. 4 for details of screening intervals, and Ch. 6.1 for details on new imaging techniques to detect dysplastic lesions).

3.4.5. Amyloidosis

Deep rectal biopsies should be performed if amyloidosis is suspected, which must include the submucosa if possible. The biopsies are stained with Congo red staining, with 50% of biopsies positive in cases of primary, idiopathic or familial amyloidosis, but are generally negative in cases of hepatorenal amyloidosis in the absence of any other disorder.

3.4.6. Solitary rectal ulcer

Biopsies should be taken from the edge of solitary rectal ulcers.

Box 5   When to biopsy colonic mucosa?

- Biopsies should always be performed in an immunosuppressed patient, particularly on the ileum and right colon, so that opportunistic infection can be detected.
- In non-immunosuppressed patients with unremarkable macroscopic colonic mucosa, biopsies should be taken from both the right and left colon if the colonoscopy is being performed for chronic diarrhea, in particular if lymphocytic or collagenous microscopic colitis is suspected. Rectal biopsies alone are not sufficient.

3.4.7. Hirschsprung's disease

Hirschsprung's disease is a developmental disorder of the enteric nervous system and is characterized by an absence of ganglion cells in the distal colon, resulting in a functional obstruction. Deep rectal biopsies involving the submucosa are indicated in such cases.

Conclusion

Only endoscopy allows access to digestive mucosa for samples. Endoscopy allows direct diagnosis and follow up of every digestive disease.

Further Reading

Axon A, Lambert R, Robaszkiewisz M, et al: The second European endoscopy forum (Sintra, Portugal, 17–18 June 1999), *Endoscopy* 32:411–418, 2000.

Kiesslich R, Neurath FM: Endoscopic confocal imaging, *Clin Gastroenterol Hepatol* 3(Suppl 1):S58–S60, 2005.

Kuramoto S, Oohara T: Flat early cancers of the large intestine, *Cancer* 64:950–955, 1989.

Schlemper RJ, Riddell RH, Kato Y, et al: The Vienna classification of gastrointestinal epithelial neoplasia, *Gut* 47:251–255, 2000.

Tsukuma H, Oshima A, Narahara H, et al: Natural history of early gastric cancer: a non concurrent long term follow up study, *Gut* 47:618–621, 2000.

CHAPTER 2

Preparation for endoscopy

2.1 Management of patients on antithrombotic therapy prior to gastrointestinal endoscopy

Ian Penman, Bertrand Napoleon, Jean Marc Canard, Jean-Christophe Létard, Laurent Palazzo

Summary

Introduction   52

1. Procedure-related bleeding   53

2. Bleeding associated with antithrombotic therapy   53

3. Risks associated with discontinuation of antithrombotic therapy   54

4. Switching from warfarin or antiplatelet drugs to alternative therapy   56

5. Resumption of antithrombotic treatment   56

6. Recommendations   56

Conclusion   57

Key Points

- Guidelines for the management of antithrombotic therapy are important but decisions must be made on a case-by-case basis.
- Bleeding is common but rarely life-threatening, while thromboembolism resulting from interruption of antithrombotic therapy may be fatal or permanently disabling.
- Low risk procedures can be undertaken in anticoagulated patients as long as treatment is within the therapeutic range.
- High-risk procedures that are non-urgent should be deferred until antithrombotic therapy has been completed or until such time as the risks of stopping therapy are low.
- For most procedures, aspirin therapy does not need to be stopped.
- If in doubt, the cardiologist or physician who prescribed antithrombotic therapy should be consulted for advice before any planned procedure.
- Where possible, low-risk procedures (e.g. biliary stenting without sphincterotomy) and measures to minimize bleeding (clips, loops), should be considered.

The editors would like to acknowledge Bernard Boneu, Luc Maillard, Charles-Marc Samama, Jean-François Sched, Gérard Gay, Thierry Ponchon, Denis Sautereau, Jean-Pierre Arput, Christian Boustière, Jean Boyer, Jean Cassigneul, Pierre-Adrien Dalbies, Jean Escourrou, René Laugier, Runo Richard-Molard, Gilbert Tucat, Bruno Vedrenne.

DOI: 10.1016/B978-0-7020-3128-1.00002-X

Introduction

The management of patients taking anticoagulant or antiplatelet drugs is an increasingly common problem prior to endoscopic procedures. The risk of bleeding must be given serious consideration, but without underestimating the risk of discontinuing antithrombotic treatment: bleeding is rarely life-threatening, whereas a thromboembolic event associated with interruption of therapy may be permanently disabling or fatal. It is not possible to formulate guidelines that cover all conceivable clinical scenarios and management of a patient's antithrombotic therapy must be individualized.

Ideally, any necessary therapeutic adjustments should be undertaken in consultation with the doctor who prescribed the treatment in question, and based on a case-by-case evaluation of the risk–benefit ratio of the planned procedure and the envisaged changes in the patient's antithrombotic therapy. Unfortunately, in most cases, these ideal conditions do not pertain, for a number of reasons: the patient may have forgotten which doctor prescribed the drug or the doctor may be unavailable; or there may be a difference of opinion or lack of knowledge regarding the respective risks entailed by the procedure and discontinuation of the medication. In deciding what to do, the following factors should be taken into account:

- The bleeding risk associated with the procedure
- The antithrombotic therapy being used

- The thromboembolic risk associated with discontinuation of therapy.

In many countries endoscopists, cardiologists, and hematologists have developed consensus recommendations, which of course are only indicative and may evolve over time, as new information emerges. Several of these guidelines are listed at the end of this chapter.

1. Procedure-related bleeding

There is little information available in the literature concerning the hemorrhagic risk associated with antithrombotic agents. It is reasonable to presume that such therapy increases the risk of bleeding above normal levels by rendering bleeding episodes symptomatic that would go unnoticed in the presence of normal coagulation. However, antithrombotics do not themselves *cause* bleeding.

Hence, antithrombotics have little impact on procedures whose bleeding risk is low. The following factors should be taken into consideration in assessing the risk of a procedure that is performed on a patient who is taking an antithrombotic:

- In the case of procedures for which the risk of spontaneous bleeding is >1%, antithrombotic therapy may exacerbate bleeding. Hence, the risk of bleeding associated with a sphincterotomy would increase by a factor of 7.8 on warfarin therapy.
- The incidence (but not severity) of bleeding may increase for bleeding that is inaccessible to endoscopic hemostasis, e.g. endoscopic ultrasound-guided FNA.
- In the presence of an elevated risk of perforation, antithrombotic therapy may complicate management should this occur.

Procedure risk may be classified as below.

1.1. Low-risk procedures (Box 1)

In these, bleeding occurs only rarely and can be managed endoscopically. In the case of colonoscopy, it is rarely known in advance whether there will be polyps requiring resection. However, the perforation risk entailed by the examination may increase the risks of maintaining antithrombotic therapy if emergency surgery turns out to be necessary. These two factors may sometimes prompt classification of colonoscopy as a risky procedure, as a precautionary measure. Taking a mucosal biopsy at these procedures (regardless of whether standard or pediatric forceps are used) does not significantly increase the risk of bleeding.

Box 1 Procedures with a low risk of bleeding
• Upper endoscopy.   • Flexible sigmoidoscopy.   • Colonoscopy without polypectomy.   • Diagnostic endoscopic ultrasound (no FNA /biopsy).   • ERCP (with ampullary or biliary dilatation, or insertion of a stent without sphincterotomy).   • Enteroscopy.   • Capsule endoscopy.   • Enteral stent placement (without dilatation).

1.2. High-risk procedures

1.2.1. High risk of bleeding

Table 1 summarizes the estimated risks of bleeding with various endoscopic procedures (1% or more), in settings where the bleeding can be managed endoscopically.

1.2.2. Low risk of bleeding (<1%) in settings where bleeding cannot be monitored endoscopically

- Endoscopic ultrasound-guided FNA
- Percutaneous gastrostomy
- Gastrointestinal stricture dilatation by bougie or balloon dilator. Insertion of a self-expanding metallic stent without dilatation
- Transnasal gastroscopy (risk of epistaxis).

2. Bleeding associated with antithrombotic therapy

2.1. Antiplatelet drugs

These drugs inhibit platelet function, particularly activation and aggregation.

Aspirin and most NSAIDs inhibit platelet aggregation. Aspirin induces irreversible inhibition of cyclooxygenase. Doses usually range from 75 to 325 mg/day (1–2 mg/kg in practice). Disturbance in clotting is not fully corrected until all platelets have been replaced, which takes 7–10 days.

However, a functional platelet level of 50×10^9/L is regarded as adequate for normal hemostatic function. Platelets are renewed at a rate of 10% per day. Thus, depending on the baseline platelet level, discontinuing treatment for 3–5 days is generally sufficient for a patient to recover their normal hemostatic function. NSAIDs also inhibit cyclooxygenase, albeit reversibly. The duration of action is temporary and is determined by the individual drug's half-life.

The limited data available suggest that standard doses of aspirin and NSAIDs do not significantly increase the risk of bleeding secondary to endoscopic biopsy, colonic snare polypectomy or biliary sphincterotomy. For snare

Table 1 The estimated risks of bleeding with various endoscopic procedures

Procedure	Estimated bleeding risk (%)
Colonic polypectomy	1–2.5
Gastric polypectomy or jumbo/snare biopsy	4
Endoscopic mucosal resection	≤22
Ampullectomy	8
Endoscopic sphincterotomy	2.5–5
Photodynamic therapy	≤6
Endoscopic treatment of esophageal or gastric varices	≤6
Endoscopic hemostasis of vascular lesions	≤5

polypectomy, use of a detachable loop is recommended in the presence of a polyp stalk >1 cm. There are no data concerning polyp resection by endoscopic mucosal resection (EMR) or other high-risk procedures in patients on aspirin therapy.

2.1.1. Thienopyridines, dipyridamole, and glycoprotein inhibitors

Thienopyridines (ticlopidine and clopidogrel) irreversibly suppress one of the adenosine diphosphate (ADP) platelet receptors. These preparations frequently prolong the bleeding time, but there is currently no test available for measurement of restoration of normal platelet function. In cases where therapy is suspended, it is recommended that 7–10 days be allowed for platelet renewal. However, as is the case with aspirin, 3–5 days may be sufficient for the return of normal hemostatic function (see above). Platelet transfusion can be beneficial for bleeding management. Ticlopidine has been largely replaced by clopidogrel because of side-effects. There is also little data available on the newer thienopyridine prasugrel. Dipyridamole has only a moderate antiplatelet effect and does not increase the risk of bleeding. Glycoprotein IIb/IIIa inhibitors, abciximab, eptifibatide, and tirofiban, are used parenterally in the short-term management of acute coronary syndromes. Endoscopy in patients receiving these agents would only occur in life-threatening situations and after careful discussion with the patient's cardiologist, and these drugs are not the subject of this chapter.

2.2. Vitamin K antagonists

Coumarin (warfarin, acenocoumarol) and phenindione are the only oral anticoagulant drugs available today. Their plasma half-lives vary but normal coagulation is usually restored 2–4 days following discontinuation of the drug. The anticoagulation effect achieved depends on the dose used and the patient's susceptibility to the drug. The International Normalized Ratio (INR) accurately reflects this effect. The risk of bleeding increases as the INR rises, an INR ranging from 2 to 3 is generally needed for effective anticoagulation and carries a low risk of bleeding.

An INR of 3–4.5 is necessary in the presence of a major thromboembolic risk. If the INR is <1.5, the bleeding risk is on a par with that of non-treated patients. In the event of an overdose (INR >6) and/or bleeding, various options are available. In the absence of bleeding, discontinuation of treatment and oral vitamin K intake may be sufficient. In the presence of major bleeding, intravenous vitamin K (5–10 mg) along with IV prothrombin complex, 30–50 units/kg or fresh frozen plasma should be considered. For minor bleeding, smaller doses of IV vitamin K should be given, e.g. 0.5–2.5 mg.

> **Warning!**
>
> Giving large doses of vitamin K can make it difficult to re-establish anticoagulation with warfarin after the bleeding episode is resolved. Discuss with Hematology and the patient's cardiologist/specialist before giving IV vitamin K.

2.3. Heparins

Heparins are the third family of antithrombotics that are widely used. The main indications for heparins are prophylaxis and therapy of venous thromboembolic disease, including deep venous thrombosis (DVT), pulmonary embolism, acute coronary syndromes, and thrombosis prophylaxis in patients with mechanical cardiac valve prostheses before switching to oral anticoagulation. Only low-molecular weight heparins (LMWHs) are used for DVT prophylaxis, in doses ranging from 2000 to 5000 U once daily according to the thrombosis risk level and the product used. The bleeding risk with these doses is low, becoming negligible 12 hour following administration. For other indications, either subcutaneous LMWHs or unfractionated heparin administered intravenously is used.

The LMWH doses in such settings vary considerably depending on the preparation used and body weight. If a LMWH is administered twice daily, it is necessary to wait 12–18 hour for the heparin level to return to a level that allows normal hemostasis. If the drug is administered once daily, 24 hour must be allowed. It should be noted that the activated partial thromboplastin time (APTT) is *not* useful in such cases as it remains normal, even in the presence of persistent heparinemia. The only way to verify the presence of residual heparinemia is the anti-Xa activity level, which should be <0.20 U/mL. The half-life for unfractionated heparin administered intravenously at a dose of 400–600 U/kg per day is 45–90 minutes and normal hemostasis returns 4–6 hour after the infusion ends. In these cases, the APTT may be useful for verifying that clotting has normalized. If unfractionated heparin is administered via two or three injections using the same dose, because of the longer half-life, it is necessary to wait 8–12 hour for normal coagulation to return. Here too the APTT may allow verification of this.

2.4. New antithrombotics

New antithrombotics are becoming available: an anti-Xa preparation known as fondaparinux (Arixtra) is available and is used for prophylaxis of deep venous thrombosis following orthopedic surgery. The bleeding risk is about the same as with LMWHs but there is no known antidote in the event of bleeding. Fondaparinux has a half-life of 15 hour and endoscopy should not be performed until the drug has been completely eliminated, which takes 4–5 half-lives.

3. Risks associated with discontinuation of antithrombotic therapy

The risk associated with discontinuation of antithrombotic therapy ranges from minor to major, depending on the specific indications involved. Cases of sudden death or coronary stent occlusion within 7 days of discontinuation have been described.

3.1. Patients receiving oral anticoagulants

3.1.1. Indications associated with acute thromboembolic risk (Table 2)

When taking a patient off warfarin, it is essential to use a specific protocol (Box 2) involving unfractionated heparin. It is also advisable to carefully weigh whether the planned procedure is truly indicated, and if so, undertake procedures associated with a low risk of bleeding (e.g. insertion of a biliary stent without sphincterotomy).

Table 2 Conditions associated with acute thromboembolic risk during interruption of antithrombotic therapy

Condition	Target INR
All prosthetic metal valves in a mitral position	3–4.5
All first-generation metal aortic valves	3–4.5
Second-generation aortic valves in patients with an additional embolic risk factor	3–4.5
Atrial fibrillation associated with other thromboembolic risk factors, particularly mitral valve disease	2–3

3.1.2. Indications associated with low or moderate thromboembolic risk (Box 3)

Temporary discontinuation of antithrombotic therapy is usually sufficient in these situations.

3.2. Patients receiving antiplatelet drugs

3.2.1. Indications associated with acute thromboembolic risk (Box 4)

- Acute coronary syndromes that began <4 weeks previously
- Insertion of a bare coronary stent <1 month previously
- Insertion of a drug-eluting coronary stent <2 months previously for sirolimus and <6 months previously for

---

Box 3 Indications associated with low or moderate thromboembolic risk

- Coronary syndromes and/or DVT management.
- Atrial fibrillation in patients over 65 years or with associated thromboembolic risk factors (history of CVA, cardiac failure <2 months previously or left ventricular dilatation with end diastolic dimension >60 mm).
- Some cases of mitral regurgitation or stenosis (with a dilated left-atrium).
- Mechanical aortic valves in the absence of embolic risk factors.

---

paclitaxel. If placed >12 months ago, the risks of stent occlusion from stopping antiplatelet therapy are much lower

- Endocoronary radiotherapy <1 year previously.

Bare (uncoated) metal coronary stents require 1 month for re-endothelialization, while this process may take at least 6 months for drug-eluting stents. Until this occurs, there is a 50% risk of acute myocardial infarction or death. A patient should only be taken off antiplatelet drugs after consulting the cardiologist or other specialist responsible for the patient and where possible, therapy should be restarted within 5 days as the thrombosis risk increases after this time. Unfractionated heparin alone or therapeutic dose LMWH should be used. Again, low-risk procedures should be used where possible if endoscopy cannot be deferred.

3.2.2. Indications associated with moderate thromboembolic risk

- Acute coronary syndromes that began >4 weeks previously; stable angina
- Secondary prophylaxis for myocardial or arterial infarction
- Secondary prophylaxis for CVA in the absence of a source of cardiac embolus

---

Box 2 Patients receiving warfarin

Switching medications in patients with acute thromboembolic risk

- Discontinuation of warfarin 3–5 days prior to the procedure.
- The day after discontinuation, begin an anticoagulant dose of heparin; monitor the patient's APTT.
- Check INR the day before the examination.
- Discontinue unfractionated IV heparin 4–6 hour prior to endoscopy or the final injection of LMWH 8 hour (three injections/day) or 12 hour before the procedure (two injections/day); resume heparin 6–8 hour post-procedure or immediately if there is no risk of bleeding.
- Resume warfarin the same evening (or later, see above).
- Discontinue heparin once two daily INR results are satisfactory.
  Switch to unfractionated heparin (or, in some countries, LMWH): same as for acute thromboembolic risk.
- Discontinue warfarin 3–5 days before the procedure.
- Begin therapeutic doses of LMWH the following day.
- Discontinue LMWH on the day before the procedure and check the INR and platelets.
- Resume LMWH 12 hour post-procedure.
- Resume warfarin the same evening (or later, see above).
- Discontinue LMWH if two INR results 2 days apart are between 2 and 3.

Taking patients off warfarin is usually undertaken using therapeutic doses of IV unfractionated heparin (400–600 IU/kg per 24 hour), which remains the reference method.

Box 4 Patients receiving antiplatelet drugs

Switching medications in patients with acute thromboembolic risk

In view of the high risk associated with the discontinuation of antiplatelet drugs and the brevity of the treatment period, high-risk procedures should be postponed if possible. If the procedure is essential, the patient's medication should only be switched after consulting with their specialist and either non-fractionated heparin or LMWH in therapeutic doses is used.

Switching to a LMWH:
- Discontinue antiplatelet agent according to the drug's half-life (7–10 days) or the time needed to restore adequate function (i.e. 50×10^9/L functional platelets, where platelets are renewed at a rate of 10% per day of the baseline platelet count).
- Begin therapeutic dose LMWH on the following day.
- Discontinue LMWH 24 hour prior to procedure and check coagulation screen.
- Resume antiplatelet agents the day post-procedure (or later; see above).

- Atrial fibrillation in patients <65 years old with no thromboembolic risk factors or source of cardiac embolus
- Peripheral vascular disease.

Temporary discontinuation of antithrombotic therapy is usually sufficient.

3.2.3. Indications associated with minor thromboembolic risk

The main goal here is primary prevention of death or myocardial infarction in patients over the age of 50 with at least one vascular risk factor. Discontinuation of the therapy may be considered.

4. Switching from warfarin or antiplatelet drugs to alternative therapy

No drug has been approved for switching from warfarin or antiplatelet therapy. The discontinuation/switching procedure takes account of the treatment currently being used and the patient's thromboembolic risk factors (Boxes 2 and 4).

Calcium heparin may also be effective. The total required dose per 24 hour (in units) is the same as or slightly higher than the dose needed for continuous infusion. The drug can be administered by two or three daily subcutaneous injections. The efficacy of therapy is assessed by the APTT. The target APTT ratio should be 2–3. If heparin levels are measured to guide results, they should be between 0.3 and 0.6 IU/L. If there is a discrepancy between the unfractionated heparin dose injected and the resulting APTT results, measurement of circulating heparin levels is recommended.

The efficacy of switching to LMWH has been validated but guidelines may vary from country to country and local practice needs to be clarified and followed. If LMWHs are used, the dose must be adjusted to the patient's weight and should be given by one or two subcutaneous daily injections.

Warning!

Heparin-induced thrombocytopenia with or without thrombosis (HITT) is a rare but serious complication of treatment with either unfractionated heparin or LMWHs and should be suspected if the platelet count drops by 50% or more. If this occurs, all heparins should be stopped and an alternative thrombin inhibitor (e.g. danaparoid) used.

A patient can be taken off antiplatelet drugs using preparations with short-term and reversible anti-thrombotic action. However, no treatment of this kind has been validated prospectively.

LMWHs are an alternative and are administered using the same protocol as for switching to warfarin.

5. Resumption of antithrombotic treatment

While most bleeding occurs within 24 hour postoperatively, it can also be delayed (for up to 3 weeks following polypectomy). Starting the patient on antithrombotic therapy too soon can provoke delayed bleeding. Following a sphincterotomy, the risk of bleeding is put at 10–15% if warfarin is resumed before the third post-procedure day. There is little hard data to guide when to resume antithrombotic therapy and each case must be decided on its individual merits.

Clinical Tip

In cases where antithrombotic therapy is temporary and an endoscopic procedure would carry a high risk of bleeding and is not urgent, the procedure should be postponed.

6. Recommendations

6.1. General recommendations

Clinical Tip

In an emergency setting or if antithrombotic therapy was not discontinued and/or is scheduled to resume at an early stage, the following, which reduce the risk of bleeding, should be used wherever possible: detachable loops; hemostatic clips; pancreatic or biliary stents without a sphincterotomy.

All equipment needed for endoscopic hemostasis should be ready to hand. Use of drugs or blood products that inhibit antithrombotic action should also be considered in light of the endoscopic alternatives and the relative thromboembolic risk.

Warning!

If an emergency situation does not allow for determination of a patient's thromboembolic risk, as a precaution the patient should be regarded as high risk.

6.2. Setting-specific therapy adjustments

6.2.1. High-risk procedures

Elevated risk of bleeding (1% or more), if the patient can be treated endoscopically (Table 3):

- In the absence of any other hemostatic abnormality, colonoscopy with snare polypectomy and sphincterotomy can be performed without stopping standard-dose aspirin or NSAIDs. A detachable loop should be used for colonic polypectomies if the stalk diameter is >1 cm. Mucosectomy (EMR) should not be performed while the patient is taking aspirin.
- Apart from these special situations, antithrombotics should be discontinued pre-procedure, for as long as necessary to deactivate them. For warfarin, confirmation that the INR has normalized should be sought.

Low risk of bleeding (<1%) in patients who cannot be monitored endoscopically:

- All antithrombotics should be discontinued prior to the procedure, for as long as necessary to deactivate them.
- For warfarin, again the INR needs to be checked pre-procedure.

Table 3 Setting-specific therapy adjustments

	Antiplatelet drugs	Vitamin K antagonists	New antithrombotics
Flexible sigmoidoscopy with or without biopsy	Yes	Recent INR	Yes
Colonoscopy without polypectomy, with or without biopsy	Yes	Recent INR	Yes
ERCP without sphincterotomy, with or without biopsy	Yes	Recent INR	Yes
Enteroscopy with or without biopsy	Yes	Recent INR	Yes
ERCP with endoscopic sphincterotomy	Yes	No	No
Gastric strip biopsy and polypectomy	No	No	No
Photodynamic therapy and radiofrequency ablation	No	No	No
Management of esophageal or gastric varices	No	No	No
Hemostasis for vascular lesions	No	No	No
Endoscopic ultrasound-guided FNA	No	No	No
Metallic stent insertion without dilatation	No	No	No
Transnasal gastroscopy	No	No	No

Yes: possible without discontinuation and without switching the patient to an alternative antithrombotic; Recent INR: possible without discontinuation and without switching the patient to a different drug if there is no INR related overdose; No: The antithrombotic must be discontinued (or replaced with a different drug), except in special cases.

6.2.2. Low-risk procedures

No adjustment of anticoagulant or antiplatelet therapy is necessary. For warfarin, a recent verification of the INR is advisable. Non-urgent procedures should be postponed if anticoagulation is outside the therapeutic range.

6.3. Treatment discontinuation and resumption

Anticoagulant treatment should be discontinued in accordance with the patient's thromboembolic risk, as follows:

- *In patients at high risk* During the discontinuation period, the patient is put on a suitable antithrombotic and monitored.
- *In patients at moderate risk* During the discontinuation period, the possibility of putting the patient on a suitable antithrombotic is considered; the patient is monitored if an antithrombotic is administered.
- *In patients at low risk* No discontinuation of therapy is necessary.

Antithrombotic therapy is resumed post-procedure. In view of the risk of delayed bleeding, the benefits of immediate resumption of antithrombotic therapy should be weighed against the increased risk of bleeding and each case must be considered on its own merits.

Conclusion

It is difficult to formulate recommendations that will cover all possible clinical scenarios that endoscopists will encounter. The bleeding risk associated with the procedure and the underlying pathology (thromboembolic risk) must be assessed on a case-by-case basis. Clear communication between the endoscopist and the prescribing physician is important in deciding the best strategy. The guidance provided in this chapter can potentially serve as a basis for such discussions but it should be borne in mind that this consensus is somewhat arbitrary in places because of lack of an evidence base for recommendations and also because guidelines differ from country to country. The British Society of Gastroenterology guidelines, for example, include a simple, practical flowchart that is a useful starting point for many of the common clinical situations (Fig. 1).

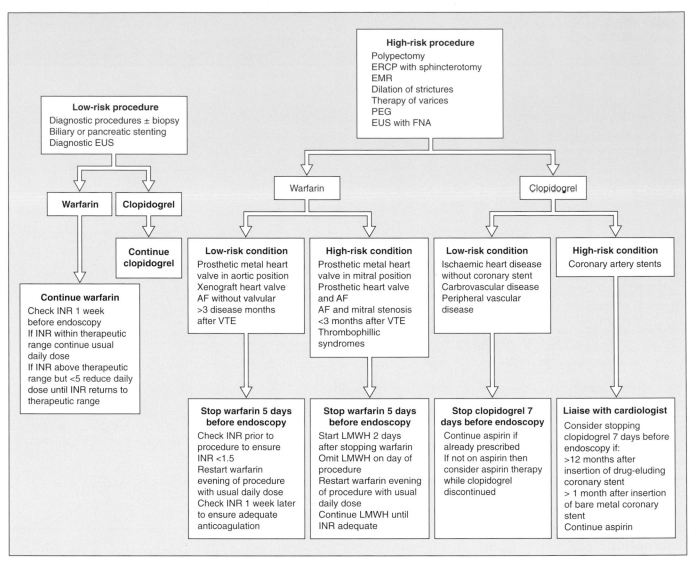

Figure 1 Guidelines for the management of patients on warfarin or clopidogrel undergoing endoscopic procedures (AF, atrial fibrillation; EMR, endoscopic mucosal resection; ERCP, endoscopic retrograde cholangiopancreatography; EUS, endoscopic ultrasound; FNA, fine needle aspiration; INR, international normalized ratio; LMWH, low molecular weight heparin; PEG, percutaneous endoscopic gastroenterostomy; VTE, venous thromboembolism) (With permission from Vietch AM *et al*. Guidelines for the management of anticoagulant and antiplatelet therapy in patients undergoing endoscopic procedures. Gut 2008; 57: 1322–1329.)

Further Reading

American Society of Gastrointestinal Endoscopy: Management of antithrombotic agents for endoscopic procedures, *Gastrointest Endosc* 70:1060–1070, 2009.

Boustière C, Veitch A, Vanbiervliet , et al: Endoscopy and antiplatelet agents. European Society of Gastrointestinal Endoscopy (ESGE) Guideline, *Endoscopy* 43(5):445–461, 2011.

Hui AJ, Wong RM, Ching JY, et al: Risk of colonoscopy polypectomy bleeding with anticoagulants and antiplatelet agents: analysis of 1657 cases, *Gastrointest Endosc* 59:44–48, 2004.

Patrono C, Coller B, Dalen JE, et al: Platelet-active drugs: the relationships among dose, effectiveness, and optimal therapeutic range, *Chest* 119(1 Suppl): 39S–63S, 2001.

Samama CM, Djoudi R, Lecompte T, et al, and the AFSSAPS Expert Group: Perioperative platelet transfusion: recommendations of the Agence française de sécurité sanitaire des produits de santé (AFSSAPS)] 2003, *Can J Anesth* 52:30–37, 2005.

Stein PD, Alpert JS, Bussey HI, et al: Antithrombotic therapy in patients with mechanical and biological prosthetic heart valves, *Chest* 119(1 Suppl):220S–227S, 2001.

Veitch AM, Baglin TP, Gershlick SH, et al: Guidelines for the management of anticoagulant and antiplatelet therapy in patients undergoing endoscopic procedures, *Gut* 57:1322–1329, 2008.

Yousfi M, Gostout CJ, Baron TH, et al: Postpolypectomy lower gastrointestinal bleeding: potential role of aspirin, *Am J Gastroenterol* 99(9):1785–1789, 2004.

Zuckerman MJ, Hirota WK, Adler DG, et al: ASGE guideline: the management of low-molecular-weight heparin and nonaspirin antiplatelet agents for endoscopic procedures, *Gastrointest Endosc* 61:189–194, 2005.

2.2 Antibiotic prophylaxis

Anne Marie Lennon

Key Points

- Prophylactic antibiotics are no longer recommended purely as prophylaxis against infective endocarditis.
- Patients with cirrhosis who present with an upper GI bleed should be given prophylactic antibiotics.
- Patients who have biliary obstruction with sepsis, or who have biliary obstruction which remains undrained following ERCP, should remain on antibiotics until the biliary obstruction is relieved.
- Patients who undergo a EUS-FNA of a cystic lesion should be given prophylactic antibiotics.
- All patients who have a PEG inserted should have pre-procedure antibiotics.
- Patients undergoing EUS or ERCP drainage of a pseudocyst require prophylactic antibiotics.

Introduction

Previously, antibiotics have been prescribed for three indications associated with endoscopic procedures:

- To prevent infective endocarditis in patients with heart disease
- To treat patients with infection prior to endoscopy (e.g. ascending cholangitis)
- As prophylaxis against infection following an endoscopic procedure.

European and American Society guidelines (Table 1) have recently changed significantly with respect to antibiotic prophylaxis against infective endocarditis. Antibiotics are no longer recommended for gastrointestinal procedures in the absence of established infection, but are still recommended for patients with evidence of infection prior to endoscopy and in patients undergoing specific procedures, which are discussed below.

Note

- It is important to have knowledge of local antibiotic resistance.
- Society guidelines for antibiotic prophylaxis vary. Ensure that you are aware of your own local guidelines.

1. Antibiotics for the prevention of infective endocarditis

European and American societies have recently significantly altered their recommendations for endocarditis prophylaxis in patients undergoing endoscopy (see Further Reading). The rationale for these changes has been summarized by the European Society of Cardiology:

- The incidence of bacteremia after endoscopic procedures versus the risk of bacteremia associated with routine daily activities.
  - The incidence of transient bacteremia varies greatly in studies. Transient bacteremia occurs frequently in daily routine activities such as brushing teeth, flossing or chewing. It therefore appears that a large proportion of cases of infective endocarditis arise from these daily activities and are not procedure related.
- Risks and benefits of prophylaxis:
  - The procedure-related risk of a patient developing infective endocarditis ranges from 1:14 000 000 for dental procedures in the average population to 1:95 000 for patients with previous infectious endocarditis. These estimates demonstrate the huge number of patients that require treatment to prevent a single case of infective endocarditis.
  - In the majority of patients, no procedure preceded the development of infective endocarditis. Therefore, infective endocarditis prophylaxis may at best protect a small proportion of patients, while the bacteremia that causes infective endocarditis in the majority of patients appears to derive from another source.
  - Antibiotic administration carries a small risk of anaphylaxis.
  - Widespread or inappropriate use of antibiotics can lead to resistant microorganisms.
- Lack of scientific evidence for the efficacy of infective endocarditis prophylaxis:
  - Studies reporting on the efficacy of antibiotic prophylaxis to prevent or alter bacteremia are contradictory, with no data demonstrating that reduced duration or frequency of bacteremia after any medical procedure leads to a reduced procedure-related risk of infective endocarditis.
  - The efficacy of antibiotic prophylaxis itself has never been investigated in a prospective randomized

Table 1 Specific society recommendations for prophylaxis of infective endocarditis in high risk patients

Society	Recommendation	Further Reading
AHA 2007	Prophylaxis against infective endocarditis is not recommended for non-dental procedures such as transesophageal echocardiogram, EGD or colonoscopy in the absence of active infection.	Wilson et al 2007; Nishimura et al 2008
NICE 2008	Antibiotic prophylaxis for gastrointestinal procedures is not recommended.	Richey et al 2008
ESC	Antibiotic prophylaxis is not recommended for gastroscopy, colonoscopy, or transesophageal echocardiography.	Habib et al 2009
BSG	Antibiotics are not indicated as prophylaxis against infective endocarditis.	Allison et al 2009
ASGE	Antibiotic prophylaxis for infectious endocarditis is not recommended.	Banerjee et al 2008

AHA, American Heart Association; NICE, National Institute for Heath and Clinical Excellence; ESC, European Society of Cardiology; BSG, British Society of Gastroenterology; ASGE, American Society of Gastrointestinal Endoscopy.

controlled trial and assumptions of efficacy are based on non-uniform expert opinion, animal experiments, case reports and contradictory observational studies.

 Note

All societies recommend that in patients with an established infection prior to endoscopy, or in patients undergoing a procedure which will require antibiotics (see below), antibiotic coverage for enterococci should be given (i.e. amoxicillin, ampicillin, piperacillin or vancomycin) in addition to the antibiotics for the specific indication.

2. Antibiotic prophylaxis in specific groups of patients

The guidelines of the American Society of Gastrointestinal Endoscopy can be found in Table 2.

2.1. Severe immunosuppression

Some societies (British Society of Gastroenterology) recommend antibiotic prophylaxis for patients with severe neutropenia ($<0.5 \times 10^9$/L) and/or advanced hematological malignancy who undergo endoscopic procedures that are known to be associated with a high risk of bacteremia.

2.2. Vascular grafts or prostheses

Antibiotic prophylaxis is not recommended for patients with vascular grafts or prostheses.

2.3. Patients with cirrhosis or portal hypertension

Patients with portal hypertension and ascites have an increased risk of bacteremia in the presence of an upper gastrointestinal bleed, while sclerotherapy is also associated with high rates of bacteremia. Patients with cirrhosis and bacterial infection have an increased risk of re-bleeding, and poor outcomes, while patients who receive antibiotic prophylaxis may have a reduced risk of variceal re-bleeding. A meta-analysis has shown that antibiotic prophylaxis in patients with variceal bleeding is associated with improved short-term survival.

Recommendation for patients with cirrhosis and upper GI bleeding:

- All patients with cirrhosis who present with an upper gastrointestinal bleed should be given prophylactic antibiotics.

3. Antibiotic prophylaxis for specific endoscopic procedures

See Table 3 for recommended antibiotics based on the British Society of Gastroenterology guidelines.

3.1. ERCP

Sepsis and cholangitis occur in 0.5–3% of ERCP procedures; however, a meta-analysis of five randomized, placebo-controlled trials failed to demonstrate a decrease in the incidence of cholangitis or sepsis with prophylactic antibiotic use. The exception to this rule is patients with incomplete biliary drainage, who have a high risk of sepsis. These patients should be given antibiotic coverage until adequate drainage is achieved. Patients with pancreatic pseudocysts are also at increased risk of infection, and should receive antibiotic cover.

Recommendations for patients undergoing ERCP:

- Patients with biliary sepsis should be given appropriate antibiotics.
- Patients with biliary obstruction with no evidence of infection do not require antibiotics, unless there is inadequate biliary drainage.
- Patients with undrained biliary systems following ERCP (cholangiocarcinoma, primary sclerosing cholangitis with failed drainage procedure) are at high risk of ascending cholangitis and sepsis and should receive antibiotic cover until adequate drainage is achieved.
- Patients with pancreatic pseudocysts are at increased risk of infection within the pseudocyst. Those patients undergoing an interventional endoscopic procedure (ERCP or EUS) should be given prophylactic antibiotics.
- Some societies (BSG) recommend antibiotic prophylaxis for patients with an orthotopic liver transplant (OLT) who undergo an ERCP.

Table 2 American Society of Gastrointestinal Endoscopy guidelines

Patient condition	Procedure contemplated	Goal of prophylaxis	Peri-procedural antibiotic prophylaxis	Grade of recommendation; comments
All cardiac conditions	Any endoscopic procedure	Prevention of infective endocarditis	Not indicated	1C+
Bile-duct obstruction in the absence of cholangitis	ERCP with complete drainage	Prevention of cholangitis	Not recommended	1C
Bile-duct obstruction in the absence of cholangitis	ERCP with anticipated incomplete drainage (e.g. PSC, hilar strictures)	Prevention of cholangitis	Recommended; continue antibiotics after the procedure	2C
Sterile pancreatic fluid collection (e.g. pseudocyst, necrosis), which communicates with pancreatic duct	ERCP	Prevention of cyst infection	Recommended	3
Sterile pancreatic fluid collection	Transmural drainage	Prevention of cyst infection	Recommended	3
Solid lesion along upper-GI tract	EUS-FNA	Prevention of local infection	Not recommended	1C; low rates of bacteremia and local infection
Solid lesion along lower-GI tract	EUS-FNA	Prevention of local infection	Insufficient data to make firm recommendation	Endoscopists may choose on a case-by-case basis; a single study indicates a low risk of infection
Cystic lesions along GI tract (including mediastinum)	EUS-FNA	Prevention of cyst infection	Recommended	1C
All patients	Percutaneous endoscopic feeding tube placement	Prevention of peristomal infection	Recommended	1A; decreases risk of soft tissue infection
Cirrhosis with acute GI bleeding	Required for all patients, regardless of endoscopic procedures	Prevention of infectious complications and reduction of mortality	Upon admission	1B; risk for bacterial infection associated with cirrhosis and GI bleeding is well established
Synthetic vascular graft and other non-valvular cardiovascular devices	Any endoscopic procedure	Prevention of graft and device infection	Not recommended	1C+; no reported cases of infection associated with endoscopy
Prosthetic joints	Any endoscopic procedure	Prevention of septic arthritis	Not recommended	1C+; very low risk of infection

From S. Banerjee, B. Shen, TH. Baron et al. Antibiotic prophylaxis for GI endoscopy. Gastrointestinal Endoscopy 2008;67:791-798.
Note: Some societies recommend prophylactic antibiotics for immunosuppressed patients or post-liver transplant patients undergoing ERCP.

3.2. EUS

The risk of infection after EUS-FNA of a solid lesion is very low (0.4%). These patients do not require antibiotic prophylaxis. There is an increased risk of infection when samples are acquired from cystic lesions. Therefore, patients undergoing endoscopic fine-needle aspiration (EUS-FNA) of cysts should receive peri-procedural antibiotics. Most endoscopists also continue oral antibiotics for 3–5 days. There is insufficient evidence to recommend antibiotics following EUS-FNA of a solid lesion in the lower gastrointestinal tract. The choice of whether or not to give antibiotics should be made on a case by case basis.

Recommendations for patients undergoing EUS:

* Patients undergoing EUS-FNA of a cystic lesion, should have prophylactic antibiotics.

* Prophylactic antibiotics are not required for EUS-FNA of solid lesions.
* Patients undergoing pancreatic pseudocyst drainage should have prophylactic antibiotics.

3.3. PEG

A large number of studies, including two meta-analyses, have shown that antibiotic prophylaxis is effective at reducing wound infection rates using a single dose of an appropriate antibiotic. PEG insertion is associated with a high risk of peristomal wound infection and patients should be given antibiotic prophylaxis.

Recommendations for patients undergoing PEG:

* Patients undergoing PEG insertion should receive antibiotic prophylaxis.

Table 3 Recommended antibiotics for prophylaxis[a]

Procedure	Antibiotic coverage
ERCP	Ciprofloxacin 750 mg PO 90 min pre-procedure
	or
	Gentamicin 1.5 mg/kg IV
OLT undergoing ERCP	Ciprofloxacin 750 mg 90 min pre-procedure
	or
	Gentamicin 1.5 mg/kg IV
	PLUS
	Amoxicillin 1 g IV or vancomycin 20 mg/kg IV infused over at least one hour
EUS FNA cystic lesion	Co-amoxiclav 1.2 g IV
	or
	Ciprofloxacin 750 mg PO 90 min pre-procedure
	3–5 day course of antibiotics post-procedure is usually given
	Antibiotics should be given prior to performing EUS-FNA
PEG	Co-amoxiclav 1.2 g IV
	or
	Second or third generation cephalosporin (i.e. cefuroxime 750 mg IV)
	Teicoplanin 400 mg IV can be used in patients who are penicillin allergic
	Antibiotics should be given prior to commencing the procedure
Cirrhosis with upper-GI bleed	Piperacillin/tazobactam 4.5 g IV three times per day
	or
	Third generation cephalosporin (i.e. cefotaxime 2 g IV three times per day)

[a]Based on British Society of Gastroenterology guidelines. Oral antibiotics should be given 60–90 min pre-procedure to allow absorption of the drug.
PEG, percutaneous endoscopic gastrostomy; ERCP, endoscopic retrograde cholangiopancreatogram; OLT, orthotopic liver transplant; EUS, endoscopic ultrasound; FNA, fine needle aspiration biopsy.

Further Reading

Allison MC, Sandoe JA, Tighe R, et al: Antibiotic prophylaxis in gastrointestinal endoscopy, *Gut* 58:869–880, 2009.
(Guidelines of the British Society of Gastroenterology)
Banerjee S, Shen B, Baron TH, et al: Antibiotic prophylaxis for GI endoscopy, *Gastrointest Endosc* 67:791–798, 2008.
(Guidelines of the American Society of Gastrointestinal Endoscopy)
Danchin N, Duval X, Leport C: Prophylaxis of infective endocarditis: French recommendation v2002, *Heart* 91:715–718, 2005.
(French Guidelines)
Habib G, Hoen B, Tornos P, et al: Guidelines on the prevention, diagnosis, and treatment of infective endocarditis. The task force on the prevention, diagnosis, and the treatment of infective endocarditis of the European Society of Cardiology, *Eur Heart J* 30:2369–2413, 2009.
Nishimura RA, Carabello BA, Faxon DP, et al: ACC/AHA 2008 Guideline update on valvular heart disease: focused update on infective endocarditis. A report of the American College of Cardiology/American Heart Association Task Force on Practice Guidelines, *Circulation* 118:887–896, 2008.
(Guidelines from the American College of Cardiology and American Heart Association)
Richey R, Wray D, Stokes T: Prophylaxis against infective endocarditis: summary of NICE guidance, *BMJ* 336:770–771, 2008.
(NICE Guidelines)
Wilson W, Taubert KA, Gewitz M, et al: Prevention of infective endocarditis. Guidelines from the American Heart Association, *Circulation* 116:1736–1754, 2007.
(Guidelines of the American Heart Association)

2.3 **Sedation**

Anne Marie Lennon, Jean-Christophe Létard, Jean Marc Canard

Key Points

- The endoscopist is ultimately responsible for sedation of a patient.
- Dose reduction is often required in the elderly or in those with renal, respiratory or hepatic impairment.
- Pre-procedure evaluation allows for assessment of sedation risk.
- Anesthetic input should be considered for patients who are ASA III or above.
- All patients should have continuous monitoring before, during, and after the procedure as standard. Visual monitoring, as well as device monitoring, is important.
- There are four levels of sedation. Most endoscopic procedures are usually undertaken under conscious sedation, although deep sedation can be obtained with propofol.
- It is essential that a member of the sedation team is capable of establishing an airway and providing positive pressure ventilation.

Box 1

- General information for patients, see Chapter 1.8.
- Management of patients on anticoagulants, see Chapter 2.1.

Introduction

Sedation is defined as a drug-induced depression. There are four levels of sedation, ranging from minimal sedation to general anesthesia (Table 1). The majority of endoscopic procedures are performed under conscious sedation, which is also known as moderate sedation. The aim of sedation is to improve patient comfort. This in turn means that the patient moves less, allowing a better assessment of the endoscopic problem. This is particularly useful where a difficult or prolonged procedure is undertaken.

There is clear variation in sedation practice in different countries, with almost all procedures undertaken in some countries under propofol sedation administered by anesthetists, while in other countries, many upper endoscopies are performed with only topical anesthesia. For any gastroenterologist involved in sedation, it is essential to have a clear understanding of the drugs used in sedation, their side-effects and how to deal with these when they occur, as it is estimated that sedation related complications account for 40–50% of endoscopy-related serious adverse events. The information given in this chapter is the authors' approach to sedation, and it is important to check local guidelines.

1. Pre-procedure assessment

Patients should be sent general information and instructions prior to the procedure, with clear instruction about medications, fasting and colonic preparation if appropriate.

1.1. Inpatient versus outpatient sedation

Patients who are suitable for outpatient sedation are as follows:

Table 1 Levels of sedation

	Level 1: Minimal sedation	**Level 2: Conscious sedation**	**Level 3: Deep sedation**	**Level 4: General anesthesia**
Responsiveness	Normal response to verbal stimulation.	Purposeful response* to verbal or tactile stimulation.	Cannot easily be aroused. Purposeful response after repeated or painful stimulation.	Unrousable even with painful stimulus.
Airway	Unaffected.	No intervention required.	Intervention may be required.	Intervention often required.
Spontaneous ventilation	Unaffected.	Adequate.	May be inadequate.	Frequently inadequate.
Cardiovascular function	Unaffected.	Usually maintained.	Usually maintained.	May be impaired.

*Reflex withdrawal from a painful stimulus is not considered a purposeful response.
Adapted from Gross JB, Bailey PL, Caplan RA, et al. Practice guidelines for sedation and analgesia by non-anesthesiologists: A report by the American Society of Anesthesiologists Task Force on Sedation and Analgesia by Non-Anesthesiologists. Anesthesiology 1996; 84:459–471.

Table 2 History and examination assessment prior to sedation

History	Physical examination
Significant cardiac or pulmonary disease. Neurological or seizure disorder. Stridor, snoring, or sleep apnea[a]. Advanced rheumatoid arthritis[a]. Previous problems with sedation or anesthesia. Chromosomal abnormality (e.g. trisomy 21)[a]. Current medications, drug and food allergies. Alcohol or drug abuse. Time of last oral intake[b]. ASA status[c].	Vital signs and weight. Body habitus – significant obesity, especially involving the neck and facial structures[a]. Auscultation of heart and lungs. Baseline level of consciousness. Assessment of airway[d] (see Cohen et al 2007 for detailed guidelines).

[a]These patients are more likely to have a difficult airway.
[b]ASA guidelines state that patients should fast a minimum of 2 hour for clear liquids and 6 hour for light meal before sedation.
[c]See Table 1 for ASA status.
[d]The following physical factors can be associated with difficult airway management: obesity, short neck, limited neck extension, hyoid-mental distance <3 cm in adult), neck mass, cervical spine disease or trauma, tracheal deviation, dysmorphic facial features (e.g. Pierre–Robin syndrome), inability to open mouth >3 cm, edentulous, protruding incisors, loose teeth, macroglossia, tonsillar hypertrophy, nonvisible uvula, micrognathia, retrognathia, trismus, significant malocclusion.

- Must live within 1 hour's drive of the institution
- Must be monitored by a competent friend or relative during the night following discharge
- The patient must have a telephone.

Patients who do not fulfill these criteria should be admitted overnight.

1.2. Pre-sedation assessment

All patients should be assessed prior to sedation. The aim of this assessment is to identify aspects of the patient's history and examination that could adversely affect endoscopic sedation. A brief history and examination are required, including airway assessment and determining ASA status (see Tables 2 and 3).

Table 3 American Society of Anesthesiology (ASA) co-morbidity status

ASA class	Description
I	The patient is normal and healthy.
II	The patient has mild systemic disease that does not limit their activities (e.g. controlled diabetes or hypertension without systemic sequelae).
III	The patient has moderate or severe systemic disease, which does limit their activities (e.g. stable angina or diabetes with systemic sequelae).
IV	The patient has a severe systemic disease that is a constant potential threat to life (i.e. decompensated heart failure, end-stage renal failure).
V	The patient is morbid and is at substantial risk of death within 24 hour.

Box 2 Key documentation for sedation

- Pre-procedure assessment.
- Informed consent.
- Doses and times of all drugs administered.
- A record of IV fluids administered.
- Oxygen administered and flow rate.
- Level of sedation, oxygenation status and hemodynamic variable must, as a minimum, be recorded before beginning the procedure, after administration of sedative-analgesic agents, at regular intervals during the procedure, during initial recovery, just before discharge.
- Level of pain should also be assessed and recorded.

From Cohen LB, Deluge MH, Isenberg J et al. AGA Institute review of endoscopic sedation. Gastroenterology 2007; 133:675–701.

Pregnant patients should be advised of the risks of sedation and the procedure deferred if possible (see ASGE Guidelines 2003 for detailed information).

1.3. Which patients should be referred for anesthetic input?

Anesthetic input should be considered for the following patients:

- Increased risk for complication because of severe co-morbidity (ASA class III or greater)
- Emergency endoscopic procedures
- Prolonged or therapeutic endoscopic procedures requiring deep sedation (e.g. EMR/ESD, pseudocyst drainage, plication of cardioesophageal junction, difficult ERCP)
- Patients with a history of: adverse reaction to sedation/ alcohol or drug abuse/inadequate response to moderate sedation/delirious or uncooperative/pregnant/ neuromuscular disorders (e.g. myasthenia gravis)/ morbid obesity
- Patients in whom airway management may be difficult (see Cohen et al 2007 for detailed guidelines).

1.4. Items which need to be documented during endoscopy and sedation

Box 2 lists the key items which must be documented during the procedure.

2. Monitoring and equipment

Patients undergoing endoscopic procedures should have continuous monitoring (both visual and devices) before, during, and after the procedure. A nurse or assistant should be present throughout the procedure. It is important that they have an understanding of the stages of sedation, monitoring, interpretation of physiologic parameters, and can initiate appropriate intervention in the event of a complication. One member of the team must be able to provide advanced cardiac life support, establish an airway and provide positive pressure ventilation if required. Emergency equipment that should be available at all times in an endoscopy unit is listed in Box 3.

Note

Visual, as well as device monitoring, is important.

2.1. Personnel and emergency equipment

A nurse or assistant with appropriate training should be present throughout the procedure. They should have a thorough understanding of the stages of sedation, monitoring,

---

Box 3   Emergency resuscitative equipment

- Assorted syringes, tourniquets, adhesive tape.
- Intravenous equipment:
  - Gloves
  - Tourniquets
  - Alcohol wipes
  - Sterile gauze pads
  - Intravenous catheters
  - Intravenous tubing
  - Intravenous fluids
  - Assorted needles for drug aspiration, intramuscular injection
  - Appropriate sized syringes
  - Tape.
- Basic airway management equipment:
  - Oxygen supply
  - Source of suction
  - Suction catheters
  - Yankauer-type suction
  - Face masks
  - Self-inflating breathing bag-valve set
  - Oral and nasal airways[a]
  - Lubricant.
- Advanced airway management equipment:
  - Laryngoscope handles and blades[a] (tested)
  - Endotracheal tubes and stylets[a]
  - Laryngeal mask airway[a].
- Cardiac equipment:
  - Pulse oximeter
  - Cardiac defibrillator.
- Pharmacologic antagonists:
  - Naloxone
  - Flumazenil.
- Emergency medications[b]:
  - Atropine
  - Diphenhydramine
  - Epinephrine
  - Ephedrine
  - 50% Dextrose
  - Hydrocortisone
  - Lidocaine
  - Naloxone
  - Sodium bicarbonate.

[a]All appropriate sizes should be available.
[b]The American Society of Anesthesiologists also suggest having nitroglycerin, amiodarone, methylprednisolone, dexamethasone, diazepam or midazolam (American Society of Anesthesiologists 2002).
Modified from Cohen LB, Deluge MH, Isenberg J et al. AGA Institute review of endoscopic sedation. Gastroenterology 2007; 133:675–701.

---

and interpretation of physiologic parameters, as well as the skills to initiate appropriate intervention in the event of a complication. One member of the team must be certified in advanced cardiac life support and be capable of establishing an airway and providing positive pressure ventilation. Emergency equipment (see Box 3) must be available at all times. AGA guidelines suggest that in moderate sedation, the assistant may perform short, interruptible tasks; however, in deep sedation, their only role is observation and monitoring of the patient (Riphaus et al 2009).

2.2. Assessment of level of consciousness

The patient's level of sedation should be documented prior to commencing sedation, during the procedure and until discharge. There are four different stages of sedation (Table 1) from minimal to general anesthesia. A combination of a benzodiazepine and an opioid is often used to provide conscious sedation, while propofol is used for deep sedation. The level of sedation required for a procedure depends on patient factors such as co-morbidity and anxiety levels, as well as procedural factors such as the complexity of the procedure and discomfort it will generate (i.e. esophageal dilatation). Usually, conscious sedation is sufficient for diagnostic upper endoscopy and colonoscopy, while deeper sedation is required for EUS and ERCP.

2.3. Hemodynamic monitoring

All patients receiving sedation should be monitored for heart rate and blood pressure. Baseline blood pressure should be checked prior to commencing the procedure, and repeated every 3–5 minutes throughout the procedure. Consider cardiac monitoring (ECG) in high-risk patients (e.g. significant cardiovascular disease or dysrhythmia).

2.4. Pulse oximetry

Pulse oximetry should be used in all patients undergoing sedation. Supplemental oxygen delays the detection of hypoventilation, thus *it is important to also monitor the patient's respiratory effort.*

2.5. Capnography

Capnography assesses respiratory function by measuring carbon dioxide non-invasively and is more sensitive than either visual observation or pulse oximetry for detecting changes in respiratory function. Capnography should not be used routinely but should be considered in patients undergoing deep sedation or where a patient's ventilation cannot be observed directly during moderate sedation.

2.6. BIS monitoring

BIS is a non-invasive method of assessing a patient's level of consciousness by monitoring electroencephalographic activity. It is not currently recommended for use in moderate sedation.

2.7. Supplemental oxygen

Supplemental oxygen should be considered for all patients undergoing moderate or deep sedation.

Table 4 FDA categorization of drugs for use in pregnancy

Category	Description
A	Adequate, well-controlled studies in pregnant women have not shown an increased risk of fetal abnormalities.
B	Animal studies have revealed no evidence of harm to the fetus; however, there are no adequate and well-controlled studies in pregnant women, or,
	Animal studies have shown an adverse effect, but adequate and well-controlled studies in pregnant women have failed to demonstrate a risk to the fetus.
C	Animal studies have shown an adverse effect and there are no adequate and well-controlled studies in pregnant women, or,
	No animal studies have been conducted and there are no adequate and well-controlled studies in pregnant women.
D	Adequate well-controlled or observational studies in pregnant women have demonstrated a risk to the fetus; however, the benefits of therapy may outweigh the potential risk.
X	Adequate well-controlled or observational studies in animals or pregnant women have demonstrated positive evidence of fetal abnormalities; use of the product is contraindicated in women who are or may become pregnant.

Adapted from Qureshi WA, Rajan E, Adler DG et al. American Society for Gastrointestinal Endoscopy. ASGE Guideline: Guidelines for endoscopy in pregnant and lactating women. Gastrointest Endosc 2005; 61(3):357–362.

2.8. Intravenous access

Intravenous access should be maintained through the procedure until the patient is no longer at risk of cardio-respiratory depression.

3. Drugs

There are several different classes of drugs commonly used in endoscopy for sedation, including, benzodiazepines, opioids and the anesthetic agent propofol. The choice of which drug to use depends on patient factors such as anxiety, co-morbidity and age, as well the properties of the drug, such as whether sedative, anxiolytic or amnesic properties are required. Regardless of which drug or combination of drugs is used, there are several key points to remember:

- Wait an appropriate time before giving additional doses of medications to avoid excessive sedation and increased side-effects
- Decrease the dose in the elderly
- Use lower doses when combining two drugs.

The most commonly used drugs are discussed below, followed by their reversal agent (Note: there is no reversal agent for propofol!). The commonest side-effects have been listed for each drug, while a complete list of side-effects associated with each drug can be found at: www.sedationfacts.org. FDA categories (Table 4) have been given for each drug for use in

pregnancy. A detailed discussion of the use of sedation medications in pregnant or lactating women can be found in Guidelines for Endoscopy in Pregnant and Lactating Women, Gastrointest Endosc, 2005.

3.1. Anesthetic agents

3.1.1. Propofol

A number of short-acting intravenous general anesthetics are used by anesthetists to provide general anesthesia, one of which is propofol. Propofol (Table 5) is an ideal drug for endoscopy with a rapid onset of action, short half-life, and amnesic properties. Recently, the use of propofol within endoscopy has increased, leading to a debate as to whether only an anesthetist is adequately trained to give propofol or whether gastroenterologist-directed propofol (GD-P) is safe and medicolegally reasonable. There is increasing evidence that propofol can safely be administered by non-anesthesiologists. A recent worldwide multicenter review of 521 000 patients given propofol for endoscopy found that between 0.1 and 0.4 per 1000 patients required assisted ventilation. Four patients required endotracheal intubation, one suffered a neurological injury and there were three deaths, which all occurred in patients with significant co-morbidity, underscoring the importance of seeking anesthetic input for any patient with an ASA >3. Currently, the decision to deliver gastroenterologist-directed propofol is often dictated by institutional guidelines or legal restrictions and it is important to check what the local gastroenterology society or legal guidelines are.

For gastroenterologists involved in propofol administration it is essential that the following criteria are followed:

Table 5 Propofol

Side-effects	Hypotension
	Respiratory depression and apnea
	Pain at the injection site
	Myoclonus
Contraindications	Children under the age of 3
	Pregnant women or nursing mothers
	Known hypersensitivity to propofol or any component of its formulation
Use with care	Patients with cardiac, respiratory, hepatic or renal impairment
	Patients with substantial blood loss or hypotension
Use in pregnant women	FDA Category B
Interactions	Drugs which will potentiate the effect of propofol
	Benzodiazepines
	Narcotics
Reversal agent	None

- There is an established protocol for drug administration.
- The sedation team must have appropriate education and training in the administration of propofol and be capable of rescuing the patient from general anesthesia.
- There is continuous patient assessment of clinical and physiologic parameters throughout the procedure.

Note

Propofol has a narrow therapeutic window with no reversal agent.

Propofol is a hypnotic with minimal analgesic effect. It produces sedation and amnesia at sub-hypnotic doses. Its mode of action is by potentiating the effects of GABA through a reduction in the rate of GABA-receptor dissociation. It is highly lipid soluble with an onset of action of 30–45 seconds, with a peak effect at 1–2 minutes. Its duration of effect is 4–8 minutes. It is metabolized in the liver by conjugation with glucuronide and sulfate followed by renal excretion. Neither cirrhosis nor renal impairment significantly affects its pharmacokinetic profile but this is potentiated if given with an opioid or benzodiazepine and its pharmacokinetics are affected by weight, sex, and age.

Propofol can either be given alone or in combination with a small dose of opioid or benzodiazepine. The rationale for

Note

Propofol must be discarded if not used within 6 hours.

the addition of a second agent is two-fold. First, propofol does not have any analgesic properties. Second, the addition of a second agent allows lower doses of both drugs to be used and has the potential for partial pharmacologic reversibility with either naloxone or flumazenil.

Clinical Tip

Decrease the dose in the elderly by 20%.

Dose

Propofol alone:

- Initial dose 10–40 mg
- Additional doses of 25–75 µg/kg per min or IV bolus dose of 10–20 mg with a minimum of 20–30 seconds between doses.

Combination dose:

- Pre-induction dose of either an opioid (fentanyl, 25–75 µg; meperidine, 25–50 mg), a benzodiazepine (midazolam 0.5–2.5 mg). A combination of both an opioid and benzodiazepine has also been used (Cohen et al. 2007).

Clinical Tip

The dose of propofol must be individualized based on the patient's total body weight.

- An induction dose of propofol is then given (5–15 mg) followed by additional boluses of 5–15 mg titrated to effect (Cohen et al. 2007).
- The dose should be decreased by 20% in patients over 60 years of age. Slower maintenance rate should be used and rapid bolus administration avoided.

Warning!

BEWARE: Combining propofol with opiod or benzodiazepine increases the risk of respiratory depression and apnea. The dose should be decreased if given in combination with benzodiazepines or narcotics.

3.1.2. Benzodiazepines

Benzodiazepines have sedative, anxiolytic and amnesic properties. The mechanism of action appears to intensify the physiologic inhibitory mechanisms mediated by γ-aminobutyric acid (GABA).

The most commonly used benzodiazepines are diazepam and midazolam. Midazolam is eliminated more rapidly and induces stronger anterograde amnesia than diazepam, allowing for rapid normalization of psychological tests (less than 4 hours). Midazolam is not associated with thrombophlebitis or histamine release, and generates a higher rate of patient satisfaction than diazepam. For these reasons diazepam is used less frequently for intravenous administration compared to midazolam.

3.1.2.1. Midazolam

Midazolam (Table 6) has a peak onset of action of 1–2 minutes, with a peak effect within 3–4 minutes. Its onset of action is more rapid if combined with an opioid (1.5 minutes), and sedation deeper. The pharmacokinetic profile is linear, over 0.05–0.4 mg/kg, allowing predictable dosage titration. Its duration of effect is 15–80 minutes. Midazolam is metabolized in the liver and secreted in the urine. Plasma clearance is reduced in the elderly, the obese, and patients with renal or hepatic impairment. The bioavailability of midazolam is increased by 30% in patients using a histamine H_2-receptor antagonist.

Dose

- The initial dose is 1 mg (or no more than 0.03 mg/kg) over 1–2 minutes
- Wait 2 minutes before giving additional doses

Clinical Tip

Decrease dose of midazolam by 30% if combining it with an opioid.

- Additional doses of 1 mg can be given to a maximum dose of 6 mg. Higher doses may be needed but should be used with caution

Warning!

BEWARE: Midazolam can cause profound respiratory depression in older patients or in those with chronic obstructive airway disease.

- The dose should be decreased by 20% for patients over 60 years of age or for patients with ASA class III or over. Patients over 70 years of age may need as little as 1 mg.

> **Clinical Tip**
>
> Midazolam should be given with care in patients on HAART, as these inhibit cytochrome P-450 and enhance its effect.

3.1.2.2. Diazepam

Diazepam (Table 7) has an onset of action of 2–3 minutes with a peak effect after 3–5 minutes, with a duration of 360 minutes. It is metabolized in the liver to active metabolites which undergo renal excretion. This half-life is increased in patients with hepatic or renal impairment.

Dose

- Initial dose 5–10 mg IV over 1 minute
- Wait 5 minutes before giving additional doses
- Usually a maximum of 10 mg is given, although 20 mg may be required if an opioid is not being co-administered.

Table 6   Midazolam

Side-effects	Respiratory depression
	Hypotension (especially when combined with an opioid)
	Cardiac dysrhythmias (rare)
	Paradoxical restlessness, agitation, disinhibition[a]
Contraindications	Narrow angle glaucoma (midazolam lowers intraocular pressure)[b]
	Myasthenia gravis
	Known hypersensitivity to diazepam or any component of its formulation
Use with care	Elderly
	Chronic obstructive airway disease (COAD)
Use in pregnant women	FDA Category D
	Increased risk of congenital malformations suggested in several studies in the 1st trimester
Interactions	Drugs which will potentiate the effect of midazolam: Alcohol, analgesics, anti-epileptics, anxiolytics, depressants, neuroleptics, tranquilizers Cytochrome P-450 inhibitors – HAART[c], erythromycin, fluconazole, diltiazem
	Drugs which will decrease the effect of midazolam: Cytochrome P-450 inducers – phenytoin, rifampicin, carbamazepine
Reversal agent	Flumazenil

[a]Consider this side-effect in patients who become increasingly agitated, despite increasing doses of midazolam.
[b]May be used in patients with open-angle glaucoma if they are on appropriate therapy.
[c]HAART, highly active anti-retroviral therapy.

Table 7   Diazepam

Side-effects	Respiratory depression, dyspnea
	Thrombophlebitis
Contraindications	Acute narrow-angle glaucoma
	Open angle glaucoma (unless on appropriate therapy)
	Myasthenia gravis
	Known hypersensitivity to diazepam or any component of its formulation
Use with care	Patients with hepatic, renal or cardiopulmonary impairment
Use in pregnant women	FDA Category D
	Increased risk of congenital malformation in the first trimester suggested in several studies
Interactions	Drugs which will potentiate the effect of diazepam: Antifungal agents (itraconazole, ketoconazole), cimetidine, disulfiram, fluvoxamine, isoniazid, non-nucleoside reverse transcriptase inhibitors (i.e. delavirdine, efavirenz), protease inhibitors (i.e. indinavir), macrolide antibiotics (i.e. erythromycin), OCP, omeprazole
	Drugs which will decrease the effect of diazepam: Rifamycin, theophyllines
	Drugs which diazepam may increase the effects of: Digoxin
Reversal agent	Flumazenil

> **Warning!**
>
> BEWARE: Respiratory depression is common in patients who receive a combination of diazepam and an opioid.

3.1.2.3. Reversal agent for benzodiazepines: Flumazenil

Flumazenil (Table 8) antagonizes benzodiazepines by competitively inhibiting GABA receptors. It antagonizes the CNS effects of benzodiazepines reversing respiratory depression, over sedation, psychomotor impairment, and memory loss. It has an onset of action of 1–2 minutes, with a peak effect after 3 minutes, and an average duration of 1 hour. It is metabolized in the liver.

Dose

- Initial dose of 0.1–0.3 mg over 15 seconds
- Additional doses of 0.2 mg can be given every minute to a maximum dose of 1 mg. Repeated doses can be administered at 20 minutes intervals if re-sedation occurs with no more than 1 mg administered at any one time and no more than 3 mg in any 1 hour.

3.2. Opioid analgesics

Most opioid analgesics have an analgesic and sedative effect without inducing amnesia. Opioid analgesics exhibit good bioavailability when administered parenterally. They act by

Table 8 Flumazenil

Side-effects	Anxiety, agitation, seizures
Contraindications	Patients who have been given a benzodiazepine for potentially life-threatening condition (e.g. control of intracranial pressure or status epilepticus)
	Patients with signs of serious tricyclic antidepressant overdose
	Known hypersensitivity to flumazenil or any component of its formulation
Use with care	Patients on long-term benzodiazepines, chloral hydrate, carbamazepine or high-dose tricyclic antidepressants, as it may precipitate withdrawal symptoms or convulsions
	Flumazenil is not recommended in epileptic patients taking benzodiazepines as it may cause convulsions
Use in pregnant women	FDA Category C
Interactions	Flumazenil will block the effects of non-benzodiazepines acting on the BDZ receptors

crossing the blood–brain barrier, and act on the specific receptors of the brain and spinal cord.

Fentanyl has a rapid, short and potent action, making it a good opioid analgesic for gastrointestinal endoscopy, where rapid recovery post-sedation is important. Pethidine (meperidine) is a less potent narcotic analgesic, and its use is declining due to its histamine release and cardiac side-effects.

3.2.1. Fentanyl

Fentanyl (Table 9) is a synthetic opioid. It is highly potent with 100 μg (0.1 mg) equivalent to 10 mg of morphine or 75 mg of pethidine (meperidine). It has a rapid onset of action of 1–2 minutes, with a peak effect within 3–5 minutes and a duration of action of 30–60 minutes. It is metabolized in the liver to active metabolites, which are excreted in the urine.

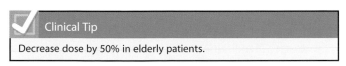

Clinical Tip

Decrease dose by 50% in elderly patients.

Dose

- Initial dose 50–100 μg. If being given with a benzodiazepine, it should be given first to allow accurate dose titration.
- Wait 2–5 minutes before giving additional doses.
- Additional doses of 25 μg can be given to a maximum dose of 200 μg.
- The dose should be decreased by 50% in elderly patients.

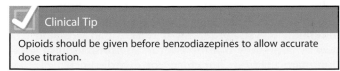

Clinical Tip

Opioids should be given before benzodiazepines to allow accurate dose titration.

3.2.2. Pethidine (meperidine)

Pethidine (Table 10) is a synthetic opioid with sedative and analgesic properties. It has an onset of action of 3–6 minutes, with a peak effect at 6–7 minutes. Its duration of effect is 60–180 minutes. It is converted into an active metabolite, normeperidine, in the liver and is excreted in the kidneys.

Dose

- Initial dose 25–50 mg
- Wait 2–5 minutes before giving additional doses
- Additional doses of 25 mg can be given to a maximum dose of 150 mg
- A reduced initial dose should be given in the elderly, debilitated patients or those with renal or hepatic impairment.

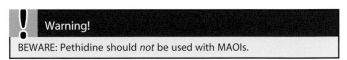

Warning!

BEWARE: Pethidine should *not* be used with MAOIs.

3.2.3. Reversal agent for opioids: naloxone

Naloxone (Table 11) has a similar structure to oxymorphone and antagonizes the CNS effects of opioids including respiratory depression, excess sedation and analgesia. It has an onset of action of 1–2 minutes, a peak effect at 5 minutes and a half-life of 30–45 minutes.

Table 9 Fentanyl

Side-effects	Respiratory depression (dose dependent)
	Hypotension
	Bradycardia (responsive to atropine)
Contraindications	Myasthenia gravis (can cause severe muscle rigidity)
	MAOIs: other narcotic analgesics have been reported to interact with MAOIs (see pethidine). Although this has not been reported for fentanyl, there are insufficient data to establish that this does not occur and fentanyl should therefore not be given to patients taking MAOIs
	Known hypersensitivity to fentanyl or any component of its formulation
Use with care	Fentanyl can cause severe bronchospasm and should be used with extreme caution in patients with asthma
	Patients with respiratory, hepatic or renal impairment
	Patients with bradycardia
Use in pregnant women	FDA Category C
Interactions	Drugs which will potentiate the effect of fentanyl:
	CNS depressants (benzodiazepines, neuroleptics, hypnotics)
Reversal agent	Naloxone

MAOIs, monoamine oxidase inhibitors.

Table 10 Pethidine

Side-effects	Respiratory depression
	Hypotension
	Irritability, tremors, agitation and convulsions
Contraindications	Myasthenia gravis
	MAOIs within the previous 14 days as pethidine may cause sweating, excitation, rigidity, hypertension, hypotension or coma
	Known hypersensitivity to pethidine or any component of its formulation
Use with care	Patients with renal impairment and the elderly
Use in pregnant women	FDA Category B
	Does not appear to be teratogenic in two studies and is preferred over morphine or fentanyl which are both Category C
Interactions	Drugs which will potentiate the effect of pethidine:
	CNS depressors (e.g. benzodiazepines, neuroleptics, hypnotics)
Reversal agent	Naloxone

MAOIs, monoamine oxidase inhibitors. These include dextroamphetamine, Emsam, iproniazid, iproclozide, isocarboxazid, linezolid, moclobemide, nialamide, phenelzine, rasagiline, selegiline, toloxatone, tranylcypromine.

Dose

- 0.2–0.4 mg (0.5–1.0 g/kg) IV every 2–3 minutes
- Additional doses may be required after 20–30 minutes.

Clinical Tip

The half-life of fentanyl is longer than naloxone, thus repeated doses of naloxone may be required.

3.3. Other drugs used for sedation

Several other drugs have been used for sedation including promethazine, dexmedetomidine, droperidol, ketamine, and nitrous oxide. Detailed information about these drugs can be found in Riphaus et al (2009).

3.4. Pharyngeal anesthesia

Topical anesthesia suppresses the gag reflex and can be used alone in cooperative patients. It can also be combined with intravenous sedation, and has been shown to be associated with improved patient tolerance and ease of endoscopy.

Table 11 Naloxone

Side-effects	Pain
	Hypertension, tachycardia
	Pulmonary edema (rare)
Contraindications	Known hypersensitivity to naloxone or any component of its formulation
Use in pregnant women	FDA Category B
Interactions	No significant interactions

However, it is important to be aware that combining pharyngeal anesthesia with intravenous sedation may increase the risk of aspiration and appropriate precautions must be taken. Other complications have been reported, including methemoglobinemia and anaphylaxis, although these are rare. The most commonly used agent is lidocaine, which is administered as an aerosol spray to the pharynx, the effect of which lasts up to 1 hour. Patients should not drink for half an hour following the procedure and their gag reflex should be checked prior to imbibing food or drink.

4. Management of the complications of sedation

A total of 50% of all endoscopy complications are sedation-related. The commonest of these are prolonged sedation and respiratory depression.

4.1. Prolonged sedation

Flumazenil should be given to counteract benzodiazepines, while naloxone should be given if opioids have been used. If both benzodiazepines and opioids have been used, then flumazenil and naloxone should be given.

Warning!

BEWARE: The half-life of flumazenil is shorter than that of midazolam and other benzodiazepines, thus repeated doses may be required.

4.2. Respiratory depression/hypoxia

The commonest cause of hypoxia is depression of the respiratory center. Other rarer causes of hypoxia include laryngospasm, obstruction of the upper airway by the tongue, aspiration or air insufflation during endoscopy, which can increase intra-abdominal pressure and alter the ventilation-perfusion ratio.

In any patient with hypoxia, the following steps should be taken:

- Encourage or stimulate the patient to breathe deeply
- Provide supplemental oxygen or increased oxygen
- Basic airway management:
  - Clear airway including suction
  - Jaw thrust maneuver
  - Insert Guedel airway if necessary
- Reverse sedation
- Give positive pressure ventilation if spontaneous ventilation is inadequate.

Warning!

BEWARE: Patients with a baseline oxygen saturation of <95% have a greater risk of hypoxia.

4.3. Circulatory insufficiency

Sedatives induce venodilatation, which can provoke circulatory collapse in hypovolemic patients secondary to an abrupt inhibition of venous return. It is essential to establish a normal circulatory volume prior to administration of sedation, particularly in the elderly or dehydrated patients, or patients who have experienced gastrointestinal bleeding.

Intravenous access should be inserted prior to commencing endoscopy in all patients. Two large bore intravenous cannulae should be inserted *prior* to commencing the endoscopy in patients at risk of circulatory insufficiency (i.e. GI bleeding). In hypotensive patients:

- Elevate patient's legs
- Give IV fluids
- Reverse sedation
- Use vasopressors if required.

Clinical Tip

Ensure that patients who are hypovolemic are fully resuscitated prior to sedation.

4.4. Quality assurance

It is essential for quality assurance that all adverse events (Box 4) should be recorded and analyzed, and appropriate changes made to sedation protocols.

Box 4   Adverse events

- Hypoxemia requiring intervention.
- Hypotension or bradycardia requiring pharmacological treatment.
- Pulmonary aspiration.
- Laryngospasm.
- Unanticipated use of reversal agents.
- Unanticipated hospitalization.

From Cohen LB, Deluge MH, Isenberg J et al. AGA Institute review of endoscopic sedation. Gastroenterology 2007; 133:675–701..

5. Recovery and discharge

5.1. Recovery monitoring

All patients should be monitored in a recovery room by a trained nurse who has appropriate training and experience, with one staff member for every six patients. The following should be measured regularly:

- Level of consciousness
- Hemodynamic parameters
- Oxygenation
- Pain/discomfort.

Standardized discharge criteria (Box 5) should be used and followed. All patients who are undergoing outpatient sedation must be driven home and have a friend or relative remain with them overnight. On discharge, patients should receive written instructions and contact numbers in case of emergency. This should include instructions on diet, activity, medication, not to consume alcohol or drive for 24 hour as well as follow-up and a telephone number to be called in case of emergency. It should be stressed to patients that no important decisions should be made during the 24 hour period.

Box 5   Aldrete scoring system

Monitoring should be discontinued and patient discharged when Aldrete score is ≥9.

Respiration
- Able to take deep breath and cough = 2.
- Dyspnea/shallow breathing = 1.
- Apnea = 0.

Oxygen saturation
- SaO_2 >95% on room air = 2.
- SaO_2 90–95% on room air = 1.
- SaO_2 <90% on supplemental air = 0.

Consciousness
- Fully awake = 2.
- Arousable on calling = 1.
- Not responding = 0.

Circulation
- BP ± 20 mmHg baseline = 2.
- BP ± 20–50 mmHg baseline = 1.
- BP ± 50 mmHg baseline = 0.

Activity
- Able to move 4 extremities = 2.
- Able to move 2 extremities = 1.
- Able to move 0 extremities = 0.

From Cohen LB, Deluge MH, Isenberg J et al. AGA Institute review of endoscopic sedation. Gastroenterology 2007; 133:675–701.

Further Reading

American Society of Anesthesiologists Task Force on Sedation and Analgesia by Non-Anesthesiologists. Practice guidelines for sedation and analgesia by Non-anesthesiologists, *Anesthesiology* 96(4):1004–1017, 2002.

Cohen LB, Deluge MH, Isenberg J, et al: AGA Institute review of endoscopic sedation, *Gastroenterology* 133:675–701, 2007.

Guidelines for conscious sedation and monitoring during gastrointestinal endoscopy, *Gastrointest Endosc* 58:317–322, 2003.

Guidelines for endoscopy in pregnant and lactating women, *Gastrointest Endosc* 61:357–362, 2005.

Guidelines for the use of deep sedation and anesthesia for gastrointestinal endoscopy procedures, *Gastrointest Endosc* 56:613–617, 2002.

Riphaus T, Wehrmann T, Weber B, et al: S3 Guidelines: sedation for gastrointestinal endoscopy 2008, *Endoscopy* 41:787–815, 2009.

Vargo JJ, Cohen LB, Rex DK, et al: Position statement: nonanesthesiologist administration of propofol for GI endoscopy, *Gastrointest Endosc* 70(6):1053–1059, 2009.

Useful Facts websites

A-Z Drug Facts. www.drugs.com/ppa/midazolam-hydrochloride.html

Safety and sedation during endoscopic procedures. http://www.bsg.org.uk/clinical-guidelines/endoscopy/

guidelines-on-safety-and-sedation-during-endoscopic-procedures.html

Sedation Facts. www.sedationfacts.org

2.4 **Chromoendoscopy and tattooing**

Christophe Cellier

Key Points

- Indigo carmine and Lugol's iodine solution should be available in all endoscopy units.
- Indigo carmine is extremely useful for relief enhancement of the mucosa.
- Lugol's iodine is used for detection of squamous esophageal dysplasia or superficial malignancies; it can be used with toluidine blue.
- Acetic acid is useful for detecting mucosal anomalies in Barrett's esophagus.
- Methylene blue stains intestinal metaplasia, but its sensitivity for identifying dysplasia is controversial.
- The histological nature of a polyp can be determined by using a magnifying endoscope in conjunction with indigo carmine or crystal violet staining.
- The following concentrations are used: indigo carmine 0.2%, acetic acid 1%, Lugol's iodine 2%, methylene blue (0.5%), toluidine blue (1%).

Introduction

In many settings, chromoendoscopy enhances diagnostic precision by bringing to light abnormalities that were not visible prior to staining. Chromoendoscopy agents are inexpensive, and with practice, it only takes a few minutes to perform. The high percentage of superficial malignancies detected in Japan is in part attributable to the widespread use of chromoendoscopy there. Contrast agents, all of which are used in an aqueous solution, fall into the following categories:

- Relief-enhancement or surface contrast agents
  - Indigo carmine
  - Acetic acid
- Contrast agents that react specifically with stained mucosa (vital stains)
  - Lugol's iodine solution
  - Methylene blue
  - Toluidine blue
  - Crystal violet.

The mucosa must always be carefully examined prior to staining, while use of a spray catheter allows for homogeneous coverage of the target area.

1. Indigo carmine

Used in concentrations ranging from 0.1 to 0.4%, indigo carmine is a surface contrast material, i.e. it is not absorbed by the mucosa. This agent brings out relief abnormalities in that it stains the bottom of an ulcer or penetrates fissures, and in so doing delineates a tumor, brings to light polyps that go undetected during standard white light examinations, or shows the central depression on the surface of a polyp that has already undergone malignant transformation (Fig. 1).

1.1. Indications

Indigo carmine is indicated in following settings:

- To delineate a sessile polyp prior to and following endoscopic resection
- To accentuate surface irregularities or visualize a surface ulceration
- To highlight areas for biopsy in Barrett's esophagus
- To assist analysis of the pit pattern of a polyp (Fig. 2)
- To detect a superficial malignancy or dysplasia of the stomach or colon

Concurrent use of a magnifying (and preferably high resolution) endoscope allows more detailed and precise images to be obtained. In the following settings, it is necessary to stain the entire colonic or duodenal mucosa:

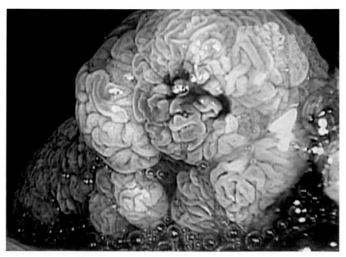

Figure 1 Indigo carmine 0.2% in a colonic polyp.

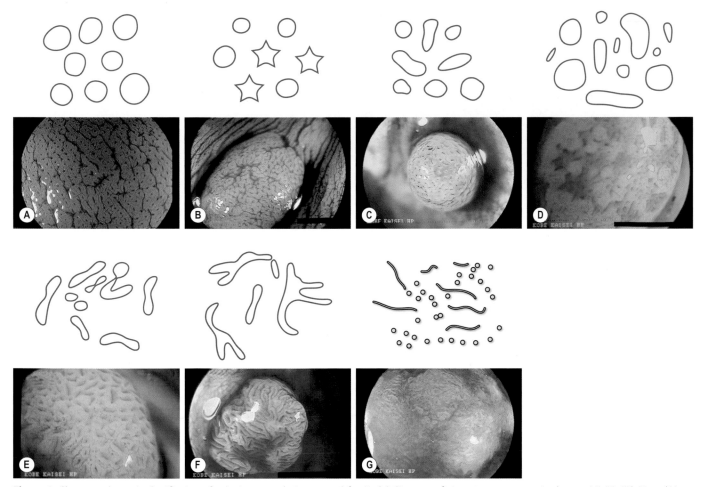

Figure 2 Chromoendoscopic classification of colonic mucosal pit patterns (after Kudo). Six types of pit pattern are recognized: types I, II, IIIL, IIIS, IV, and V. (A) Type I small round pits seen in normal mucosa. (B) Larger, symmetrical type II stellar pits seen in hyperplastic polyps. (C,D) Type IIIS, small tubular pits. (E) Type IIIL, large tubular, non-branching pits. (F) Type IV, gyrus or branched pits. (G) Type V, loss of pit pattern or irregular, non-structured pits. Types IIIL, IIIS, IV, and V correlate closely with neoplasia. Most adenomas have type IIIL pits, while type IIIS is associated with depressed lesions. Type V pattern is strongly associated with the presence of malignancy.

- HNPCC syndrome, where polyps may only appear if they are stained
- Long standing ulcerative colitis, during surveillance colonoscopy
- Celiac disease (Fig. 3).

1.2. Preparation

To obtain 25 mL of 0.4% indigo carmine solution, transfer 10 mL of 1% indigo carmine to a 30 mL syringe and add 15 mL of water. To obtain 50 mL of a 0.2% indigo carmine solution, add 40 mL of water to a 50 cc syringe after transferring 10 mL of 1% indigo carmine to it.

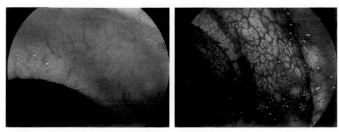

Figure 3 Celiac disease seen with white light endoscopy (right) and after application of 0.2% indigo carmine.

1.3. Staining procedure

The area can be sprayed either using a spray catheter or by adding 10 mL of solution with 40 mL of air in a 50 mL syringe directly in the working channel. The contrast material may disappear quickly, and it is sometimes necessary to re-spray.

1.4. Precautionary measures

There are no contraindications for the use of indigo carmine.

2. Acetic acid

Acetic acid, which has long been used to diagnose cervical cancer at colposcopy, has recently come into use for assessment of Barrett's esophagus. The chemical whitens inflammatory and dysplastic areas, provoking edema that allows for more precise assessment of the mucosal surface (Fig. 4).

2.1. Indications

When sprayed on Barrett's esophagus, acetic acid enhances relief structures and brings to light the villous characteristics of intestinal metaplasias and mucosal irregularities for biopsy.

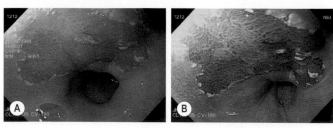

Figure 4 Acetic acid staining of Barrett's esophagus. (A) White light endoscopy. (B) NBI following acetic acid spray (Courtesy of Dr Marcia Canto, Johns Hopkins Hospital).

2.2. Preparation

A 1% acetic acid solution is prepared (20 mL are needed for a 5 cm segment of Barrett's esophagus).

2.3. Staining procedure

Spray the acetic acid on the entire Barrett's esophagus. Biopsy areas with relief abnormalities.

3. Lugol's iodine

Lugol's iodine solution stains normal non-keratinized squamous epithelium of the esophagus, and does not stain the following:

- Malignant tissue
- Dysplasia
- Inflammatory or eroded mucosa
- Gastric metaplasia

The brownish-black staining obtained with Lugol's iodine is not homogenous because of the variable concentrations of glycogen in the epithelium. Glycogenic acanthosis accentuates the coloration. Non-stained areas exceeding 5 mm in diameter should be biopsied (Fig. 5).

 Clinical Tip

It is the *non-staining* areas that are abnormal with Lugol's iodine.

3.1. Indications

When used solely in the squamous epithelium of the esophagus, Lugol's iodine allows:

- Detection of early malignancy
- Accurate delineation of a malignancy prior to endoscopic treatment
- Determination of synchronous areas of dysplasia or malignancy.

Numerous studies, particularly from Japan, have reported using Lugol's iodine solution for the detection of early esophageal neoplasia. A study by Dawsey et al (1998) is particularly informative in this regard. In this study, 225 Chinese patients underwent chromoendoscopy using Lugol's iodine. Prior to staining, all visible lesions were biopsied. After staining, biopsies were taken from areas that exhibited abnormal or no coloration. The sensitivity of endoscopy for the detection of an early malignancy or dysplasia was 62% without staining and 96% with staining, with specificities of 79% and 63%, respectively.

3.2. Preparation

25 mL of a 2% Lugol solution is required.

3.3. Staining procedure

The patient should be intubated prior to the procedure so as to allow for staining up to the upper esophageal sphincter.

- Starting from the cardia, spray the esophagus with 25 mL of the Lugol's iodine while gradually withdrawing the endoscope.
- Wait 2 minutes. Then biopsy all non-stained areas whose diameter exceeds 5 mm, bearing in mind the following:
  - Specificity is lower for non-stained areas that are <5 mm in diameter.
  - Non-stained benign areas tend to be round, whereas malignant areas generally exhibit irregular margins and are >1 cm in diameter.

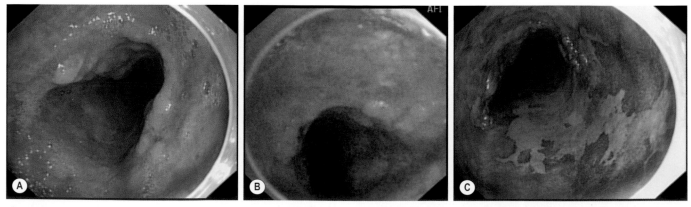

Figure 5 Lugol's iodine staining. (A) White light image showing Paris type 0–IIa lesion, which is nearly circumferential. High-grade dysplasia was found on histology following endoscopic mucosal resection. (B) The same lesion seen with autofluorescence. (C) The same lesion following application of 2% Lugol's iodine. Note how much more extensive proximal high-grade dysplasia (non-staining) is visible with Lugol's iodine.

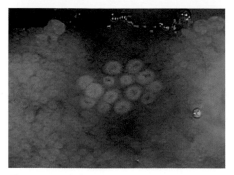

Figure 6 Methylene blue staining.

3.4. Precautionary measures

To minimize the risk of burns, make sure that Lugol's iodine does not come into contact with the patient's or user's face. This can be done by placing a covering over the patient's left cheek and mouth. Classical allergy to iodine is not a contraindication for use of Lugol's iodine, which also has little or no effect on thyroid function. Spraying from the upper oesophageal sphincter while moving distally to the cardia may help to avoid regurgitation in the absence of intubation.

4. Methylene blue

Methylene blue, which is absorbed by the mucosa in the colon and small intestine, allows the detection of abnormal intestinal epithelium and for more detailed visualization of the intestinal mucosa (Fig. 6).

4.1. Indications

To detect dysplasia in Barrett's esophagus and chronic gastritis. For the stomach, intestinal metaplasia staining displays 96% sensitivity and 95% specificity. For Barrett's esophagus, Canto et al (2002) demonstrated that specific intestinal metaplasia staining displays 95% sensitivity and 97% specificity. It has also been reported that less intense and somewhat irregular methylene blue impregnation in a stained area suggests the presence of dysplasia (the dysplastic cells do not absorb the contrast material as readily) and can be used to guide biopsies. This latter finding has been contested by other authors.

4.2. Preparation

To obtain 20 mL of a 0.5% methylene blue solution (the volume needed for a 5 cm long Barrett's segment):

- Draw up ×10 1 mL vials of 1% methylene blue into a 30 mL syringe.
- Add 10 mL of water for an injectable solution.

To obtain 20 mL of a 1% acetylcysteine solution (used to remove mucus prior to methylene blue staining):

- Proceed as above, but using 1 mL 20% acetylcysteine (Mucomyst)
- Add 19 mL of water for an injectable solution.

4.3. Staining procedure

Spray the acetylcysteine solution on the target area (Barrett's esophagus or gastric atrophy). Wait 1 minute and then spray

methylene blue on the area. Wait 2 minutes. Irrigate abundantly using ×3 50 mL syringes while suctioning the fluid regularly to avoid pulmonary aspiration. Biopsy the blue areas, i.e. areas that exhibit irregular coloration (Fig. 7).

4.4. Colon and small intestine relief enhancement

The indications here are the same as those for indigo carmine. However, a mucolytic solution is unnecessary, as this procedure does not entail exact delineation of the mucosa of the abnormal area. Spray the target area (using a spray catheter) with 0.5% methylene blue solution.

4.5. Precautionary measures

There are no contraindications for the use of methylene blue.

5. Toluidine blue

As it is absorbed by nucleic acids, toluidine blue stains malignant or dysplastic lesions with elevated mitotic activity.

5.1. Indications

Toluidine blue stains esophageal malignancies and dysplasia, although Lugol's iodine solution has supplanted it to a great extent. Nonetheless, it is useful as an adjunct to Lugol's, particularly in cases where it is essential to clearly delineate the limits of a superficial malignancy before performing endoscopic mucosal resection. In such a case, toluidine blue staining should be performed first, as otherwise the product will stain not only the lesion but also normal epithelium that was altered by Lugol's iodine solution.

5.2. Preparation

25 mL of each of the following solutions are needed:

- 1% toluidine blue solution
- 1% N-acetylcysteine acid solution for mucus removal.

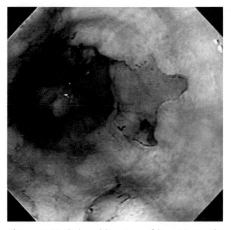

Figure 7 Methylene blue stain of Barrett's esophagus secondary to cleaning using acetylcysteine solution.

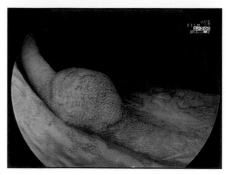

Figure 8 Crystal violet.

5.3. Staining procedure (Monnier technique)

Spray the target area with 1% *N*-acetylcysteine solution. Wait 1 minute. Then spray the area with toluidine blue solution. Wait 2 minutes. Irrigate abundantly using 50 mL syringes while suctioning the fluid regularly to avoid inhalation. Biopsy the bluish areas.

5.4. Precautionary measures

Toluidine blue is contraindicated in the presence of abnormally low G6PD enzyme activity, because of the risk of precipitating hemolysis.

6. Crystal violet

Crystal violet is absorbed by intestinal gland orifices (Fig. 8).

6.1. Indications

Used alone or in association with indigo carmine, crystal violet enhances detail of the intestinal crypts and allows prediction of polyp histology, particularly if a magnifying endoscope is also used.

6.2. Preparation

0.5% crystal violet solution is used. Only a few milliliters are needed.

6.3. Staining procedure

Crystal violet can be used secondary to indigo carmine, by spraying a few drops onto the polyp surface, or it can be used in lieu of indigo carmine, up to a maximum of 3 mL.

6.4. Precautionary measures

Crystal violet can induce mucosal ulceration and should only be used in small amounts.

7. Tattooing

Tattooing of the gastrointestinal wall (usually the colon) is useful for marking the location of a lesion or for endoscopic surveillance of an area where, for example, a large or malignant polyp has been removed (Fig. 9). A sterile carbon suspension (e.g. Sterimark; GI Spot), rather than India ink should be used.

7.1. Tattooing procedure

Agitate the syringe vigorously for 15–20 seconds, so as to suspend the solution evenly. Insert a sclerotherapy needle into the submucosa at an oblique angle (30–45°). The needle should not be inserted at right angles, as this could result in serosal penetration and extensive black discoloration of the peritoneum. Inject 0.5–0.75 mL of the marker in each of the four quadrants just distal to the lesion in the right colon and just proximal to the lesion in the rectosigmoid. Should surgery be performed, the surgeon can use the site of tattoo for planning the appropriate surgical resection margin. Do not inject more than 5 mL of the marker.

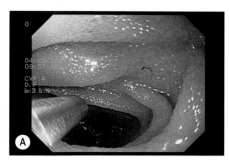
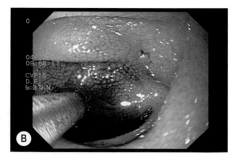

Figure 9 Tattooing. (A) Injection needle is inserted into the submucosa and tattoo is injected. (B) Following tattoo.

Further Reading

ASGE Technology Committee: Technology Status Evaluation Report. Endoscopic tattooing, *Gastrointest Endosc* 55:811–814, 2002.

Askin MP, Waye JD, Fiedler L, et al: Tattoo of colonic neoplasm in 113 patients with a new sterile carbon compound, *Gastrointest Endosc* 56(3):339–342, 2002.

Canto MI, Yoshida, T, Gossner L, et al: Chromoscopy of intestinal metaplasia in Barrett's esophagus, *Endoscopy* 34:330–336, 2002.

Dawsey SM, Fleisher DE, Wang GQ, et al: Mucosal iodine staining improves endoscopic visualization of squamous dysplasia and squamous cell carcinoma of the esophagus in Linxian, China, *Cancer* 83(2):220–231, 1998.

Fennerty MB, Sampliner RE, McGee DL, et al: Intestinal metaplasia of the stomach: identification by a selective mucosal staining technique, *Gastrointest Endosc* 38(6):696–698, 1992.

Kiesslich R, Von Bergh M, Hahn M, et al: Chromoendoscopy with indigo carmine improves the detection of adenomatous and nonadenomatous lesions in the colon, *Endoscopy* 33(12):1001–1006, 2001.

Nakamura A, Honma T, Suzyki Y, et al: The usefulness of crystal violet solution for the magnifying observation of colorectal neoplasm, *Gastrointest Endosc* 49(4 Part 2): AB64, 1999.

2.5 Pre-endoscopy checklist

Geneviève Obel

Summary

Introduction   77

1. Examination room and equipment check   77

2. Equipment that should be present   77

3. Troubleshooting   78

> ### Key Points
>
> - It is essential to check that all equipment that may be required for a procedure is available and working prior to commencing with the procedure.
> - All equipment should be available in duplicate.

Introduction

The equipment should be checked to ensure that it is in working order prior to commencing with any procedure. All endoscopes must be disinfected prior to use (see Ch. 1.10 for a detailed description of disinfection guidelines).

1. Examination room and equipment check

Each examination room should keep a log in which the following is recorded: the time at which the room is first opened each day; the activities that are carried out in the room (listed chronologically); the names of the patients who undergo procedures in the room; the drugs and personnel that are present during each procedure.

1.1. Video console check

- Verify that the screen is tuned to the correct channel
- Verify that all cables are properly plugged into the rear panel.

1.2. Cold-light source

- Activate the lamp
- Activate the air.

1.3. Suction

- Check that a new suction tube is attached for each patient. Check that the suction is working by placing the tip of the endoscope into water and suctioning.

1.4. Recording

- Ensure that the recording instrument is correctly attached and that the correct channel is selected to record images.

1.5. Electrosurgical generator

- An electrosurgical generator should be available for each room. Check that it is working appropriately. Ensure that grounding pads are available.

- Ensure that the active cord (this is the cord which is attached from the electrosurgical generator to the cautery instrument) is present. Active cords come in different sizes. Make sure that it fits the cautery instruments that you are likely to use.

1.6. Endoscope

- Check white balance
- Check that the endoscope is suctioning and blowing air appropriately by placing the tip in water. Air bubbles should be seen clearly flowing from the tip, while water can be seen on suctioning, running through the suction tubing. Then test that the water function is working properly to clean the lens
- Check that the angulation (right/left, up/down) is working
- For ERCP and linear EUS endoscopes check that the elevator is working.

2. Equipment that should be present

The following is a list of equipment which should be present in each endoscopy suite.

2.1. Patient-related

- Bite-block.

2.2. Endoscope-related

- All purpose cloth
- Lubricating gel
- Foot pump for water (check that you also have the water pump, appropriate tubing to connect the water pump to the endoscope and a 1 L bottle of normal saline).

2.3. General equipment

- Syringes and sterile water
- Spray catheters
- Stains
- Contrast agent (if fluoroscopy is to be used)
- Simethicone or other anti-foaming agent.

2.4. Polypectomy

- Biopsy forceps
- Foreign-body forceps

- Snares in various forms and diameters
- Straight and side firing APC probes
- Polyp trap filters
- Tripod
- Roth net or equivalent.

2.5. Dilation and stenting equipment

- Selection of esophageal, pyloric and colonic balloons
- Savary wire and dilators
- In complex strictures fluoroscopy, contrast agent, catheter and guidewires may be required
- Selection of esophageal, enteric, and colonic stents (covered, uncovered, and plastic)
- Sclerotherapy needle with contrast or external markers (i.e. paper clip) to mark the upper and lower extent to be stented.

2.6. Bleeding equipment

- Sclerotherapy needles
- Adrenaline (epinephrine) 1 : 10 000
- Cyanoacrylate or thrombin. This is determined by local expertise
- Endoloop
- Clips
- Banding kit
- APC catheter (side and forward firing)
- Hydrogen peroxide and simethicone
- Water pump
- Sengstaken Blakemore tube.

3. Troubleshooting

3.1. The air is not working

- Water bottle is:
  - Not properly connected to the endoscope
  - Not properly closed
  - Empty
  - Overfilled (check that it is not over the black line)
  - Cracked or leaking
  - The O ring valve is worn or defective.

Check that there is water in the bottle. Take it off and make sure that it is tightly closed. Check that it is correctly attached to the box. In Pentax machines there is an up/down valve. Check that this is correctly orientated. If necessary, replace the water bottle with a new one.

- The air/water valve:
  - is defective
  - not watertight.

Take the valve off, dip it in some water and see if this helps. Lubricate the O ring with silicone gel. If this does not work, get a new valve.

- Instrument channel valve is leaking: This can occur if the valve has been used multiple times. Replace it with a new valve
- Air function deactivated at the source: Check that the air is on and is on the correct setting (position 2–3)

- Endoscope channel blocked: Clear out the channel by flushing it with 60 mL sterile water or by pushing a biopsy forceps or equivalent through it.

3.2. The suction is not working

Disconnect the suction where it joins the endoscope. Place your finger over the suction tubing. If there is suction, then the problem is within the endoscope. If there is no suction, then the problem is the suction tubing or the wall filter.

The following can be the cause:

- The wall filter is not on
- The wall filter is full
- The liner is defective (replace)
- Ensure that the top of the wall filter and any caps are tightly sealed
- The suction tubing is disconnected. Reinsert the tubing. Sometimes the tubing may not have a good seal. In these cases cut the end off the tubing to improve the seal
- Suction channel is blocked by debris, mucus, coagulated blood, etc. Clean out the suction channel using a 50 cc syringe filled with sterile water. If this fails, you can remove the suction button and attach the suction tubing directly to the suction channel.

3.3. The visibility is poor

- Debris or secretions on lens:
  - Remove the debris by gently rubbing the tip of the endoscope off the mucosa
  - Flush the lens by forcefully injecting 50 mL saline through the instrument channel. If this fails and visibility is still poor, the endoscope should be removed, and the lens cleaned with a sterile alcohol swab.
- Lens fogged:
  - Clean the lens with anti-fog solution.

3.4. Image is too dark

- Too little light: Verify that the light source is in the automatic rather than the manual position
- Lamp burned out: Suspect this if the image is dim or there is no light. The lamp will need to be replaced
- Monitor controls set incorrectly: Check the monitor setting and adjust the light, contrast and colors using the control-panel buttons.

3.5. The image is too bright

- Check that the light level is on automatic and not manual
- Defective electrical contacts: The image is usually distorted. Clean the endoscope's electrical contacts before plugging it in. Clean the connector contacts using a cotton swab soaked in alcohol.

3.6. The image has a pink tinge

- White balance not set: Repeat white balance
- Faulty BNC cable connection: Verify that each cable is plugged and screwed in all the way on the rear panel of the screen.

3.7. There is no image on the screen

- A console element is not powered: Check that the monitor, processor and light source are all on
- Endoscope not plugged in properly: Take the endoscope out and ensure that it is fully inserted

- Defective electrical contacts at the source connector: Carefully clean the contacts
- Frozen image: Unfreeze
- Processor cable not connected to endoscope: Check the connections and reconnect the cable
- Lamp burned out: Change the lamp
- Screen control panel switches not activated properly (can occur if there are multiple input channels): Select the correct channel on the screen control panel
- Defective connecting cable between the screen and processor: Check the connections (if possible, make a connection diagram showing all cable connections).

Jean-Christophe Létard

Key Points

- An endoscopy report should be legible and clearly written.
- It should incorporate an administrative and clinical section.
- A minimum number of images should be included in the report to document key sections of the procedure and any abnormality detected.
- Well-structured endoscopy reporting databases are an important source of data for audit, quality assurance, training, research, and service improvement.

Introduction

Endoscopy reports should be legible, clearly written, and for archiving reasons, should not be more than one page long. An endoscopy report is composed of an administrative and clinical section. The former relates to the patient, the attending physician and endoscopy assistant who performed the procedure, and the endoscopy unit; the latter relates to the indication for the procedure, the technique used, anesthesia, medical devices, procedure time, and a precise description of the relevant diagnoses and any therapeutic procedures.

1. Administrative section

This section should provide the following information:
- Contact details for the unit where the endoscopy procedure was performed
- Patient's name, date of birth, gender, address and telephone number
- Patient's insurance number and insurer (if relevant) or unique hospital identifier
- Type of examination (e.g. gastroscopy, colonoscopy, etc.)
- Date and time of the procedure
- Name, address, telephone number and credentials of any doctor to whom the report is to be sent
- Name and credentials of the endoscopist
- Name and credentials of the endoscopy assistants who disinfected the endoscope(s) used
- Name of the endoscopy assistant(s) involved
- Name and credentials of the anesthesiologist
- Name of any other staff member, e.g. any other doctor, anesthesia nurse, or technician who participated in the procedure
- The initials of the secretary who typed up the report (if appropriate).

It is useful to indicate in the report that the patient was given information describing the risks, benefits, and alternatives to the procedure.

It is important to indicate the patient's risk of harboring vCJD, as follows:

- Patients without any specific risk factors
- Patients with individual risk factors for prion diseases (treatment with human growth hormone; familial prion diseases; neurosurgery prior to 1995)
- Patients with Creutzfeldt–Jakob disease.

2. Clinical section

This section should provide the following information:

- Indication for the procedure, in accordance with local guidelines; or the reasons and indications for the procedure if they do not fall within the scope of the guidelines
- The manner in which the patient was prepared for the procedure, including the quality of the preparation if undergoing colonoscopy
- The nature of the examination (diagnostic or therapeutic endoscopy)
- The instruments used and their serial numbers; the endoscope/endoscope accessory cleaning and disinfection procedures
- The following anesthesia data: ASA score, drugs used (benzodiazepine, morphine, propofol); intubation in cases of therapeutic endoscopy for the upper GI tract
- The following examination-specific parameters: examination time, any problems encountered during the examination, the anatomic extent of the examination as defined by the most distal point to which the endoscope was inserted. The quality of the pre-procedure preparation and any limitation in the examination must be documented
- A comprehensive descriptive analysis of any lesions observed. Each report should:
  - Use the minimal standard terminology (MST) for gastrointestinal endoscopy, which is recommended by the European Society of Digestive Endoscopy (ESDE) and the World Organization of Digestive Endoscopy (OMED) (www.omed.org/index.php/resources/re_mst/)
  - The dimensions of a lesion should be indicated in mm or cm
- A description of any additional diagnostic procedures (biopsies and staining) or therapeutic procedures (e.g. polypectomy, sphincterotomy, etc.) that were

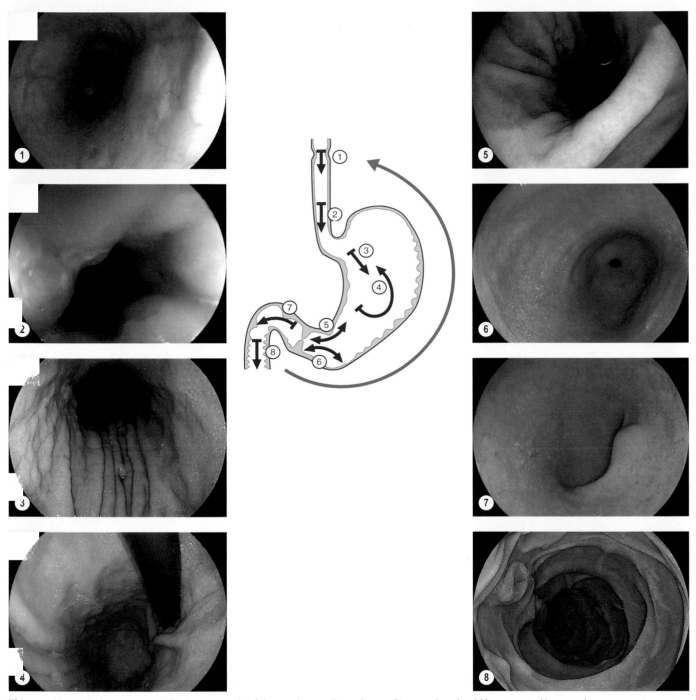

Figure 1 Upper endoscopy report. This is an example of the number, quality and type of images that should be presented in an endoscopy report (European Society of Digestive Endoscopy, ESDE). (1) View into the upper esophagus from above, 20 cm from the dental arches; (2) lower esophagus, 2 cm above the Z line; (3) upper part of the body, following stomach insufflation; (4) retroverted endoscopic view of the cardia, and fundus; (5) angle of the lesser curvature (reverse view); (6) gastric antrum with the pylorus in the center; (7) centered view of the duodenal bulb (D1); (8) view into the second portion of the duodenum, from above.

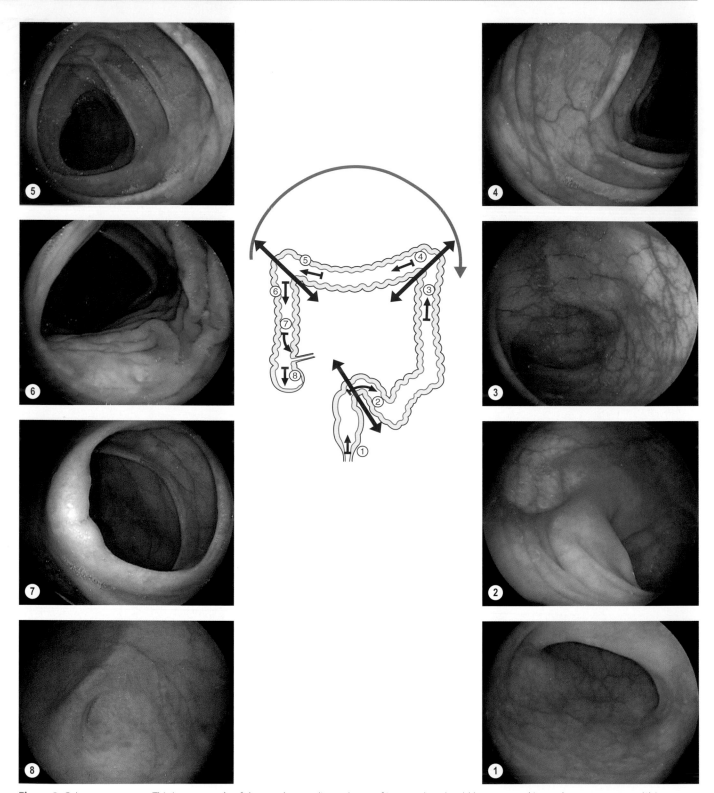

Figure 2 Colonoscopy report. This is an example of the number, quality and type of images that should be presented in a colonoscopy report. (1) Lower rectum, 2 cm above the pectineal line; (2) med segment of the sigmoid colon; (3) descending colon, below the splenic flexure; (4) transverse colon proximal to the splenic flexure; (5) transverse colon anterior to the hepatic flexure; (6) ascending colon proximal to the hepatic flexure; (7) ileocecal valve; (8) cecum with appendicular orifice.

performed, including the number of procedures, their exact locations, and the number of the specimen jar into which the specimens were placed

- The conclusion should provide a summary of the examination, including the endoscopic diagnosis indicated by the examination findings. However, no new lesions should be described in this section. The interpretation of the findings should not include any unrelated data, unless a valid explanation for these data is provided
- Codes should be used in the report, based on the International Classification of Diseases
- The images from the examination. This documents the extent of the areas examined, illustrates the pathology that was identified, and provides an impression of the image quality obtained (see Figs 1, 2)
- Comments may be added, particularly if difficulties were encountered during the examination, for example, if abdominal compression or position changes were required or any failure or complication associated with the examination. Diagrams should have captions to indicate lesion characteristics, the examination images (eight images are recommended by the European Society of Gastrointestinal Endoscopy (ESGE); the European Society of Gastroenterology and Endoscopy Nurses and Associates (ESGENA).

Endoscopy reports can either be printed, or may be available as digital endoscopy reports, depending on the system used in the endoscopy unit.

Report findings should be communicated orally to patients on completion of the examination. The patient should be given a definitive printed version of the report before leaving the endoscopy unit, or at a later time. The definitive version that is provided immediately should contain sufficient information to allow the patient to undergo any further therapy within the timescales indicated in the report. The definitive endoscopy report can also be sent to the referring physician.

3. Endoscopy reports

3.1. Upper endoscopy

Figure 1 is an example of the number and quality of images which should be provided.

3.2. Colonoscopy

Figure 2 is an example of the number and quality of images which should be provided. The photographs on this page were taken while the endoscope was being withdrawn.

CHAPTER 3

Diagnostic upper endoscopy

Jean Marc Canard, Jean-Christophe Létard, Anne Marie Lennon

Summary

Key Points

- Upper endoscopy is a commonly performed procedure.
- Always intubate under direct vision and never push.
- Be aware of 'blind' areas, which can be easily missed.
- Cancers should be classified using the Paris classification system.

Introduction

Esophagogastroduodenoscopy (EGD) is one of the commonest procedures that a gastroenterologist performs. This chapter covers how to perform a diagnostic upper endoscopy. Therapeutic interventions in upper endoscopy are discussed in Chapter 7.

1. Upper gastrointestinal anatomy

1.1. The esophagus

The cervical segment of the esophagus begins at the upper esophageal sphincter, which is 15 cm from the incisors and is 6 mm long (Fig. 1). The thoracic segment of the esophagus is approximately 19 cm long. Its lumen is open during inspiration and closed during expiration. The imprint of the arch of the aorta is sometimes apparent at 25 cm from the incisors on the left. How to describe where a lesion is in terms of anterior, posterior, right, left, is very important and is shown in Figure 2. The transition between the esophagus and gastric epithelium (Z line) is identified by the change in color of the mucosa from pale-pink to reddish-pink.

1.2. The stomach

The stomach extends from the cardia to the pylorus (Fig. 3). The fundus is the portion of the stomach above the horizontal line that passes through the cardia and that is visible in a retroflexed endoscopic view. The body is the remainder of the upper part of the stomach and is delimited at its lower edge by the line that passes through the angular notch. Endoscopically, the transition from the body to the antrum is seen as a transition from rugae to flat mucosa (Fig. 4). The pylorus is a circular orifice, which leads to the first part of the duodenum.

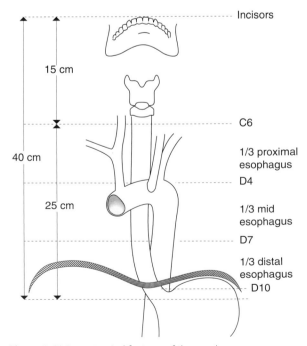

Incisors

15 cm

C6

40 cm

1/3 proximal esophagus

D4

25 cm

1/3 mid esophagus

D7

1/3 distal esophagus

D10

Figure 1 Main anatomical features of the esophagus.

DOI: 10.1016/B978-0-7020-3128-1.00003-1

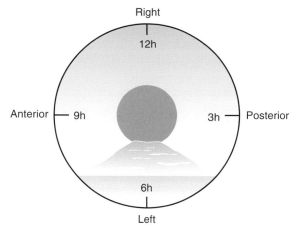

Figure 2 Orientation in the esophagus. It is very important to understand your orientation in the esophagus so that you can describe where a lesion is. This figure demonstrates the orientation of the esophagus when the patient is in the left lateral decubitus position, water naturally stays in the left side of the esophagus.

☑ **Clinical Tip**

Always consider linitis plastica if the stomach fails to distend normally.

When the patient is in the lateral left decubitus position, the greater curvature is at the bottom, the lesser curvature at the top, the posterior stomach wall on the right, and the anterior stomach wall is on the left (Fig. 4). The anterior wall can be visualized with transillumination, a technique used for PEG insertion (see Ch. 4). A normal stomach distends fully with insufflation, with the rugae flattening out (Fig. 5).

1.3. The duodenum

The duodenum extends from the pylorus to the duodeno-jejunal angle. The duodenal bulb extends from the pylorus to the genu superius. The second portion (D2) extends from

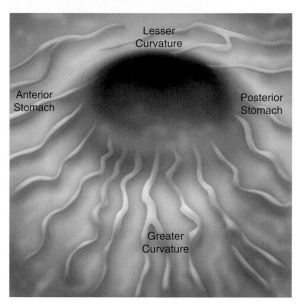

Figure 4 Orientation in the stomach. When the patient is in the lateral left decubitus position, the greater curvature is at the bottom, the lesser curvature at the top, the posterior stomach wall on the right, and the anterior stomach wall on the left.

the genu superius to the genu inferius. The ampulla of Vater is usually found in a horizontal fold in the middle of the second portion of the duodenum (Fig. 6). The accessory papilla is a small protuberance, which is usually found just superior and proximal to the ampulla of Vater.

1.4. Postoperative endoscopy of the stomach and duodenum

Common post-surgical anatomy includes a Billroth I (Fig. 7), where only one lumen is present. In a Polya or Billroth II (Fig. 7), two gastrojejunal orifices are visible. The afferent limb leads to the duodenum, while the efferent limb leads to the colon.

☑ **Clinical Tip**

The afferent limb is usually the more difficult limb to enter.

---

2. Indications

Upper endoscopy (EGD) is indicated for investigation of the following presentations or for screening for pre-malignant lesions.

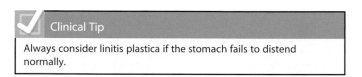

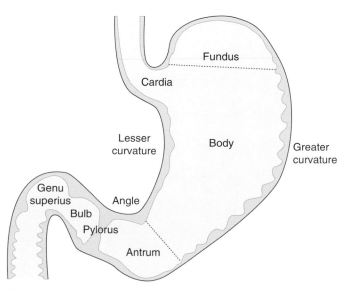

Figure 3 Gastric anatomy.

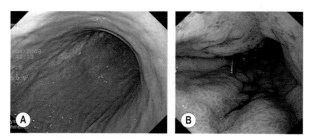

Figure 5 Insufflation of the stomach. (A) Normal insufflations of the stomach. (B) Non-distention of the stomach in a patient with linitis plastica.

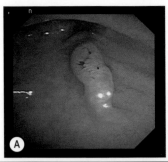

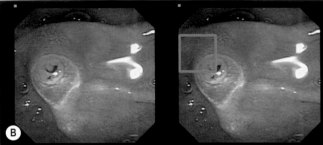

Figure 6 (A) Normal ampulla of Vater. (B) Biopsies should be taken AWAY from the pancreatic orifice to avoid pancreatitis. A safe area to biopsy is the upper left quadrant in the area within the box.

2.1. Dyspepsia

Age ≥50 with new onset dyspepsia:

- Should undergo EGD regardless of whether they have alarm symptoms.

Age <50 with dyspepsia:

- Patients with alarm symptoms should undergo EGD
- Those without alarm symptoms should undergo an initial test-and-treat approach for *H. pylori*
- Patients who are *H. pylori*-negative should be offered a short trial of PPI therapy
- Patients who do not respond to empiric PPI therapy or have recurrent symptoms after an adequate trial should undergo endoscopy.

 Clinical Tips

Upper GI alarm symptoms

- Age ≥50 with new onset symptoms.
- Family history of upper GI malignancy.
- Unintended weight loss >6 lb (2.7 kg).
- GI bleeding or iron deficiency anemia.
- Progressive dysphagia.
- Odynophagia.
- Persistent vomiting.
- Palpable mass or lymphadenopathy.
- Jaundice.

Box 1   Indications for upper endoscopy

- Dyspepsia associated with alarm symptoms at any age.
- New onset dyspepsia in a patient ≥50.
- Dysphagia or odynophagia.
- Symptoms of GERD that persist or recur despite appropriate therapy.
- Persistent vomiting of unknown cause.
- Diseases in which the presence of upper GI pathology may affect planned management, e.g. decision to anticoagulate.
- Confirmation of radiological abnormalities.
- Suspected neoplasia.
- Assessment and treatment of GI bleeding (acute or chronic).
- Sampling of tissue or fluid.
- To document or treat esophageal varices.
- Surveillance for malignancy in high risk groups, e.g. Barrett's esophagus, hereditary gastric cancer families.
- Follow-up of gastric ulcer.
- Follow-up of patients who undergo endoscopic mucosal resection (EMR) or endoscopic submucosal dissection (ESD) of an early cancer.

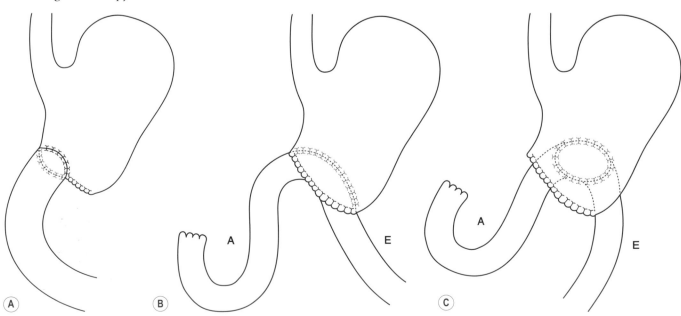

Figure 7 (A) Billroth I. (B) Polya. (C) Billroth II. A, afferent limb. B, efferent limb.

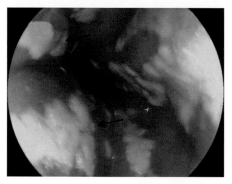

Figure 8 Odynophagia. *Candida* esophagitis causing dysphagia and odynophagia. Note the white plaques (arrows).

2.2. Dysphagia or odynophagia

Unless there is a clear history pointing to a neurological cause or ENT origin for dysphagia, all patients should undergo urgent EGD as their first investigation (Fig. 8). Note, patients with GERD can present with atypical symptoms including laryngitis, chronic cough or bronchospasm.

2.3. Gastroesophageal reflux

- Gastroesophageal reflux (GERD) can be diagnosed on the basis of typical symptoms without the need for EGD
- In patients with uncomplicated GERD an initial trial of empiric medical therapy is appropriate
- EGD should be performed if patients have alarm symptoms or symptoms suggesting complicated GERD or in patients who fail to respond to empiric medical therapy.

Box 2 Upper endoscopy is not indicated

- Symptoms felt to be functional in origin.
- 'Simple' dyspepsia <50 years of age.
- Metastatic adenocarcinoma of unknown primary site when the results will not alter management.
- Radiographic findings of an asymptomatic/uncomplicated sliding hiatal hernia, uncomplicated duodenal ulcer or deformed duodenal bulb when symptoms are absent or respond to ulcer therapy.
- Surveillance of *healed* benign disease.
- Surveillance during repeated dilations of benign strictures unless there is a change in status.

2.4. Persistent vomiting

EGD is indicated for isolated vomiting persisting for over 48 hours after acute intestinal obstruction and non-digestive causes have been excluded.

2.5. Assessment and treatment of upper gastrointestinal bleeding

- EGD is indicated in patients suspected of having an acute upper gastrointestinal bleed (hematemesis or melena) (see Ch. 7 for how to treat upper GI bleeding.)
- EGD should be repeated if bleeding persists when an initial examination including upper endoscopy and colonoscopy has been inconclusive (Fig. 9).

2.6. Investigation of chronic anemia and/or iron deficiency

- All patients should be screened for celiac disease (Fig. 10f)

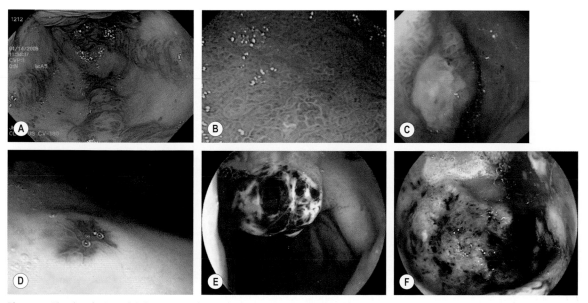

Figure 9 Bleeding lesions. (A) Gastric Antral Vascular Ectasia (GAVE); (B) portal hypertensive gastropathy; (C) duodenal ulcer; (D) gastric arterio-venous malformation (AVM); (E) ulcer with adherent clot in the duodenum; (F) large benign necrotic gastric ulcer.

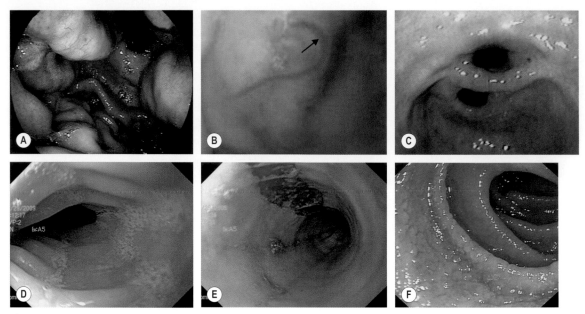

Figure 10 Miscellaneous. (A) Hypertrophic gastric folds in Zollinger–Ellison syndrome. (B) Anisakis worm (arrow). (C) Pyloric duplication. (D) Eosinophilic esophagitis with classic ridges. *Beware* dilating strictures in these patients as there is an increased risk of perforation. (E) Esophageal mucosal tear in a patient with eosinophilic esophagitis. (F) Celiac disease with scalloping of the edges of the mucosa.

 Clinical Tip

The optimum number of duodenal biopsies for accurate diagnosis of celiac disease is four.

- EGD and colonoscopy should be considered in all male patients, unless there is a history of overt non-GI blood loss
- EGD and colonoscopy should be considered for female patients who are post-menopausal, ≥50 years of age, or have a strong family history of colorectal cancer
- The presence of esophagitis, erosions or peptic ulcer disease should not be accepted as the cause of anemia until colonoscopy is performed and is normal.

2.7. When to obtain duodenal biopsies

Duodenal biopsies during upper endoscopy are indicated in the following situations:

- Iron-deficiency anemia with no identified cause
- Folate deficiency (combined with gastric biopsies)
- Other nutritional deficiencies
- Isolated chronic diarrhea
- Dermatitis herpetiformis
- Confirmation of celiac disease in patients with positive serology
- If parasitic diseases are suspected when a parasitological stool examination has been negative (giardiasis, strongyloidosis).

2.8. To assess portal hypertension

- To detect esophagogastric varices in patients with cirrhosis or non-cirrhotic portal hypertension (Figs 9A,B, Figure 11) (see Ch. 7.8 for information on grading and treatment of varices)

- Repeat EGD every 2 years in patients with cirrhosis in whom initial upper endoscopy showed no varices
- After endoscopic treatment of esophageal varices to confirm their eradication (see Ch. 7.8 for schedule for follow up of patients with varices).

2.9. Screening or surveillance in patients at risk of upper GI malignancy

Upper endoscopy is also indicated for screening premalignant lesions.

2.9.1. Gastroduodenal ulcers

- Multiple biopsies should be performed routinely in patients with gastric ulcer with endoscopic and histological follow-up after 4–6 weeks of antisecretory treatment.
- Follow-up upper endoscopy is not indicated in an asymptomatic patient after treatment of a duodenal ulcer.
- Patients who undergo resection of an early cancer with endoscopic mucosal resection (EMR) or endoscopic submucosal dissection (ESD) should have close follow-up.

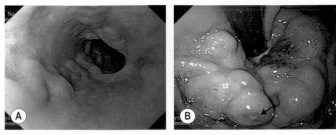

Figure 11 Esophageal and gastric varices. (A) Small esophageal varices. (B) This image is taken in retroflexion, where multiple gastric varices are present with an erosion over one (arrow).

Clinical Tip

All patients with a gastric ulcer should undergo repeat EGD after 4–6 weeks of antisecretory therapy to ensure ulcer healing and for biopsies if healing is incomplete.

2.9.2. Achalasia

- These patients are at increased risk of developing squamous cell cancer
- It is reasonable to commence surveillance 15 years after symptoms began. Subsequent surveillance intervals are not clear but every 2–3 years is reasonable.

2.9.3. Caustic injury

- Increased risk of squamous carcinoma, especially after lye ingestion.
- Have a low threshold to investigate dysphagia with endoscopy.
- Begin surveillance 15–20 years after caustic injury.
- Repeat EGD every 1–3 years.

2.9.4. Tylosis

- There are two types of tylosis:
  - Type A tylosis presents between the ages of 5 and 15 years and is associated with increased risk of esophageal cancer.
  - Type B tylosis is associated with onset by age 1 and is not associated with increased risk of esophageal cancer.
- Begin surveillance at age 30.
- Repeat EGD every 1–3 years.

2.10. Patients with a history of squamous cancer of the head, neck, pharynx, lung or esophagus

There are insufficient data to support screening; however, some authors advocate a single endoscopy with Lugol's iodine chromoendoscopy to look for squamous esophageal cancer.

2.11. Gastric epithelial polyps

- All gastric polyps should be biopsied to determine whether they are hyperplastic or adenomatous (Fig. 12)
- Adenomatous polyps are at risk of malignant transformation and should be resected
- Surveillance endoscopy should be performed 1 year after removing an adenomatous gastric polyp. If

surveillance is negative, EGD should be repeated at 3–5 years. Surveillance in patients with high-grade dysplasia or early gastric cancer should be individualized.

2.12. Gastric intestinal metaplasia

- Is associated with >10 fold increased risk of gastric cancer in high risk parts of the world and in patients infected with *H. pylori*
- In Western countries, endoscopic surveillance is not uniformly recommended
- If surveillance is performed, a topographic mapping of the entire stomach is necessary
- Patients with high-grade dysplasia are at significant risk for progressing to cancer and should be considered for either endoscopic resection or gastrectomy. Following endoscopic therapy, these patients (with high-grade dysplasia or cancer on histology) require close follow-up a minimum of every 6 months to 1 year.

2.13. Pernicious anemia

- There may be an increased risk of gastric cancer or gastric carcinoid
- A single EGD should be performed to identify gastric cancer or carcinoid tumor in patients with pernicious anemia
- Surveillance of carcinoid tumors is controversial and should be individualized.

2.14. Gastric/bariatric surgery patient

2.14.1. Pre-surgery

An EGD should be performed in all patients with upper GI tract symptoms who are to undergo bariatric surgery.

- An EGD should be considered in all patients who are going to undergo a Roux-en-Y gastric bypass regardless of the presence of symptoms
- An EGD should be considered in patients who are undergoing gastric banding to exclude large hernias (Fig. 13A), which could alter the surgical approach
- Patients without symptoms who opt not have an EGD should have non-invasive testing for *H. pylori*, followed by treatment if positive.

2.14.2. Post-gastric surgery

- There are insufficient data to support routine endoscopic surveillance for patients with previous partial gastrectomy for peptic ulcer disease
- There should be a low threshold for investigating upper GI symptoms in patients, post-gastric surgery.

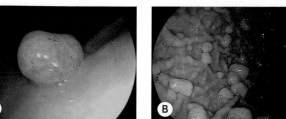
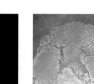
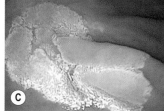

Figure 12 Polyps. (A) and (B) Fundic gland polyps. (C) Adenomas of the duodenum.

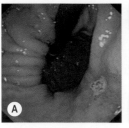 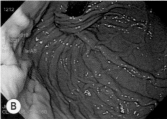

Figure 13 Retroflexed view of the fundus and cardia in (A) patient with a hiatus hernia (arrow), (B) post-Nissen's fundoplication.

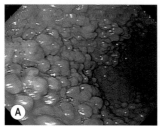 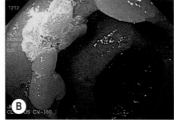

Figure 14 Familial adenomatous polyposis (FAP). (A) Image of multiple fundic gland polyps in a patient with FAP. (B) Duodenal adenoma in patient with FAP.

2.15. Familial adenomatous polyposis (See Box 4 in Chapter 1.11)

- Fundic gland polyps are found in 88% of patients with FAP (Figure 14a)
- Adenomas occur in 2–50%. They are usually solitary, sessile and located in antrum
- Duodenal adenomas occur in 90% of patients (Fig. 14b)
- Jejunal and ileal polyps are present in 50–90% of patients
- Patients should undergo screening with both forward and side-viewing endoscopes between the ages of 25 to 30
- Biopsies should be taken from the largest duodenal polyps and from the ampulla
- Subsequent follow-up should be determined based on the Spigelman score (Tables 1, 2).

Table 1 Spigelman classification of duodenal polyps in patients with FAP

Polyp (n)	1–4	1 point
	5–20	2 points
	>20	3 points
Size (mm)	1–4	1 point
	5–10	2 points
	>10	3 points
Histology	Tubulous	1 point
	Tubulovillous	2 points
	Villous	3 points
Degree of dysplasia	Low	1 point
	High	3 points

Table 2 Spigelman score

Spigelman stage	Management	Endoscopic surveillance
0 (0 points)	Endoscopic surveillance	4 years
I (1–4 points)	Endoscopic surveillance	2–3 years
II (5–6 points)	Endoscopic surveillance	2–3 years
III (7–8 points)	Surgery or endoscopic management	6–12 months
IV (9–12 points)	Consider referral for surgery	3–6 months

> **! Warning!**
> Biopsying the ampulla.
> Biopsies should be taken AWAY from the pancreatic orifice to avoid pancreatitis. A safe area to biopsy is the upper left quadrant (see Fig. 6B).

2.16. Hereditary non-polyposis colorectal cancer (HNPCC)

- Patients with HNPCC are at increased risk of gastric and small bowel cancer
- Endoscopic surveillance should be considered commencing at age 30.

3. Contraindications

There are no absolute contraindications to EGD.

- The examination, however, may be dangerous in the following cases:
  - Known or suspected perforation. EGD should not be performed unless to insert a covered stent to treat the perforation (see Ch. 7.3)
  - Massive gastrointestinal hemorrhage suggesting an aortoduodenal fistula
  - Acute cardiorespiratory failure not responding to medical therapy
  - Hypovolemic shock not responding to aggressive resuscitation
- EGD should be performed with caution in the following situations:
  - Large Zenker's diverticulum
  - Severe respiratory failure
  - Thoracic aortic aneurysm
  - Strictures of the cervical esophagus.

4. Equipment

4.1. Gastroscope

- Standard gastroscopes have a diameter of ≤10 mm with an instrument channel of 2.8 mm
- A gastroscope with a large operating channel measuring 3.8–4.2 mm is useful in severe acute upper GI bleeding
- A gastroscope with double instrument channel is also useful in patients with an acute upper GI bleed (see

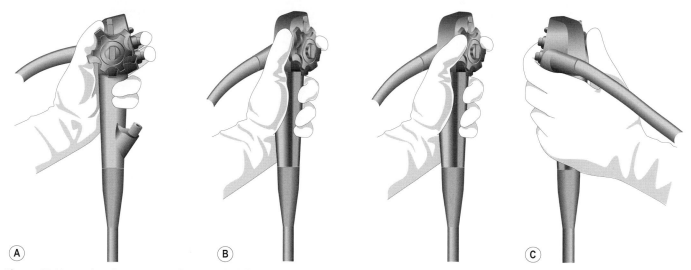

A   B   C

Figure 15 How to handle an upper endoscope. The left hand controls up/down (large wheel), right/left angulation (small wheel), insufflation, water, and suction buttons.

Ch. 7.8). It can also be used with a miniprobe to assess submucosal lesions (Chapter 9)

- High-definition gastroscopes with optical zoom should be available to assess Barrett's esophagus, or when screening for pre-malignant gastric or duodenal lesions
- Small caliber gastroscopes are useful to pass through strictures. These can either be transnasal videoendoscopes or slim caliber gastroscopes (4.9–5.9 mm).

4.2. Accessories

- Biopsy forceps (standard and jumbo)
- Dye spray catheter
- Chromoendoscopy stains (see Ch. 2.4)
  - 1% acetic acid (Barrett's esophagus assessment)
  - 0.5% methylene blue (intestinal metaplasia in stomach, adenomatous polyps, Barrett's esophagus)
  - 2% (range 1.5–3%) Lugol's iodine (squamous esophageal dysplasia or cancer)
  - 0.2% (range 0.1–0.8%) indigo carmine (Barrett's esophagus or adenocarcinoma)

- Additional equipment may be required if therapeutic procedures are anticipated (see Ch. 7 for details).

5. Endoscopy technique

5.1. Handling the endoscope

The control section of the endoscope should rest comfortably in the palm of the left hand, in the V formed between the thumb and index finger (Fig. 15). The left hand controls up/down (large wheel), right/left angulation (small wheel), insufflation, water, and suction buttons, while the right hand is responsible for advancing and withdrawing the endoscope, and its axial rotation.

- Hold the endoscope approximately 30 cm from its distal end with your right hand. Your left hand should control the up/down angulation (Fig. 16)
- Check that the endoscope is correctly angulated (so that it curves down over the tongue when you insert it)
- Advance the endoscope into the mouth and to the base of the tongue

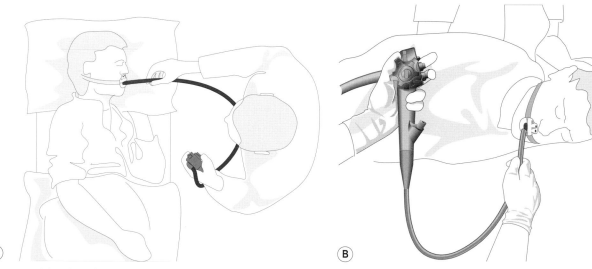

A   B

Figure 16 (A) Right and (B) left hand positioning for upper endoscopy. Hold the endoscope approximately 30 cm from its distal end with your right hand. Your left hand should control the up/down angulation.

- Gently angle the tip of the gastroscope downward until the vocal cords, epiglottis and cricoarytenoid cartilage become visible
- Pass behind and to the right of the arytenoid
- Ask the patient to swallow and apply *gentle* pressure while insufflating air
- The upper esophageal sphincter relaxes and the endoscope should be inserted under direct vision into the esophagus
- In the past, blind intubation has been used where the base of the tongue is pressed down with the index and middle finger of the left hand, and the endoscope is advanced blindly into the esophagus. However, we recommend that the esophagus should be intubated under direct vision rather than using this technique.

5.1.1. Problems with intubating the esophagus (Table 3)

- If you meet any resistance DO NOT PUSH. This will cause trauma, edema and spasm, which will make intubation more difficult. It can also cause perforation. Withdraw the endoscope slightly and confirm that you are in the correct position. If it is not possible to pass to the right of the arytenoid, try passing on the left. If

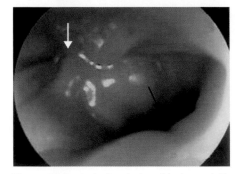

Figure 17 Zenker's diverticulum (black arrow). The true esophagus is highlighted with the white arrow.

this fails, check the patient's position. They should be fully in the left lateral position with slight, but not severe, neck flexion. If it does not work, ask the nurse assistant to provide chin lift.
- Intubated patients may sometimes need the tracheal tube balloon to be deflated to allow intubation of the esophagus.
- A Zenker's diverticulum can be recognized immediately (Fig. 17). It is important to determine which is the true esophageal lumen and which is the diverticulum. If there

Table 3 Potential problems faced in upper endoscopy and how to manage them

Problem	Cause	Action required
Respiratory distress, cyanosis	Incorrect endoscopy path with intubation of the trachea	Remove endoscope

	Desaturation associated with the following
	    Respiratory insufficiency
	    Cardiac insufficiency
	    Or abnormal cardiac rhythm
	    Or laryngeal spasm
		Remedy the respiratory problem by the following:
		    Remove endoscope
		    Clear out airways
		    Aspirate buccal cavity
		    Oxygenation (mask ventilation, intubation if necessary)

	Regurgitation of gastric contents	Elevate the patient's head
		Place them in the recovery position
		Assess for bronchial aspiration
		Consider chest X-ray
Unable to intubate the upper esophagus	Zenker diverticulum	Withdraw the endoscope and reinsert it under visual control; if necessary use a wire guide under fluoroscopy to direct the endoscope
	High esophageal stricture	Dilate
Looping in esophagus	Diverticulum	Withdraw. If necessary, pass a guidewire to the cardia under fluroscopic guidance
	Hiatal hernia	
	Achalasia or stenosis (benign, malignant or due to external compression)	Gentle dilation or use a small caliber gastroscope
Looping in stomach	J-shaped stomach	Withdraw to the GEJ and follow the lesser curve
	Altered anatomy post-surgery	Exert external pressure on the stomach
	Pyloric stenosis	Insert a guide wire through the pylorus and use this to guide the endoscope passage. This may require fluoroscopy if there is a complex stricture
		Dilation is sometimes required

is any doubt, a guidewire with an atraumatic tip can gently be guided under fluoroscopic or visual control into the esophagus and then followed with the endoscope.

- The same technique can be used with a high tight esophageal stricture. Advance a guidewire into the esophagus and follow it with the endoscope (see Ch. 7.1 for dilation of strictures). Alternatively, a small caliber gastroscope can be used.

Warning!

Never force the endoscope against resistance. If there is resistance, the esophagus MUST be intubated under direct vision.

5.1.2. Advancing the gastroscope

- The gastroscope should be advanced under visual control, applying moderate insufflation. If there are positioning problems, always withdraw and never advance blindly.
- Any fluid should be aspirated before advancing the endoscope to minimize the risk of aspiration and to ensure that all areas have been visualized. Note the appearance of the fluid (e.g. the presence of altered blood). Anti-bubble solution (simethicone) is sometimes helpful.
- The esophagus is examined while inserting the endoscope. Once the cardia is reached, pause and examine the gastroesophageal junction. The proximal margin of the gastric folds is commonly accepted as the junction of the stomach and esophagus. The level of the squamocolumnar junction should be noted. If the squamocolumnar junction is displaced proximal to the gastroesophageal junction, biopsies should be taken to look for Barrett's esophagus.
- The gastroesophageal junction should remain closed unless a swallow is initiated or air is insufflated. A patulous junction suggests the presence of reflux.
- The level of the diaphragmatic hiatus should be noted.
- Once in the gastric cavity (Fig. 18A), follow the lesser curvature as far as the pylorus without waiting for maximum inflation of the stomach (where there is disappearance of folds), as the gastric cavity will be examined on the way back.
- Antral peristalsis may prevent approach to the pylorus; simply wait a few moments before continuing to advance.
- To pass through the pylorus, position the endoscope just in front of the pylorus (Fig. 18B,C). Apply a little air and gentle constant pressure against the orifice using only up/down angulation.
- The duodenal bulb is examined on insertion, advancing and withdrawing the gastroscope until the bulb is fully visualized. If endoscope is expelled into the gastric antrum during these maneuvers, simply re-intubate the pylorus.
- To pass the superior flexure of the duodenum and enter the second part of the duodenum, position the endoscope at the apex of the bulb and perform the following maneuver: angulation to the right; right axial

rotation through 90° and angulation upwards (Fig. 18D). This is achieved by clockwise rotation of small wheel with anticlockwise rotation of big wheel. The superior flexure of the duodenum is often passed blindly and examined on the way back.

- The lower part of the second part of the duodenum is reached by 'straightening the endoscope', i.e. by withdrawing the instrument until the 70 cm marker (approximately) is visible at the incisors. In practice, this maneuver reduces the loop along the greater curve of the stomach (Fig. 18E).
- On withdrawal, insufflate the gastric lumen so that it can be examined fully.
- The endoscope should be placed in the 'retroflexed' position to visualize the fundus and cardia. To retroflex, position the endoscope in the antrum facing the pylorus, angle upwards (big wheel anticlockwise) and advance the endoscope (Fig. 18F).
- The endoscope is next withdrawn in the retroflexed position, rotating it axially through 180° to examine the fundus and the cardia (Fig. 18G).
- The endoscope is then returned to a neutral position in the body; then withdrawn.
- Once the stomach has been fully inspected, intragastric air should be removed by suctioning.
- The esophagus is again examined on withdrawal of the endoscope.
- The cervical esophagus, which is often not clearly viewed as the endoscope advances, is examined carefully on withdrawal.
- The average duration of a diagnostic upper endoscopy is 5–10 min under optimal sedation conditions.
- All lesions identified are biopsied, except for vascular malformations and duodenal ulcers.

5.2. Special situations

5.2.1. Gastroesophageal reflux disease

Gastroesophageal reflux disease (GERD) should be classified using the Savary–Miller (Table 5) or Los Angeles (Table 4) classification (Fig. 19). Longstanding or severe GERD can result in peptic stricture formation (Fig. 20) and is associated with the development of Barrett's esophagus (Fig. 21).

Table 4 Los Angeles classification of GERD

Grade	Description
A	≥1 mucosal break ≤5 mm that does not extend between the tops of two mucosal folds
B	≥1 mucosal break >5 mm that does not extend between the tops of two mucosal folds
C	≥1 mucosal break that is continuous between the tops of ≥2 mucosal folds but involves <75% of the circumference
D	mucosal break that involves ≥75% of the esophageal circumference

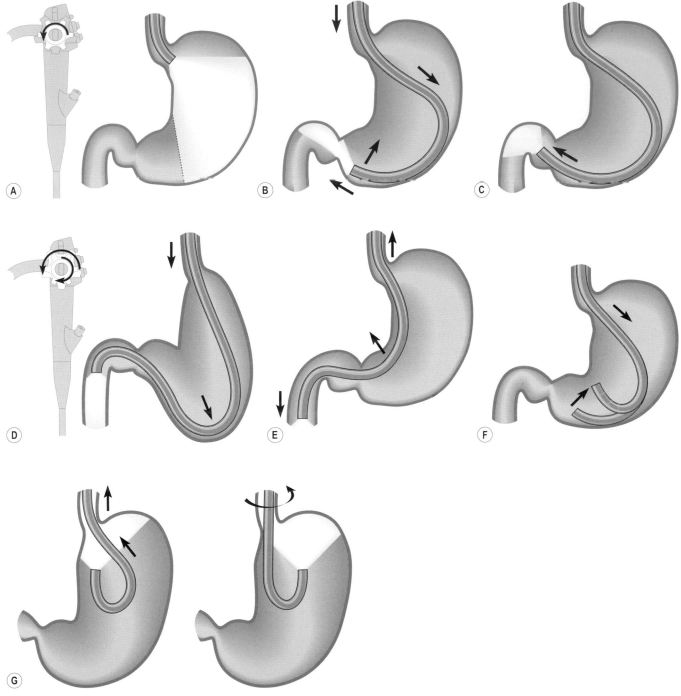

Figure 18 Steps to perform a complete examination of the upper GIT.

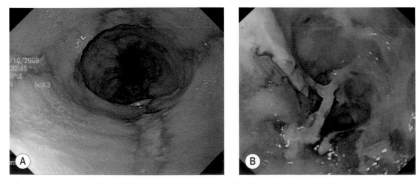

Figure 19 Esophagitis. (A) LA grade B esophagitis. (B) LA grade D esophagitis.

Table 5 Savary–Miller classification of GERD

Grade I	Single or isolated erosive lesion, oval or linear, only affecting one longitudinal fold
Grade II	Eerosive and exudative lesions in the distal esophagus that may be confluent, but not circumferential
Grade III	Circumferential erosions in the distal esophagus, covered by hemorrhagic and pseudomembranous exudate
Grade IV	Chronic lesions including ulcer, stricture ± short esophagus, or associated with lesions of grades I–III

5.2.2. Barrett's esophagus

Patients with longstanding GERD symptoms, particularly Caucasian males aged over 50, should be considered for an upper endoscopy to assess for Barrett's esophagus (Fig. 21).

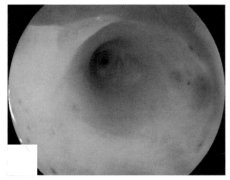

Figure 20 Peptic esophageal stricture associated with GERD.

- Screening should ideally be performed using a high resolution endoscope
- Chromoendoscopy with methylene blue or acetic acid can be used (see Ch. 2.4)
- Advanced imaging techniques such as confocal endomicroscopy have been shown to decrease the numbers of biopsies required (see Ch. 6.1)
- Barrett's esophagus can appear as circumferential (i.e. the entire width of the esophagus is Barrett's) or as tongues (a segment of the esophagus contains Barrett's) or as islands (where there is an isolated area of Barrett's separate from the main area affected by Barrett's)

Warning!

The following areas may not be viewed clearly. They should be examined *carefully* by the endoscopist:
1. The cervical esophagus.
2. Cardia.
3. Incisura.
4. Posterior wall of the body.
5. Pylorus.
6. Immediate post-pyloric area of the duodenal bulb.
7. Superior flexure of the duodenum.
8. Medial wall of the second part of the duodenum.

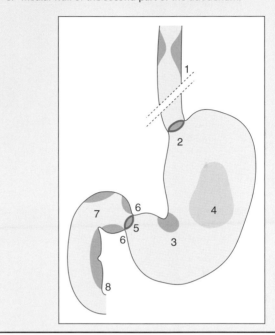

- Barrett's should be classified using the Prague classification, where the length of Barrett's that is circumferential (C) and the total length of the esophagus affected by Barrett's (M), that is the distance from the most proximal extent of the Barrett's (whether this is an island, tongue or circumferential) to the most distal extent, is measured. These data are then presented as Barrett's CM. For example if a patient has circumferential Barrett's esophagus from 38 to 40 cm with a tongue from 36 to 38 cm, this patient is C2 (38–40 cm) M4 (36–38 cm).

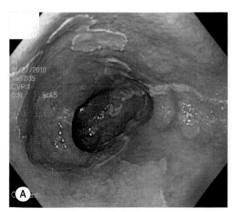
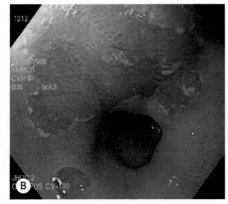
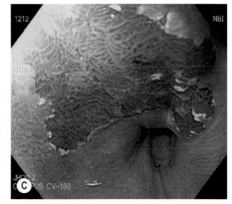

Figure 21 Barrett's esophagus. (A) Long segment Barrett's esophagus. (B) and (C) Barrett's esophagus seen under white light and following acetic acid application using NBI. (Courtesy of Dr Marcia Canto, Johns Hopkins Hospital, Baltimore).

Clinical Tip

How to biopsy the esophagus

A Advance the biopsy forceps through the instrument channel and into the lumen.

B Ask the assistant to open the forceps.

C Withdraw the open forceps until they abut the endoscope.

D Turn the tip of the endoscope with the forceps onto the area of interest using torque.

E Suction slightly and close the forceps.

F Blow a little air and confirm that the biopsy forceps are closed on the area of interest. If they are in the correct place, withdraw the biopsy forceps with the tissue sample.

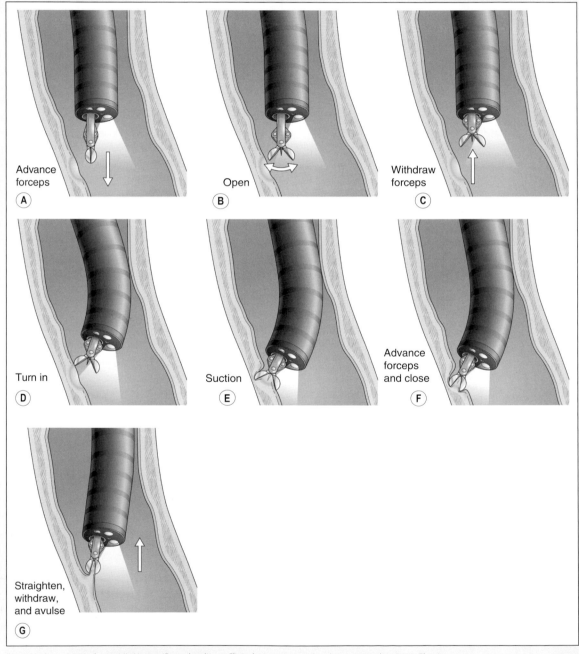

From Ginsberg GG, Kochman ML, Norton ID, et al., editors: Clinical gastrointestinal endoscopy. London, 2005, Elsevier.

- Screening should ideally be performed using a high definition endoscope.
- The Barrett's should be assessed using the Prague classification.
- Four quadrant biopsies should be obtained in every 2 cm of the Barrett's mucosa.
- Where dysplasia is detected, endoscopy should be repeated after 2 months of double-dose proton pump inhibitor therapy and repeat biopsies taken.

Low-grade dysplasia

- Follow-up endoscopy within 6 months to ensure that no higher grade of dysplasia is present.
- If no high-grade dysplasia, perform yearly endoscopy until no dysplasia is present on two consecutive annual endoscopies.

High-grade dysplasia

- Confirm the presence of high-grade dysplasia by an expert GI pathologist.
- Patients with high-grade dysplasia with mucosal irregularity should undergo endoscopic mucosal resection.
- Patients with confirmed high-grade dysplasia, even if unifocal, should be counseled regarding therapeutic options, including intensive surveillance, esophagectomy or ablative therapies.

Box 3 gives guidelines for screening and follow-up of Barrett's esophagus.

5.2.3. Eosinophilic esophagitis

Eosinophilic esophagitis should be suspected in an atopic patient with dysphagia or food bolus obstruction, in whom no cause for the obstruction or dysphagia is evident. It can also present with GERD-like symptoms, esophageal dysmotility or abdominal pain. Endoscopically, the esophagus can be normal or sometimes esophageal rings or stricture can be seen (Fig. 10d). Biopsies should be taken along the length of the esophagus. Great care should be taken with strictures associated with eosinophilic esophagitis as they are at increased risk of perforation (Fig. 10e).

5.2.4. Gastritis

The stomach should be examined for evidence of gastritis which is characterized by edema, erythema, friability, exudates, flat erosions, protruded erosions, fold hyperplasia, fold atrophy, loss of the vascular network, mucosal hemorrhagic points or nodularity.

The affected portion of the stomach should be documented (antrum, body, pangastritis) and the severity of the gastritis (absent, slight, moderate or severe) described.

5.3. Endoscopic classification of early or superficial cancers

Cancers should be classified endoscopically using the Paris classification as Type 0–5 (Table 6). Type 0 are superficial cancers, whose endoscopic appearance suggests that the depth of penetration into the wall is not more than into the submucosa (Figs 22). Type 0 are subdivided further into I, II and III. Lesions can combine several different types of lesions which are shown in Figures 23 and 24). The clinical relevance of classifying these lesions is that it predicts the likelihood of submucosal invasion and lymph node metastases.

6. Complications

A detailed discussion of the management of complications of endoscopy can be found in Chapter 8.

Complications (Table 3) associated with upper endoscopy include:

- Hypoxemia
- Heart rhythm disturbance

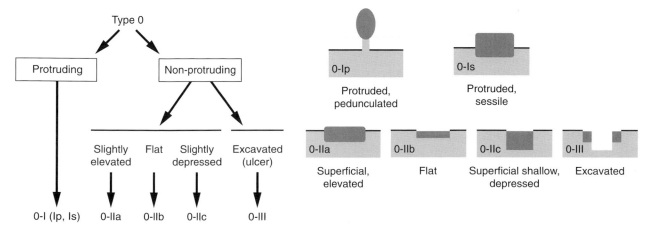

Figure 22 How to subdivide a Type 0 lesion. Examine the lesion and decide if it is protruding or non-protruding. Protruding lesions are either pedunculated (0–Ip) or sessile (0–Is) as documented on the right. If the lesion is non-polypoid, decide if it is slightly elevated (0–IIa), flat (0–IIb) or depressed (0–IIc). An excavated, or ulcerated lesion is classified as 0–III. (Modified from The Paris endoscopic classification of superficial neoplastic lesion. Paris Workshop Participants. Gastrointestinal Endoscopy 2003: 58(6); S5.)

Table 6 Paris endoscopic classification of tumors

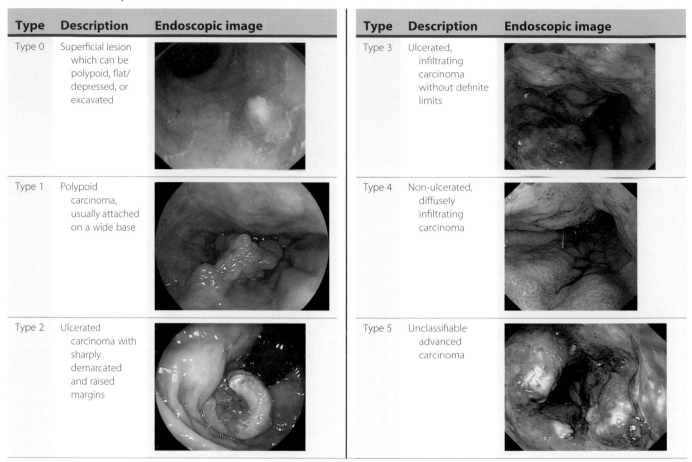

Type	Description	Endoscopic image	Type	Description	Endoscopic image
Type 0	Superficial lesion which can be polypoid, flat/depressed, or excavated		Type 3	Ulcerated, infiltrating carcinoma without definite limits	
Type 1	Polypoid carcinoma, usually attached on a wide base		Type 4	Non-ulcerated, diffusely infiltrating carcinoma	
Type 2	Ulcerated carcinoma with sharply demarcated and raised margins		Type 5	Unclassifiable advanced carcinoma	

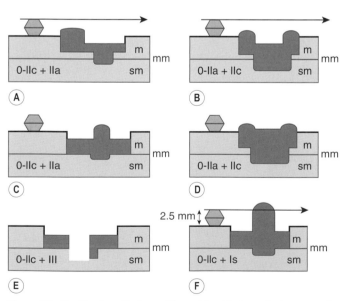

Figure 23 Classification of lesions with combined features. Lesions sometimes combine more than one endoscopic feature. These lesions are classified by whatever features are present. (A,B) The lesion protrudes less than the closed biopsy forceps (Type 0–II), and has a slight depression (0–IIc) as well as an elevation (0–IIa). (C) The lesion is depressed (Type 0–IIc) but also has an elevation within the depression (Type 0–IIa), the reverse is found in (D) where an elevated lesion (Type 0–IIa) has a central depression (Type 0–IIc). (E) A large excavated lesion (0–III contains a central depressed zone (0–IIc), while in (F), there is a central section which protrudes above the closed biopsy forceps (type 0–Is), associated with a depression on either side (Type 0–IIc). (Modified from the Paris Workshop Participants. The Paris Endoscopic classification of superficial neoplastic lesion. Gastrointest Endosc 58(6):S6 and S8, 2003.)

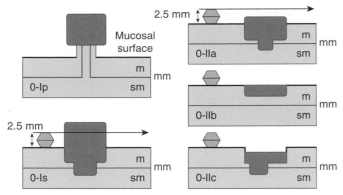

Figure 24 How to differentiate between Type 0–I and Type 0–II. Protruding lesions (Type 0–I), seen on the right, protrude higher than the cups of a closed biopsy forceps (2.5 mm). Non-protruding lesions (Type 0–II) can be differentiated from protruding (Type 0–I) as they protrude less than the height of a closed biopsy forceps (2.5 mm). The endoscopic appearance of the lesion is associated with the depth of penetration into the bowel wall (m, mucosa; mm, muscularis mucosae; sm, submucosa). (Modified from The Paris endoscopic classification of superficial neoplastic lesion. Paris Workshop Participants. Gastrointestinal Endoscopy 2003: 58(6); S6.)

- Perforation
  - Risk 0.03%
  - Associated with Zenker's diverticulum, esophageal stricture, anterior cervical osteophytes, malignancy
- Abdominal distension
- Suffusion of submucosal air with or without pneumoperitoneum and pneumomediastinum without evident perforation (resolves spontaneously)
- Infection
  - Aspiration pneumonia
  - Transient bacteremia
  - Retropharyngeal/retroesophageal abscess (rare)
  - Infection from contaminated equipment.

7. Upper endoscopy in children

7.1. Equipment

A pediatric gastroscope can be used from birth to 7 years old. A nasogastroscope should be used in premature infants weighing <2 kg. Adult equipment can be used from the age of 7 upwards.

7.2. Preparation for upper endoscopy

- Fasting: children over 6 months old – at least 6 h. Neonates under 6 months old – 2–4 hours
- Anesthesia: sedation and oropharyngeal anesthesia are not generally used before the age of 6 months, in view of good tolerance (the baby sucks the endoscope) and the risk of inhaling saliva after the examination
- Atropine is used intramuscularly, subcutaneously or sublingually to prevent vasovagal syncope
- Therapeutic endoscopy is performed in all cases under general anesthesia
- The psychological approach is key in children old enough to understand the examination; it is essential to gain their confidence
- After the examination, the child is placed in the recovery position and monitored. Whenever the pharynx and larynx have been anesthetized, normal swallowing should be confirmed before restarting feeding.

7.3. Indications

- Assessment of neonatal esophagogastritis manifested by hematemesis, general discomfort, bradycardia and refusing the bottle during the first few days of life
- Diagnosis of reflux esophagitis (failure to thrive for more than 1 month, heartburn or dysphagia,

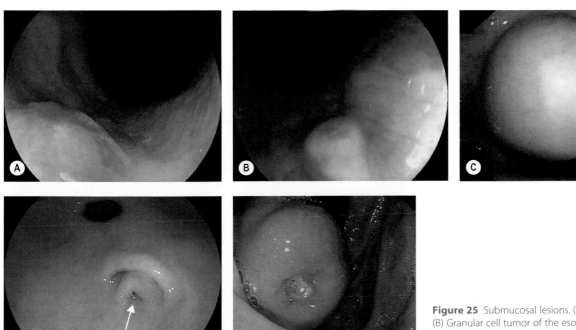

Figure 25 Submucosal lesions. (A) Carcinoid tumor. (B) Granular cell tumor of the esophagus (Abrikossoff tumor). (C) Lipoma. (D) Ectopic pancreas (white arrow). (E) GIST.

regurgitation or vomiting of blood, and anemia). Biopsies are performed on the lower esophagus if there are no macroscopic lesions from which to obtain histological evidence of reflux, or if Barrett's is suspected. If esophagitis is obvious, biopsies are not routinely required

- Diagnosis and dilation of esophageal strictures (peptic, caustic or following surgery for esophageal atresia)
- Diagnosis and banding of esophageal varices
- Gastroduodenal ulcers: upper endoscopy is indicated when there is hematemesis or melena
- Recurrent abdominal pain:
    - If it is cyclical
    - If the pain occurs at night or very early in the morning
    - If it is associated with repeated vomiting
    - If the pain is accompanied by anemia
    - In adolescents, if the pain is atypical
- Duodenal biopsies in patients with malabsorption syndrome or protein-losing enteropathy (in this case, gastric biopsies are routinely required)
- Suspected Crohn's disease
- GI bleeding
- Caustic burns (except those caused by dilute bleach)
- Removal of esophageal foreign bodies trapped for more than 6 hours
- Intragastric foreign bodies are removed only if they are caustic, measure >5 cm at their largest diameter, are likely to perforate (a needle, for example) or if they have been present for more than 10 days.

7.4. Technique

- The technique is similar to that used in adults, with the endoscope introduced and advanced under direct vision
- Insufflation should be kept to a minimum
- The gastroesophageal junction is located, depending on age, between 20 and 40 cm from the incisors. The Z line is not always identifiable in neonates and young infants
- Gastric air and saliva from the oropharynx are aspirated on withdrawal of the apparatus.

7.5. Complications

In addition to the complications listed above, the following can occur:

- Episode of cyanosis with apnea, resolving on immediate withdrawal of the fibroscope after desufflating the stomach (gastric insufflation rapidly desaturates babies and the presence of the endoscope in the esophagus may compress the trachea). This complication is observed more frequently in children under 6 months old, particularly if the head is hyperextended
- Epistaxis
- Longitudinal fissuring of the cardia after retroversion on the stomach
- Duodenal hematoma after biopsy.

Further Reading

ASGE Standards of Practice Committee: The role of endoscopy in the assessment and treatment of esophageal cancer, *Gastrointest Endosc* 57:817–822, 2003.

ASGE Standards of Practice Committee: ASGE guideline: the role of endoscopy in the surveillance of premalignant conditions of the upper GI tract, *Gastrointest Endosc* 63:570–580, 2006.

ASGE Standards of Practice Committee: The role of endoscopy in dyspepsia, *Gastrointest Endosc* 66:1071–1075, 2007.

ASGE Standards of Practice Committee: Role of endoscopy in the bariatric surgery patient, *Gastrointest Endosc* 68:1–10, 2008.

Cohen J, Safdi MA, Deal SE, et al: ASGE/ACG Taskforce on Quality in Endoscopy. Quality indicators for esophagogastroduodenoscopy, *Am J Gastroenterol* 101:886–891, 2006.

Eisen GM, Baron TH, Dominitz JA, et al: ASGE. Complications of upper GI endoscopy, *Gastrointest Endosc* 55:784–793, 2002.

Goddard AF, James MW, McIntyre AS, et al: Guidelines for the management of iron deficiency anemia, *Gut* 46(Suppl 4):iv1–iv5, 2000.

Jacobson BC, Hirota W, Baron TH, et al: ASGE. Obscure gastrointestinal bleeding, *Gastrointest Endosc* 57:817–822, 2003.

Paris Workshop Participants: The Paris endoscopic classification of superficial neoplastic lesion, *Gastrointest Endosc* 58:S1–S43, 2003.

Standards of Practice Committee: Role of endoscopy in the management of GERD, *Gastrointest Endosc* 66:219–224, 2007.

CHAPTER 4

Diagnostic colonoscopy

Jean Marc Canard, Jean-Christophe Létard, Ian Penman

Summary

Key Points

- High quality colonic preparation is essential.
- Good technique is the key to allowing a rapid, complete examination of the colon.
- The colonoscope should be advanced under visual control.
- The colonoscope should be shortened frequently to ensure a short, straight endoscope.
- Abdominal palpation and patient position changes are useful adjuncts.
- Confirmation that the cecum has been reached should be made by identifying the ileocecal valve, appendix or entering the ileum and visualizing the small bowel.
- Withdrawing the colonoscope should take a minimum of 6 minutes.
- Retroflex gently in the rectum to avoid missing distal lesions.
- Audit of colonoscopy outcomes should be performed regularly.

Introduction

Optical colonoscopy is the gold standard method for examining the colon, is widely available, and offers the potential for biopsy and/or therapy during the same procedure. It is commonly performed for the evaluation of patients with lower GI symptoms and for screening/surveillance in people at risk of colorectal cancer. While colonoscopy has been an established technique for over 30 years, it can be technically difficult and is associated with a small but real risk of major complications. For these reasons, a good, careful technique, combined with a sound knowledge of polypectomy procedures is essential.

1. Anatomy

The colon is an elastic tube that extends from the rectum to the ileocecal valve and whose normal mucosa is pale-pink in color. The submucosal vascular network is visible, as are the rather large submucosal veins.

The colon comprises mobile segments (Fig. 1) (cecum, transverse colon, sigmoid colon) whose length depends on the size of the mesocolon, which attaches these segments to the posterior abdominal wall and the fixed segments (ascending colon, hepatic flexure, descending colon, rectum). The splenic flexure is partially attached by the phrenocolic ligament, the length and rigidity of which enable it to descend and become rounded on insertion of a colonoscope.

However, there are numerous anatomic variations resulting from the absence of mesorectal stickiness during gestation, which in turn induces variable mobility in the ascending and descending colon. In some cases, the cecum is incompletely rotated (cecum recurvatum).

The rectum is 12–15 cm long beginning from the anal margin. It is the shape of an elongated ampulla and is

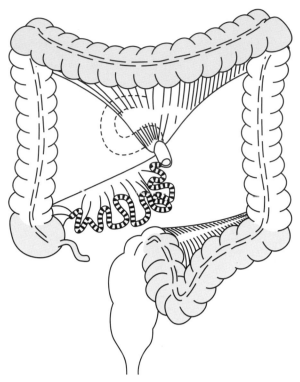

Figure 1 Mobile colonic segments: cecum; transverse colon; sigmoid colon.

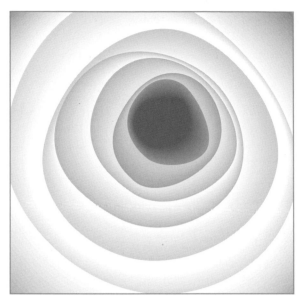

Figure 2 Circular haustrations in the descending and sigmoid colon.

segmented by three or four mucosal folds (valves of Houston). The sigmoid varies in length, depending on the length of its mesocolon. The colonic lumen and haustrations in the descending or sigmoid colon are generally circular (Fig. 2). The splenic flexure exhibits a blue area that is attributable to the impression of the spleen. The lumen of the transverse colon is triangular (Fig. 3).

The indentation of the liver at the hepatic flexure can be recognized by its bluish color but note that this may also be visible from the descending colon or in the middle of the transverse colon. The hepatic flexure is easily confused with the cecal pole (one of the lips of the ileocecal valve may be confused with the thickened fold viewed tangentially above a flexure). The only reliable reference points are the terminal ileum, ileocecal valve and the appendicular orifice.

The internal aspect of the cecal pole, which typically exhibits a 'crow's foot' shape, is the point of convergence of the three longitudinal bands of colonic muscle that extend to the appendicular orifice, which generally takes the form of a very narrow slit. An operated appendix looks the same, except that the stump has been buried and may resemble a polyp (can be biopsied but not resected).

The ileocecal valve is 5 cm above the cecal pole, on the medial wall of the right colon, usually on the left side of the colonoscopic field of vision. The valve takes the form of a transversally elongated mouth and is generally situated on the margin of one of the crow's foot folds. The orifice of the ileocecal valve can rarely be viewed right away as it is normally located on the upper lip. Once the lower and upper lips of the ileocecal valve have been identified, it is possible to enter its orifice and examine the terminal ileum, where the submucosal vascular network is far more visible than in the colon. In children and adolescents, Peyer's patches are often observed in the terminal ileum, where they constitute 2–3 mm white or translucent sessile protrusions and villi are also seen.

1.1. Postoperative colonic anatomy

The most prevalent types of colonic surgery are left hemicolectomy (anastomosis between the rectum and transverse colon), right hemicolectomy (anastomosis between the small intestine and transverse colon), subtotal colectomy (anastomosis between the ileum and rectum), and total colectomy with ileo-anal anastomosis. Anastomoses involving the small intestine, colon or rectum can either be end-to-side or end-to-end. Hence, it is necessary to be able to recognize the cul-de-sac and withdraw the endoscope in order to progress in the right direction. In cases of colostomy, colonoscopy can be performed via the stoma.

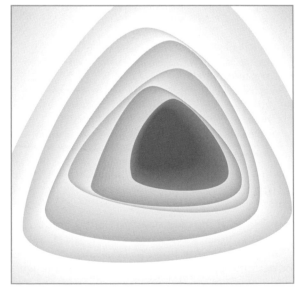

Figure 3 Triangular haustrations in the transverse colon.

2. Indications for colonoscopy (TC)

These are general indications but specific guidelines exist in many countries and may vary. Readers should be familiar with the guidelines of the country in which they are practicing. References to some of these guidelines can be found elsewhere in this text. The following are the guidelines from the Société Française d'Endoscopie Digestive (SFED).

2.1. Patients at average risk of colorectal cancer (CRC)*

- Asymptomatic patients with a positive occult blood test (performed as part of a screening program, not on an individual basis)
- Patients with abdominal pain associated with a change in bowel habit to looser for >6 weeks
  - Over the age of 50
  - Under the age of 50, if there is no response to symptomatic treatment
- Patients with overt rectal bleeding
  - Repeated episodes of dark red bleeding, irrespective of age
  - Repeated isolated episodes of bright red bleeding in patients over 50 (flexible sigmoidoscopy or TC in patients under 50)
  - Profuse bleeding, as soon as the patient's condition allows
- Patients with symptomatic diverticulosis
- TC is contraindicated in suspected acute diverticulitis, but should be undertaken at a later date (~6 weeks) if surgery is being considered or the diagnosis is in doubt
- Patients with endocarditis caused by *Streptococcus bovis* or group D streptococci.

2.2. Surveillance of asymptomatic patients at high risk of CRC

- Patients with a family history of CRC with a 1st-degree relative under 60 or several 1st-degree relatives with CRC:
  - TC at age 45 or 5 years younger than the age at diagnosis of the index case; if he/she was under 50 then TC at 5 and 10 years
  - For adenoma including non-advanced forms: follow-up colonoscopy at 3 years
- Family history of colonic adenoma in a 1st-degree relative under 60:
  - TC at the age of 45 or 5 years younger than the age at diagnosis of the index case; if he/she was under 50, then TC at 5 and 10 years.
- After surgery for colorectal cancer:
  - Incomplete colonic examination before surgery: TC at 6 months
  - Complete colonic examination before surgery: TC at 2–3 years then at 7–8 years

- Patients with acromegaly:
  - At diagnosis, then depending on the findings. If normal, every 5 years until biochemical evidence of 'cure'.

2.3. Surveillance of asymptomatic patients at very high risk of CRC

- FAP (familial adenomatous polyposis) (see Ch. 1.11, Box 4)
  - Member of a family with FAP: flexible sigmoidoscopy annually from the age 10–12 years
  - Member of a family with attenuated FAP: TC annually from the age of 30
  - FAP after colectomy: flexible sigmoidoscopy annually.
- Hereditary non-polyposis colon cancer (HNPCC)
  - Member of a family with HNPCC: TC every other year from the age of 20–25
  - HNPCC after surgery: TC every other year
- Juvenile polyposis (JP) family member: TC every 2–3 years from the age of 10–15
- Peutz–Jeghers syndrome family member: TC every 2–3 years from the age of 18
- Inflammatory bowel disease: pancolitis (> 10 years) or left-side colitis (> 15 years): TC every 2 (pancolitis) to 3 years (left-side colitis) and biopsies every 10 cm. Recent studies recommend routine use of indigo carmine or methylene blue chromoendoscopy with fewer, targeted biopsies of subtle abnormalities of colonic crypts or vessel pattern.

2.4. Surveillance of patients after resection of one or more colonic polyps

- Hyperplastic polyps (size ≥1 cm, ≥5 in number, location in the proximal colon with a family history of hyperplastic polyposis): TC at 5, and 15 years
- Low-risk adenomas (V3) or advanced adenomas (size ≥1 cm, ≥25% villous component, high-grade dysplasia (HGD) or *in situ* carcinoma) or V4.1/V4.2 adenomas:
  - Incomplete resection: TC at 3 months
  - Complete resection: advanced adenoma or ≥3 in number, or a family history of CRC; TC at 3, 8, 13, and 23 years
  - Complete resection: non-advanced adenoma, <3 in number and no family history of CRC; TC at 5, 10, and 20 years
- Malignancy in an adenoma (V4.3, V4.4, V5, 'polyp-cancers')
  - Incomplete resection (V4.3, V4.4): TC at 3 months then at 3 years if nothing at 3 months

---

Box 1   Amsterdam II criteria for HNPCC

- Three or more relatives with HNPCC associated cancers (colorectal cancer, endometrial cancer, small bowel, ureter, or renal pelvis), one of whom is a 1st-degree relative to the other two.
- At least two generations must be affected.
- One individual from the family must have been diagnosed with one or more cancers before the age of 50.
- FAP must be excluded.

---

*Defined as the average population risk.

Box 2 Vienna classification of gastrointestinal epithelial neoplasia and superficial gastrointestinal cancers

- Category V1: negative for neoplasia.
- Category V2: indefinite for neoplasia.
- Category V3: low-grade neoplasia (LGIN).
- Category V4: high-grade neoplasia (HGIN).
  - V4.1: high-grade dysplasia.
  - V4.2: *in situ* (non-invasive) carcinoma.
  - V4.3: suspicious for invasive carcinoma.
  - V4.4: intramucosal carcinoma.
- Category V5: submucosal invasion by carcinoma.

- Complete resection (V4.3/4.4): TC at 3 years
- Complete resection (V5): TC at 3 months if patient does not undergo colectomy.

3. Contraindications

- Colonic perforation
- Peritonitis
- Acute cardiorespiratory failure
- Recent myocardial infarction
- Recent colonic surgery
- Major aneurysm of the abdominal aorta or its branches.

4. Equipment

The standard, multipurpose colonoscope used routinely measures 130 cm in length. The long colonoscope (170 cm) is more fragile, more expensive and less practical. Flexible sigmoidoscopes (60 cm long) are also available but are less useful, except in young adults with bright red rectal bleeding, or bloody diarrhea.

The more flexible pediatric colonoscope (130 cm long, 11 mm in diameter) is used in children from the age of 2 years upwards. It may be useful in adults for passing through strictures or in patients with a narrow, tortuous or acutely angulated sigmoid colon.

The following accessories are required: cold biopsy forceps, hot biopsy forceps, foreign body forceps, tripod grasper forceps, polypectomy snares, lavage catheter, injection needles, endoscopic clips, detachable loops dilating balloons, polyp retrieval ('Roth') nets, fixative containers.

5. Preparation of the examination room (Box 3)

5.1. Setting up and testing endoscopes

- Set up the video colonoscope on the console
- Check that the colonoscope is working properly (angulation, aspiration, insufflation, clear image)
- Check the connections with the monitor, the printer and the image capturing equipment
- Test the white balance for any endoscopes that still require this function
- Check the image storage equipment, computer switched on, patient data entered.

5.2. Setting up and testing additional equipment

- Suction bottle and connections: (single use disposable)
- Examination couch: correctly insulated with a disposable protective covering and cot sides to prevent falls
- Instrument trolley with labeled drawers or tiers containing all the instruments. It must be carefully checked before each examination and should match the type of examination
- Accessories
- Dyes and tattoos: to detect, delineate and mark small mucosal lesions (flat polyps, etc.)
  - 0.2% indigo carmine. It should be ready for use in a 50 mL syringe; colitis surveillance requires 150–200 mL, so it is useful to make it up in a bag of 0.9% saline
  - 0.5 or 0.7% methylene blue
  - Pure carbon black ('Spot', GI Supply Inc., Camp Hill, PA, USA) can be used to mark the site of a lesion before surgery, or for marking where a polyp was removed so that the area can easily be identified during subsequent screening colonoscopy. Sterile India ink suspension is an alternative but has been associated with immunological reactions
- Anti-foaming agent (simethicone)
- Lavage catheter
- Disposable gloves
- Gauze swabs
- Lubricant for rectal examination and for lubricating the colonoscope
- Washing equipment: sterile water, 50 mL syringes, connector tubing, and power wash pump.

6. Handling the colonoscope

The endoscopist may work seated or standing, but must be in a comfortable position to keep the instrument as straight as possible.

Colonoscopy is performed by a single endoscopist who holds the control handles in their left hand (insufflation, aspiration, washing with the index and middle fingers, lever for up/down angulation between the thumb and index

Box 3 The minimum equipment required for a colonoscopy room

- 1 cold light source.
- 1 video processor.
- 1 or more television monitors. These should ideally be high definition.
- 1 bottle full of sterile water for irrigation.
- 1 diathermy unit.
- 1 argon plasma coagulation (APC) generator.
- Additional imaging equipment: DVD recorder and discs; computer.
- There should be at least four videocolonoscopes for one room to allow for cleaning, disinfection, maintenance and repair.
- CO_2 insufflator.
- Powered washing pump to clear adherent fecal matter.

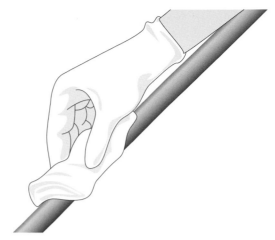

Figure 4 The lubricated endoscope is held between the thumb and index finger of the right hand with a compress.

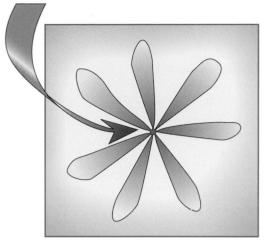

Figure 5 The lumen of the colon is at the centre of the convergence of folds.

finger). The right hand advances or withdraws the apparatus, and introduces instruments into the biopsy channel. As it advances, the lubricated colonoscope is held between the thumb and index finger (Fig. 4).

6.1. General principles

- The parts of the colonoscope that have not been introduced into the patient should be kept straight and not allowed to form loops.
- Avoid excess air insufflation. Excessive air is uncomfortable for the patient as well as distending the proximal colon, which can make reaching the cecum more difficult.
- Advance gently under visual control, avoiding the formation of loops by reducing them as they occur and preventing their reappearance by abdominal palpation (see Clinical Tips, below).
- The instrument should be withdrawn to shorten the colon whenever possible. This is usually performed after navigating through the sigmoid, again after negotiating the splenic flexure, once or twice in the transverse colon and again once the instrument is in the ascending colon.
- It is usually better to withdraw the instrument than to push it in blindly. If it is necessary to insert the colonoscope without a view of the lumen, the mucosal vascular network should pass in front of the lens. If the mucosa appears blanched, then there is excessive pressure on the colonic wall and a risk of perforation. Insertion must stop and the luminal view re-established.
- Any polyp discovered during insertion should be removed because it may not be found during withdrawal.
- Residues unlikely to obstruct the colonoscope should be aspirated during insertion so that the mucosa can be examined completely during withdrawal.
- The procedure is usually performed with the patient lying in the left lateral position or supine, the latter usually when it is performed under general anesthesia. If there are problems advancing the colonoscope,

consider moving the patient. In general, the following patient positions often facilitate scope passage if difficulty is encountered:
  - Rectosigmoid – supine or right lateral
  - Splenic flexure – right lateral
  - Hepatic flexure – supine or left lateral.
- The lumen of the colon is at the center of the convergence of folds if the colon is not insufflated or in spasm (Fig. 5).
- The instrument should be directed at the areas in shadow (Fig. 6A) and towards the center of the arcs formed by the folds so as to advance in the direction of the lumen (Fig. 6B).
- On withdrawal, which is done slowly to examine the whole mucosa, it may be necessary to re-advance to see areas difficult to observe (beyond the ileocecal valve, hepatic flexure, splenic flexure, sigmoid colon and rectosigmoid junction, and the distal rectum) (Fig. 7). Longer withdrawal times are associated with increased adenoma detection rates. Current recommendations suggest that the colonoscope should be withdrawn over at least 6 minute.
- The report should specify whether the bowel preparation was adequate (to determine the reliability of the examination); any problems with advancing and the maneuvers used should also be noted. This may be useful in a subsequent examination.

6.2. Bowel preparation score

The Ottawa bowel preparation quality score is determined by scoring the right, mid and left colon as well as the score for the quantity of fluid within the entire colon and adding the four scores together (Table 1), the range being 0-14.

7. Examination technique

7.1. Preparation of the colon

The colon must be scrupulously clean in order to perform reliable colonoscopy and polypectomy safely. Up to 23% of

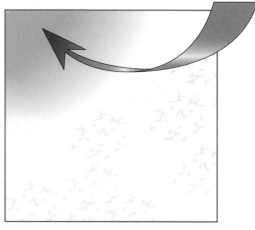

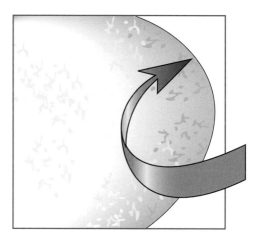

Figure 6 (A,B) The colonoscope should be directed at the areas in shadow and the concave area of the arcs formed by the folds.

Loop management

What is a loop?

A loop forms if the tip of the colonoscope does not advance at the same rate as the shaft during insertion. One-to-one movement is lost and paradoxical movement can be seen where the tip appears to fall backwards as the scope is inserted.

What types of loops are there?

- Alpha loop (Fig. 9) (see full discussion below).
- Omega loop (Fig. 10).

How do I know if I have a loop?

Suspect a loop if there is loss of one-to-one movement as you advance the colonoscope.

How do I reduce a loop?

The endoscope is torqued clockwise or in rare cases anticlockwise and then withdrawn.

How do I know if I have successfully reduced the loop?

Loops are reduced correctly when the tip of the endoscope advances during scope withdrawal. If the tip falls backwards, the loop reducing maneuver is incorrect and should be repeated with torque in the opposite direction.

Do I have to reduce every loop?

An alpha loop does not always have to be reduced. If the patient is comfortable and the endoscopist is making good progress, you can push through an alpha loop and then reduce it after you have passed the splenic flexure.

How do I stop it recurring?

Reduce the loop as described above. Once you have one-to-one movement, advance the scope with gentle clockwise torque and use abdominal pressure to keep the scope straight and to prevent the loop recurring. If it does recur, reduce the loop and apply abdominal pressure on another area.

Table 1 Ottawa bowel preparation quality score

	Score
Score right (R), mid (M) and left (L) colon separately (quality of preparation)	
No liquid	0
Minimal liquid, no suction required	1
Suction required to see mucosa	2
Wash and suction	3
Solid stool, not washable	4
Score the entire colon (overall quantity of fluid)	
Minimal	0
Moderate	1
Large	2
Total score: R + M + L + Fluid = __ / 14	

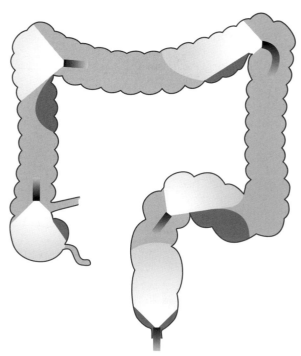

Figure 7 Blind areas difficult to observe: behind the ileocecal valve, hepatic flexure, splenic flexure, sigmoid colon and rectosigmoid junction, lower part of the rectum.

colonoscopies are reported to have inadequate preparation. This is associated with increased risk of missing polyps or small cancers, prolonged procedures and may increase the risk of complications. Preparation is carried out at home except for elderly, frail patients who may require hospitalization.

Various preparations are available including:

- Macrogols: polyethylene glycol (PEG e.g. Klean-Prep, Moviprep). These are isosmotic and do not cause net shift of large amounts of fluid across the intestinal epithelium. They require large volumes of 2–4 L for efficacy and can be unpalatable. Dividing the dose may facilitate dosing, so that half is taken the night before and half on the morning of the procedure. Electrolyte shifts are rare.
- Sodium phosphate (sodium dihydrogen phosphate, e.g. Fleet Phospho-Soda) is hyperosmotic and works by causing net secretion of large volumes of water into the intestinal tract. It is better tolerated than PEG solutions with equal or better cleansing. Hypovolemia, electrolyte disturbances and renal failure are more common with NaP in patients with risk factors (see Warning, below).
- Sodium picosulphate and magnesium citrate (e.g. Picolax) in combination: picosulphate is metabolized in the gut and stimulates peristalsis. The ingested volume is low and bowel cleansing is usually adequate. Dehydration, electrolyte shifts, and renal failure are rare.
- Magnesium carbonate and citric acid (e.g. Citramag) are low volume osmotic stimulants, mainly used for bowel preparation prior to barium enema or CT colonography.

In general, there is little to choose among them in terms of efficacy and all require clear, careful explanation to patients beforehand and full compliance if good results are to be achieved. Serious reports of major complications, particularly with sodium phosphate preparations, have recently led to many countries issuing safety notices regarding the use of bowel preparation in general and NaP in particular (see Warning and Table 2).

Most centers therefore now use polyethylene glycol solution (PEG) or sodium picosulphate rather than NaP. Splitting the dosing of polyethylene glycol, with half of the dose on the day before the colonoscopy and the second half on the morning of the procedure, is associated with improved bowel preparation quality.

Table 2 Comparison of sodium phosphate (NaP) and polyethylene glycol (PEG) bowel preparation solutions

	NaP	PEG
Volume	Low	High
Palatability	+	±
Cost	Low	Low
Side-effects	Cramps; caution in patients with cardiac or renal failure; hypovolemia and electrolyte shifts	Bloating and vomiting secondary to large volume
Bowel cleansing	+++	++

Warning!

Contraindications to bowel preparation

Absolute
- Intestinal obstruction, ileus or perforation.
- Acute severe IBD or toxic megacolon.
- Ileostomy.
- Reduced conscious level or other risk of pulmonary aspiration.
- Hypersensitivity to bowel preparation agents.

Relative (NaP)
- Chronic kidney disease (stage 3, 4, or 5, see below).
- Congestive cardiac failure.
- Liver cirrhosis with ascites.
- Concomitant treatment with ACE inhibitors, angiotensin II receptor blockers, high-dose diuretics, NSAIDs (see below).

PEG-electrolyte solutions are generally used unless the colon is obstructed in which case repeated enemas (3 L of physiological saline or tepid water) are preferred. It is well tolerated clinically (risk of nausea, vomiting, bloating, and anal irritation) and does not cause serum electrolyte disturbances). A prokinetic (metoclopramide, domperidone) may be useful if there is nausea or vomiting. PEG solutions may be used in children and in patients with inflammatory bowel disease.

Warning!

Side-effects of bowel preparation include hypovolemia, which may in turn lead to syncope, myocardial ischemia and acute renal injury. Hypokalemia, phosphate nephropathy, hyponatremia (from ingestion of excess water during preparation) and hypernatremia can also occur.

Preparation may be repeated over several days in very constipated patients and those with chronic intestinal pseudo-obstruction or incomplete obstruction. If the patient is unable to ingest a large quantity of fluid, it may be administered via nasogastric tube.

Mannitol (risk of dehydration or explosion during polypectomy), physiological saline (risk of sodium and water retention in patients with heart, liver or renal failure), and purgative-enema combinations are no longer used.

7.2. Bowel preparation in specific situations

7.2.1. Chronic kidney disease (CKD)

Renal function should be measured in all patients and only PEG solutions or sodium picosulphate used if there is CKD

Box 4 PEG-electrolyte solution contents
- Polyethylene glycol: 4000–64 g/L.
- Anhydrous sodium sulphate: 5.7 g/L.
- Sodium bicarbonate: 1.68 g/L.
- Sodium chloride: 1.46 g/L.
- Potassium chloride: 0.75 g/L.
- Flavorings.

stage 3 or greater (eGFR is <60 mL/min). PEG should be used for patients with CKD stage 4 or 5. Hypovolemia in patients undergoing hemodialysis may result in thrombosis of the vascular access and must be avoided. Admission to hospital for supervision, continuation of dialysis and for intravenous fluids is advised. Careful communication with the patient's nephrologists is essential to optimize bowel preparation and avoid complications.

7.2.2. Congestive cardiac failure

PEG solutions are preferred in this patient group and NaP must be avoided in patients with NYHA Class III or IV heart failure.

7.2.3. Therapy with ACE inhibitors, renin-angiotensin blockers or diuretics

These should be omitted on the day of bowel cleansing and not restarted for 72 hour post-procedure. If in doubt, the patient's cardiologist should be consulted for advice.

 Clinical Tips

Consider the following questions when prescribing bowel preparation:

- Are there absolute contraindications (see Warnings box, above)?
- Have serum electrolytes and eGFR been checked recently?
- Is the patient taking ACE inhibitors, renin-angiotensin blockers, diuretics, NSAIDs?
- Does the patient have other co-morbidities, e.g. renal, cardiac or liver failure?
- Will the patient be able to ingest a large volume of fluid?
- Will the patient be able to understand and undertake bowel preparation safely at home?
- Have written instructions and advice been given to the patient?

7.3. Taking PEG solution bowel preparation

7.3.1. Ingestion in one amount (best suited to an afternoon procedure)

3 L is taken over 2 hour, 6 hour before the examination. The preparation should have been ingested at least 4 hour before the start of the colonoscopy. Fluid passed should be clear at the end of preparation.

7.3.2. Ingestion in two amounts (best suited to an examination performed in the morning)

2 L is taken the previous evening and at least 1 L on the morning of the examination, 4 hour before the start of the colonoscopy. This results in less nausea with superior efficacy. The liter of solution consumed in the morning is essential because, if preparation is completed too early the previous day, the right colon will be coated with secretions, especially bile.

 Clinical Tips

Achieving good bowel preparation

- Clear instructions and careful explanation are necessary to ensure compliance.
- Fiber-free diet for at least 3 days beforehand. Note: omit fiber supplements, e.g. ispaghula for at least 1 week.
- Stop iron/charcoal preparations for at least 1 week beforehand.
- Minimize use of drugs that inhibit colonic motility, e.g. opioids, calcium-antagonists, amitriptyline, ondansetron, etc. (consider additional preparation if these cannot be stopped).
- 'split-dosing', taking part of the preparation on the morning of the procedure, may improve right colon cleansing.

7.4. Colonoscopy technique

The patient normally lies in the left lateral decubitus position. The first stage of the procedure is a careful rectal examination, using transparent water-soluble gel or local anesthetic ointment such as lidocaine. This lubricates the anus, allows an assessment of the bowel preparation and detection of rectal masses or strictures. The lubricated tip of the endoscope is introduced through the anus by pressing it against the orifice with the index finger.

Examination of the rectum presents few problems. The presence of residue is normal. It is important to examine the low rectum in retroflexion (Fig. 8). This is performed by inserting the colonoscope to approximately 20 cm and then tipping up with the big wheel. The small wheel occasionally needs to be moved slightly to the right or left to fully visualize the low rectum. It is essential to be gentle and attempts should cease if there is resistance or pain.

The first problem is to pass through the sigmoid loop. Passage of the colonoscope into the sigmoid may result in two spatial configurations.

7.4.1. Alpha loop

Alpha loop (Fig. 9). The colonoscope passes along the concave part of the sacrum in the pelvis (rectum). In

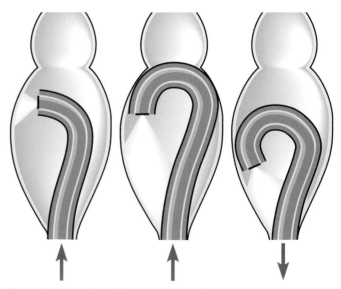

Figure 8 Examination of the rectum in retroflexion.

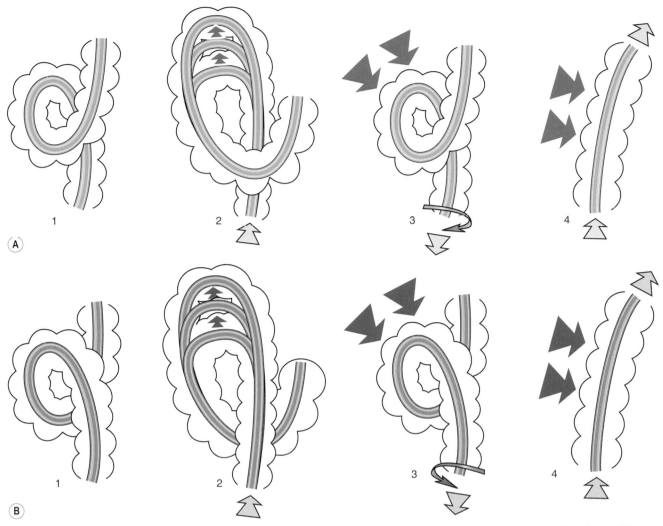

Figure 9 (A) Sigmoid alpha loop (1–2), clockwise rotation (3), palpation (4). (B) Sigmoid alpha loop (1–2), anticlockwise rotation (3), palpation (4).

the abdomen (sigmoid colon), it passes upwards and forwards then turns downwards and backwards to enter the descending colon, resulting in the formation of a spiral anteroposterior loop. In this case, there are usually no problems passing through the sigmoid-descending colon junction.

Once the colonoscope has passed this area and/or the splenic flexure, the sigmoid alpha loop must be reduced. The endoscope should be torqued clockwise or, in rare cases, anticlockwise, and then withdrawn. Reinsertion with torque still applied and/or palpation of the umbilical region in the direction of the left iliac spine as the colonoscope advances usually further prevents the loop reappearing.

7.4.2. Omega loop

Omega loop (Fig. 10). Sometimes the colonoscope creates an acute flexure in the sigmoid colon during insertion. The sigmoid-descending junction, between 40 and 70 cm from the anal margin, appears as an arc of mucosa against a duller background. It may be closed and give the impression of a pouch.

The colonoscope may be withdrawn, excess air aspirated and the colonoscope advanced by palpating the left iliac

fossa to prevent the formation of an omega loop and an acute flexure. The patient may also be moved (supine or right lateral position). Sometimes instillation of 200–300 mL of water at body temperature relaxes the sigmoid colon and opens up the acute angle.

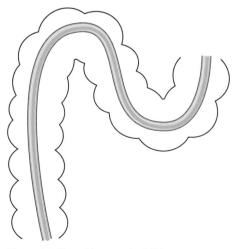

Figure 10 Sigmoid omega (or 'N') loop.

Box 5   All patients should undertake the following

Fiber-free diet

For 3 days before the examination, the patient should only eat the following foods:

- White meat: veal, pork.
- Poultry: chicken, turkey (white meat) cooked without fat.
- Pork products: lean ham, knuckle, brawn.
- Eggs: soft-boiled, hard-boiled, fried (in a non-stick pan).
- Fish: cod, haddock, plaice, skate, sole, trout, hake (poached or baked).
- Cereal products: crackers, toast, pasta, rice, tapioca, semolina, cornflour.
- Vegetables: vegetable stock, clear soup (no vegetables allowed).
- Hard cheeses (Cheddar, Gruyère, Edam, Emmental).
- Fruit: peeled, grated or stewed apple.
- Fat: 15–20 g butter or margarine, a soup-spoon of soya or sunflower oil.
- Sweet products: jellies (not red-coloured and no jam or marmalade).
- Biscuits, meringue, milk puddings.
- Condiments: salt, vanilla.
- Drinks: still water, weak tea and coffee, fruit juice without pulp.

Not allowed:

Fat, bread, vegetables, raw or cooked fruit, milk, fizzy drinks.

Stop taking any medications containing iron or charcoal 1 week before colonoscopy. Omit fiber supplements, e.g. ispaghula for at least 1 week

Example of colonic preparation with PEG for colonoscopy in the *morning*

3 days before the examination: fiber-free diet as documented above.

On the eve of the examination, take the following in the morning on an empty stomach and again in the evening before dinner:

- ◦ 2 × 10 g of magnesium sulphate (10 g in the morning, 10 g in the evening).
- ◦ 2 × 4 tablets of Cascara (4 tablets in the morning and 4 tablets in the evening).
- Take 2 L of PEG 4000 solution (dissolve 1 sachet per liter of water) after dinner.
- On the day of the examination, on an empty stomach:
  - ◦ 4 hourbefore the examination, drink 1 L of PEG 4000 solution over 1 hour.

Example of colonic preparation with PEG for colonoscopy in the *afternoon*

3 days before the examination: fiber-free diet as documented above.

On the eve of the examination, take the following once in the morning on an empty stomach and once in the evening before dinner:

- ◦ 2 × 10 g of magnesium sulphate (10 g in the morning, 10 g in the evening).
- ◦ 2 × 4 tablets of Cascara (4 tablets in the morning and 4 tablets in the evening).
- On the day of the examination, on an empty stomach:
  - ◦ 6 hour before the examination, drink 3 L of PEG 4000 solution over 2 hour.

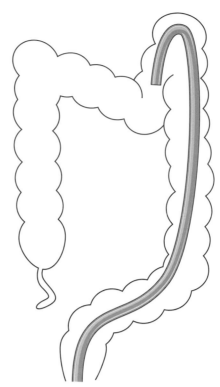

Figure 11 (1) Closed splenic flexure: patient supine. (2) Open splenic flexure: patient in right lateral position.

- Passing through the left colon does not normally present problems
- If there are problems passing around the splenic flexure (Fig. 11), it may help to position the patient in right lateral decubitus, which tends to open the flexure.

A reversed splenic flexure (Fig. 12) combined with a mobile descending colon is the commonest cause of unexplained problems advancing the colonoscope. If a loop of this type is suspected, reducing it by anticlockwise rotation should be considered. To prevent the loop reappearing, compress the splenic flexure and pass through it.

Passing through the transverse colon (Fig. 13) may be the cause of a new problem if there is a long mesocolon (formation of an omega or alpha loop as in the sigmoid, requiring the same maneuvers to reduce it). After passing the midline, it is then necessary to repeatedly straighten the transverse loop so as to concertina the colon onto the colonoscope. Aspiration, changing the patient's position and abdominal compression (left iliac fossa to keep the sigmoid in position, left hypochondrium to lower the splenic flexure, umbilical palpation to keep the transverse colon in position) will help with this.

If there are problems passing through the hepatic flexure, it may be helpful to position the patient in left lateral decubitus to open the flexure. Once past the hepatic flexure (the optimum maneuver (Fig. 14) is a combination of aspiration, angulation, withdrawal of the endoscope and abdominal compression), descent into the ascending colon is usually straightforward. The colonoscope should then be advanced as far as the cecum (Fig. 15) with the aid of aspiration and compression of the transverse colon and/or sigmoid colon, lifting the right lumbar fossa or changing the patient's position (right lateral decubitus).

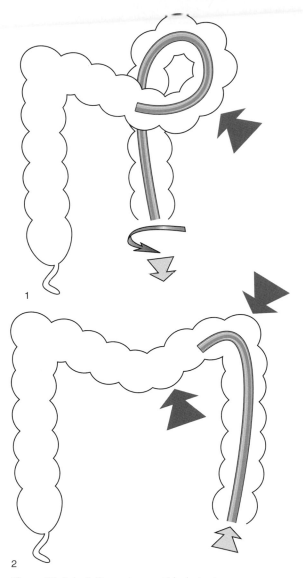

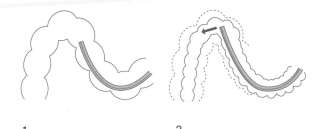

Figure 14 (1) The colonoscope stops before the hepatic flexure. (2) It passes through the hepatic flexure by means of aspiration and angulation.

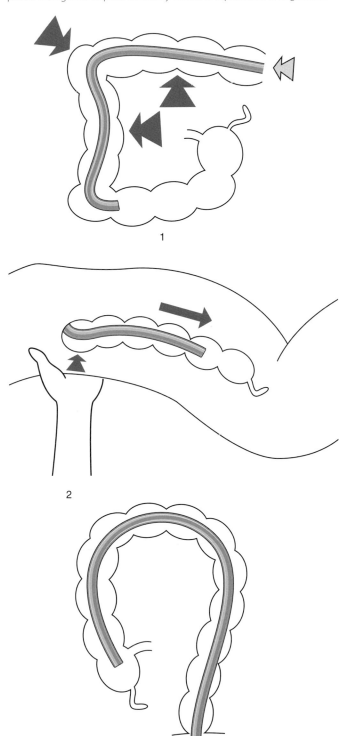

Figure 12 Splenic flexure loop: anticlockwise torque.

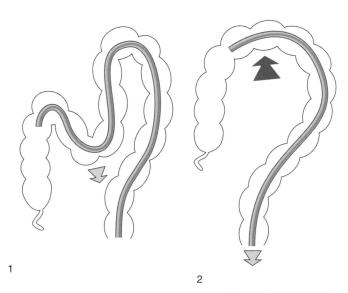

Figure 13 (1) Loop in the transverse colon. (2) Umbilical palpation upwards to keep the transverse colon in position.

Figure 15 (1) Advancing the colonoscope into the cecum with the aid of palpation of the sigmoid and transverse colon; positioning the patient in right lateral position will maintain the splenic flexure open. (2) Lift the right lumbar fossa to advance the colonoscope into the cecum. (3) Apparatus straightened in the cecum.

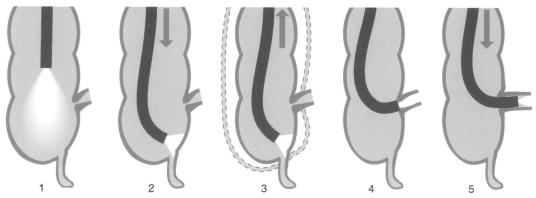

Figure 16 Passing through the ileocecal valve.

7.5. Four maneuvers may be used to intubate the ileocecal valve

- The commonest maneuver (as shown in Fig. 16) is to:
  - Place the colonoscope under the ileocecal valve (1, 2); usually with the patient supine the valve will be seen in the 7–9 o'clock position
  - Slightly deflating the cecum (3)
  - Withdrawing as far as the lower lip of the valve (4)
  - Angulating the tip towards the expected location of the orifice (usually upwards), torquing counterclockwise and insufflating air to open the orifice when it begins to appear (5)
  - The small intestine is easily recognized from its granular or pseudopolypoid appearance (lymphoid hyperplasia). With careful observation, villi can be seen, instillation of water often makes them more readily apparent
- Direct passage when the valve is viewed from the front
- Retroflexed maneuver (Fig. 17) in the cecum and withdrawal of the endoscope until it meets the entrance to the ileocecal valve
- Introduction of biopsy forceps, which serve as a guide over which the colonoscope is advanced.

Advancing the colonoscope through the small intestine is facilitated by angulation and aspiration. The intestine slides by itself onto the endoscope without needing to be pushed.

7.6. There may be problems advancing the colonoscope

- After gynecological surgery, the sigmoid colon may be affected by adhesions
- In patients with diverticulosis complicated by diverticulitis and pericolic inflammation (Fig. 18)
- In patients with anatomical anomalies (long mesocolon), or in obese patients, abdominal compression may be impossible or ineffective. Abdominal compression may also be ineffective when complex loops form in small, thin patients. The endoscope should be withdrawn as far as the rectum and a new attempt made.

In such problematic cases, a magnetic imager system or using a pediatric colonoscope may be useful.

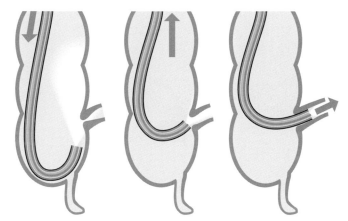

Figure 17 Passing through the ileocecal valve: retroflex maneuver.

7.7. Locating the tip of the colonoscope

Knowledge of the endoscopic anatomy of the colon will help to locate the endoscope in the colon. The length of colonoscope introduced after reducing all the loops is useful for giving the endoscopist an idea of the location of the colonoscope but cannot be used to confirm cecal intubation. With a straight scope, the descending colon/sigmoid junction is 40 cm from the anal margin, the splenic flexure is at 50 cm, the hepatic flexure is 60–65 cm from the anal margin, and the cecum is approximately 70–80 cm.

Previously finger indentations in the region of the right iliac fossa and viewing the colonoscope through the abdom-

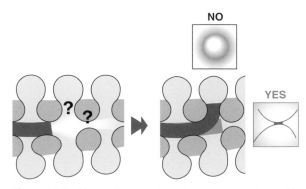

Figure 18 Problems advancing the colonoscope in patients with diverticulosis of the colon.

inal wall (transillumination) were used to identify the cecum. These two techniques are no longer used, as they are unreliable. Only the ileocecal valve, appendix or visualization of the terminal ileum should be used to confirm that the cecum has been reached.

> **Clinical Tip**
>
> **Useful cecal landmarks**
> - Ileal intubation: visualization of typical small intestinal mucosal villi.
> - Ileocecal valve: a smooth, subtle bulge usually in the 6–9 o'clock position. If difficult to find, locate the appendix orifice and imagine its crescentic shape as a 'bow-and-arrow'. The arrow will usually point at the ileocecal valve.
> - Appendix orifice.
> - Convergence of the colonic taenia coli ('triradiate fold').

7.8. Abdominal palpation

The aim of abdominal palpation is to prevent the formation of a loop, or its recurrence (after being reduced). It is therefore useful for keeping mobile areas of the colon in position. The sigmoid is kept in position by palpating the left iliac fossa, while for the transverse colon, the periumbilical region is palpated.

To advance the colonoscope through the hepatic flexure, it is sometimes useful to place the hand flat over the liver, moving it slightly up under the ribs, which opens the flexure. To advance the colonoscope through the transverse colon, it is sometimes useful to lower the splenic flexure. To reach the cecum, the right lumbar fossa can be lifted. In problematic cases, the area of the colon which should be palpated can be determined as follows: press the hand on the various parts of the abdomen while watching the position of the endoscope light. When the endoscope advances, the optimum place for palpation has been located. Many units using Olympus instruments possess a magnetic imager system ('Scopeguide') and this is often valuable in negotiating difficult loops. An adjustable shaft stiffener is present on some

colonoscopes (Olympus) and is useful when looping in a 'floppy' colon is a problem. If the sigmoid loop reappears despite abdominal compression and changes of position, this should be used by turning it to the 3 position. The stiffener is particularly useful in the sigmoid and transverse colon. External stiffening overtubes are very rarely used.

7.9. The approach to the patient with a very difficult colon

Patients with a very difficult colon are patients in whom other experienced colonoscopists have failed to reach the cecum. A flowchart for the approach to use in this group of patients is shown in Figure 19. We recommend using a magnetic imager (Scopeguide) in this group of patients if it is available.

Narrowed or angulated sigmoid colon:
- Commence with a pediatric colonoscope
- If this is unsuccessful an upper endoscope can be used
- If this fails, insert a guidewire of at least 360 cm through the upper endoscope and into the colon. Exchange the upper endoscope over the wire. Backload a pediatric colonoscope onto the guidewire. A polypectomy snare is often useful to grasp the wire and pull it through the instrument channel.

Redundant colon:
- Commence with a colonoscope with variable stiffness. This resists looping more than a pediatric colonoscope. The colonoscopy is commenced with the variable stiffener off. If looping occurs, the stiffener is set to 3 and the insertion tried again in combination with abdominal pressure. Once the segment is passed, the stiffener is returned to normal position.
- Avoid over insufflations and suction regularly.
- Shorten the endoscope frequently and remove all loops. Failure to withdraw sufficiently is the commonest mistake made in a redundant colon.
- Position change is important. Moving the patient to the right lateral decubitus position often propels the endoscope from the ascending colon and into cecal pole.

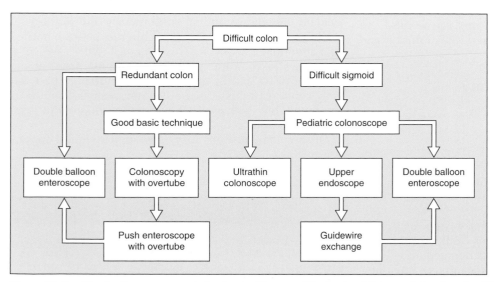

Figure 19 Algorithm for the management of patients with a very difficult colon. (With permission from Rex DK. Gastrointest Endosc 2008;67:938-944.)

- If these maneuvers fail, a stiffening overtube may be used. Overtubes are available from Olympus, USGI Medical ShapeLock, Spirus Endo-Ease. It is backloaded onto the endoscope before starting the colonoscopy and introduced into the colon after straightening the sigmoid loop. Overtubes are potentially dangerous and should not be used in angulated or narrowed sigmoid colons. They should be well lubricated before being introduced and should not be forced against resistance.
- Using a double-balloon enteroscope (DBE) will often facilitate total colonoscopy in a redundant colon. Inflating the balloon, once the scope tip has negotiated the sigmoid allows adequate traction to advance without looping.

7.10. Third eye retroscope

The third eye retroscope is an auxiliary imaging device that is designed to allow visualization of 'hidden areas' during colonoscopy by providing an additional, retrograde view that complements the antegrade view of the colonoscope. It allows visualization of the proximal aspect of haustral folds and rectal valves, as well as the areas behind flexures and the ileocecal valve.

7.10.1. Third eye technique

To use the third eye, it is important that the colonoscopic preparation is as good as possible. The colonoscopy is undertaken with a water pump. All debris is removed by washing and suctioning on insertion of the endoscope, as suctioning is diminished once the third eye is in place. Once the cecum is reached, the endoscope is withdrawn until it is just distal to the ileocecal valve. The third eye is advanced through the instrument channel. As it emerges from the distal tip of the colonoscope, the third eye retroscope automatically bends 180° to form a 'J' shape. Once the two bars (image) appear, the third eye is gently rotated until it is at the 11 o'clock position. The water jet is then tested. The third eye should be positioned so that the water jet cleans it. The endoscope is then withdrawn keeping the third eye and the endoscope in the middle of the lumen (image). There is a learning curve for the third eye with decreasing time and increased polyp detection after 10–20 cases. The results of randomized prospective studies of routine colonoscopy versus third eye colonoscopy are awaited to see the exact role of third eye in screening colonoscopy.

8. Colonoscopy in inflammatory bowel disease

8.1. Endoscopic appearance

A variety of lesions occur and often co-exist:

- Ulceration is the commonest lesion, and may be superficial, erosive (a sign of severity) or aphthoid (specific to Crohn's disease)
- Non-ulcerated mucosal lesions: mucosa appears friable, erythematous, edematous or bleeds easily on contact
- Stricturing due to ulceration or scarring: requires multiple biopsies, after balloon dilatation, to rule out cancer

- Fistulae: specific to Crohn's disease, rarely visible endoscopically
- Scarring: ulcer related scarring appears whitish and vascularized
- Pseudopolyps: may simulate a polyp or cancer and may be ulcerated or hemorrhagic (biopsies are routinely required).

8.2. Endoscopic assessment of severity

- Extensive erosive ulceration. Craters with a white base, sometimes surrounded by an inflammatory ridge, bleeding on contact with forceps. Pitted ulcers have an orifice a few millimeters in diameter, they are deep and often communicate with one another since the mucosa connecting them has detached completely. The ulceration may form longitudinal bands along the colon, sometimes connected by transverse ulcers giving it a *cobblestone* appearance. This may expose the muscular layer
- Mucosal detachments between ulcers can be readily observed by raising the mucosa at the edge of an ulcer with closed biopsy forceps
- Almost total abrasion of the mucosa leaving only a few islands of erythematous mucosa.

8.3. Differential diagnosis

Lesions specific to Crohn's disease are aphthoid ulceration, 'skip' lesions and terminal ileal lesions.

> **Note**
>
> There is sometimes rectal sparing in ulcerative colitis in patients who have been treated with rectal steroids or 5-ASA.

Lesions suggestive of ulcerative colitis but which can be seen in Crohn's disease: mucosal lesions starting from the dentate line and extending continuously and homogeneously upwards with a distinct upper border between normal and abnormal mucosa.

Biopsies taken from normal and affected areas, at the edges of ulcers and in the upper gastrointestinal tract can only confirm Crohn's disease if non-caseating granulomas are found, but their presence is inconsistent, even in cases of definite Crohn's.

Other colonic diseases may yield similar clinical appearances (Box 6).

> **Note**
>
> The colonic mucosa appears normal in collagenous or microscopic colitis. In patients who present with diarrhea or anemia but have an endoscopically normal colon, biopsies should be taken from the right and left colon to assess for microscopic colitis.

- Inflammatory bowel disease: UC, Crohn's disease.
- Infections:
  - Bacterial: *Salmonella, Shigella, Campylobacter, Yersinia, Mycobacteria* tuberculosis.
  - Viral: cytomegalovirus, chlamydia.
  - Parasitic: amoebiasis, schistosomiasis.
- Acute diverticulitis.
- Drugs, e.g. NSAIDs.
- Ischemic colitis.
- Radiation colitis.
- Solitary rectal ulcer syndrome.

- Postoperative or post-radiation adhesions.
- Severe diverticulosis.
- Severe inflammation or stricturing of the colon.
- Use of excessive force to pass an anatomical problem.
- Inexperienced endoscopist.
- Polypectomy.

9. Complications of colonoscopy

Colonoscopy is generally very safe but the potential for harm always exists. Careful patient selection and consent are vital and the endoscopist and endoscopy staff must be ever vigilant to the possibility of complications.

Mortality is rare, although the exact incidence is difficult to define. Figures of 0–0.02% and even 0.07% are quoted. Most deaths occur in frail, elderly patients with major co-morbidity and result from myocardial infarction, strokes or pneumonia. Approximately 5% of colonoscopic perforations are fatal. Complications are classified below (see also Table 3).

9.1. Perforation

The incidence of perforation is approximately 1 in 1000–2000 procedures but in some studies, is higher in patients undergoing biopsy or polypectomy. Other studies have found that perforation risk is related to polyp size (especially >2 cm) and location (right colon) rather than the overall number of polypectomies performed. Perforation can be pneumatic, mechanical or intervention-related. Pneumatic perforation is more likely in the cecum or when inflammation causes bowel wall-thinning, e.g. in severe colitis. Mechanical perforation results from forceful insertion of the colonoscope lacerating the wall. It is more likely when the bowel wall is weakened by inflammation, ischemia or diverticulosis. Interventional-related perforation results from thermal injury during polypectomy. Other factors contributing to perforation are listed in Box 7.

Several scenarios are possible:

- Instrument insertion in the wrong direction
- A tear at the insertion point of an adhesion
- Pneumatic perforation due to a combination of excessive air insufflation in a pathological or fragile colon, usually the right colon. A plain abdominal X-ray may show a combination of air in the colon wall and pneumoperitoneum). The appearance of the mucosa is characteristic, with tears in the muscle layer in parallel bands, like striae, with bloody serous fluid (Fig. 20)
- Diverticular perforation: this may result from excess insufflation in a fragile area or from reopening of a spontaneously sealed perforation.

Perforation may be immediately obvious during the procedure but in 50% of cases it is only apparent afterwards and can be delayed for up to 30 days or more. Its occurrence should be suspected if there is increasing pain, distension, inability to pass flatus or the development of tenderness, signs of peritonitis, fever, tachycardia and distress. Perforation may be difficult to recognize if it is small, localized and plain X-rays do not show free air.

Table 3 Complications of colonoscopy

Timing	Comments
Pre-colonoscopy	
Bowel preparation	Incontinence
	Fluid and electrolyte shifts, dehydration
	Renal failure (NaP)
	More common in elderly with cardiac or renal disease
During colonoscopy	
Sedation-related	See Chapter 2.3
Instrumentation-related	Cardiovascular-arrhythmias, hypertension due to autonomic responses to stretching mesentery/viscus
	Pain – excess air insufflation or loop formation
	Perforation: see text
	Incarceration in hernia sac
	Splenic hematoma/rupture
	Cecal/sigmoid volvulus
	Pneumatosis coli
Intervention-related	Perforation: see text
	Post-polypectomy syndrome
	Bleeding (acute or delayed)

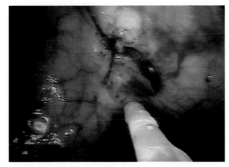

Figure 20 Post-colonoscopy fissure syndrome.

 Clinical Tips

Minimize the risk of colonic perforation

Good patient selection:

- Caution in the elderly, frail; severe diverticulosis, severe active UC, extensive prior surgery/adhesions or radiotherapy.

Careful technique:

- Minimize air insufflation
- Early recognition and reduction of loops
- Use of palpation, changing patient position
- Understanding safe use of electrocautery (avoid hot biopsy without good technique)
- Use of submucosal injection for resection of sessile polyps (± endoscopic clipping).

Treatment is surgical, except for pneumatic perforation, for which conservative medical treatment may be attempted, but only if the colon is perfectly clean. Application of one or more endoscopic clips following resection of sessile polyps or EMR can be effective in closing small perforations but surgery remains the gold standard. Conservative treatment consists of analgesia, nasogastric aspiration, antibiotic therapy, and parenteral nutrition. In the absence of a rapid clinical improvement and an improvement in laboratory tests, surgery will be required. Similarly, should fever, signs of peritonitis or a worsening leucocytosis develop, surgery is mandatory.

! Warning!

Use of hot biopsy techniques

These effectively destroy and remove polyps <5 mm. Use of hot biopsy has been associated with an increased risk of perforation, especially in the cecum and right colon. 'Cold' snaring of small lesions is usually preferable but if hot biopsy is used, good technique and care are vital: lesions should be gently 'tented up' into the lumen, low-power settings (e.g. 20 W) should be used and current applied only until whitening of the base begins to appear ('Mount Fuji effect'). The superficial tissue can then be removed.

The prognosis for these types of perforation depends on the patient's age, the underlying state of the colon and how early treatment is started. This emphasizes how important it is that any patients who have undergone colonoscopy should have a clinical assessment before discharge. Post-procedural pain should never be attributed simply to 'gas' and needs to be evaluated. If there is any doubt, plain abdominal and erect chest X-rays should be performed immediately. Patients should be ambulant, pain-free and have normal pulse, blood pressure and temperature before being allowed home.

 Clinical Tip

Endoscopic closure of colonoscopic perforations

This can be attempted when a small defect or perforation is noted at the time of polypectomy or EMR/ESD. It should not be attempted where a large perforation has occurred, e.g. the instrument has entered the peritoneum, as it is unlikely to be successful. Rotatable clips are useful and closure should begin at one lateral margin of the defect, progressing in a zip-like manner. Patients must be carefully monitored and surgery considered promptly if there is clinical deterioration.

9.1.1. Post-polypectomy syndrome

Patients who have undergone polypectomy may develop 'post-polypectomy syndrome' in which a transmural thermal burn leads to pain, tenderness and fever but no free air is seen on radiology: most cases settle conservatively. The approach to a patient complaining of pain after colonoscopy is shown in Figure 21 and steps to minimize the chances of perforation are outlined in the Clinical Tips box above.

9.2. Bacteremia

Bacteremia is common (up to 27% of cases) but clinical infection is rare and antibiotic prophylaxis is only required in patients at high risk of endocarditis.

9.3. Severe abdominal distension

Rule out perforation (as above).

 Clinical Tips

Removal of polyps <10 mm

- Electrocautery causes almost all polypectomy related perforations and most delayed bleeding.
- 1–3 mm polyps should be removed with cold forceps.
- 3–7 mm polyps can often be removed 'cold' with a small snare.

9.4. Hemorrhage

This is the most common complication following polypectomy, with a bleeding rate of <1%. Polyp size and anticoagulation are both risk factors. Patients on aspirin do not need to stop the drug before colonoscopy but patients on clopidogrel should stop taking it 7 days pre-procedure or be deferred if ongoing therapy is essential (see Chapter 2.1). Diagnostic colonoscopy can be performed in warfarinized patients if the INR is in the therapeutic range but biopsies, polypectomy and other interventions require reversal of anticoagulation. Hemorrhage is rare following diagnostic colonoscopy, including cold 'pinch' biopsy. It more frequently complicates hot biopsy or snare polypectomy. The use of low-power coagulation current is associated with an increased risk of delayed bleeding, while blended and cutting current are associated with increased risk of immediate bleeding.

Bleeding after polypectomy (Fig. 22) is more common with polyps >2 cm, thick-stalked polyps and after EMR or endoscopic submucosal dissection (ESD). Mechanical transaction of the stalk ('cheese-wiring') before effective thermal effect occurs is a significant contributory factor. Bleeding may be immediately apparent but can be 'secondary', occurring up to 14 days later. Most bleeding is minor and stops spontaneously but severe bleeding requires intervention (Box 8).

9.5. Missed adenomas

The miss rate for adenomas is as high as 27%, with a miss rate for adenomas ≥1 cm of between 12% and 17%. Miss rates vary widely among even senior endoscopists, ranging from 17 to 48%. The miss rate can be decreased by ensuring a high quality colonic preparation and a withdrawal time of at least 6 minute from cecum to rectosigmoid junction. Particular care must be taken in the right colon as flat or serrated adenomas may be subtle, pale and difficult to detect.

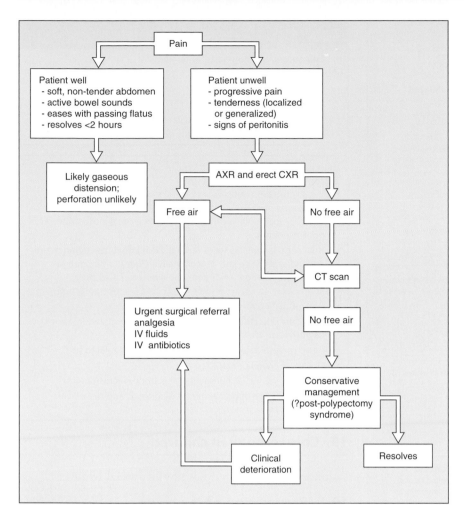

Figure 21 Assessment of patients with pain post-colonoscopy.

Box 8   Bleeding following polypectomy

Prevention

- Appropriate use of electrocoagulation.
- Submucosal epinephrine injection (decreases the risk of immediate, but not delayed bleeding).
- Detachable loops.
- Place clip if high-risk patient (i.e. on anticoagulation following a large polypectomy).

Immediate hemorrhage

- Quickly grasp or clip stalk before view is obscured by blood; immersing the area with water and viewing underwater often allows identification of the exact bleeding point.
- Injection of 1 : 10 000 epinephrine.
- Local electrocoagulation or APC.
- For severe bleeding:
  ○ Grasp stalk tightly with snare for 5–10 minute and wait.
  ○ Use clips or detachable loops.
  ○ Instill large volumes of cold water with 1 : 100 000 epinephrine to the bleeding point.
- If bleeding continues, refer for surgery or interventional radiology.

Delayed hemorrhage

- Resuscitate.
- Repeat colonoscopy.
- Consider angiography or surgery if severe.

Take care to inspect the proximal side of folds. Some evidence suggests that more polyps can be detected if a programmed series of position changes is used during extubation and examination of the colon:

- Cecum to hepatic flexure: left lateral position
- Hepatic flexure to descending colon: supine position
- Sigmoid and rectum: right lateral position.

9.6. Incomplete removal of neoplasia

Approximately 21% of interval cancers are believed to result from previous incomplete removal of neoplastic tissue. It is essential to ensure that the polyp has been completely removed. Hot biopsy forceps should not be used for polyps >5 mm, as these leave residual polyp in 16–28% of cases. If there is a suspicion that adenomatous tissue remains, the edges of the polypectomy site should be treated with APC (low-power with short pulses), or biopsied. The site should be marked with a tattoo (see Clinical Tip below) to allow easy identification in subsequent colonoscopies. Patients who undergo large sessile polyp resection in piecemeal fashion should have short follow-up intervals, usually 3–6 months after initial resection, to ensure adequacy of resection.

9.7. Quality assurance in colonoscopy

The miss rate for colorectal cancer is <1%. Studies suggest that incomplete colonoscopy may be responsible for many

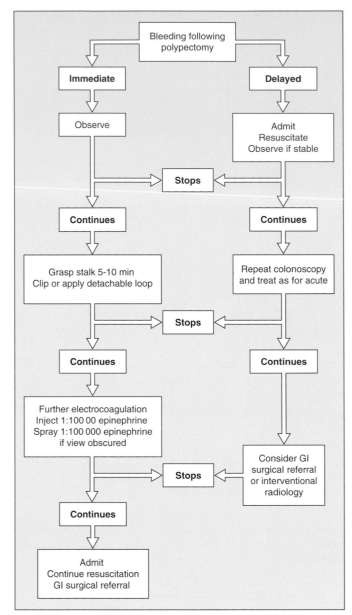

Figure 22 Management of bleeding following polypectomy.

Box 9 Risk factors for interval cancers

- Colonoscopy by non-gastroenterologists.
- Diverticular disease.
- Older patient age.
- In office colonoscopy.
- Right-sided or transverse colon cancer.
- Low-quality bowel preparation.

Units and endoscopists should regularly audit their colonoscopy practice and assess the following:

- Cecal intubation rate should be ≥90% of all colonoscopies and ≥95% screening colonoscopies (this excludes cases with poor bowel preparation, severe colitis or where cecal intubation was not the intention)
- How cecal landmarks were verified. Photo documentation of the appendiceal orifice and ileocecal valve. Transillumination or 'finger' indentation is not acceptable and can lead the endoscopist to falsely assume the cecum has been reached
- Ileal intubation rate (>40%)
- Adenoma detection rate (in an average mix population, should be >10% and ideally 25%)
- Polyp retrieval rate >90%
- Quality of bowel preparation
- Withdrawal time (≥6 minute from cecum to rectosigmoid)
- Appropriate use of guidelines for diagnostic and surveillance colonoscopy.

10. Colonoscopy in children

Colonoscopy in children has several special features.

10.1. Preparation of the colon

PEG solution should be attempted first, but children are sometimes unable to swallow large quantities of fluid. PEG should be administered by the parents or carers over two 2-hour periods with a total dose corresponding to twice the body surface area. If the child cannot manage the volume, a nasogastric tube can be used. The alternative is a combination of a phosphate or sodium citrate enema (dose adjusted for age) and a laxative (e.g. lactulose or senna). Administration of enemas can be distressing for children and sedation may be required.

10.2. Sedation or anesthesia

Intravenous sedation or general anesthesia is essential in children.

10.3. Equipment

A pediatric gastroscope can be used in infants under 2 years old, since suitable colonoscopes do not yet exist; a pediatric colonoscope can be used in children over 2; and a standard colonoscope in children aged 10 and over.

10.4. Technique

This is the same as in adults. It should be performed very carefully. The creation of an alpha loop by the endoscopist is common practice in patients under 12 to negotiate the sigmoid colon. Polypectomy is performed in the same way as for adults.

of these cases, while others result from missed or incompletely removed polyps. This may be especially so for sessile serrated adenomas in the right colon.

 Clinical Tips

Tattooing in the colon

- Use a commercially available sterile, inert carbon particle solution where possible rather than India ink.
- Shake solution before use to ensure evenly suspended in solution.
- Use a 22–25 G sclerotherapy needle.
- Inject 0.5–0.75 mL submucosally into each of four quadrants at site of lesion or just proximally. This ensures at least one site will be visible at surgery.
- Inject tangentially and try to avoid intraperitoneal injection: this will blacken the peritoneal cavity and may obscure the view at surgery.

10.5. Complications

Complications are the same as in adults. Preparation of the colon in infants can occasionally be followed by the appearance of blisters on the buttocks. This can be avoided by changing nappies frequently and use of a barrier ointment such as zinc oxide.

10.6. Indications

These are summarized in Box 10.

10.7. Contraindications

Severe acute fulminant colitis, because of the risk of perforation or toxic megacolon.

Box 10 Indications for colonoscopy in children
• Recurrent rectal bleeding. After ruling out anal lesions (fissures or anal cryptitis), by far the most frequent cause is juvenile polyps (between the ages of 2 and 8), followed by lymphoid nodular hyperplasia of the colon. Other causes are rare: thermometer-induced ulceration; solitary rectal ulcer; vascular malformation; colorectal cancer; or Meckel's diverticulum. • Suspected inflammatory bowel disease. • Gastrointestinal polyposis syndromes. • Colitis in immunosuppressed patients: 　◦ HIV-AIDS 　◦ Graft-versus-host disease 　◦ Cytomegalovirus.

11. Images

11.1. Colon cancer

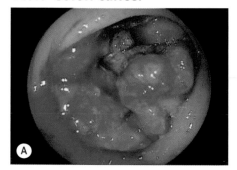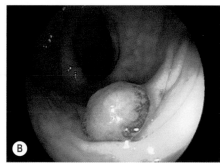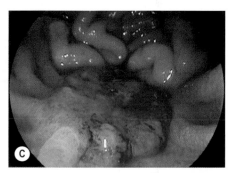

Figure 23 Colon cancer. (A) Fungating adenocarcinoma. (B) *In-situ* adenocarcinoma arising in a villous adenoma. (C) Superficial colon cancer.

11.2. Colon polyps

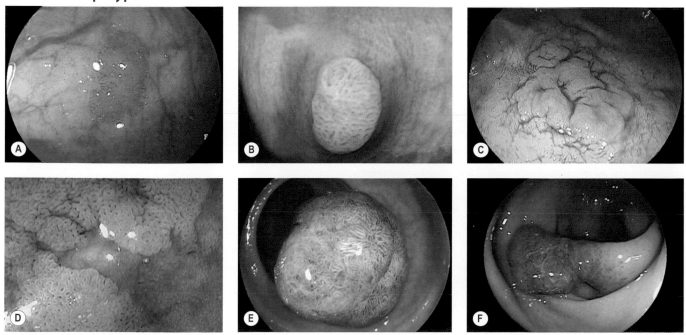

Figure 24 Colon polyps. (A) Flat adenoma. (B) Sessile flat adenoma. (C) Extensive flat adenoma after staining with 0.2% indigo carmine. (D) Borderline serrated adenoma with normal surrounding mucosa. (E) Sessile polyp. (F) Pedunculated polyp.

11.3. Miscellaneous colonic images

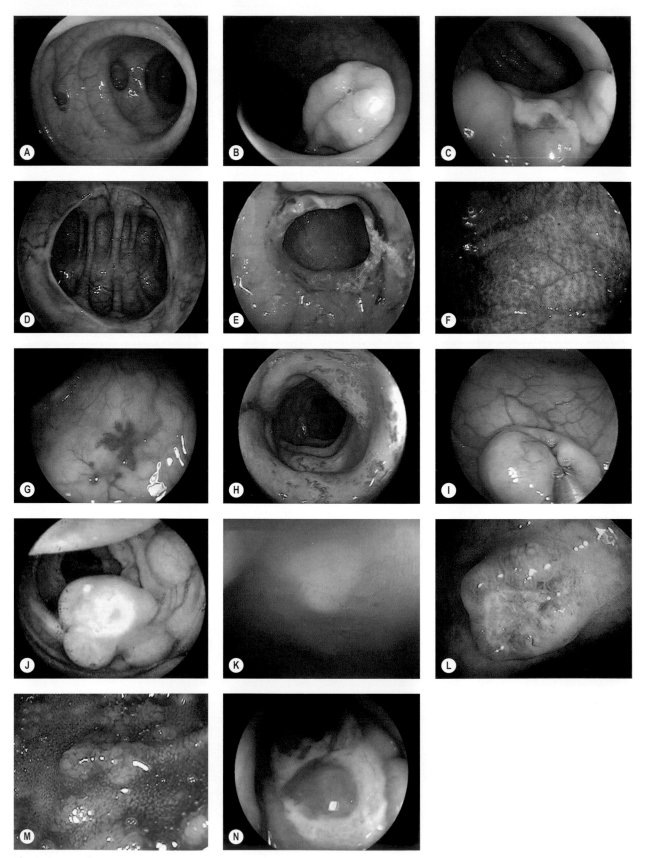

Figure 25 Miscellaneous colonic images. (A) Diverticula of the sigmoid colon. (B) Prolapsed diverticulum of the colon resembling a pseudopolyp. (C) Pus discharging from an infected sigmoid diverticulum. (D) 'J' or side-to-end colorectal anastomosis. (E) Benign stenosis of a colorectal anastomosis. (F) Melanosis coli due to laxative abuse. (G) Colonic angiodysplasia. (H) Rectal radiation 'proctitis'. (I) Colonic GIST. (J) Pneumatosis cystoides of the colon. (K) Carcinoid tumour of the rectum. (L) Ulcerated carcinoid tumour of the rectum. (M) Peutz–Jeghers syndrome. (N) Solitary rectal ulcer.

11.4. Colitis

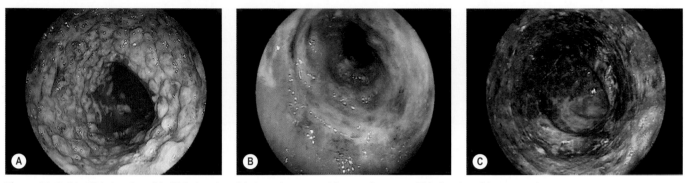

Figure 26 Colitis. (A) Ischemic colitis. (B) Ischemic colitis, boundary zone with normal mucosa. (C) Ischemic colitis at necrotic stage.

11.5. Crohn's disease

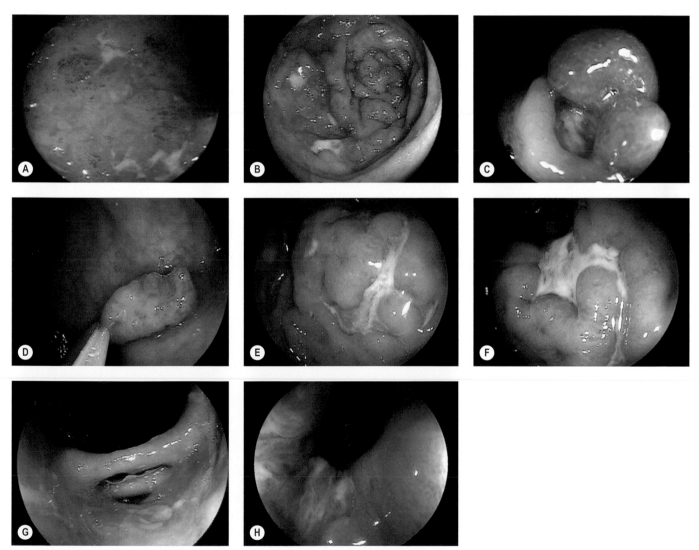

Figure 27 Crohn's disease. (A) Terminal ileal Crohn's disease, superficial ulceration. (B) Ileal Crohn's disease, ulceration. (C) Crohn's disease, erosive ulceration of the ileocecal valve. (D) Crohn's disease in remission, colonic pseudopolyp. (E) Rectal Crohn's disease. (F) Rectal Crohn's disease. (G) Crohn's disease, with mucosal bridges of scar tissue after an acute episode. (H) Anal canal ulcer in Crohn's disease.

11.6. Ulcerative colitis

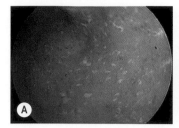 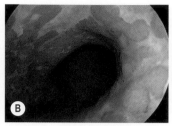 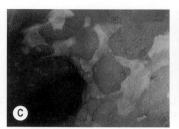 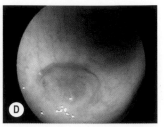

Figure 28 Ulcerative colitis. (A) Aphthoid erosions of the sigmoid colon. (B) Multiple geographic ulcers at the splenic flexure. (C) Multiple geographic ulcers seen with magnification. (D) Invasive colonic adenocarcinoma in ulcerative colitis (in remission).

Further Reading

Barclay RL, Vicari JJ, Doughty AS, et al: Colonoscopic withdrawal times and adenoma detection during screening colonoscopy, *N Engl J Med* 355(24): 2533–2541, 2006.

Barthet M, Gay G, Sautereau D, et al: Endoscopic surveillance of chronic inflammatory bowel disease, *Endoscopy* 37(6):597–599, 2005.

Belsey J, Epstein O, Heresbach D: Systematic review: adverse event reports for oral sodium phosphate and polyethylene glycol, *Aliment Pharmacol Ther* 29(1):15–28, 2009.

Belsey J, Epstein O, Heresbach D: Systematic review: oral bowel preparation for colonoscopy, *Aliment Pharmacol Ther* 25(4):373–384, 2007.

Cairns SR, Scholefield JH, Steele RJ, et al: (on behalf of the British Society of Gastroenterology and the Association of Coloproctology for Great Britain and Ireland). Guidelines for colorectal cancer screening and surveillance in moderate and high risk groups, *Gut* 2010; 59:666–690.

Heresbach D, Barrioz T, Lapalus MG, et al: Miss rate for colorectal neoplastic polyps: a prospective multicenter study of back-to-back video colonoscopies, *Endoscopy* 40(4):284–290, 2008.

Levin B, Lieberman DA, McFarland B, et al: Screening and surveillance for early detection of colorectal cancer and adenomatous polyps, 2008: Joint guidelines from the American Cancer Society, the US Multi-Society Task Force on Colorectal Cancer, and the American College of Radiology, *Gastroenterology* 134:1570–1595, 2008.

Levin TR, Zhao W, Conell C, et al: Complications of colonoscopy in an integrated health care delivery system, *Ann Intern Med* 145(12):880–886, 2006.

Napoleon B, Ponchon T, Lefebvre RR, et al: French Society of Digestive Endoscopy (SFED) Guidelines on performing a colonoscopy, *Endoscopy* 38(11):1152–1155, 2006.

Qureshi WA, Zuckerman MJ, Adler DG, et al: ASGE guideline: modifications in endoscopic practice for the elderly, *Gastrointest Endosc* 63(4):566–569, 2006.

Rex DK, Petrini JL, Baron TH, et al: Quality indicators for colonoscopy, *Gastrointest Endosc* 63:S16–S28, 2006.

Rex DK: Achieving cecal intubation in the very difficult colon, *Gastrointest Endosc* 67:938–944, 2008.

US Preventive Services Task Force: Screening for colorectal cancer: US Preventive Services Task Force Recommendation Statement, *Ann Intern Med* 149:627–637, 2008.

Whitlock EP, Lin JS, Liles E, et al: Screening for colorectal cancer: a targeted, updated systematic review for the US Preventive Services Task Force, *Ann Intern Med* 149:638–658, 2008.

CHAPTER 5

Small bowel endoscopy: indications and technique

5.1 **Video capsule endoscopy**

Gérard Gay, Michel Delvaux, Isaac Fassler, Muriel Frédéric, Ian Penman

Summary

Key Points

- Video capsule endoscopy (VCE) plays an important role in the investigation of small intestinal disease.
- The diagnostic yield in obscure GI bleeding is approximately 60%.
- Other indications include unexplained iron deficiency anemia, assessment of Crohn's disease, NSAID toxicity and suspected small bowel malignancy.
- Purgative bowel preparation improves the diagnostic yield but not the completion rate.
- VCE and single or double balloon enteroscopy are complementary techniques.
- VCE should be undertaken with caution in patients with suspected small intestinal strictures or obstruction.
- Capsule retention occurs in approximately 3% of cases.
- Specific esophageal and colonic capsules have been developed but remain experimental at present.

Introduction

The first endoscopic video capsule was initially developed by Iddan and Meron, two Israeli engineers. The capsule and the workstation for processing images were originally marketed by Given Imaging Ltd (Yoqneam, Israel). It was approved for clinical use by the FDA in August 2001, and EC approval followed in May 2002. Since then, other manufacturers have produced similar systems. Olympus (Olympus Optical Co., Ltd, Tokyo, Japan) markets the 'Endocapsule' system, while more recently IntroMedic (Seoul, South Korea) have developed the 'MiRoCam' and the Chonqing Jinshan Science and Technology Group from China have developed the 'OMOM' capsule.

1. Technical principles

Development of the first capsule (Fig. 1) was based on three scientific advances: a CMOS (complementary metal oxide silicone) microchip capable of producing an image comparable with that obtained with a CCD camera; an ASIC (application-specific integrated circuit) system, which allows integration of a small, low-energy video transmitter; and miniature high-power lighting such as an LED (light-emitting diode). These three components are placed in a capsule measuring $1.1 \text{ cm} \times 2.6 \text{ cm}$ that can be swallowed. The field of vision obtained is $140°$. It is weighted so that it retains its longitudinal orientation for approximately 80% of its intestinal journey, and it passes through the body naturally. The system also comprises a series of sensors which are placed on the surface of the patient's abdomen and detect signals emitted by the capsule. These are transmitted to a high-frequency tape recorder, contained in a case and worn

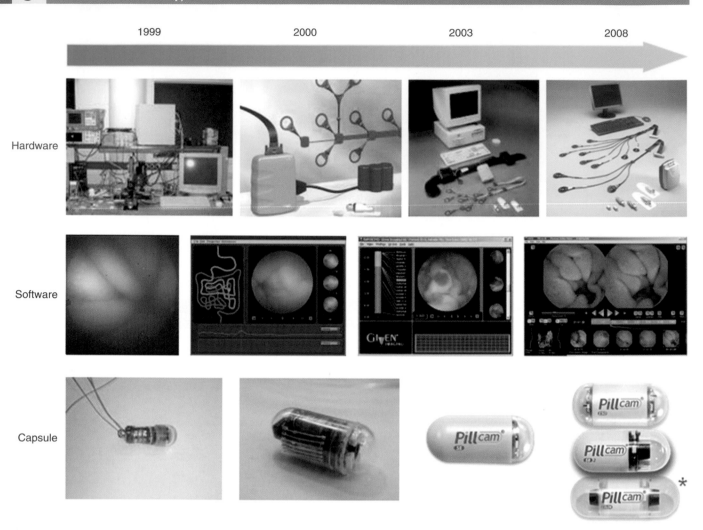

Figure 1 Development of the Given Imaging system. (Courtesy of Given Imaging Ltd.)

on a belt by the patient, before transfer to a workstation. The capsule is eliminated in the stools and is a single-use device. This description corresponds to the system developed by Given Imaging Ltd. Since then, the capsule has been improved and is available under the name 'PillCam SB', characterized by a wider angle of vision (156°), better resolution (65 536 pixels), and an increased depth of field. The 'EndoCapsule', 'MiRoCam' and 'OMOM' capsules differ in using a CCD rather than CMOS sensor (Fig. 2) to capture images. Studies comparing the 'Pillcam' and 'Endoscapsule'

have not demonstrated any differences in diagnostic yield in patients with obscure gastrointestinal bleeding. The 'MiroCam' capsule (Fig. 3) has longer-life batteries (11 h), is smaller in size (11 × 24 mm), has a larger number of pixels (102,400), takes three images per second, and transmits data using conduction through body tissues. This requires constant contact with the mucosa, which may be a limiting factor. Comparative studies with the other two systems are

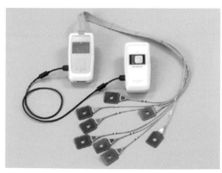

Figure 2 Olympus Endo-cap system: antennae and case. (Courtesy of Olympus.)

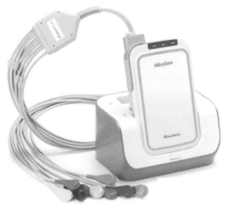

Figure 3 Intromedic MiroCam system. (Courtesy of IntroMedic.)

currently underway. The 'OMOM' capsule (27.9 mm long, 13 mm diameter, and 6 g weight) is significantly bigger than the others (24–26 × 11 mm and 3.4–3.6 g weight).

2. Examination procedure

The patient fasts for 12 h before swallowing the capsule. The five 1.2 V nickel batteries are worn by the patient on a belt, along with the 305 GB data recorder for storing the images. The patient may move around freely after swallowing the capsule. It is eliminated in stools in 24–48 h, depending on gut transit. Air bubbles and food residue may impair image quality and in fit patients, bowel preparation is recommended, as it improves mucosal visualization and diagnostic yield. Polyethylene glycol (PEG) solutions or sodium picosulphate can be used. There is some evidence that simethicone reduces air bubbles and improves views. Transit of the VCE capsule may be slower in diabetic patients or those in poor health and, for them, a prokinetic such as erythromycin is recommended.

3. Safety of VCE and contraindications

No harmful effects have been reported in cases of prolonged capsule retention. The presence of a capsule for 2 years in one individual had no adverse consequences. There is, however, a real risk of small intestinal obstruction as a result of stricturing, especially in inflammatory disorders. This risk is approximately 3.6% in large-scale studies and is offset by the fact that capsule retention is often caused by the lesion or lesions requiring examination by VCE in the first place. Surgery with or without endoscopy usually resolves both the problem of retention and the underlying disease at the same time.

To solve the problem of retention, Given Imaging Ltd has developed a calibration capsule, called the 'M2A Patency Capsule'. If it has not been expelled after 2–3 days, this breaks down spontaneously into small fragments, which easily pass through a narrowed segment. Latest modifications have incorporated two openings at each end of the capsule (the Agile Patency Capsule, Fig. 4), to enhance capsule breakdown. It is important to remember that neither small intestine barium studies nor CT or MR enteroclysis can detect all strictures. It is therefore essential to enquire about the patient's medical history (complex surgery, use of NSAIDs, radiotherapy of the abdomen, and recent episodes of obstructive symptoms) before carrying out an examination by VCE. The risk of obstruction should be explained clearly before VCE, along with the possibility that a retained capsule may have to be removed endoscopically or surgically. CT or MR enteroclysis or the use of an Agile Patency Capsule is recommended before performing VCE in patients felt to be at risk of small bowel strictures.

Clinical Tip

VCE should be performed with caution in patients at high risk of, or suspected of having, intestinal strictures or obstruction. If VCE is undertaken, a patency capsule study or small bowel imaging should be performed first.

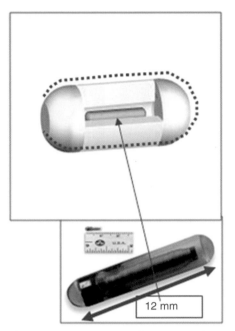

12 mm

Figure 4 Agile patency capsule. (Courtesy of Given Imaging Ltd.)

! Warning!

VCE is not approved for use in pregnant women because of the microwaves emitted. It is contraindicated in patients with swallowing disorders or signs of gastrointestinal obstruction. VCE does not interfere with cardiac pacemaker function. MRI studies should not be undertaken until it is clear that the capsule has been expelled.

4. Indications and results

VCE has already changed the management of patients in the following disorders:

4.1. Chronic obscure gastrointestinal bleeding

This is defined as isolated or recurrent melena, rectal bleeding or iron deficiency anemia with evidence of gastrointestinal bleeding. Patients should have undergone negative upper endoscopy and total colonoscopy before VCE is considered. A positive diagnosis may be found in 55–81% of patients, the yield being higher in those with overt as opposed to obscure bleeding. VCE is superior in detecting lesions responsible for bleeding compared with push enteroscopy (PE), particularly in patients with overt bleeding. Studies have also emphasized the need for examination by VCE as soon as possible after the bleeding episode, the diagnostic yield dropping as time elapses. Finally, the use of a repeat study in patients in whom VCE had initially been negative will yield a diagnosis in a significant number of patients. Two meta-analyses of 14 and 17 studies, respectively, demonstrate that VCE yields a positive diagnosis in 63% of patients compared with 28% for push-enteroscopy. The lesions detected are usually, in decreasing frequency, arteriovenous malformations (Fig. 5), ulceration secondary to NSAIDs, and tumors. When compared with double balloon enteroscopy (DBE), both methods have similar diagnostic yields in obscure gastrointestinal bleeding: 43–60% for DBE and 59–80% for VCE.

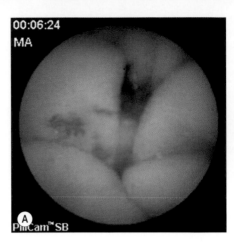

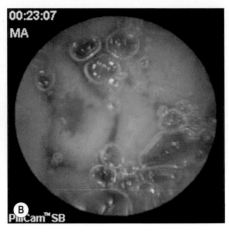

Figure 5 (A,B) Arteriovenous malformation.

Box 1 The role of VCE in Crohn's disease

- VCE is not indicated for diagnosis in patients with Crohn's confirmed by other radiological or endoscopic investigations.
- VCE is useful if Crohn's disease is suspected clinically or from laboratory tests or during recurrence if the radiological and endoscopic picture is normal.
- VCE is useful in patients with indeterminate colitis to detect small intestinal lesions.
- VCE is recommended in a patient with known disease if the discovery of small intestine lesions will influence the long-term management strategy.
- Detection of jejunal ulcerative lesions may predict early recurrence in a patient who has undergone ileocecal resection.

4.2. Recurrent iron deficiency anemia

VCE is associated with a diagnostic yield of approximately 50–60% of patients with a negative upper and lower gastrointestinal work-up and is superior to small bowel radiology.

4.3. Crohn's disease

VCE detects more intestinal lesions in patients with Crohn's disease (Fig. 6) than conventional radiological imaging. The lesions usually detected are mucosal: erosions, purpuric lesions, ulceration, aphthoid lesions, and strictures. Some practical conclusions are shown in Box 1.

One of the problems in evaluating VCE in Crohn's disease is the lack of reliable objective criteria for diagnosis. Scoring indices are under evaluation, based on three parameters: edematous appearance of villi, the presence of ulcers and the presence of strictures. Although these scores provide a common language to try and quantify the disease activity in the small intestine, they need further validation. Ulcers in the small bowel are not always due to Crohn's – NSAIDs, lymphoma, radiation, and vasculitis can all cause similar appearances. The risk of capsule retention in CD patients is 5–13% and so small bowel imaging or patency capsule studies should be performed to exclude strictures before VCE is undertaken.

4.4. Celiac disease

Some authors have suggested that VCE could be an alternative to endoscopic duodenal biopsies obtained at OGD, particularly in patients unwilling to undergo the procedure, and could be carried out for: chronic iron-deficiency anemia, children with clinical evidence and laboratory results suggesting celiac disease, patients with anti-transglutaminase antibodies, and atypical symptoms in elderly patients (Fig. 7A,B).

VCE in combination with DBE is, moreover, the best way of examining patients with celiac disease who have warning symptoms (weight loss, anemia and abdominal pain), while adhering closely a gluten-free diet. VCE is a useful tool for monitoring patients with celiac disease to detect malignant

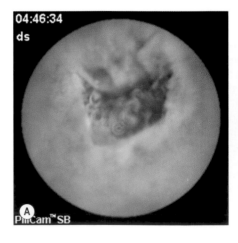

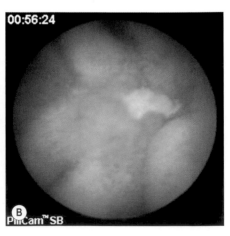

Figure 6 Crohn's disease of the small intestine. (A) Stenosis. (B) Ulcer.

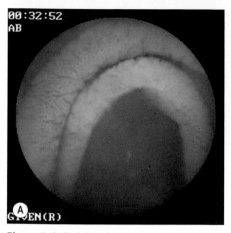
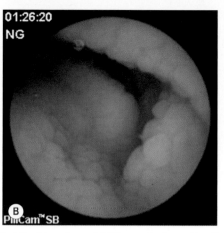
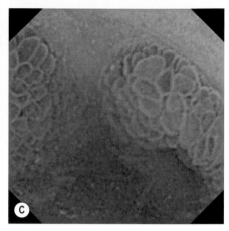

Figure 7 (A,B) Celiac disease. (C) Enteropathy associated T-cell lymphoma (EATL) complicating celiac disease.

lesions, i.e. adenocarcinoma or lymphoma (Fig. 7C), particularly if ulcerative jejunitis is present.

4.5. NSAID enteropathy

Ulcers, erosions and stenotic diaphragms or webs are usually found (Fig. 8). The clinical significance of minor lesions accompanying the use of NSAIDs is uncertain, as they are also detected in up to 22% of healthy volunteers participating in the control group in studies of NSAID toxicity.

4.6. Detection of intestinal tumors

The frequency of these tumors (Fig. 9) in patients examined by VCE for chronic obscure gastrointestinal bleeding is approximately 6–12%, and 60% of these are malignant. Since the introduction of VCE, it has been noted that the most frequent presentation of these intestinal tumors is chronic obscure bleeding rather than abdominal pain, weight loss or obstruction. This means that VCE has the potential to detect these tumors at an earlier stage.

4.7. Surveillance of familial polyposis

VCE is capable of demonstrating the existence of polyposis (Fig. 10) along the small intestine. Although it may miss

duodenal lesions in comparison with PE and DBE, it performs better in the jejunum and ileum. Its use is even more impressive in Peutz–Jeghers syndrome in which it can detect lesions capable of causing intussusception, and demonstrate ulcerated polyps responsible for chronic anemia. Its use is now widely accepted in the surveillance of familial adenomatous polyposis (FAP) associated with duodenal polyps. The same applies in juvenile polyposis. If VCE is used to monitor patients with FAP, it should be kept in mind that it does not detect all lesions in the duodenum, particularly the periampullary region. The duodenum must be investigated by a side-viewing endoscope in these patients. Finally, VCE cannot accurately assess the size of tumors in patients with familial polyposis, and often overestimates this. MR-enteroclysis appears to be better for assessing the size of these lesions.

Box 2 summarizes the role of VCE in small intestinal disorders.

5. Specific situations

5.1. Children

VCE may be used in children over the age of 9 years. It is specifically indicated in this age group for the diagnosis of chronic anemia, and can detect ulcerated or intussuscepting polyps in Peutz–Jeghers syndrome. It is also useful in the diagnosis of Crohn's disease when it is suspected from the clinical presentation.

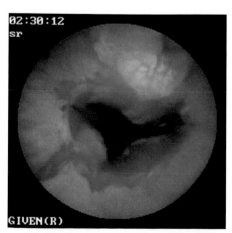

Figure 8 NSAID toxicity.

Box 2 Indications for VCE
• Chronic obscure gastrointestinal bleeding.
• Recurrent iron deficiency anemia.
• Crohn's disease.
• Celiac disease.
• NSAID enteropathy.
• Small intestinal tumors.
• Surveillance of familial polyposis.
• Other disorders: gastrointestinal amyloidosis, Waldmann's disease, common variable hypogammaglobulinemia, graft-versus-host disease, radiation enteritis, Whipple's disease (Fig. 11).

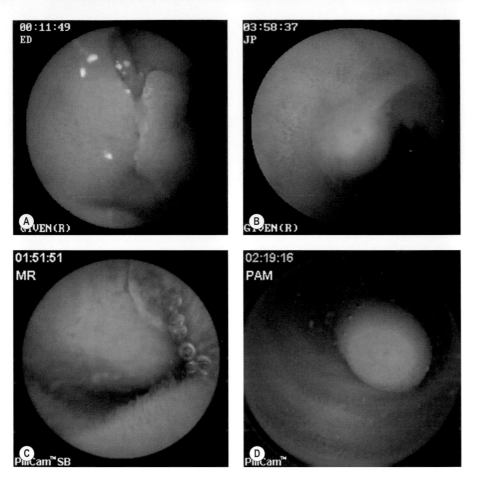

Figure 9 (A) Adenocarcinoma of the small intestine. (B) Carcinoid tumor. (C) Gastrointestinal stromal tumor (GIST). (D) Lipoma.

5.2. Other situations

In diabetic patients with gastroparesis, a capsule can be placed in the stomach using an enteroscope overtube or in the duodenum using a device that releases the capsule mechanically. Esophageal VCE (Pillcam ESO, Given) is available and may be useful in screening patients for Barrett's esophagus or esophageal varices but its role has not yet become established. A colon capsule (PillCam Colon, Given) is under evaluation at present.

6. Technical aids to reading images obtained by VCE

Precise anatomic localization of the capsule (Figs. 12, 13) remains too inaccurate to be used in practice, regardless of the electronic means of detection used. The capsule is, in fact, located based on differentiation between the appearance of the jejunum and the ileum and the time elapsed in relation to passage through the pylorus and the caecum. The

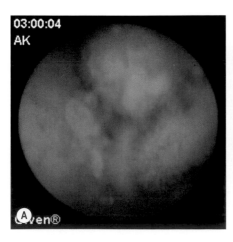
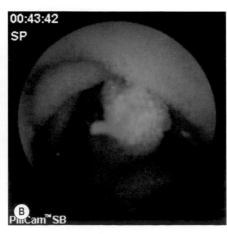

Figure 10 (A) Peutz–Jeghers syndrome with ulceration. (B) Familial adenomatous polyposis.

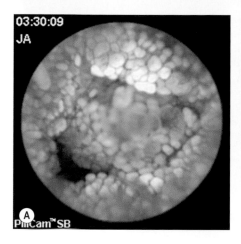
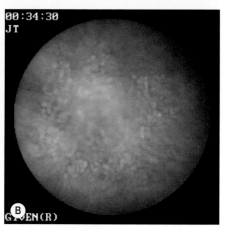

Figure 11 (A) Radiation enteritis. (B) Whipple's disease.

Real-Time Viewer, which is available from Olympus, Given Imaging Ltd and MiroCam, allows the images observed by the capsule to be read directly in real-time. These three systems are similar in principle and can be used at the patient's bedside. It is useful for determining whether the capsule has passed through the pylorus and for deciding to administer an erythromycin infusion to make sure the small intestinal examination is completed within the battery's life. It may be particularly useful for locating the site of active gastrointestinal bleeding, thereby allowing targeted therapeutic endoscopy.

7. Discussion

VCE has had a major impact on the examination of the small intestine in recent years. It is superior to other radiological examinations in the detection of mucosal, and particularly vascular, lesions. The same applies to tumors, particularly those measuring <1 cm. Its limitations relate to inferior image quality than classic endoscopy and to its inability to be manipulated in order to examine the small intestine more completely, or to be stopped over a suspicious lesion. Inability to take biopsies is another limitation at present.

Furthermore, the combined use of VCE and DBE to examine the small intestine has radically transformed the investigation and treatment of diseases of the small intestine. Strategies can be developed by combining the initial use of VCE followed by DBE. VCE is capable of indicating the route of insertion (oral or anal), which should then be carried out at DBE, thus allowing the correct management of patients. DBE should, nevertheless, still be considered the examination of choice if intestinal stricturing is strongly suspected or there is severe active bleeding known to be of intestinal origin.

8. Recent developments in VCE: esophagus and colon

8.1. The esophagus (Fig. 14)

A new VCE method has been developed by Given Imaging Ltd (PillCam™ ESO) for detecting esophageal mucosal abnormalities. It is a double-domed capsule which produces seven images per second at each end. The patient fasts for 2 h before the examination and the transit of the PillCam ESO is slowed after the patient swallows the device while lying down and then gets up gradually from this position over a period of 7 min. The images of the esophageal mucosa obtained with this capsule are comparable with those obtained at OGD. The reading time varies from 5–15 min. A recent modification allows a string to be attached to the capsule, which can then be withdrawn back up the esophagus in a controlled manner with better imaging results.

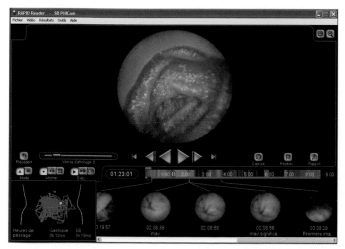

Figure 12 Location system. (Courtesy of Given Imaging Ltd.)

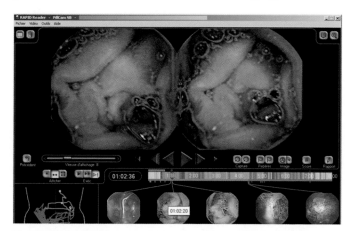

Figure 13 Red detection system. (Courtesy of Given Imaging Ltd.)

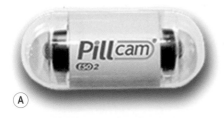

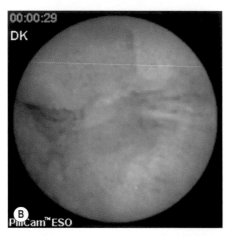

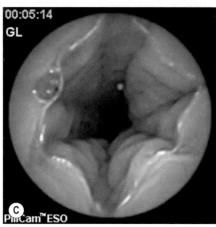

Figure 14 (A) Esophageal capsule. (B) LA-grade A esophagitis. (C) Esophageal varices grade II.

The sensitivity of VCE is between 60% and 100% for the detection of Barrett's esophagus and 50–89% for the detection of different grades of esophagitis. Matters are simpler as regards detection of esophageal varices. VCE has a sensitivity of 100% and a specificity of 80% for detecting esophageal varices. There is, moreover, a good correlation between the lesions detected during VCE and OGD for estimating variceal size, although small varices are more difficult to assess. Esophageal VCE may therefore be useful for detecting and monitoring portal hypertension in patients with cirrhosis, and it could replace OGD as the first-line investigation for this. VCE is not appropriate as the first-line endoscopic examination in the investigation of the upper gastrointestinal tract in symptomatic patients.

8.2. The colon

This is a recent development proposed by Given Imaging Ltd. The PillCam Colon (Fig. 15) is a capsule measuring

11 mm by 32 mm with two domes and two cameras. Images are acquired at a rate of 4/s. The batteries have a life of approximately 10 h. This capsule first examines the esophagus, stomach and duodenum, then switches off. It is programmed to switch on again when it reaches the terminal

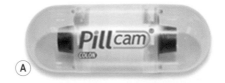

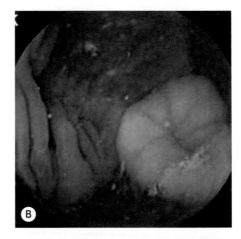

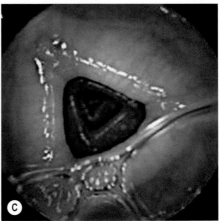

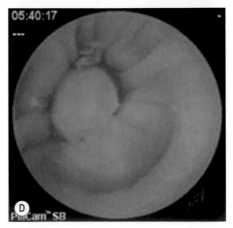

Figure 15 (A) Colon VCE. (B) Ileocecal valve. (C) Transverse colon. (D) Colonic polyp.

ileum. Patients require intensive preparation before the introduction of the colon capsule since exquisite cleanliness is required for a complete and careful examination of the mucosa, and passage of the capsule must also be facilitated. Stimulant agents (sodium phosphate) and laxatives (bisacodyl) are therefore used. This type of preparation, which is therefore slightly harsher than typical colonic preparation, can be used to obtain a clean colon.

One of the main potential indications for the use of this colon video capsule is the detection of colorectal cancer. Two studies show good correlation for the detection of colon polyps between the colon capsule and colonoscopy. Sensitivity and specificity of 56% and 76% for the colon capsule increase to 69% and 100%, respectively if the recording tapes for colon VCE are reviewed by an expert panel.

The difficulties encountered in our personal experience when reading colon VCE recordings are: difficulty detecting polyps owing to fluid in the colonic lumen; too rapid progression of the capsule in some colonic segments, particularly the rectum, and difficulty localizing and measuring the size of lesions found. Other indications are currently being considered for the colon capsule, particularly in patients in whom colonoscopy is incomplete and in monitoring patients at high risk of colorectal cancer, for example those with ulcerative colitis.

Conclusion

VCE is a now a key method of gastrointestinal investigation. It is constantly improving in terms of illumination, angle of view, and resolution. Numerous studies have confirmed its value in the examination of the small intestine, in which it has revolutionized the diagnostic approach. Its role in esophageal and colonic disorders remains to be determined.

Further Reading

American Gastroenterological Association: Medical position statement: evaluation and management of occult and obscure gastrointestinal bleeding, *Gastroenterology* 118:197–200, 2000.

Cellier C, Green PH, Collin P, et al: ICCE consensus for celiac disease, *Endoscopy* 37:1055–1059, 2005.

Delvaux M, Fassler I, Gay G: Clinical usefulness of the endoscopic video capsule as the initial intestinal investigation in patients with obscure gastrointestinal bleeding: validation of a diagnostic strategy based on the patient outcome after 12 months, *Endoscopy* 36:1067–1073, 2004.

Delvaux M, Gay G: Capsule endoscopy: technique and indications, *Best Pract Res Clin Gastroenterol* 20:813–837, 2008.

Galmiche JP, Coron E, Sacher-Huvelin S: Recent developments in capsule endoscopy, *Gut* 57:695–703, 2008.

Gay G, Delvaux M, Fassler I: Outcome of capsule endoscopy in determining indication and route for push-and-pull enteroscopy, *Endoscopy* 38:49–58, 2006.

Hartmann D, Eickhoff A, Damian U, et al: Diagnosis of small-bowel pathology using paired capsule endoscopy with two different devices: a randomized study, *Endoscopy* 39:1041–1045, 2007.

Iddan G, Meron G, Glukhovsky A, et al: Wireless capsule endoscopy, *Nature* 405:417, 2000.

Jones BH, Fleischer DE, Scharma VK, et al: Yield of repeat wireless video capsule endoscopy in patients with obscure gastrointestinal bleeding, *Am J Gastroenterol* 100:1058–1064, 2005.

Ladas SD, Triantafyllou K, Spada C, et al; ESGE Clinical Guidelines Committee: European Society of Gastrointestinal Endoscopy (ESGE): recommendations (2009) on clinical use of video capsule endoscopy to investigate small-bowel, esophageal and colonic diseases, *Endoscopy* 42(3):220–227, 2010.

Solem CA, Loftus JR, Fletcher JG, et al: Small-bowel imaging in Crohn's disease: a prospective, blinded, 4-way comparison trial, *Gastrointest Endosc* 68:255–266, 2008.

Gérard Gay, Michel Delvaux, Isaac Fassler, Muriel Frédéric

Key Points

- Overtube-assisted enteroscopy allows much greater depth of insertion into the small bowel than previously achieved with push enteroscopy.
- Total enteroscopy can be achieved by combining anterograde and retrograde approaches. Total enteroscopy using only anterograde or retrograde approach is very rare.
- Overtube-assisted enteroscopy can be used to access the afferent limb in patients with altered anatomy who require an ERCP.
- Double balloon enteroscopy and/or colonoscopy can be used in patients in whom conventional colonoscopy fails.
- Double balloon enteroscopy is the most established form of overtube-assisted enteroscopy, providing the deepest depth of insertion.
- Single balloon enteroscopy and spiral enteroscopy are new techniques, the roles of which are being evaluated.

Introduction

Enteroscopy is the endoscopic examination of the small intestinal mucosa. Endoscopic investigation of the small bowel has been dominated for the last 20 years by push enteroscopy, which has many diagnostic and therapeutic capabilities but is limited in its depth of insertion. Recent advances in overtube-assisted enteroscopy, with the development of the double balloon enteroscopy (DBE) (Fuji Photo Optical Co, Ltd, Saitama, Japan), single balloon (SBE) (Olympus Ltd, Tokyo, Japan) and spiral enteroscopy (Spirus Medical, Inc, Stoughton, MA, USA) systems, allow much greater depth of insertion than previously possible with push enteroscopy. If retrograde enteroscopy is performed in addition to anterograde enteroscopy, total enteroscopy is possible, allowing visualization of the entire small bowel.

DBE, SBE or spiral enteroscopy?

DBE is the most established technique, with the greatest evidence in the literature supporting its use. One study has shown increased depth of insertion of with DBE compared with SBE. The diagnostic accuracy of DBE and SBE have been compared in a prospective study by May et al (2010), in 100 patients with suspected small intestine pathology. Total enteroscopy was achieved in 66% of the patients undergoing DBE and 22% of the patients undergoing SBE ($p < 0.001$). A total of 72% of the patients who underwent DBE had a significant diagnostic finding or therapeutic intervention compared with 48% in the SBE group ($p = 0.025$). Based on the results of this study, DBE should be considered the gold standard for investigation of the small bowel. Initial studies of spiral enteroscopy have not altered this position.

Side-effect profiles appear to be similar, although data are limited for SBE and spiral enteroscopy. SBE can be performed by a single endoscopist, while spiral enteroscopy requires two endoscopists. DBE requires two endoscopists when initially learning the technique; however, with experience, particularly with the oral approach, a single endoscopist and trained nurse are sufficient. Both DBE and SBE can be used for both anterograde and retrograde enteroscopy. A colonic spiral enteroscopy overtube has been developed but experience with it is limited.

1. Indications and contraindications

Indications for enteroscopy:

- Assessment of abnormality detected on cross-sectional imaging, contrast studies or capsule endoscopy.
- Assessment of obscure GI bleeding or iron deficiency anemia.
- Assessment of chronic diarrhea.
- Diagnosis and assessment of Crohn's disease.
- Diagnosis and treatment of small bowel strictures (dilation or stenting).
- Diagnosis and treatment of small bowel polyps, tumor or lymphoma.
- Miniprobes can be placed through the enteroscope to assess submucosal lesions.
- Assessment of refractory celiac disease.
- Assessment of the afferent limb and excluded stomach in patients with altered anatomy (Roux-en-Y), including placement of PEG (Fig. 1).
- ERCP in patients with altered anatomy (Fig. 2) (see Ch. 10.6 for further details).
- Removal of retained foreign bodies.
- Colonoscopy in patients in whom convention colonoscopy has failed.

✓ Clinical Tip

Performing altered anatomy ERCP

Regular ERCP accessories can be used with the DBE colonoscope (Fujinon EC-540 B15), which has a working length of 152 cm.

Contraindications to overtube-assisted enteroscopy:

- Contraindications are the same as those of endoscopy of the upper and lower digestive tract.

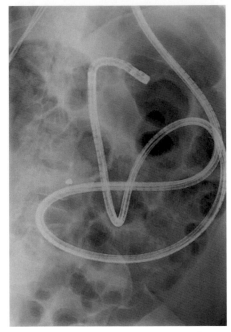

Figure 1 Radiological image of DBE in the bypassed gastric pouch.

- Retrograde enteroscopy in patients with ileoanal anastomoses is a relative contraindication.

2. General enterosocpy technique

- Overtube-assisted enteroscopy can be performed using conscious sedation, monitored anesthesia care (MAC) with propofol or general anesthesia.
- An anterograde procedure to the proximal ileum takes approximately 1 h. Retrograde examination to the mid-ileum may take up to 1.5 h. If a long anterograde procedure is envisioned, intubation may be necessary.
- Fluoroscopy is useful when learning any of the overtube-assisted enteroscopy techniques. As endoscopists gain experience with a technique, fluoroscopy requirements decrease.
- Use of CO_2 instead of air, may allow deeper insertion and decreases post-procedure pain.

 Clinical Tip

Anterograde or retrograde approach?

If the transit time from ingestion of a capsule at VCE to arrival at the lesion is ≥75% of the total time from ingestion to arrival at the cecum, a retrograde approach should be performed.

3. Double balloon enteroscopy

3.1. Principles

DBE was initially developed by Yamamoto, based on the principle of gathering the small intestine on the enteroscope overtube. The endoscope and the overtube are equipped with latex balloons at their distal end, which are alternately inflated and deflated. By withdrawing the enteroscope and the overtube with their balloons inflated, the small intestine can be pleated onto the overtube. It is possible to reach the jejunum and proximal ileum by an oral approach. Total enteroscopy can be performed by performing retrograde enteroscopy (via the colon), which allows visualization of the distal ileum.

 Clinical Tip

How do you know if total enteroscopy has been performed?

- The most distal extent of an anterograde procedure is marked with a tattoo.
- A retrograde procedure is then performed. Once the tattoo is reached, a total enteroscopy has been performed.

3.2. Equipment

The DBE (see Table 1) consists of a thin endoscope 8.5 mm in diameter and 2300 mm long, with a flexible overtube measuring 1450 mm with an external diameter of 12.2 mm. The two latex balloons attach to the end of the overtube and the endoscope, respectively, and are inflated and deflated by a pump, which maintains constant pressure in the balloons (Fig. 3).

3.3. Technique (Fig. 4)

DBE is performed with two endoscopists (at least one of whom is experienced). Anterograde (Fig. 5) and retrograde

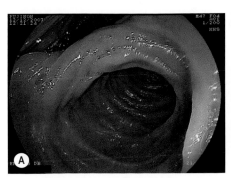
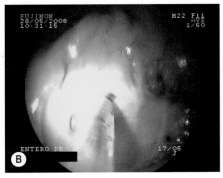
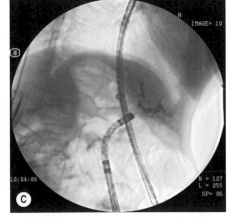

Figure 2 (A) Small intestine anastomosis (Roux-en-Y, bariatric surgery). (B) Dilation of a hepaticojejunal anastomosis. (C) Radiological image of the dilation of the hepaticojejunal anastomosis. (DBE Fujinon.)

(Fig. 6) approaches are usually required to visualize the entire small bowel.

Regardless of the route chosen, pleating of the small bowel over the overtube is obtained by the combined withdrawal of the enteroscope and the overtube repeatedly. A total of 12

Box 1   Overtube-assisted enteroscopy

- Overtube-assisted enteroscopy is when an enteroscope is used with an overtube.
- There are currently three types of overtube-assisted enteroscopy systems available: DBE, SBE, and spiral enteroscopy.
- Anterograde enteroscopy is where the enteroscope and overtube are advanced through the mouth and into the small bowel.
- Retrograde enteroscopy is where the enteroscope and overtube are advanced through the colon, with intubation of the terminal ileum, and then advancement into the small bowel.
- Total enteroscopy is where the entire small bowel is visualized. This is sometimes possible with anterograde DBE, but is rarely achieved with either SBE or spiral enteroscopy. The combination of anterograde and retrograde enteroscopy allows total enteroscopy in many cases.

Table 1   Specification of enteroscopes and overtubes used for DBE and SBE

	DBE		SBE
Endoscope	Fujinon EN-450P5	Fujinon EN-450T5	Olympus SIF-Q180
Working length (cm)	200	200	200
External diameter (mm)	8.5	9.4	9.2
Operating channel diameter (mm)	2.2	2.8	2.8
Overtube external diameter (mm)	12.2	13.2	13.2

Clinical Tip

Technique for DBE

- Insert endoscope.
- Inflate endoscope balloon.
- Deflate overtube balloon.
- Advance overtube.
- Inflate overtube.
- Pull back endoscope and overtube.
- Deflate endoscope balloon.

Box 2   Overtube-assisted enteroscopy, VCE or cross-sectional imaging as a first test?

Obscure GI bleeding

Video capsule endoscopy (VCE) should be used as the initial diagnostic test. DBE should be the initial test if an abnormality has already been detected (i.e. CT or MRI) or a therapeutic intervention is required. It should also be used first if a lesion of the small intestine is strongly suspected or in a patient with active bleeding known to originate in the small intestine, particularly if an ileal location is suspected.

Suspected small tumor (<1 cm)

- DBE combined with VCE is superior to radiological techniques for identifying tumors <1 cm.

Larger tumor (>1 cm)

Cross-sectional imaging is useful for identifying tumors >1 cm, and provides information about the lesion and its environment. Overtube-assisted enteroscopy is used to confirm a histological diagnosis or perform a therapeutic intervention.

Inflammatory diseases

Cross-sectional imaging provides information on the wall, determines the topography of lesions and provides information on the surrounding tissues, e.g. fat-wrapping, and even on the degree of inflammation (functional MRI). VCE is useful in this type of disease for locating very small ulcers which cannot be detected by cross-sectional imaging. Overtube-assisted enteroscopy allows histological confirmation or therapeutic intervention.

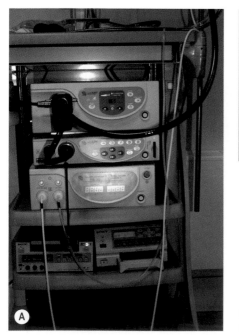

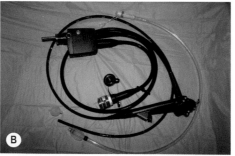

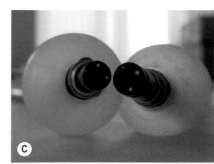

Figure 3 (A) Processor and peristaltic pump, Fujinon. (B) Fujinon therapeutic enteroscope. (C) Fujinon enteroscopes with balloons inflated.

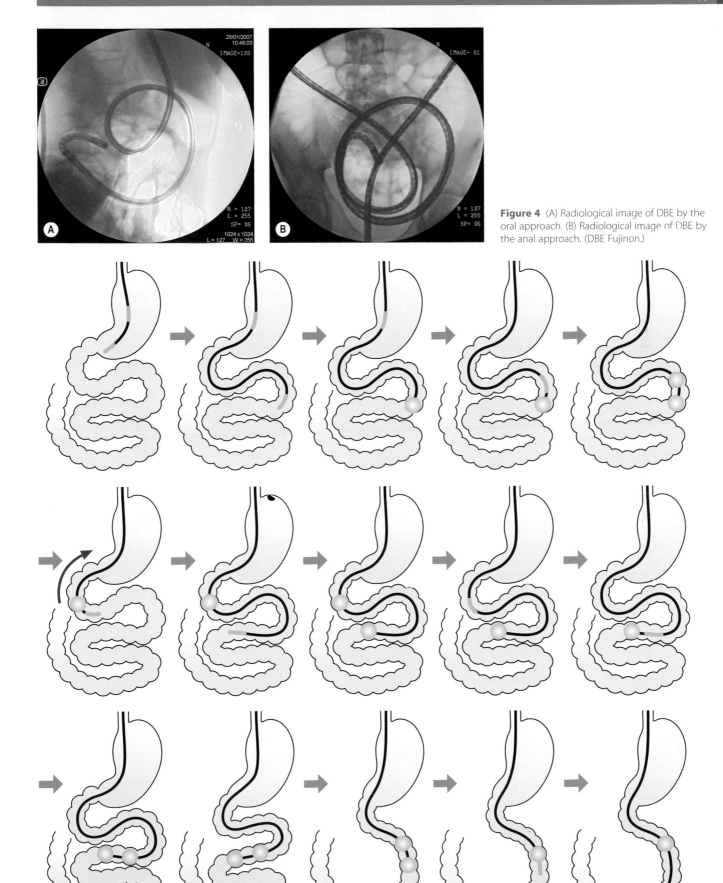

Figure 4 (A) Radiological image of DBE by the oral approach. (B) Radiological image of DBE by the anal approach. (DBE Fujinon.)

Figure 5 Anterograde double balloon enteroscopy.

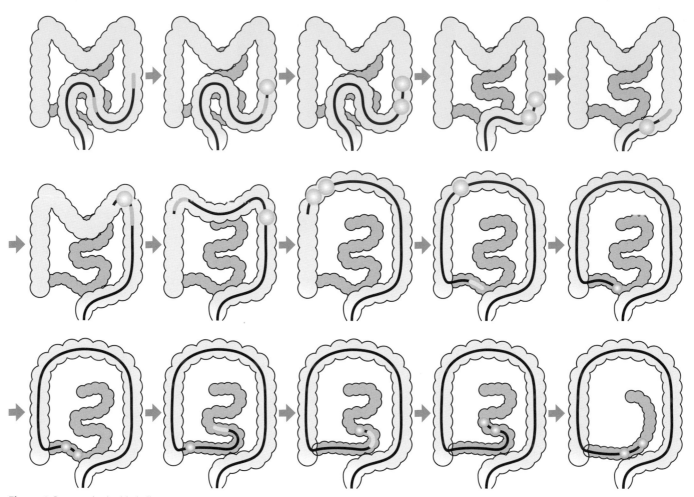

Figure 6 Retrograde double balloon enteroscopy.

maneuvers are generally performed in succession, resulting in a significant shortening of the small intestine. The successive withdrawal of the enteroscope and the overtube results in the endoscope being inserted deep into the small intestine. The anal approach is more difficult than the oral approach. Problems may arise as a result of a very long sigmoid colon which requires reduction of loops. Intubation of the ileocecal valve can also be tricky, and requires careful positioning of the endoscope and overtube in the area of the cecum to avoid being too perpendicular to the ileocecal valve.

Anterograde DBE enteroscopy is performed as follows:

The enteroscope is advanced using the following series of maneuvers (Fig. 5). The enteroscope is advanced. The scope balloon is inflated. The overtube is advanced. The overtube balloon is inflated. A 'short endoscope' position is achieved by pulling back on the endoscope and overtube together. The scope balloon is then deflated and the enteroscope advanced. The process is then repeated.

Retrograde DBE enteroscopy is performed as follows:

The enteroscope is advanced using a series of maneuvers similar to those described above. The enteroscope is inserted as far as the descending colon (Fig. 6). The scope balloon is inflated. The overtube is advanced and the overtube balloon inflated. The enteroscope and overtube are withdrawn, straightening the sigmoid colon. The enteroscope is then advanced by repeating these maneuvers.

> **Clinical Tip**
>
> **Increasing the depth of insertion**
> - Ensure the overtube remains filled with water to reduce friction.
> - Minimize use of air/CO_2.
> - Abdominal compression in the center or left lower quadrant.
> - Patients can be placed prone, using their weight to provide abdominal compression.
> - In retrograde procedure, placing the patient on their back can assist intubation of the ileocecal valve.

3.4. Complications of DBE

Procedure-related complications in DBE: The rate of complications related to the procedure is low: 0.4–0.8%. The most serious complication associated with anterograde enteroscopy is acute pancreatitis. This is thought to be due to inflation of the balloons in the region of the major papilla, but may also be due to excessively rough push and pull maneuvers, causing pancreatic ischemia. To avoid this complication, the double balloon should not be inflated until the enteroscope is beyond the angle of Treitz.

The complication rate related to therapeutic intervention with DBE is approximately 3–4%, comprising mainly instances of perforation and bleeding. Although this rate appears slightly higher than for endoscopic procedures, it must be acknowledged that the small bowel is a more

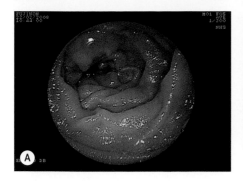
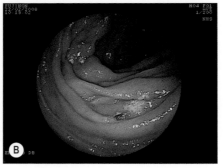

Figure 7 (A) AVM of the small intestine. (B) Treatment with APC of an AVM of the small intestine. (DBE Fujinon.)

difficult area for endoscopic therapy because the lesions are often large (i.e. polyps associated with Peutz–Jeghers syndrome), and the manipulation of accessories is less straightforward. Perforation rates of up to 10% have been reported in specific situations.

The risk of complications, in particular perforation, is higher in patients with altered anatomy (i.e. Roux-en-Y).

Anesthesia-related complications in DBE: The complications related to anesthesia are less than 1% and usually consist of respiratory depression and aspiration pneumonia.

3.5. Results of DBE

The first results were published by Yamamoto. An initial retrospective study of 178 enteroscopy procedures, including 89 anterograde and 89 retrograde procedures, performed in 123 patients, 66 of whom had obscure gastrointestinal bleeding. Total examination of the small intestine by the oral approach was possible in two patients. In 22 patients, a combination of the two approaches achieved examination of the whole small intestine. The lesions found included angiodysplasia, ulcers related to the use of NSAID or secondary to Crohn's disease, polyps, and tumors. The source of the bleeding was identified in 50 of the 66 patients who had been referred for obscure digestive bleeding. DBE was never preceded by VCE in this study.

Three European studies confirmed these initial results. DBE allowed treatment in 62% of the 100 patients examined, of whom 42% had APC, polypectomy or dilation. Medical treatment was implemented as a result of DBE in 12% of cases and the patient was referred for surgery in 8% of cases.

3.6. Obscure GI bleeding

The diagnostic superiority of DBE over push enteroscopy in obscure digestive bleeding was demonstrated in a series of 52 patients with obscure GI bleeding in whom anterograde DBE

found lesions in 38 patients, compared with 23 patients who underwent push enteroscopy (Fig. 7).

3.7. Crohn's disease

DBE is the method of choice for obtaining endoscopic and histological confirmation of Crohn's disease affecting the small intestine (Fig. 8A,B). DBE should be performed only if it alters patient management either by assessing the severity of mucosal lesions and their extent, or to determine whether they are fibrostenotic or inflammatory in nature. DBE should be used if a short fibrous stenotic stricture requires dilation. DBE should never be performed in active Crohn's disease (Fig. 8C). Some 50% of dilated patients retain the benefit of this endoscopic procedure at 6 months.

3.8 Tumors

DBE and VCE are comparable for detecting tumors. DBE is useful for the detection and removal of polyps in both familial adenomatous polyposis (FAP) and Peutz–Jeghers syndrome (PJS) (Fig. 9A). DBE should be used as the first procedure if polypectomy is envisaged. Use caution when performing polypectomies in this group of patients, particularly for large polyps or those with a broad stalk (Fig. 9B). Submucosal injection with dilute adrenaline (epinephrine) should be used to decrease the risk of bleeding or perforation.

4. Single balloon enteroscopy

The single balloon enteroscopy (SBE) system (Fig. 10) was developed by Olympus. It can be used to perform both anterograde and retrograde examinations. Total enteroscopy rates appear to be lower in SBE (15%) compared with DBE (40%). The overtube is coated with silicone and measures

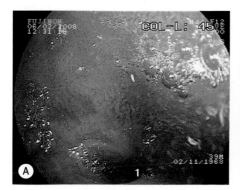
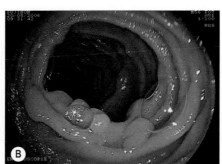
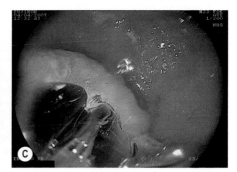

Figure 8 (A) Crohn's disease, with stricture. (B) Crohn's disease with pseudo polyps. (C) Dilation of a stricture in Crohn's disease. (DBE Fujinon.)

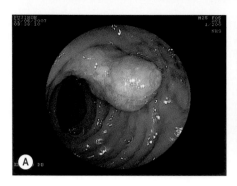

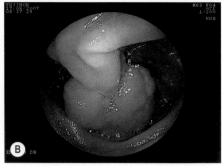

Figure 9 (A) A polyp in a patient with Peutz–Jeghers syndrome. (B) Pediculated polyp of small intestine. (DBE Fujinon.)

140 cm (ST-SB1 Olympus) with an external diameter of 13 mm (see Table 1). The balloon is made of silicone and is attached to the end of the overtube.

> **Clinical Tip**
>
> **How do you know what distance the enteroscope has been inserted?**
>
> Several techniques have been proposed including:
> - Adding the centimeters of scope inserted during each cycle of passage and using this number to estimate the total depth of insertion
> - Measuring the distance during the withdrawal phase of the procedure
> - Fluoroscopy has been used to assess the depth of insertion, assuming that the left upper quadrant correlates with the proximal jejunum, the left lower quadrant with the proximal ileum, the pelvis with the mid-ileum and the right lower abdomen with the terminal ileum.

4.1. Technique

The sequence of maneuvers is slightly different from DBE. As with DBE the small intestine is pleated onto the overtube when the balloon at its tip is inflated. The main difference from the DBE technique is the use of the endoscope tip to secure the small intestine by retroflexion and angulation maneuvers. It is then possible to pleat the small intestine over the overtube with the endoscope in this position and the balloon inflated.

> **Clinical Tip**
>
> **Technique for SBE**
> - Insert enteroscope.
> - Deflate overtube balloon.
> - Suction and deflect enteroscope tip.
> - Advance overtube.
> - Inflate overtube.
> - Pull back enteroscope and overtube.

4.2. Results

The method is relatively easy to perform and allows the same high quality examination of the jejunum as DBE.

4.3. Complications

Lacerations have been described, possibly related to the positioning of the endoscope tip during pulling maneuvers of the overtube with its balloon inflated. Cases of perforation have also been reported.

5. Spiral enteroscopy

The Spirus system (Fig. 11), developed by Endo-Ease Discovery SB (Table 2), is based on a different principle from the previous two systems. The small intestine is concertinaed by rotating the overtube.

5.1. Technique

The overtube is turned using a rubber handle, which causes rotational movement of the overtube. It is advanced through the small intestine by rotating in a clockwise direction over the enteroscope until the duodenum is reached. Once in place in the second portion of the duodenum, rotation continues in a clockwise direction so that the small intestine is gathered on the system. The Discovery SB system is then rotated anticlockwise to release it from the retracted intestine. Once released from the spiral system, retraction from the small intestine is possible, and the endoscope can be moved and advanced in the traditional manner. This technique requires a substantial amount of training, with ten procedures required before sufficient mastery of the technique can be acquired. Fluoroscopy is useful initially to understand the maneuvers applied to the Spirus system and the effects of rotation in the opposite direction in the small intestine.

Table 2 Spiral enteroscopy overtubes.
Two spiral overtube diameters are available, with the standard profile used in the majority of patients

Type of device	Length (cm)	Spiral height (mm)	Product name
Endo-Ease Discovery SB (Standard profile)	118	5.5	EED-300
Endo-Ease Discovery SB (Low profile)	118	4.5	EED-250

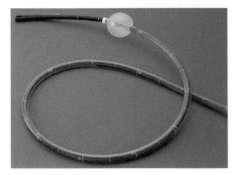

Figure 10 Single balloon enteroscope. (Olympus.)

5.2. Complications

To date, six cases of perforation were reported, in 1750 patients. To date, no cases of pancreatitis have been reported. Mucosal abrasion or laceration can occur.

6. Intraoperative enteroscopy

The role of intraoperative enteroscopy has been reduced by the performance of VCE and augmented enteroscopy. However, it still has two exclusive indications:

- Bleeding originating in the small intestine which, owing to its massive nature, renders both VCE and DBE

Clinical Tips

Technical tips for spiral enteroscopy

- Take care to lubricate the overtube fully and test it before insertion into the patient. The enteroscope should move easily within the overtube.
- Advance the overtube over the enteroscope and lock it in place so that the distal end of the overtube is at the 40 cm mark on the enteroscope.
- Lubricate the spirals to avoid trauma in the esophagus.
- Take time advancing through the stomach to prevent gastric loop formation.
- If a gastric loop is present, remove this as soon as possible by counterclockwise rotation of the overtube. You will know that the loop has been removed as there is rapid re-engagement of the overtube with the small bowel on clockwise rotation.
- Once the deepest insertion of the overtube has been reached, deeper intubation of the small bowel can be achieved by advancing with the enteroscope alone. Once the enteroscope is advanced as deep as possible, turn the tip of the scope into the mucosa and gently apply suction. While maintaining suction, rotate the overtube clockwise over the enteroscope. This maneuver allows deeper depth of insertion to be achieved.
- Once the deepest point of insertion has been reached, withdraw the enteroscope slowly until the proximal end of the overtube is at 140 cm on the enteroscope. Lock the overtube in this position, and then withdraw the overtube and enteroscope together by turning the overtube counterclockwise.

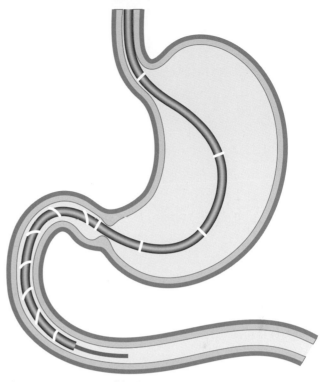
Figure 11 Description of the Spirus system.

impossible. Patients with this type of clinical picture should be transferred directly from the recovery room to the operating theatre. It should be emphasized that DBE used perioperatively will facilitate the endoscopic analysis of the small intestine during surgery.

- DBE has a similar role in perioperative enteroscopy for the removal of multiple polyps in Peutz–Jeghers syndrome. The polyps are often large, numerous, and scattered through the small intestine. Perioperative surgical enteroscopy can be performed via a laparoscopic route using DBE which can be used to detect the polyps. It should be emphasized that this combined procedure requires medical and surgical teams used to working together with careful planning of how the procedure will be carried out.

Further Reading

Ell C, May A, Nachbar L, et al: Push and pull enteroscopy in the small bowel using the double balloon technique: results of a prospective European multicenter study, *Endoscopy* 37:613–616, 2005.

Gay G, Delvaux M, Fassler I: Outcome of capsule endoscopy in determining indication and route for push-and-pull enteroscopy, *Endoscopy* 38:49–58, 2006.

Lo SK: Technical matters in double balloon enteroscopy, *Gastro Intest Endosc* 66:S15–S18, 2007.

May A, Farber M, Aschmoneit I, et al: Prospective multicenter trial comparing push-and-pull enteroscopy with the single- and double-balloon techniques in patients with small-bowel disorders, *Am J Gastroenterol* 105:575–581, 2010.

May A, Nachbar L, Pohl J, et al: Endoscopic interventions in the small bowel using double-balloon enteroscopy: feasibility and limitations, *Am J Gastroenterol* 102:527–535, 2007.

Mensink P, Haringsma J, Kucharzik TF, et al: Complications of double balloon enteroscopy: a multicenter survey, *Endoscopy* 39:613–615, 2007.

Monkemuller K, Bellutti M, Neumann H, et al: Therapeutic ERCP with the double-balloon enteroscope in patients with Roux-en-Y anastomosis, *Gastrointest Endosc* 67:992–996, 2008.

Sidhu R, Sanders DS, Morris AJ, McAlindon ME: Guidelines on small bowel enteroscopy and capsule endoscopy in adults, *Gut* 57:125-136, 2008.

Teshima CW, Kuipers EJ, Van Zanten SV, Mensink PB: Double balloon enteroscopy and capsule endoscopy for obscure gastrointestinal bleeding: an updated meta-analysis, *J Gastroenterol Hepatol* 2010 Oct 18. doi: 10.1111/j.1440-1746.2010. 06530.x. [Epub ahead of print]

Tsujikawa T, Saitoh Y, Andoh A, et al: Novel single-balloon enteroscopy for diagnosis and treatment of the small intestine: preliminary experiences, *Endoscopy* 40:11–15, 2008.

Yamamoto H, Kita H, Sunada K, et al: Clinical outcomes of double-balloon endoscopy for the diagnosis and treatment of small-intestinal diseases, *Clin Gastroenterol Hepatol* 2:1010–1016, 2004.

CHAPTER 6

Advanced imaging

6.1 Confocal endomicroscopy

Kerry B. Dunbar

Summary

<table>
<tr><td>Introduction 140</td><td>4. Technique 142</td></tr>
<tr><td>1. Indications 140</td><td>5. Complications 142</td></tr>
<tr><td>2. Equipment 140</td><td>6. Special considerations 142</td></tr>
<tr><td>3. Contrast agents 142</td><td></td></tr>
</table>

Key Points

- Confocal laser endomicroscopy has been used to image many disorders of the gastrointestinal tract.
- Intravenous fluorescein sodium is the most commonly used contrast agent when performing endomicroscopy.
- Obtaining a stable position is key when using either the confocal endoscope or confocal probes to obtain clear microscopic images.
- When learning endomicroscopy, it is helpful to work with someone already trained in endomicroscopy and to study image atlases.
- When learning endomicroscopy, confirmation of the microscopic imaging findings with a mucosal biopsy is essential, until competence is achieved.

Introduction

Confocal laser endomicroscopy (CLE) is one of the newer advanced imaging methods for the gastrointestinal tract. Microscopic images of the gastrointestinal mucosa are obtained by illuminating the mucosa with blue laser light (488 nm), which causes fluorescence. The light reflected is collected through a pinhole-sized aperture and processed, creating a microscopic image. The laser light and collected light are 'confocal', meaning they are in the same focal plane. The images produced allow visualization of small structures, such as capillaries and colonic crypts and gastric pits (Figs 1–4), as well as individual cells, such as epithelial cells and red blood cells.

1. Indications

Endomicroscopy has been used to study many gastrointestinal disorders. Several of the earliest studies looked at patients undergoing colorectal cancer screening and examined polyps with endoscope-based endomicroscopy (eCLE). Other colonic disorders studied include patients with inflammatory bowel disease undergoing surveillance for dysplasia, collagenous colitis, and pouchitis. Small bowel disorders investigated with endomicroscopy include celiac disease and graft-versus-host disease. Gastric cancer and *Helicobacter pylori* gastritis have been imaged with CLE. In the esophagus, Barrett's esophagus and squamous cell esophageal cancer have been studied. Endomicroscopy has been used to help target biopsies in all these disorders as well, and may also reduce the number of biopsies needed to achieve a diagnosis. Examination of biliary strictures at ERCP to differentiate cholangiocarcinomas from benign strictures has recently been reported.

2. Equipment

There are currently two endomicroscopy systems available (Table 1). One is an endoscope-based endomicroscopy (eCLE) system, the EC-3870CIFK colonoscope, and EG-3870CIK upper endoscope (Pentax, Tokyo, Japan). A probe-based endomicroscopy (pCLE) system, the Cellvizio (Mauna Kea Technologies, Paris, France) is also available. Both systems allow standard endoscopic imaging while

DOI: 10.1016/B978-0-7020-3128-1.00006-7

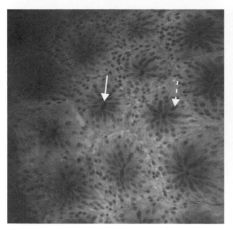

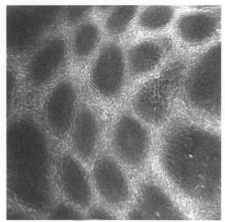

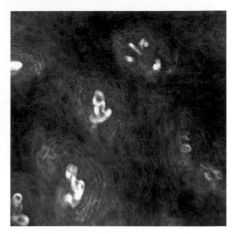

Figure 1 Endomicroscopy of the colonic mucosa. The colonic crypts (solid arrow) and goblet cells (dashed arrow) can be seen.

Figure 2 Normal gastric mucosa seen by endomicroscopy.

Figure 3 Mucosa of the squamous esophagus. Intrapapillary capillary loops are visible.

Table 1 Endomicroscopy systems

	Confocal endoscope (eCLE)	Confocal probe		
		Gastro/Coloflex	Gastro/Coloflex UHD	Cholangioflex
Depth of imaging (µm)	0–250	70–130	55–65	40–70
Field of view (µm)	475 × 475	600	240	320
Lateral resolution (µm)	0.7	3.5	1	3.5
Axial resolution (µm)	7	15	5	
Diameter (mm)	12.8 (scope diameter)	2.7	2.5	1
Imaging rate (images/second)	0.8 (1024 × 1024 pixels) 1.6 (1024 × 512 pixels)	12	12	12

providing the ability to obtain microscopic views of the mucosa, but there are several differences between the two systems. Each system has an endomicroscopic image processor and separate screen for viewing endomicroscopic images. The confocal endoscope comes in lengths appropriate for colonoscopy and one for upper endoscopy, although the colonoscope-length endoscope can also be used for investigation of the upper GI tract. The confocal endoscope has the standard wheels, air, water, suction and photo buttons, and

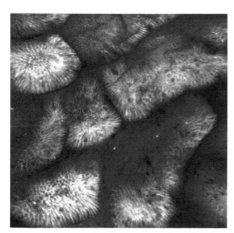

Figure 4 Normal duodenal mucosa. Small goblet cells (dark) are visible.

a standard-size biopsy channel. The miniprobes for pCLE can be used with a standard endoscope that has a 2.8 mm channel and the probes are attached to a special processor. They come in lengths appropriate for upper endoscopy, colonoscopy, and cholangioscopy. Both systems require a contrast agent to be used to collect images. The confocal endoscope can image sequentially from the surface, down to a depth of 250 µm, while the confocal probes have set ranges of imaging depth, ranging from 55–65 µm from the surface for the Gastroflex UHD probe to 70–130 µm for the Gastroflex probe. The resolution of the images is higher with the confocal endoscope than the probes, with a lateral resolution of 0.7 µm compared with 1–3.5 µm. The imaging rate for the confocal probe is higher than the confocal endoscope, with an imaging rate of 12 images per second compared with 0.8–1.6 images per second. The pCLE system also creates a 'mosaic' of images collected together to show a larger portion of the mucosa. Both systems allow image capture and export.

3. Contrast agents

Several contrast agents can be used for imaging with the confocal endoscope and the confocal probe systems. Fluorescein sodium is the most commonly used contrast agent and is used in ophthalmology for retinal vascular imaging.

The standard dosing with the confocal endoscope is 5 mL of 10% fluorescein sodium, given intravenously. In studies using the confocal probe, 2.5–10 mL of 10% fluorescein sodium is used. Fluorescein highlights the vessels and intracellular spaces, and lamina propria of tissues, but does not stain nuclei. Goblet cells in the colon, small bowel, and in Barrett's esophagus appear dark when fluorescein is used for contrast. Capillaries appear bright, with individual red blood cells visible. All patients who receive fluorescein sodium intravenously will have yellowing of the skin, eyes, and urine that lasts several hours. Rare allergic reactions have been reported with fluorescein sodium and some patients may have nausea. Topical acriflavine 0.05% has also been used as a contrast agent during endomicroscopy and stains the nuclei of cells. However, acriflavine is used less frequently, as it binds nuclei and there is concern for potential mutagenicity. Topical cresyl violet 0.25–1% has been used in a few studies and is also helpful as it functions as a surface chromoendoscopy agent. Cresyl violet highlights the cytoplasm, thus some nuclei can be seen and appear dark.

4. Technique

When performing either eCLE or pCLE, complete the white light portion of the endoscopic exam before proceeding with endomicroscopy. This will allow you to select areas to image and will ensure that your contrast agent is still present when you are ready to begin imaging. If you are using topical contrast, clearing the mucosa with water may help you get more even staining of the mucosa. In the colon, a poor bowel preparation will significantly limit the use of topical contrast agents as they will not reach the mucosa and will also limit imaging with intravenous contrast, due to the presence of stool on the imaging window.

When ready to obtain eCLE images, place the tip of the confocal endoscope directly on the mucosa. The imaging window is located on the lower left portion of the tip and can be seen on the edge of the endoscopic image (Fig. 5). Applying suction using the endoscope can help stabilize your position. Once a stable position is obtained, press the home button (button 3), which will return the imaging to

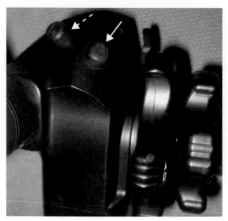

Figure 6 The handle of the confocal endomicroscope. Button 3 (solid arrow) and button 4 (dashed arrow) are used to return the imaging plane to the surface and to section down and up through the mucosa.

the surface (Fig. 6). Press button 4 to begin sectioning down through the mucosa. Depressing the button moves the imaging plane 4 μm deeper. The direction of imaging can be reversed towards the surface by quickly depressing button 4 twice. Microscopic images can be captured using the foot pedal, the mouse, or the touch screen.

To use the pCLE system, the probes are attached to the processor and passed through the instrument channel of a standard endoscope. The tip of the probe is placed directly on the surface of the mucosa and images are acquired. To obtain a stable image with the confocal probe system, a plastic cap on the end of the endoscope can be helpful, such as the plastic caps that come with the endoscopic mucosal resection (EMR) kits. Images can be obtained and saved, as can mosaic video sequences.

5. Complications

Complications during endomicroscopy are rare. The standard risks of endoscopy are present and the additional risk is related to the contrast agent used. All patients who receive fluorescein should be alerted that they will have yellow skin, eyes, and urine for several hours after the procedure.

In one review of 2272 eCLE and pCLE endomicroscopy cases performed at 16 academic medical centers, no serious adverse events were reported. The most common mild adverse reactions reported (1.4% of patients) were nausea and vomiting, transient hypotension, rash, injection site erythema, and epigastric discomfort. However, the package insert for fluorescein sodium and ophthalmologic reviews list several other reported complications, such as seizures, hypotension, syncope, wheezing, thrombophlebitis, and anaphylaxis.

6. Special considerations

6.1. Learning

There are two components needed to acquire competence in endomicroscopy: the technical ability to acquire good quality images and the cognitive ability to interpret the

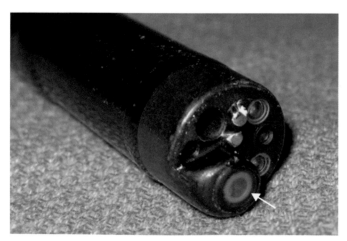

Figure 5 The tip of the confocal endoscope has the normal light channel, and air and water channel, but also has the confocal microscope built into the tip (arrow).

images properly. To learn endomicroscopy, it is ideal to perform cases supervised by an endoscopist already trained in endomicroscopy. This can be very helpful when learning to use the imaging systems and acquire stable images. When beginning your endomicroscopy career, start by collecting images in the colon and stomach, as these organs are the easiest to obtain stable images. The esophagus is most challenging, due to the movement of the heart, lungs, and esophageal peristalsis, which can make obtaining a stable image difficult. To track your own learning, record your interpretation for each imaging site and then obtain a mucosal biopsy so you can determine if your endomicroscopic interpretation is correct. Studying endomicroscopic images to become familiar with normal and abnormal microscopic images is also helpful and some resources are listed below.

6.2. Research and informed consent issues

Both the confocal endoscope and confocal probes are commercially available in the USA and Europe. Depending on the planned use at your institution, whether clinical or research or both, you will need to obtain consent from patients for endomicroscopy. The consent forms should include language discussing the risks of the contrast agent used, which typically is fluorescein sodium.

6.3. Further research

Studying endomicroscopic images and learning the tissue patterns is important. Review articles summarizing the latest endomicroscopic research are readily available. The references below have multiple images for review.

- *Atlas of Endomicroscopy*. Kiesslich R, Galle PR, Neurath MF, editors (Springer Medezin Verlag, 2008, Heidelberg). The first book of endomicroscopy, which contains numerous endomicroscopic images, with corresponding pathology and endoscopic images. Discusses endomicroscopic technique in detail, and has sections on normal and abnormal conditions of the GI tract.
- www.endomicroscopy.org A website which includes more information about technique, and case studies that include eCLE images with corresponding histopathology and endoscopic photos.
- www.maunakeatech.com/atlas/atlasmedgi A website which includes an image library of pCLE cases.
- http://daveproject.org Search 'endomicroscopy' and several videos of endomicroscopy are available.

Further Reading

Bojarski C, Gunther U, Rieger K, et al: In vivo diagnosis of acute intestinal graft-versus-host disease by confocal endomicroscopy, *Endoscopy* 41:433–438, 2009.

Dunbar KB, Okolo P 3rd, Montgomery E, et al: Confocal laser endomicroscopy in Barrett's esophagus and endoscopically inapparent Barrett's neoplasia: a prospective, randomized, double-blind, controlled, crossover trial, *Gastrointest Endosc* 70:645–654, 2009.

Kiesslich R, Burg J, Vieth M, et al: Confocal laser endoscopy for diagnosing intraepithelial neoplasias and colorectal cancer in vivo, *Gastroenterology* 127:706–713, 2004.

Kiesslich R, Goetz M, Burg J, et al: Diagnosing Helicobacter pylori in vivo by confocal laser endoscopy, *Gastroenterology* 128:2119–2123, 2005.

Kiesslich R, Goetz M, Lammersdorf K, et al: Chromoscopy-guided endomicroscopy increases the diagnostic yield of intraepithelial neoplasia in ulcerative colitis, *Gastroenterology* 132:874–882, 2007.

Kiesslich R, Hoffman A, Goetz M, et al: In vivo diagnosis of collagenous colitis by confocal endomicroscopy, *Gut* 55: 591–592, 2006.

Kitabatake S, Niwa Y, Miyahara R, et al: Confocal endomicroscopy for the diagnosis of gastric cancer in vivo, *Endoscopy* 38:1110–1114, 2006.

Leong RW, Nguyen NQ, Meredith CG, et al: In vivo confocal endomicroscopy in the diagnosis and evaluation of celiac disease, *Gastroenterology* 135:1870–1876, 2008.

Lipson BK, Yannuzzi LA: Complications of intravenous fluorescein injections, *Int Ophthalmol Clin* 29:200–205, 1989.

Pech O, Rabenstein T, Manner H, et al: Confocal laser endomicroscopy for in vivo diagnosis of early squamous cell carcinoma in the esophagus, *Clin Gastroenterol Hepatol* 6:89–94, 2008.

Trovato C, Sonzogni A, Fiori G, et al: Confocal laser endomicroscopy for the detection of mucosal changes in ileal pouch after restorative proctocolectomy, *Dig Liver Dis* 41:578–585, 2009.

Wallace MB, Meining A, Canto MI, et al: The safety of intravenous fluorescein for confocal laser endomicroscopy in the gastrointestinal tract, *Aliment Pharmacol Ther* 31:548–552, 2010.

6.2 New endoscopic imaging modalities

Ian Penman, Denis Heresbach

Key Points

- Many novel imaging modalities have been developed in recent years to improve detection and characterization of early neoplasia in the upper and lower GI tract.

- Although several such systems are now commercially available, definite evidence of their superiority over high-resolution white light endoscopy is lacking for most indications.

- Narrow band imaging (NBI) endoscopy, combined with magnification and targeted biopsies, may be superior to systematic or random biopsy protocols for detection of dysplasia in Barrett's esophagus or ulcerative colitis.

- Autofluorescence systems are not yet adequate for detection of early neoplasia and suffer from high false-positive rates but are likely to improve in the near future.

- Other modalities such as optical coherence tomography and spectroscopic methods remain investigational at present.

Introduction

The prognosis of gastrointestinal cancers depends upon their stage at presentation and most recent improvements in diagnostic endoscopy have therefore focused on earlier diagnosis. The introduction of videoendoscopy over 20 years ago was considered a major advance but merely hinted at the technological improvements that were possible in endoscopy. Progress since then has focused on improving image resolution, particularly by using optical or electronic magnification and by increasing the number of pixels and photodiodes per pixel. Monochromatic light or light containing only certain wavelengths or narrow spectral bands and use of wavelengths outside the visible light spectrum (ultraviolet or near infrared) have all recently been developed for endoscopy, as alternatives to standard white light of the visible spectrum. Combined with improvements in image definition and magnification, these novel imaging modalities offer enormous possibilities for diagnosis of early neoplasia. Multiple systems exist either commercially or as prototypes: narrow band imaging (NBI) endoscopy; confocal laser endomicroscopy (CLE); autofluorescence (AFI); optical coherence tomography (OCT); endocytoscopy; spectral fluorescence, and Raman effect or light-scattering spectroscopy.

Two strategies are evolving beyond the impressive technological progress in miniaturizing the charge coupled devices (CCDs) at the tip of a flexible videoendoscope:

- Improving visualization of small lesions, which may not be detectable by white light videoendoscopy
- Determining the architecture and, if possible, the dysplastic nature of a lesion previously detected by videoendoscopy.

To achieve the first of these objectives, NBI and AFI techniques are undergoing clinical validation, while for the second, methods involving CLE, endocytoscopy, OCT or elastic or non-elastic light-scattering spectroscopy (LSS) are being developed. NBI, AFI and CLE methods are currently available commercially, while OCT and other methods are only at the prototype stage of development. The use of these technologies is set to expand, but there are currently few controlled, randomized comparative studies to determine precisely the utility of these new tools in endoscopy. The range of potential applications is wide, but for the moment the main focus is on areas as outlined in Box 1.

1. Technical principles

White light of the visible light spectrum is characterized by a wavelength of 400–700 nm. This light beam is partly absorbed in its tissue target depending on the wavelength but also on the composition of naturally occurring tissue fluorophores and chromophores, and on their vascularity.

1.1. Principle of narrow band imaging (FICE or NBI system)

The penetration of the mucosa and submucosa by light depends on its wavelength and increases as the wavelength approaches infrared. Target tissues can be illuminated by specific wavelengths or a spectral band corresponding to the absorption spectrum of specific structures in the illuminated tissue. Preference may be given to wavelengths with known absorption by certain tissue components. NBI endoscopy conventionally uses three wavelengths at around 430, 460, and 575 nm; the shorter (blue) wavelengths provide better visualization of vascular structures, particularly in the mucosa and, to a lesser degree, the submucosa (Fig. 1). There are several ways of preferentially using these wavelengths and their narrow spectral band (usually 30 or 50 nm), which

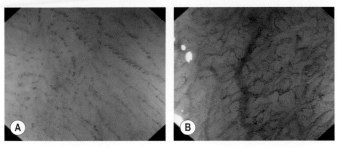

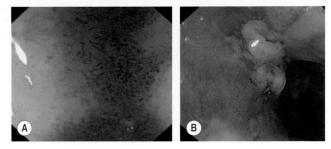

Figure 1 (A) NBI (×115) of squamous esophageal mucosa showing normal IPCL and obliquely running vessels. (B) NBI (×115) image of distal esophagus in a patient with Barrett's. No crypt pattern can be observed but long, thin, regular vessels are noted, consistent with intestinal metaplasia but without dysplasia.

Figure 2 (A) NBI (×115) showing crowded, thickened and irregular IPCLs in a patient with high grade squamous esophageal dysplasia. (B) NBI image of early squamous esophageal carcinoma. Abnormal IPCL vessel pattern and an irregular raised lesion are seen.

can be limited to three bands or, by contrast, a range of 9–12 narrow spectral bands can be offered; a combination of these predetermined (by the manufacturer) or chosen (by the gastroenterologist) provides a wider palette of virtual color and enhancement of the vascular structures and mucosal crypt orifices. Of the methods currently available, the one developed by Fujinon offers a choice of nine narrow bands (FICE system); the method developed by Olympus uses three fixed narrow bands (NBI system); and the iSCAN system from Pentax similarly has nine 'tone enhancement' modes. These are obtained using a mechanical light filter (NBI) or an electronic selection technique based on spectral analysis of the pixels forming the image in each spectral band, which are then reallocated (selected or deleted) to reconstitute an image corresponding to the narrow band

selected (FICE). These selections are made for each of the narrow bands and are then fused to produce a single image. One of the current advantages of FICE technology is that it can be used with a standard endoscope or a high resolution videoendoscope with zoom (>400 000 or up to 800 000–1 million pixels), whereas the advantage of the NBI system is that the narrow band imaging endoscopy can be connected to high definition television (HDTV), which doubles the number of horizontal lines of pixels, producing better horizontal resolution. The drawback of the FICE technique is that it needs a light source and a 4400 series processor, whereas the drawback of the NBI system is that it uses the Exera II system, i.e. a dedicated light source, processor, and specific videoendoscopes. Magnifying videoendoscopes are required in both cases, since fine structures can be enhanced for analysis of fourth-order vessels in the mucosa or the crypt orifice pattern (Figs 2, 3). There is no universally agreed classification system specifically for mucosal lesions using narrow band imaging but most have used magnifying videoendoscopes to examine the superficial vessel networks and crypt openings in the lower esophagus or colon (Table 1).

Box 1 Established and investigational uses of advanced endoscopic imaging modalities

- Detection of intestinal metaplasia, dysplasia or early cancer in Barrett's esophagus.
- Detection of early squamous esophageal neoplasia in high-risk groups.
- Detecting dysplasia during surveillance of chronic ulcerative colitis.
- Detection of flat colonic polyps – reducing miss-rates at colonoscopy.
- Characterization of colonic polyps as hyperplastic or adenomatous.

Clinical Tip

While technical details differ among manufacturers of narrow band imaging systems, all rely on the principle of restricting the spectral bandwidths used for imaging to enhance visualization of surface structures – mucosal crypt patterns and superficial vessel networks.

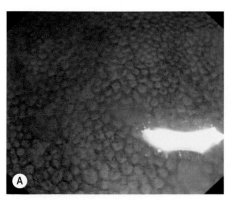

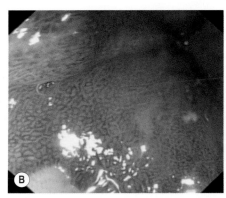

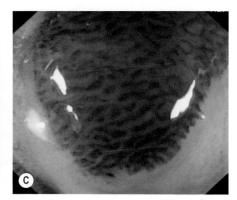

Figure 3 Barrett's esophagus seen at NBI. (A) Type 1–2 round and oval pits. (B) Regular round and oval pits. (C) Type 3 villous/ridged pits.

Table 1 Classification used in narrow band imaging endoscopy or electronic, optical chromoendoscopy (without staining)

Narrow band imaging endoscopy of the esophagus

Squamous cancer of the esophagus

According to Kumagai et al 2002:

IPCL: intrapapillary capillary loops, from fourth-order branching vessels (×80) in the lamina propria of comparable homogeneous appearance.

Spread of squamous cancers of the esophagus.

m1: Thick, irregular pattern, intertwined with the IPCL.
m2: As m1 but with thicker and longer IPCL.
m3: Partial disappearance of the IPCL, partly replaced by thick, dilated vessels.
sm: IPCL entirely absent.

According to Yoshida et al 2004:

IPCL anomaly: (1) dilation or (2) tortuosity or (3) bead-like variation of diameter or (4) of variable appearance and heterogeneous form.

Inflammation and dysplasia of the esophageal mucosa.

Type 1: Normal IPCL (lugol + = normal mucosa).
Type 2: Stretching and moderate elongation of the IPCL (lugol + = esophagitis).
Type 3: 3 of the 4 IPCL anomalies (lugol − = low-grade dysplasia).
Type 4: 4 IPCL anomalies (lugol − = high-grade dysplasia)..

Barrett's esophagus and dysplasia

According to Kara et al 2005:

Type 1: Crypts showing a villous and gyrus-shaped pattern, homogeneous in size and distribution (= intestinal metaplasia).
Type 2: Rounded, circular or oval crypts with regular distribution (= columnar mucosa).
Type 3: Crypts showing a gyrus-shaped pattern, unequal in size and with irregular distribution (= high-grade dysplasia).

According to modified classification of Kara et al 2005:

Mucosal crypt pattern: regular or irregular.
Vascular pattern: regular or irregular.
Abnormal vessels: present/absent (likelihood of early neoplasia increases with increasing number of abnormalities present).

According to modified classification based on Singh et al 2008:

(A) Round pits and regular microvasculature (= columnar mucosa, no intestinal metaplasia).
(B) Villous/ridge pits with regular microvasculature (= intestinal metaplasia).
(C) Absent pits with regular microvasculature (= intestinal metaplasia).
(D) Distorted pits with irregular microvasculature (= HGD)..

Narrow band imaging endoscopy of the stomach

Gastritis

According to Yagi et al 2002: (see Fig. 11)

Z–0: Regular hexagonal capillary network surrounding the crypts and collecting veins spaced and distributed homogeneously.
Z–1: Irregular capillary network and disappearance of collecting veins.
Z–2: Disappearance of the capillary network and presence of pale dilated, elongated crypts.
Z–3: As Z–2, with whitish, dilated crypts surrounded by an erythematous halo.

According to Yao and Oishi 2001:

R: Regular polygonal capillary network surrounding the necks of crypts distributed homogeneously and in the antral region, capillaries resembling springs at the top of islands of mucosa separated by grooves.
I: Irregular capillary network, corkscrew or twig pattern, distributed heterogeneously.
D: Disappearance of the capillary network and a few collecting veins.

According to Sakaki et al 1978:

Stages – FP: Foveolar pattern with round crypts.
FIP: Foveolar intermediate pattern with round, oval crypts.
FSP: Foveolar/sulcus pattern with horseshoe- or doughnut-shaped crypts.
SP: Sulcus pattern with crypts in a groove or convoluted.
MP: Mesh pattern.
Stage distribution.
SP, MP: Pyloric gland area.
FP, FSP: Fundic gland and intermediate area.
FIP: Intermediate area and gastritis with intense cell infiltration.
SP: Severe atrophic gastritis.

Table 1 Continued

Gastric carcinoma

According to Yao et al 2002; Endo et al 2005: (see Fig. 12)

Differentiated mucosal carcinoma:

Hypervascularized capillary network, irregular in size and with a trellis pattern, combining branched and loop patterns.

Undifferentiated mucosal carcinoma:

Few, short capillaries without interconnections, twig pattern.

According to Nakayoshi et al 2004:

Differentiated depressed early cancer (type IIc): fine, dense capillary network.
Undifferentiated depressed early cancer (type IIc): capillary network that is not particularly dense, with a twig or corkscrew pattern.

Narrow band imaging endoscopy of the colon

Colon polyps

According to Machida et al 2004, based on Kudo et al 1994, 2001: (see Fig. 6)

Crypt patterns

Type I: Round crypts, homogeneous in distribution.
Type II: Stellar crypts, homogeneous in distribution.
Type III–L: Tubular, enlarged, curved crypts.
Type III–S: Small round, curved crypts, with dense distribution.
Type IV: Gyrus-shaped convoluted crypts.
Type V: Absence of any classifiable crypt structure.

According to type I and II patterns = normal mucosa or hyperplastic polyp, type III–L or IV = tubular or tubulovillous adenoma, type III–S and V = adenoma with high-grade dysplasia or carcinoma.

According to Machida et al 2004, based on Konerding et al 2001; and Sano et al 2006:

Vascular network pattern (see Fig. 9).

Normal and hyperplastic polyps: regular, hexagonal, honeycomb vascular network around the mucosal glands and crypts with visible first- to fourth-order branching.

Adenomatous polyp: part of the hexagonal vascular network is associated with a denser, shorter capillary pattern, without third- or fourth-order branches or with interrupted blind branches distributed heterogeneously.

Carcinoma: increased density of disorganized vessels with nodular clusters of capillaries.

Note: there is no universally agreed or validated classification specifically for narrow band imaging using FICE or NBI. Most of the classifications described are based on using magnifying videoendoscopes.

1.2. Principle of confocal laser endomicroscopy and endocytoscopy

Confocal laser endomicroscopy is discussed in Chapter 6.1. Endocytoscopy is a contact microscopy technique. After dye spraying with methylene blue, a probe is passed through the operating channel of a standard videoendoscope, with approximately ×1100 magnification and this allows cytological analysis and visualization of the density of cell nuclei.

1.3. Principles of optical coherence tomography

Optical coherence tomography is based on the principle of interferometry, which uses a light beam of a specific wavelength and a defined spectral width. This spectral band is split so that it can be simultaneously directed at the tissue target and at a reference mirror. The two beams thus reflected are recombined and form an interference wave when the distances covered between the source and these two targets are identical. By moving the reference mirror, the reflection of the tissue target can thus be received at variable distances or depths. The wider the spectral band used, the greater the interference wavelength that defines the axial resolution, and the better the definition. Only photons in the light beam from a plane in the tissue target will thus interfere and the intensity of the interference signal will then correspond to a slice image (tomography). If there is a difference in the refractive index between two environments or types of tissue, in this section located equidistantly from the reference mirror, the reflection will be greater and interference intense between the bundle of photons reflected by the slice plane and by the mirror located at the same distance. This measurement, repeated for different reference mirror positions, can be used to obtain an image at the depth of the tissue target analysed. With a source wavelength of 1270 nm and a spectral width of 210 nm, the lateral resolution is approximately 4 μm, but the axial resolution varies between 5 and 15 μm. This wavelength is chosen in the near infrared range so that the light beam penetrates the tissue target deeply enough, to approximately 2 mm.

Optical coherence tomography has an advantage over high-resolution endoscopic ultrasound, since it does not require contact with the tissue target, and it has a resolution of approximately 10 μm compared with 110 μm for 20–30 MHz probes; it nevertheless has the drawback of examining the tissue target to a depth of 2 mm, whereas high-frequency endoscopic ultrasound can examine it to about 20 mm depth. Several optical coherence tomography probes with a diameter of 2.0 and 2.4 mm have been developed using longitudinal or circular scanning. These two methods have a comparable lateral resolution of 10 μm and a field of view of 5.5 × 2.5 mm for the former and 7 mm in diameter for the latter.

1.4. Principle of autofluorescence imaging

Most fluorescence studies originally consisted of point spectral analysis focused on a lesion or a mucosal irregularity detected by other means. It involved the measurement, after laser excitation, of a difference in spectral amplitude for a given wavelength (500 or 630 nm), or of the time taken to observe a reduction in the intensity of the fluorescence emitted (relaxation time). It is only subsequently that autofluorescence has been used for a full inspection of the tissue surface (esophagus or colon), in particular by means of the LIFE-GI (Light-induced Fluorescence Endoscopy for the GastroIntestinal tract) system developed by Xillix Technologies.

Autofluorescence is based on the stimulation of endogenous fluorophores (e.g. NADPH, flavones and collagen) with a short wavelength or ultraviolet light beam that is reflected by fluorophores with a longer wavelength. Some biological processes and changes in tissue composition are associated with specific autofluorescence, with mucosal and submucosal collagen showing green autofluorescence, while dysplastic or neoplastic changes show red or purple autofluorescence (Fig. 4). Early studies with autofluorescence used an excitation probe through the operating channel of a fiberoptic endoscope, using a spectral filter, to emit and receive the fluorescent beams. This approach has been replaced more recently by endoscopic detection of the autofluorescence, using a CCD detector with a simultaneous increase in image resolution and, above all, detection of fluorescence emitted in proximity to its reflection. In this way a good signal:noise ratio can be obtained and signal intensity loss due to photon transmission by the optical fibers can be prevented. In videoendoscopy, by using a single CCD, the conventional image can first be visualized in white light, then detected in autofluorescence, whereas the use of an optical fiber probe requires a filter upstream of the fibers as well as two separate CCDs to capture a conventional image and an autofluorescence image. The only advantage of using optical fibers and spectral filters is that a choice can be made from a larger sample of filters. This is currently more of a theoretical than clinical advantage.

Two autofluorescence detection systems have been developed and tested: the LIFE-GI system and a system from

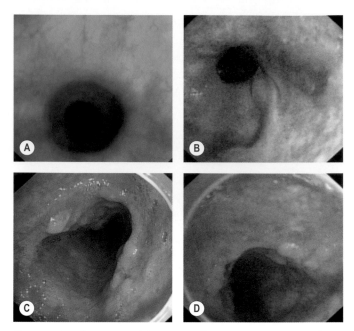

Figure 4 Autofluorescence. (A) Green autofluorescence appearance of normal esophagus (Olympus AFI). (B) Abnormal pale-pink/purple signal can be seen at the top right and bottom left of the image. High-grade dysplasia was confirmed on biopsy of these areas. (C) White light image of squamous carcinoma *in situ*. (D) AFI image demonstrate the lesion as an extensive area of pink signal.

Olympus incorporating two CCDs at the endoscope tip, one for white light and one for autofluorescence. In autofluorescent mode, the excitation light beam emitted by a xenon lamp and monochromatic illumination for the green and red light (550 and 610 nm, respectively) are selected from a rotating filter. For detection, the CCD is connected to a filter, which allows only wavelengths between 490 and 625 nm to pass when the excitation light beam is in autofluorescence, and wavelengths of between 395 and 475 nm for monochromatic illuminations. During detection, the reflection following excitation with blue light is eliminated and the sequential detection of images in autofluorescent mode or from green and red monochromatic excitation beams are integrated to reconstruct an image composed from these three modes of illumination. Clinically, in autofluorescent mode, normal squamous mucosa and non-dysplastic Barrett's esophagus appear green, while tissues containing dysplastic areas or early carcinoma appear purple. Tissue contents rich in hemoglobin appear purple because absorption of a light beam with a wavelength characterizing green light (550 nm) is greater than that of a light beam characterized by the wavelength of red light (610 nm).

> ### ✓ Clinical Tip
>
> Autofluorescence systems offer the possibility of acting as a 'red-flag' system for screening wide areas of mucosa for abnormalities. Inflammation and non-specific tissue thickening are responsible for high false-positivity rates for the detection of neoplasia – use of magnifying narrow band imaging of AFI-positive lesions can significantly improve its positive predictive value.

2. Clinical applications of new imaging techniques

These new imaging techniques have been investigated by 'open-label' studies and case series with few published randomized controlled studies.

2.1. Clinical studies (FICE or NBI system)

Most clinical studies relate to Barrett's esophagus or characterization of colonic polyps. Narrow band imaging in the esophagus examines the vascular network of the lower esophagus and the appearance of mucosal crypts based on descriptions of glands seen during studies of chromoendoscopy. This method was better able to visualize the gastroesophageal junction than standard endoscopy (58% and 17% good quality images, respectively) and was more powerful for detecting areas of intestinal metaplasia with sensitivities of 56% and 24%, and specificities of 95% and 67%, respectively. Numerous other studies have shown that, in Barrett's esophagus, NBI endoscopy can define intestinal metaplasia and detect low- or high-grade dysplasia or early cancer (Fig. 5) with comparable accuracy to chromoendoscopy. For squamous esophageal neoplasia, NBI can detect high-grade dysplasia (Fig. 2) and differentiate mucosal from submucosal involvement as accurately as high resolution magnifying endoscopy. These studies suggest that narrow band imaging endoscopy is an alternative to systematic four-quadrant biopsy protocols for Barrett's surveillance; targeted biopsies of abnormal areas may increase the yield of dysplasia with fewer biopsies.

In the colon, narrow band imaging endoscopy analyses the crypt pattern (Figs 6–8) in a manner similar to chromoendoscopy but also allows definition of vascular network changes (Fig. 9). It has been compared with conventional colonoscopy with chromoendoscopy using 0.2% indigo carmine in 34 patients with 43 polyps to distinguish hyperplastic polyps from adenomas. These two methods had equivalent sensitivity and specificity (100% and 75%, respectively) for diagnosing colonic neoplasia. Both techniques were superior to conventional endoscopy alone, with sensitivity and specificity of 83% and 44%, compared with histological examination. In two further studies, including 43 and 30 patients with 32 and 30 polyps, narrow band imaging endoscopy had a sensitivity and a positive predictive value (PPV) of 94% and 83%, respectively, for the diagnosis of

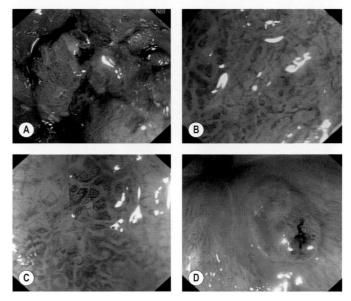

Figure 5 NBI images of early Barrett's neoplasia. (A) Intramucosal carcinoma – irregular pits and irregular and thickened vessels. (B) Magnified image showing absence of crypts and thickened irregular vessel pattern (×115). (C) Irregular crypts and vessel pattern in a patient with low-grade dysplasia (×115). (D) Small intramucosal carcinoma. Absent crypts and thick, irregular vessels can be seen.

adenoma, whereas the PPV and NPV were 74% and 81% in a study of 31 patients, eight of whom had 18 adenomas.

In ulcerative colitis (UC), NBI with targeted biopsies was compared with a systematic biopsy protocol in 11 patients (7 and 42 biopsies on average performed by the two strategies). Both strategies were equivalent and found no dysplasia in seven patients, an 'indefinite dysplasia' lesion in one patient and dysplasia or carcinoma in three patients, suggesting that NBI with targeted biopsies was an alternative to systematic biopsy protocols that require 33–56 biopsies per patient.

In the stomach, NBI can recognize normal crypts (Fig. 10A), vascular changes in gastritis (Fig. 11) but also well- or poorly-differentiated gastric carcinomas (Figs 12, 10B). Few studies have been published but NBI is used mainly by experts in assessment of lesions prior to endoscopic mucosal resection or submucosal dissection of early gastric cancers.

These studies show that for the diagnosis of high-grade dysplasia or early cancer in Barrett's esophagus, NBI is more than simply a clinical practice aid and could be an

Crypts pattern

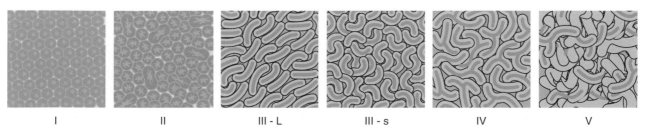

| I | II | III - L | III - s | IV | V |

Figure 6 Colonic polyps Crypts pattern. Type I, evenly distributed, small round crypts; Type II, evenly distributed, star-shaped crypts; Type III–L, tubular crypts, enlarged and curved; Type III–S, round, curved, densely packed crypts with small tails; Type IV, convoluted, cerebriform crypts; Type V, absence of classifiable crypt structures.

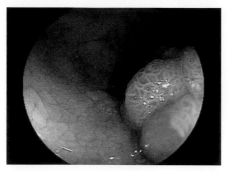

Figure 7 Type III–L pit pattern on the surface of a colonic tubulovillous adenoma.

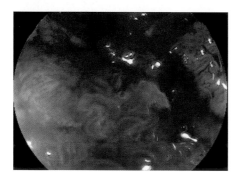

Figure 8 Cerebriform pattern of type IV pits in a villous adenoma.

alternative to the Seattle protocol of systematic four-quadrant biopsies every 1–2 cm. For the detection of dysplasia in UC, emerging data could also support this method as an alternative to multiple random biopsies every 10 cm. For the characterization of polyps, particularly adenomas, NBI is equivalent to chromoendoscopy but, like the latter, its NPV is too low to replace pathological analysis. Recently, a group of international experts has reached a consensus on the relevance of NBI or FICE in daily endoscopic practice (Table 2).

2.2. Clinical application of endoscopy with autofluorescence

Most studies have been conducted with the first-generation LIFE-I system for the examination of the esophagus. In an initial study of 34 patients with short-segment Barrett's esophagus, the yield of 136 biopsies performed after standard esophageal fiberoptic endoscopy was compared with that of

Schematic micro-vascular architecture

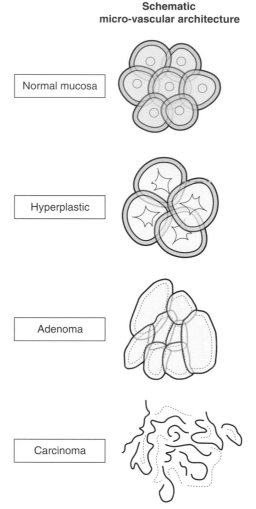

Normal mucosa

Hyperplastic

Adenoma

Carcinoma

Figure 9 Microvascular network of colonic mucosa and polyps at narrow band imaging (NBI). (Modified from Sano Y, Horimatsu T, Fu KI, Katagiri A, Muto M, Ishikawa H. Magnifying observation of microvascular architecture of colorectal lesions using a narrow-band imaging system. Digestive Endoscopy 2006; 18 (Suppl. 1): S44-S51.)

109 targeted biopsies after location by autofluorescence using an optical probe (excitation at 442 nm) through the operating channel of a fiberoptic endoscope. High-grade dysplasia was detected in these two groups in one and seven patients (3% vs 21%), respectively. Per-sample analysis found low-grade dysplasia in 19 and 27% (significant difference) of the samples and high-grade dysplasia in 0.7 and 8.3%

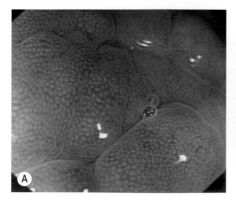

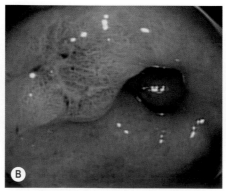

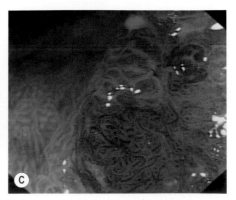

Figure 10 (A) Low magnification NBI image of normal gastric pits. (B) Paris type 0–IIa+c early gastric cancer. (C) The pit pattern is irregular and distorted.

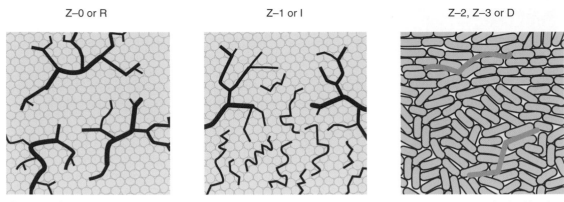

Figure 11 Gastritis. Irregular capillary network and disappearance of collecting veins (type Z–1 or D), presence of pale, dilated and elongated crypts at the level of the gastric mucosa (type Z–2).

Table 2 Statement regarding the usefulness of narrow band imaging endoscopy technology (NBI or FICE)

Condition	Statement	Final expert consensus and evidence grading	
		NBI	FICE
A. Barrett's esophagus	1. NBI and FICE have a high sensitivity and specificity for characterizing esophageal lesions as with and without high-grade dysplasia or cancer, with similar accuracy to chromoendoscopy.	2a, Grade B	2a, Grade C
	2. Random biopsies are still useful after NBI or FICE targeted biopsies for surveillance of Barrett's esophagus to detect flat dysplasia.	2a, Grade B	2a, Grade B
B. Squamous cell carcinoma of the esophagus	3. NBI is helpful for detecting squamous cell carcinoma of the esophagus in high-risk groups compared with standard endoscopy with or without iodine staining.	3b, Grade C	nd
C. Colon	4. NBI or FICE has a high sensitivity and specificity for classifying colonic lesions as neoplastic or non-neoplastic.	1a, Grade A	2b, Grade B
	5. NBI or FICE is equivalent to chromoendoscopy for characterizing colonic lesions.	2b, Grade B	2b Grade B
	6. Neither NBI nor FICE significantly increases adenoma detection rates at colonoscopy in average risk populations.	1b, Grade A	2b, Grade B
D. Ulcerative colitis	7. Random biopsies or chromoendoscopy is still useful after NBI targeted biopsies for surveillance of ulcerative colitis.	2a Grade B	nd

nd, not defined. Responses graded according to the Oxford Centre for Evidence-based Medicine – Levels of Evidence (March 2009). www.cebm.net/index.aspx.

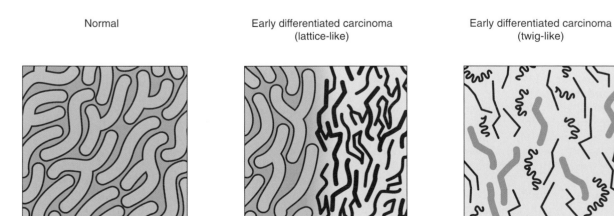

Figure 12 Gastric carcinoma. Normal mucosa (left panel). Well-differentiated early carcinoma: hypervascular capillary network with an irregular mesh pattern (middle panel). Poorly-differentiated early carcinoma sparse, short twig-like capillaries without branching (right panel).

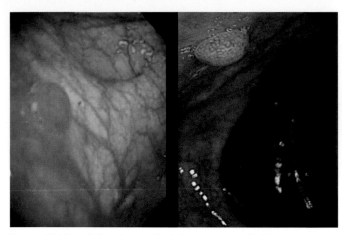

Figure 13 View of dilated, curved tubular crypts (type III–L) in a colonic tubulovillous adenoma. The left-hand panel shows the magenta colour of the polyp with autofluorescence.

(significant difference). A second study compared AFI via an optical probe used through an operating channel with methylene blue chromoendoscopy during fiberoptic videoendoscopy and videoendoscopy with four-quadrant staged biopsies. PPVs for the diagnosis of any grade of dysplasia or cancer were 49% and 58% for AFI and chromoendoscopy, respectively, whereas their NPVs were 69% and 72%, respectively. Per-patient analysis showed that the sensitivity and specificity for this diagnosis were 59% and 78% using AFI, and 71% and 50% using methylene blue chromoendoscopy. A later study tested the second generation LIFE-II system which uses a fiberoptic endoscope with two CCDs in the optical fiber to detect green (490–550 nm) and red (>590 nm) fluorescence. An 'intra-patient' comparison in 50 patients with Barrett's esophagus between LIFE-II autofluorescence and systematic four-quadrant biopsies shows that the sensitivity for the diagnosis of high-grade dysplasia or early cancer was comparable, at 62%. The PPVs for the diagnosis of high-grade dysplasia or early cancer were 41% and 28%, respectively.

These studies show that for the diagnosis of high-grade dysplasia or early cancer in Barrett's esophagus, the LIFE-I or LIFE-II system cannot replace the Seattle protocol of systematic four-quadrant biopsies in clinical practice. The OncoLife system, the latest version of LIFE-II (excluding reflectance interference), is undergoing trials and data are awaited.

In the colon, first-generation LIFE-I system autofluorescence has been compared with standard fiberoptic colonoscopy in 20 patients, six of whom had chronic inflammatory bowel disease. A total of 22 of the 42 samples showed flat dysplasia or a polyp with a PPV for AFI and for standard endoscopy, 91% and 85%, respectively, and a NPV of 90% and 100%. The principle of AFI with image reconstitution has been developed more recently using a videoendoscope in the esophagus and colon (Fig. 13). The CCD detected the various fluorescences, while the filter was positioned at the tip of the videoendoscope (prototype developed by Olympus).

Compared with a standard videoendoscopy in the examination of 23 patients with high-grade dysplasia or early cancer and 18 patients after endoscopic treatment of these lesions, the PPV and NPV of videoendoscopy with AFI were 49% and 89%, respectively. If low-grade dysplasia lesions were included, the PPV increased to 59% and the NPV remained the same. The false positives responsible for a low PPV resulted from acute inflammation. A final study used a prototype Olympus videocolonoscope with AFI to characterize 168 colon polyps as hyperplastic or adenomatous. The sensitivity and specificity of AFI were 89% and 81%, with the adenomas appearing magenta against a green colonic mucosa (Fig. 13), whereas hyperplastic polyps appeared pink: 37 of the 168 polyps were examined using the LIFE-II system with a sensitivity and specificity for the diagnosis of adenoma of 87% and 71%. Color and contrast intensity were better with the videoendoscopy AFI system, compared with optical fibers, accounting for the difference in specificity of 10%.

Overall, AFI by videoendoscopy has a positive and negative predictive value for the diagnosis of dysplasia or early cancer complicating Barrett's esophagus that is comparable with that of systematic four-quadrant biopsy protocols, but it should probably be carried out after antisecretory treatment to minimize false positive results related to acute inflammation and to obtain a NPV applicable in clinical practice. Using magnification with NBI to examine AFI-positive areas can reduce the number of false-positive results considerably and this 'trimodality' imaging may offer significant advantages in the evaluation of Barrett's esophagus. The image contrast and its ease of use make it a technique for the future to reduce the miss-rate for colonic adenomas or to characterize the nature of polyps; the first published results indicate a sensitivity of 90%.

2.3. Clinical application of confocal laser endoscopy (CLE) or endocytoscopy

See Chapter 6.1 for a discussion on the results of confocal laser endomicroscopy studies. This technique will probably have more of a future for CLE probes used through the operating channel of a videoendoscope, additionally equipped with a detection system such as autofluorescence or narrow band imaging endoscopy. Endocytoscopy, even although it uses a vital stain (methylene blue) instead of a fluorochrome injection, can be likened to confocal laser endoscopy. This technique has been tested in 87 patients with neoplasia (38 of the esophagus, 18 of the stomach, and 35 of the colon). Visualization of cell nucleus size and the nuclear-cytoplasmic ratio was of very good quality in 95% of cases. There are currently no clinical or comparative studies that define its positive and negative predictive value in comparison with chromoendoscopy or standard histology.

2.4. Clinical application of optical coherence tomography (OCT)

As regards the esophagus, OCT succeeded in diagnosing intestinal metaplasia in 121 patients with Barrett's esophagus with a sensitivity and specificity of 97% and 92%, respectively, and a PPV of 84%. Another study has reported a PPV and NPV for the diagnosis of dysplasia in Barrett's esophagus, of 53% and 89%, respectively. The sensitivity and specificity for the diagnosis of dysplasia were 68 and 82%, and 50 and 72% for high-grade dysplasia only and 58 and 71% for carcinoma. There was, however, significant inter-observer variation among the endoscopists in their ability to detect dysplasia or early cancer. The technique of optical coherence tomography with longitudinal scanning has also been used to characterize the mucosa of 46 patients with Barrett's esophagus, assigning a score between 0 and 2 to describe reflected wave intensity, mucosal gland irregularity and epithelial layer thickness; by correlating 177 sites biopsied and examined by OCT, a multifactorial score was determined based on the signal intensity of the surface, and on the regularity and dilation of the mucosal glands. By using an integrated score, it was possible to diagnose intramucosal carcinoma or high-grade dysplasias versus other metaplastic lesions or normal mucosa with a sensitivity and specificity of 83% and 75%, respectively.

Examination of the colon by optical coherence tomography using a radial probe has been used to determine criteria in order to characterize and differentiate them. This technology seems promising, particularly when the incident beam is produced by high-power lasers with a resolution, not of 10 µm, but of 1 µm. This technique achieves good visualization of the mucosa with a correlation of 0.84 between measurement of mucosal thickness by histology and by optical coherence tomography with a mean overestimation of 9%. There are, however, no clinical studies in the literature to recommend its use.

2.5. Other methods

Finally, other new endoscopic imaging methods are undergoing validation *ex vivo* or *in vivo* using prototypes which are mainly methods for the focal or point characterization (spectroscopy) of lesions detected by other means. For example, fluorescence with spectral measurement and analysis has yielded useful results for differentiating between neoplastic polyps and hyperplastic polyps in the colon using a short-wavelength monochromatic light for excitation, but other methods such as measurement of the RAMAN effect using a long-wavelength light beam (near infrared) can already characterize *in vitro* the composition and nature of intermolecular bonds in tissue samples and differentiate between hyperplastic polyps and adenomas. Measurement of the scattering of a light beam with a wavelength belonging to the visible spectrum (400–700 nm) with an identical wavelength (elastic scattering) or an increased wavelength (non-elastic scattering) has also been used alone or combined with reflecting measures to characterize cell nucleus density and size in the mucosa or submucosa in previously identified lesions or areas of mucosal irregularity.

Conclusion

Narrow band imaging endoscopy with the FICE or NBI system could be an alternative to systematic four-quadrant biopsy protocols for the diagnosis of high-grade dysplasia or early cancer in Barrett's esophagus. This method could also be effective as an alternative to multiple random biopsies to detect dysplasia in UC. It cannot, however, replace chromoendoscopy for detecting or characterizing polyps. Autofluorescence cannot replace systematic biopsies in Barrett's esophagus and is no better than iodine staining for detecting squamous esophageal carcinomas, but it should prove useful in the future for reducing the number of adenomas missed at colonoscopy or for characterizing the nature of polyps with 90% sensitivity. Confocal laser endomicroscopy is a histological approach, which has the drawback of requiring intravenous injection of contrast medium and previous location of the lesion. If combined with NBI and AFI, it could replace chromoendoscopy and biopsy for the diagnosis of hyperplastic polyps or low-grade dysplasia in Barrett's esophagus.

Further Reading

Adler A, Aschenbeck J, Yenerim T, et al: Narrow-band versus white-light high definition television endoscopic imaging for screening colonoscopy: a prospective randomised trial, *Gastroenterology* 136:410–416, 2009.

Curvers W, Baak L, Kiesslich R, et al: Chromoendoscopy and narrow-band imaging compared with high-resolution magnification endoscopy in Barrett's esophagus, *Gastroenterology* 134:670–679, 2008.

Curvers WL, van den Broek FJ, Reitsma JB, et al: Systematic review of narrow-band imaging for the detection and differentiation of abnormalities in the esophagus and stomach, *Gastrointest Endosc* 69:307–317, 2009.

East JE, Suzuki N, Bassett P, et al: Narrow band imaging with magnification for the characterization of small and diminutive colonic polyps: pit pattern and vascular pattern intensity, *Endoscopy* 40:811–817, 2008.

East JE, Tan EK, Bergman JJ, et al: Meta-analysis: narrow band imaging for lesion characterization in the colon, esophagus, duodenal ampulla and lung, *Aliment Pharmacol Ther* 28:854–867, 2008.

Endo T, Nosho K, Arimura Y, et al: Study of the tumor vessels in depressed-type early gastric cancers using narrow band imaging magnifying endoscopy and cDNA array analysis, *Digest Endosc* 17:210–217, 2005.

Evans JA, Poneros JM, Bouma BE, et al: Optical coherence tomography to identify intramucosal carcinoma and high-grade dysplasia in Barrett's esophagus, *Clin Gastroenterol Hepatol* 4:38–43, 2006.

Haringsma J, Tytgat GN, Yano H, et al: Autofluorescence endoscopy: feasibility of detection of GI neoplasms unapparent to white light endoscopy with an evolving technology, *Gastrointest Endosc* 53:642–650, 2001.

Inoue H, Cho JY, Satodate H, et al: Development of virtual histology and virtual biopsy using laser-scanning confocal microscopy, *Scand J Gastroenterol* 38:37–39, 2003.

Kara MA, Peters FP, Rosmolen WD, et al: High-resolution endoscopy plus chromoendoscopy or narrow-band imaging in Barrett's esophagus: a prospective randomised crossover study, *Endoscopy* 37:929–936, 2005a.

Kara MA, Peters FP, Ten Kate FJ, et al: Endoscopic video autofluorescence imaging may improve the detection of early neoplasia in patients with Barrett's esophagus, *Gastrointest Endosc* 61:679–685, 2005b.

Kara MA, Smits ME, Rosmolen WD, et al: A randomised crossover study comparing light-induced fluorescence endoscopy with standard videoendoscopy for the detection of early neoplasia in Barrett's esophagus, *Gastrointest Endosc* 61:671–678, 2005c.

Kiesslich R, Burg J, Vieth M, et al: Confocal laser endoscopy for diagnosing intraepithelial neoplasias and colorectal cancer in vivo, *Gastroenterology* 127:706–713, 2004.

Konerding MA, Fait E, Gaumann A. 3D microvascular architecture of pre-cancerous lesions and invasive carcinomas of the colon, *Br J Cancer* 84:1354–1362, 2001.

Kudo S, Hirota S, Nakajima T, et al: Colorectal tumors and pit-pattern, *J Clin Pathol* 47(10):880–885, 1994.

Kudo S, Rubio CA, Teixeira CR, et al: Pit pattern in colorectal neoplasia: endoscopic magnifying view, *Endoscopy* 33:367–373, 2001.

Kumagai Y, Inoue H, Nagai K, et al: Magnifying endoscopy, stereoscopic microscopy, and the microvascular architecture of superficial esophageal carcinoma, *Endoscopy* 45:369–375, 2002.

Machida H, Sano Y, Hamamoto Y, et al: Narrow-band imaging in the diagnosis of colorectal mucosal lesions: a pilot study, *Endoscopy* 36:1094–1098, 2004.

Nakayoshi T, Tajiri H, Matsuda K, et al: Magnifying endoscopy combined with narrow band imaging system for early gastric cancer: correlation of vascular pattern with histopathology, *Endoscopy* 36:1080–1084, 2004.

Poneros JM, Brand S, Bouma BE, et al: Diagnosis of specialized intestinal metaplasia by optical coherence tomography, *Gastroenterology* 120:7–12, 2001.

Sakaki N, Iida Y, Okazaki Y, et al: Magnifying endoscopic observation of the gastric mucosa, particularly in patients with atrophic gastritis, *Endoscopy* 10:269–274, 1978.

Sakashita M, Inoue H, Kashida H, et al: Virtual histology of colorectal lesions using laser-scanning confocal microscopy, *Endoscopy* 35:1033–1038, 2003.

Sano Y, Horimatsu T, Fu KI, et al: Magnifying observation of microvascular architecture of colorectal lesions using a narrow-band imaging system, *Dig Endosc* 18(Suppl. 1): S44–S51, 2006.

Sharma P, Weston AP, Topalovski M, et al: Magnification chromoendoscopy for the detection of intestinal metaplasia and dysplasia in Barrett's esophagus, *Gut* 52:24–27, 2003.

Singh R, Anagnostopoulos GK, Yao K, et al: Narrow-band imaging with magnification in Barrett's esophagus: validation of a simplified grading system of mucosal morphology patterns against histology, *Endoscopy* 40:457–463, 2008.

Sivak MV Jr, Kobayashi K, Izatt JA, et al: Narrow-band imaging with magnification in Barrett's esophagus: validation of a simplified grading system of mucosal morphology patterns against histology, *Gastrointest Endosc* 51:474–479, 2000.

Song LM, Adler DG, Conway JD, et al: Narrow band imaging and multiband imaging. ASGE Technology Committee, *Gastrointest Endosc* 67:581–589, 2008.

Tischendorf JJ, Wasmuth HE, Koch A, et al: Value of magnifying chromoendoscopy and narrow band imaging (NBI) in classifying colorectal polyps: a prospective controlled study, *Endoscopy* 39:1092–1096, 2007.

Uedo N, Iishi H, Tatsuta M, et al: A novel videoendoscopy system by using autofluorescence and reflectance imaging for diagnosis of oesophagogastric cancers, *Gastrointest Endosc* 62:521–528, 2005.

van den Broek FJ, Fockens P, Dekker E: Review article. New developments in colonic imaging, *Aliment Pharmacol Ther* 26(Suppl 2):91–99, 2007.

van den Broek FJ, Fockens P, van Eeden S, et al: Endoscopic tri-modal imaging for surveillance in ulcerative colitis: randomised comparison of high-resolution endoscopy and autofluorescence imaging for neoplasia detection; and evaluation of narrow-band imaging for classification of lesions, *Gut* 57(8):1083–1089, 2008.

van den Broek FJ, Reitsma JL, Curvers WL, et al: Systematic review of narrow-band imaging for detection and differentiation of neoplastic and non neoplastic lesion in the colon, *Gastrointest Endosc* 69(1):124–135, 2009.

Wolfsen HC, Crook JE, Krishna M, et al: Prospective, controlled tandem endoscopy study of narrow band imaging for dysplasia detection in Barrett's esophagus, *Gastroenterology* 135:24–31, 2008.

Yagi K, Nakamura A, Sekine A: Comparison between magnifying endoscopy and histological, culture and urease test findings from the gastric mucosa of the corpus, *Endoscopy* 34:376–381, 2002.

Yao K, Oishi T: Microgastroscopic findings of mucosal microvascular architecture as visualized by magnifying endoscopy, *Digest Endosc* 13:S27–S33, 2001.

Yao K, Oishi T, Matsui T, et al: Novel magnified endoscopic findings of microvascular architecture in intramucosal gastric cancer, *Gastrointest Endosc* 56:279–278, 2002.

Yoshida T, Inoue H, Usui S, et al: Narrow-band imaging system with magnifying endoscopy for superficial esophageal lesions, *Gastrointest Endosc* 59:288–295, 2004.

CHAPTER 7

Interventional endoscopy

Mouen Khashab, François Cessot, Sanjay Jagannath

Summary

Key Points

- Apply the 'rule of 3' as a guideline when using bougie dilation to dilate esophageal strictures.
- Do not perform pneumatic dilation in achalasia patients who are not fit for surgery because if perforation occurs, it may require surgical management. Alternative therapeutic options, such as Botox injection, may be better choices.
- Esophageal dilation in the setting of eosinophilic esophagitis (EE) carries a high risk for deep tears and esophageal perforation. Dysphagia due to EE is best treated with topical steroids.
- Use an upper endoscope for high-grade left-sided colonic strictures and a pediatric colonoscope for more proximal strictures.

Introduction

Strictures, both benign and malignant, occur in all regions of the gastrointestinal (GI) tract, but are most common in the esophagus. Dilation of benign strictures is considered definitive therapy, while dilation of malignant strictures is considered palliative therapy, primarily because the response to dilation is short-lived. Malignant strictures are dilated primarily to aid in the successful completion of other endoscopic procedures such as palliative stent placement or endoscopic ultrasonographic tumor staging.

An understanding of the various tools and techniques used to perform safe and effective GI stricture dilation is essential because: (1) strictures are commonly encountered in daily practice and (2) potential serious complications can occur when performing stricture dilation.

1. Clinical and endoscopic assessment

1.1. Esophageal strictures

- Esophagogastroduodenoscopy (EGD) should be the initial diagnostic test in patients who (1) present with dysphagia consistent with an esophageal obstruction; (2) are at least 40 years of age with new onset dysphagia, and (3) in any patient with dysphagia and alarm symptoms (e.g. odynophagia, weight loss, anemia, etc).
- Box 1 depicts the etiologies of mechanical esophageal obstruction.
- Anticoagulants should be discontinued for the procedure, based on existing recommendations (see Ch. 1).
- The risk of bacteremia after esophageal bougienage is 12–22%, which is less than that associated with brushing of teeth. Antibiotic prophylaxis solely to prevent infectious endocarditis is not recommended prior to luminal stricture dilation.
- Patients should fast for at least 4 h prior to the procedure, and ideally 8 h for patients who have eaten food. In certain clinical scenarios, such as achalasia dilation, patients should fast for longer time periods (see below).
- Strictures are anatomically classified into simple or complex strictures. Complex strictures have at least one of the following features: asymmetry, diameter ≤12 mm, or inability to pass the endoscope. Complex strictures that are long or too tight to allow passage of

Box 1 Causes of esophageal strictures

- Peptic injury.
- Schatzki's ring.
- Esophageal webs.
- Esophageal cancer.
- Corrosive injury.
- Radiation therapy.
- Esophageal surgery.
- Eosinophilic esophagitis.
- Sclerotherapy.
- Photodynamic therapy (PDT).
- Endoscopic mucosal resection (EMR).
- Radiofrequency ablation (RFA).
- Cryotherapy.
- Sclerotherapy.
- Infectious esophagitis.
- Pill-induced esophagitis.

an endoscope can be safely dilated under fluoroscopic guidance.
- The esophageal mucosa should be examined for endoscopic features of eosinophilic esophagitis (EE). Esophageal dilation in the setting of EE carries a high risk for deep tears and esophageal perforation. Dysphagia in the setting of EE responds well to topical steroid therapy, and dilation may not be necessary.
- For patients who complain of dysphagia, but do not have an endoscopically visible stricture, empiric esophageal dilation is discouraged. This technique has not been shown to be clinically effective. In addition, the patients may have undiagnosed EE, and dilation in this clinical scenario carries an extremely high risk of complication.

Clinical Tips

- Patients with achalasia may need a prolonged fast prior to dilation because of a higher risk of aspiration due to esophageal stasis.
- Look for endoscopic features of eosinophilic esophagitis: ringed esophagus and mucosal furrows. If EE is suspected, a total of five biopsy specimens must be obtained from the proximal and distal esophagus.
- Do not perform empiric dilation for esophageal dysphagia when a stricture is not identified: it is clinically ineffective and has the potential risk of serious complications.
- Biopsy specimens of the stricture should be obtained to exclude malignancy when the clinical presentation (such as rapid progression of dysphagia or significant weight loss) or the endoscopic appearance (such as the presence of a mass) is suggestive.
- Biopsy specimens of a stricture to rule out occult malignancy should be obtained in patients with strictures that are refractory to dilation.

Box 2 Causes of non-esophageal upper GI strictures

- Peptic ulcer disease.
- Corrosive injury.
- Crohn's disease.
- Radiation therapy.
- Postoperative.

1.2. Gastric, pyloric, and small bowel strictures

- Non-esophageal upper GI (UGI) strictures occur most commonly at the pylorus and manifest as gastric outlet obstruction. Etiologies of gastric or pyloric strictures are illustrated in Box 2. Peptic ulcer disease (PUD) is the most common cause of gastric outlet obstruction.
- Endoscopic dilation of UGI strictures due to Crohn's disease often do not respond long term due to the high recurrence rate.
- The use of fluoroscopy is advocated for strictures that cannot be traversed with the scope.
- Roux-en-Y gastrojejunal bypass (RYGB) is one of the most common surgeries performed today for the treatment of morbid obesity. Gastrojejunal stomas are generally 10–12 mm in diameter. Anastomotic strictures are defined as stomas with diameter <10 mm and occur in 3–28% of these patients.

Clinical Tips

- History of non-steroidal anti-inflammatory drugs (NSAIDs) intake needs to be elucidated in these patients and *Helicobacter pylori* infection needs to be ruled out.
- Prolonged gastric outlet obstruction may result in gastric atony. Response to endoscopic therapy is not immediate in these patients.
- Suspicious strictures must be biopsied to rule out malignancy.

1.3. Ileocolonic and colonic strictures

- Etiologies of ileocolonic and colonic strictures are depicted in Box 3. The most common site for these strictures is at surgical anastomoses.
- Dilation of colonic strictures should only be performed if the patient is symptomatic.
- NSAID colopathy most commonly manifest in the right colon and may lead to colonic strictures with a pathognomonic 'diaphragm type' appearance.

Box 3 Causes of ileocolonic and colonic strictures

- Postoperative.
- Crohn's disease.
- Radiation injury.
- NSAID colopathy.
- Diverticular disease.
- Ischemia.
- Malignancy.

Table 1 Esophageal dilators

	Mercury or tungsten-filled bougies	Wire-guided polyvinyl bougies	Balloon dilators
Dilator type	Maloney Hurst	Savary American Endoscopy Celestin	Through the scope (TTS) Controlled radial expansion (CRE) TTS
Characteristics	Maloney has tapered tip and Hurst has blunt tip	Passed over a guidewire Available diameters 5–20 mm (15–60 French)	May pass over a guidewire Available length 3–8 cm and diameter 6–20 mm (18–60 French)
Advantages	Blind self-home dilation performed by patients	Widely available Inexpensive Relatively safe	Widely available TTS Relatively safe
Disadvantages	Higher perforation rate with blind passage	Endoscope needs to be removed before introducing the dilator	Expensive

2. Equipment

- Diagnostic upper endoscope
- Pediatric colonoscope (for proximal colonic strictures)
- Dilators (Table 1)
- Guidewires
- Fluoroscopy
- Achalasia Rigiflex balloon dilator.

3. Endoscopic techniques

3.1. General principles

3.1.1. Dilation using bougies

- Bougies exert both shearing and radial force and dilate progressively from the proximal to the distal end of the stricture (Fig. 1).
- The initial dilator size chosen should equal the estimated diameter of the stricture.
- Apply the 'rule of 3': Use no more than three dilators successively larger than the first dilator to meet moderate resistance when passed. This rule is a general guideline, and physicians should use their clinical discretion when dilating strictures.
- Savary dilation involves passage of spring-tipped guidewire via the working channel of the endoscope, followed by withdrawal of the endoscope while leaving the guidewire in place (Fig. 2).
- If the stricture is not traversable by the endoscope, then the guidewire is passed through the stricture under fluoroscopic guidance, with the tip of the endoscope placed just above the stricture. The endoscope is then withdrawn leaving the guidewire in place. One should not advance the guidewire if firm resistance is met.
- A conservative approach to dilation is recommended to reduce the risk of perforation. Patients are usually brought back in 1–2 weeks for repeat sessions to achieve sufficient dilation.

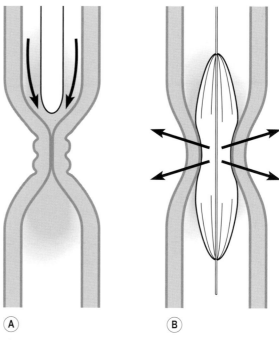

Figure 1 Radial and longitudinal forces. Bougies are associated with longitudinal dilation forces (A), while balloon dilation is associated with radial dilation forces (B).

✓ **Clinical Tips**

- Do not try to accomplish too much dilating in one setting.
- Apply the 'rule of 3' as a guideline when using bougie dilation. Use no more than three dilators successively larger than the first dilator to meet moderate resistance when passed.

3.1.2. Dilation using balloons

- Balloons exert radial force only and the force is applied simultaneously to the entire length of the stricture (Fig. 1).
- The 'rule of 3' does not apply to balloon dilators.

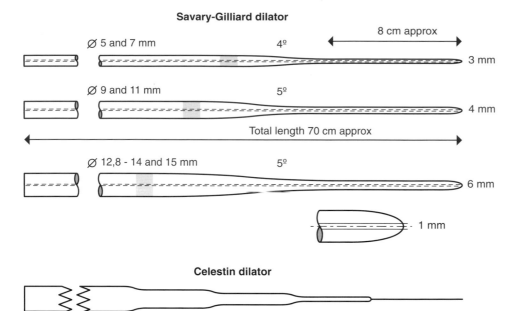

Savary-Gilliard dilator

Ø 5 and 7 mm 4º

8 cm approx

3 mm

Ø 9 and 11 mm 5º

4 mm

Total length 70 cm approx

Ø 12,8 - 14 and 15 mm 5º

6 mm

1 mm

Celestin dilator

Figure 2 Bougies.

- There are multiple TTS balloons that are available in either single or multiple diameters. The balloons may be passed with or without wire guidance (Fig. 3).
- The balloon is advanced through the working channel of an endoscope and then through the stricture under direct endoscopic visualization (Figs 4, 5).
- The balloon should remain inflated for 30–60 s although the optimal duration is not known.
- Fluoroscopic and wire guidance may be used for tight strictures that are not traversable with the endoscope.
- Most widely used balloons are the controlled radial expansion (CRE) TTS balloons, which have three different inflation steps that achieve graded dilation.

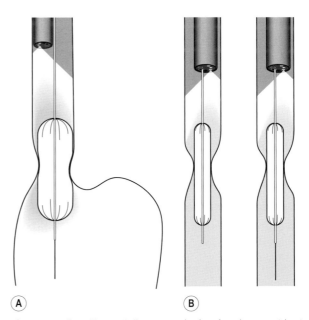

Ⓐ Ⓑ

Figure 3 Balloon dilation. Balloons can also be placed on a guidewire outside the endoscope (A). Through the scope (TTS) esophageal balloons can be non-wire guided (B) or wire guided (C).

Clinical Tips

- It is of the utmost importance to maintain balloon position through the stricture during balloon inflation. The proximal portion of the catheter remaining outside of the endoscope should be held firmly against the endoscope using the endoscopist's left little finger in order to prevent the balloon from slipping out of the stricture as it is inflated. Failure to do so may cause the balloon to slip out of the stricture and only part of the stricture may be dilated. In general, a slow inflation of the balloon to anchor to its initial diameter will secure it in the stricture and minimize the risk of migration. In addition, use of the longer balloon will help to minimize slipping out of the stricture.
- You cannot apply the 'rule of 3' to balloon dilation.
- Inflate the balloon using water and with radiologic product of contrast rather than air, because liquid is less compressible than gas in tight strictures.

symptom relief after dilation, dysphagia recurs in 90% of patients within 3 years. Repeat dilation is advised on a needed basis. There is some evidence that acid suppression may prevent recurrence of Schatzki's rings.
- Webs occur in the upper and mid-esophagus and respond well to bougie dilation.

3.2. Esophageal strictures

- No difference in outcome has been observed between bougie and balloon dilation.
- Schatzki's rings are best treated with passage of single large diameter bougie (16–20 mm) to achieve rupture of the ring. Although most patients experience

Warning!

Do not mistake eosinophilic esophagitis for multiple esophageal webs. These are different pathologies. Eosinophilic esophagitis carries a high risk of perforation, especially if dilation is performed with a single large diameter bougie.

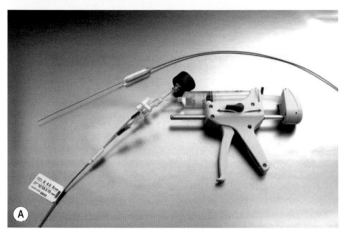
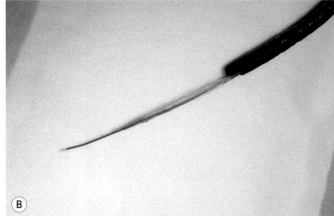
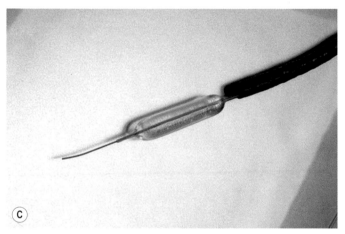
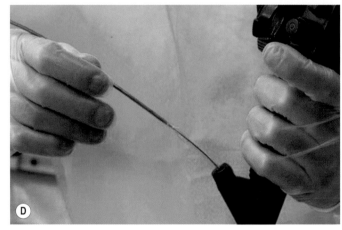

Figure 4 Balloon dilation. Syringe gun, manometer and balloon (A).Through the scope (TTS) balloon (B), and following inflation (C). TTS balloon is inserted into the operating channel (D).

- Peptic strictures may be treated with bougienage (using the 'rule of 3') or balloon dilation. Patients should be placed on proton pump inhibitor (PPI) therapy and strictures will recur in as few as 30% of these patients.
- Corrosive strictures require more dilation sessions and are associated with a higher recurrence rate as compared to peptic strictures. The use of bougies seems most suitable for these strictures.
- Anastomotic strictures are common after esophagectomy, and are most commonly treated with balloon dilation.
- Radiation-induced strictures are best treated with bougie dilation.
- Injection of steroids into benign recurrent or refractory esophageal strictures may improve the outcome of dilation.

✓ Clinical Tips

Steroid injection technique

The procedure involves using 200 mg of triamcinolone (40 mg/mL). Using a standard sclerotherapy catheter, 1 mL aliquots are injected into the distal margin of the stricture in a four-quadrant fashion.

- Dilation of malignant strictures provides only temporary relief of dysphagia that lasts from a few days to 2 weeks and it may be performed using either bougie or balloon dilation. Dilation is usually performed to

Box 4 ASGE guidelines for the performance of esophageal dilation

- Fluoroscopy can be used when using non-wire guided dilators during dilation of complex esophageal strictures or in patients with a tortuous esophagus.
- Bougie and balloon dilators are equally effective in patients with esophageal strictures.
- The 'rule of 3' should be followed when dilation of esophageal strictures is performed with bougie dilators.
- Steroid injection into recurrent or refractory benign esophageal strictures may improve the outcome after esophageal dilation.
- Administration of PPIs is effective in preventing recurrence of esophageal strictures and the need for repeat esophageal dilation.

allow passage of echoendoscope to perform tumor staging, stent placement, or laser therapy.
- ASGE guidelines for the performance of esophageal dilation are summarized in Box 4.

✓ Clinical Tips

- If you are not sure if the stricture is peptic or a Schatzki's ring, treat it as a peptic stricture by using the 'rule of 3'.
- Remember that you only need to dilate the stricture to 13–15 mm diameter to relieve dysphagia.
- PPI therapy improves outcome of peptic stricture dilation. This may also apply to Schatzki's rings.

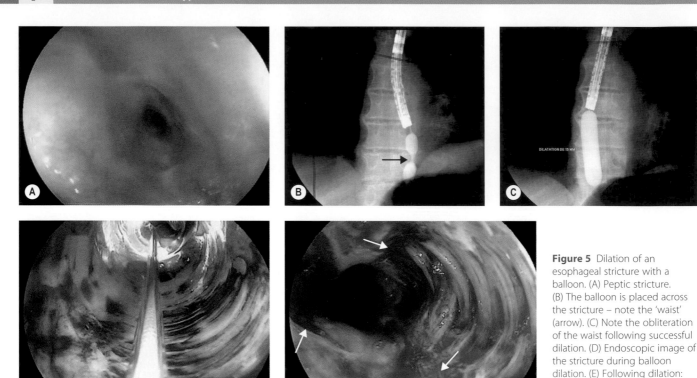

Figure 5 Dilation of an esophageal stricture with a balloon. (A) Peptic stricture. (B) The balloon is placed across the stricture – note the 'waist' (arrow). (C) Note the obliteration of the waist following successful dilation. (D) Endoscopic image of the stricture during balloon dilation. (E) Following dilation: note the presence of several mucosal tears (white arrows).

3.3. Achalasia

- A thorough EGD examination is performed first to clear the esophagus of luminal contents, exclude esophageal or proximal gastric cancer (causing secondary achalasia), determine the extent of esophageal tortuosity, and identify the presence and localization of a hiatal hernia for appropriate localization of the LES fluoroscopically.
- Pneumatic dilation is performed using Rigiflex balloon dilators with balloon diameters of 30 mm, 35 mm, or 40 mm.
- Dilation is generally performed over a guidewire under fluoroscopic guidance initially using a 30 mm balloon. Non-fluoroscopically guided dilation using endoscopic visualization alone is feasible and can be performed safely in expert hands.
- The balloon is first inflated to 3 pounds per square inch (PSI) to confirm appropriate localization of the balloon and looking for a waist in its center. The balloon is then inflated slowly up to a limit of 10 PSI. Complete obliteration of the waist should be noted fluoroscopically.
- A water-soluble contrast esophagram should be obtained after the patient has awakened to rule out procedural perforation.
- Fluoroscopy before and after dilatation should be performed to check for the presence of air in the mediastinum. If this is present it suggests that a perforation has occurred.
- If the initial treatment is unsuccessful, repeat dilation with a larger balloon may be performed at a later setting.
- Patients usually require 2–3 dilations over a 5-year period to remain in symptomatic remission.

Box 5 ASGE guidelines for the performance of pneumatic dilation in achalasia

- Pneumatic dilation with large-diameter balloons is effective for the treatment of achalasia.
- Botulinum toxin therapy is the preferred endoscopic treatment for achalasia in poor operative and non-operative patients.

- Gastroesophageal reflux disease develops in some patients after pneumatic dilation, but it responds readily to PPI therapy.
- ASGE guidelines for the performance of pneumatic dilation in achalasia are summarized in Box 5.

✓ Clinical Tips

- Do not exceed a balloon pressure of 10 PSI because of an increased chance of perforation above this limit.
- Do not perform pneumatic dilation in achalasia patients who are not fit for surgery because if perforation occurs, it may require surgical management. Alternative therapeutic options, such as Botox injection, may be better choices (see below).

3.4. Gastric/pyloric strictures

- Pyloric strictures are mostly treated with balloon dilation although successful treatment using Savary dilators has also been reported in the literature.
- A non-surgical approach for the treatment of these strictures is associated with high failure or recurrence rate. Repeat dilations every 1–2 weeks may be required to try to avoid surgery.

- Long fibrous Crohn's strictures are best treated surgically.
- Pyloric strictures that are not traversable and those that are long and extend to the C loop of the duodenum are best dilated by passing the balloon over a guidewire under fluoroscopic guidance.
- Gastrojejunal anastomotic strictures in RYGB patients can be treated effectively by using either balloon or bougie dilators. Dilation to 15 mm only is recommended to avoid weight regain.

3.5. Small intestinal/colonic strictures

- Use an upper endoscope for high-grade left-sided strictures and a pediatric colonoscope for more proximal strictures. Enteroscopy (push or balloon) can be used to access and dilate strictures beyond the reach of an upper endoscope or colonoscope.
- These strictures are usually treated using balloon dilators. Bougie dilation may be suitable for distal colonic or rectal strictures.
- There is data to suggest that dilating colonic strictures to a diameter larger than 51 French is associated with better outcome. Large diameter balloons (up to 25 mm in size) are available for the treatment of colonic anastomotic strictures.

 Clinical Tip

Most Crohn's strictures occur at previous surgical anastomoses, although de novo stricture may occur and are also amenable to balloon dilation. However, only symptomatic strictures need to be treated!

- Once the stricture is dilated allowing passage of the endoscope, the remaining proximal colon should be examined to evaluate for more proximal strictures. If there is any concern for malignancy, the stricture should be biopsied.
- Colocolonic anastomotic strictures can be dilated to 15–18 mm in one treatment setting. In the setting of ileal or neo-terminal strictures, the initial dilation is taken to 10–12 mm. If there is no symptomatic response, a second dilation to 15 mm is undertaken during a later session. Strictures stemming from Crohn's disease, diverticulitis, ischemia, or radiation therapy are rarely taken past 10–12 mm during the first treatment session.

Clinical Tip

If the colonic stricture cannot be traversed with an endoscope, fluoroscopy is used. Placement of the balloon over a guidewire is helpful for high-grade strictures and those associated with an end-to-side anastomosis. If difficulty is encountered in passing the guidewire across the stricture, a more flexible hydrophilic 0.021 or 0.035 mm ERCP guidewire may be helpful. In the case of near total colonic obstruction, a standard ERCP catheter may be placed over the guidewire and standard contrast will be used to determine the length and geometry of the stricture.

4. Complications

- The most serious complication of esophageal dilation is perforation which occurs in 0.1–0.4% of procedures (Box 6).
- The published rate of perforation following dilation of malignant esophageal strictures is 10%. However, the actual rate in the hands of experienced endoscopists may be as low as 1–2%.
- The risk of perforation with balloon dilation in achalasia is in the range of 3–4% with a mortality of <1%.
- Perforation rate of 4–7% is reported in small series of balloon dilation of pyloric stenosis.
- Most series describing colonic stricture dilation depicted a complication rate of about 5%.

Box 6   Esophageal perforation

- Occurs in 0.1–0.4% of patients undergoing dilation.
- Risk is higher in complex strictures and radiation induced strictures.
- Perforation should be suspected with symptoms and signs of fever, tachycardia, persistent pain, dyspnea or subcutaneous crepitus.
- Confirm diagnosis with water-soluble contrast esophagram or contrast chest CT.
- Many patients may be managed conservatively with nasogastric tube placement and intravenous antibiotics.
- Some perforations are amenable to treatment with placement of an esophageal stent.

Further Reading

Borotto E, Gaudric M, Danel B, et al: Risk factors of oesophageal perforation during pneumatic dilatation for achalasia, *Gut* 39:9–12, 1996.

Hernandez LV, Jacobson JW, Harris MS: Comparison among the perforation rates of Maloney, balloon, and savary dilation of esophageal strictures, *Gastrointest Endosc* 51:460–462, 2000.

Kochhar R, Makharia GK: Usefulness of intralesional triamcinolone in treatment of benign esophageal strictures, *Gastrointest Endosc* 56:829–834, 2002.

Kuwada SK, Alexander GL: Long-term outcome of endoscopic dilation of nonmalignant pyloric stenosis, *Gastrointest Endosc* 41:15–17, 1995.

Lemberg B, Vargo JJ: Balloon dilation of colonic strictures, *Am J Gastroenterol* 102:2123–2125, 2007.

Pereira-Lima JC, Ramires RP, Zamin I Jr, et al: Endoscopic dilation of benign esophageal strictures: report on 1043 procedures, *Am J Gastroenterol* 94:1497–1501, 1999.

Sgouros SN, Bergele C, Mantides A: Eosinophilic esophagitis in adults: what is the clinical significance? *Endoscopy* 38:515–520, 2006.

7.2 Emergency endoscopy in benign gastrointestinal obstruction

Mouen Khashab, Anne Le Sidaner, Sanjay Jagannath

Key Points

- Patients with acute gastric volvulus may present with Borchardt's triad of pain, unproductive retching, and the inability to pass a nasogastric tube.
- Acute endoscopic reduction of gastric volvulus can be performed using the alpha-loop maneuver.
- An initial attempt at endoscopic detorsion can be followed in stable patients with sigmoid volvulus. Placement of a decompression tube decreases early recurrence.
- Majority of patients with acute colonic pseudo-obstruction (ACPO) respond to neostigmine therapy. Placement of a decompression tube decreases recurrence.
- Patients with ACPO who fail medical and endoscopic therapy should undergo surgical therapy.

Information about the emergency management of gastroduodenal or colonic obstruction due to stricture or malignancy can be found in Chapter 7.3.

Introduction

Gastroduodenal and colonic obstructions are common clinical entities treated by gastroenterologists and surgeons. It is critical to recognize those disease states that are better treated endoscopically and thus avoid the morbidity and mortality of a more invasive approach, e.g. surgery. Gastrointestinal obstruction may result from either mechanical cause or failure of intestinal motility in the absence of obstructing lesions (ileus, pseudo-obstruction). The obstruction should be classified as simple or strangulated, depending on whether there is absence or presence of intestinal ischemia, respectively. Strangulated obstructions have worse outcomes and treatment is generally surgical. Interventional gastroenterologists play a crucial role in the management of simple obstructions.

1. Volvulus

1.1. Gastric volvulus

Gastric volvulus is a rare, potentially life-threatening entity that occurs when the stomach twists upon itself (Fig. 1). By definition, gastric volvulus is rotation of the entire or part of the stomach more than 180°. It is supra-diaphragmatic and associated with a paraesophageal or a mixed diaphragmatic hernia in two-thirds of the cases, and is subdiaphragmatic in the remaining one third. The volvulus is organoaxial in 60%

of cases where the axis passes through the gastroesophageal and gastropyloric junctions, and mesenteroaxial in 40% of cases where the axis bisects the lesser and greater curvatures.

Gastric volvulus can present as: (1) transient event with mild short-lived upper abdominal symptoms; (2) chronic volvulus with mild and non-specific symptoms such as dysphagia, hiccups, early satiety, bloating, heartburn, and upper abdominal discomfort, with symptoms being worse after meals; or (3) acute gastric volvulus which presents with sudden onset of severe pain in the upper abdomen or lower chest and unproductive retching. Some patients present with Borchardt's triad of pain, unproductive retching, and the inability to pass a nasogastric tube.

Although strangulation is more common in organoaxial volvulus, it only occurs in 5–28% of these cases due to the rich blood supply of the stomach. Mesenteroaxial volvulus usually causes incomplete obstruction that may be intermittent in nature.

If gastric volvulus is associated with a diaphragmatic hernia, physical examination may reveal evidence of the stomach in the left chest. Chest X-ray will reveal a gas-filled viscus in the chest. The diagnosis is usually confirmed with a barium upper gastrointestinal study. Upper endoscopy will show twisting of gastric folds at the point of torsion.

! Warning!

- EGD should be avoided if there is suspicion of gastric ischemia or perforation, such as in patients with rebound abdominal tenderness.
- If EGD is performed, the endoscope should be advanced forward gently and air insufflation should be kept to a minimum.

Acute gastric volvulus carries a high mortality risk if not recognized early. Early diagnosis and surgical correction remain the mainstays of therapy. Nonetheless, gastroenterologists still play a crucial role in the diagnosis and management of acute and chronic gastric volvulus.

- Chronic gastric volvulus presents with mild and non-specific symptoms. The endoscopist performing the EGD can recognize the presence of twisted gastric folds, which establishes the diagnosis.
- An endoscopist may diagnose acute gastric volvulus when performing upper endoscopy on a patient with more severe and acute symptoms. Stomach decompression with a nasogastric tube may be attempted. Reduction of an acute volvulus may be achieved with this intervention alone.

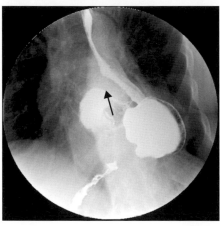

Figure 1 Barium contrast study showing organoaxial gastric volvulus (arrow).

 Clinical Tip

Placement of a nasogastric tube in acute gastric volvulus may be unsuccessful in patients with organoaxial rotation due to complete obstruction at the cardia.

- The gastric mucosa should be inspected carefully for signs of ischemia and necrosis. The examination should be aborted if these signs are present because such patients are at higher risk of perforation with air insufflation.
- If signs of gastric infarction are not present, acute endoscopic reduction of the volvulus may be

 Clinical Tips

The alpha-loop maneuver (Fig. 2)

- The endoscope is slowly advanced through the narrow lumen formed by the twisted gastric folds of the fundus or body into the antrum. Once the antrum is entered, a J-turn maneuver is performed to confirm the passage of the endoscope through the gastric volvulus.
- The endoscope is then withdrawn back into the fundus. The endoscope is retroflexed and advanced with gentle pressure in the proximal stomach to form an alpha-loop. The tip of the endoscope is passed anterior to the retroflexed portion and re-advanced through the narrowed lumen into the antrum.
- The endoscope is then torqued in a clockwise manner to allow untwisting of the alpha-loop and reduction of the gastric volvulus.

considered using the alpha-loop maneuver, which should be performed under fluoroscopic guidance.
- In surgically fit patients, semi-elective laparoscopic gastropexy should follow the reduction of gastric torsion after the patient is stabilized. Associated diaphragmatic hernias should also be repaired.
- In surgically unfit patients, simple endoscopic gastropexy may be performed by placement of one or two percutaneous gastrostomy (PEG) tubes.
- A management algorithm for patients with gastric volvulus is illustrated in Figure 3.

1.2. Colonic volvulus

Colonic volvulus is the third most frequent cause of large bowel obstruction after neoplasms and diverticulitis. Whereas colonic neoplasms and diverticulitis usually result in an open-loop obstruction where the lumen is occluded at a single point along the bowel segment, colonic volvulus occurs when a colonic segment becomes twisted on its mesenteric axis and occludes both ends of the bowel segment resulting in a closed-loop obstruction (Fig. 4). The mesentery gets trapped and the blood supply to the bowel segment becomes strangulated, potentially leading to gut ischemia, necrosis and perforation. Delay in diagnosis and decompression compromises viability of the bowel and is a major cause of mortality.

The sigmoid colon (Fig. 4) and cecum (Fig. 5) are the most frequent sites of colonic volvulus, accounting for 75% and 22% of all cases, respectively. Patients with acute colonic volvulus present most commonly with acute abdominal distension and may have other non-specific symptoms of abdominal pain, nausea, vomiting, and constipation. The diagnosis of colonic volvulus can be made with plain abdominal films (supine and upright) or water-soluble contrast enemas in 85% of the cases.

 Clinical Tips

- The use of barium as the contrast medium during contrast enema studies in patients with suspected colonic volvulus is discouraged because of risk of severe peritonitis in case of bowel perforation.
- A contrast-enema study may occasionally cause volvulus detorsion.

Acute colonic volvulus should be managed on an emergent basis. Patients with colonic necrosis/perforation should be managed surgically. A more conservative approach with an initial attempt at endoscopic detorsion and decompression can be followed in more stable patients (Fig. 6). The benefits of such a strategy are:

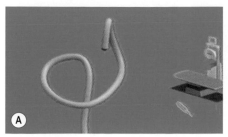 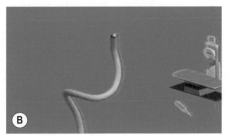 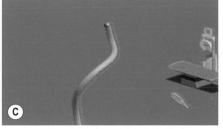

Figure 2 Alpha-loop maneuver. (A) An Olympus magnetic imager showing an alpha loop and (B,C) the reduction of the volvulus, with straightening of the colonoscope.

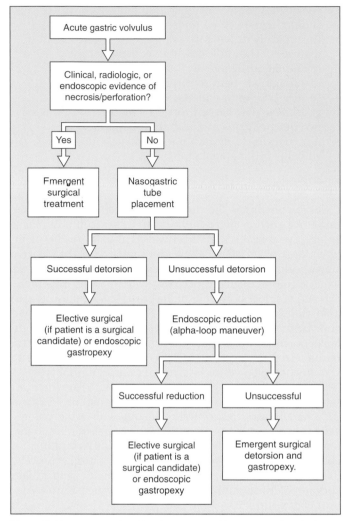

Figure 3   Management algorithm for patients with acute gastric volvulus.

- Avoid emergency surgery on an un-prepped colon with risk of field contamination
- Avoid colostomy and its associated morbidity and mortality
- Improve quality of life by avoiding colostomy
- Allow a one stage semi-elective surgery with the possibility of a laparoscopic approach
- Assess the viability of colonic mucosa.

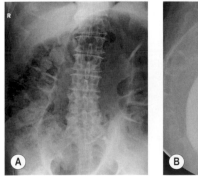
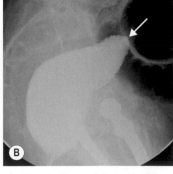

Figure 4 (A) Plain AXR showing grossly distended loop of sigmoid colon. (B) Contrast radiology shows typical 'bird's beak' occlusion at site of volvulus (arrow).

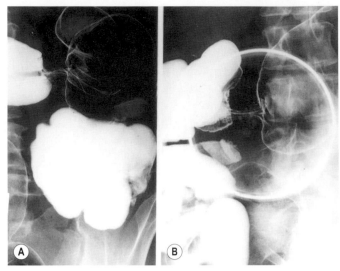

Figure 5   Cecal volvulus. (A) Contrast enema study showing a cecal volvulus. (B) Reduction of the cecal volvulus with rectal tube inserted.

✓ Clinical Tips

Endoscopic treatment of colonic volvulus

- Consult with your surgical colleagues before any attempt at endoscopic management of colonic volvulus.
- Avoid excessive air insufflation to minimize risk of perforation.
- Consider using carbon dioxide, if available, for colonic insufflation.
- Examination should be aborted if there is any evidence of colonic gangrene (e.g. the presence of bloody effluent in the colonic lumen is an indication of bowel gangrene); detorsion should be avoided in these cases as it can precipitate an irreversible septic shock.
- The volvulus should be traversed slowly with a flexible endoscope in the usual manner. A gush of stool is expected after successful detorsion.
- Place a decompression tube over a guidewire to decompress the distended colon and to decrease the early recurrence risk. Early recurrence rate is unacceptably high without tube placement. The tube should be placed on low intermittent suction and should be flushed with 20–30 mL of water or normal saline solution every 6 hours to maintain patency.
- Perform supine and upright abdominal radiography to confirm successful detorsion and to exclude pneumoperitoneum.
- Endoscopic treatment of colonic volvulus is only a temporizing measure.

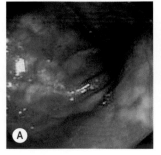
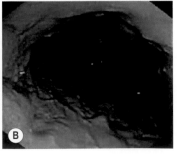

Figure 6   Endoscopic view of a sigmoid volvulus. (A) Before reduction. (B) Following endoscopic reduction.

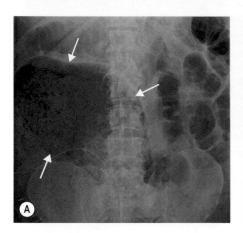

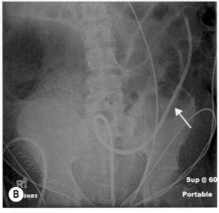

Figure 7 Acute colonic pseudo-obstruction. (A) A large dilated loop of bowel (white arrows). (B) A colonic decompression tube (white arrow) has been inserted as far as the splenic flexure.

> **Warning!**
>
> Endoscopic management of cecal volvulus is less well defined than sigmoid volvulus because of a lower success rate (<33%) and a heightened cecal perforation rate because of the thinned-wall cecum.

Colonic segmental resection and primary anastomosis is considered the treatment modality of choice of colonic volvulus after successful endoscopic detorsion. Non-resectional techniques such as colonopexy and colonostomy carry a substantial risk of recurrence, but may be considered in high-risk patients.

2. Acute colonic pseudo-obstruction

Acute colonic pseudo-obstruction, also known as Ogilvie's syndrome, is a disorder characterized by massive colonic dilation in the absence of colon obstruction. This definition excludes toxic colitis, which occurs in the setting of severe colitis secondary to inflammatory bowel disease or infection. It occurs most often in the setting of surgery and severe medical illnesses, and thus is a disorder of institutionalized patients. Acute colonic pseudo-obstruction is believed to result from autonomic imbalance with suppressed large bowel parasympathetic tone. This results in decreased colonic motility, accumulation of gas and fluid in the colon, increased intraluminal pressure, colonic distension and rising wall tension. Wall tension is highest in the cecum where the

colonic diameter is the largest. This may result in the impediment of cecal capillary circulation and lead to ischemia, gangrene, and subsequent perforation. Plain abdominal radiographs show diffuse dilatation of the colon. A cutoff in the colonic gas is often seen at the hepatic flexure, splenic flexure, or sigmoid region with minimal air distal to the cutoff (collapsed left colon). Unlike toxic colitis, preserved haustral markings, smooth inner colonic contour, and thin colonic wall are present. In contrast to mechanical obstruction, air fluid levels are absent and distension is gaseous (Figs 7, 8). Water-soluble contrast enema is usually needed to rule out a true mechanical obstruction.

> **Clinical Tips**
>
> - Radiographic contrast enemas are frequently needed in patients with acute colonic pseudo-obstruction to rule out mechanical obstruction.
> - Avoid using barium as the contrast medium because of peritonitis risk if perforation occurs.
> - The use of water-soluble contrast enema has a therapeutic effect in some patients by stimulating colonic motility, which sometimes speeds recovery.
> - There is a small risk of colonic perforation with the use of enemas in patients with acute colonic pseudo-obstruction.
> - Computed tomography scan may be needed in some patients to rule out a true mechanical obstruction.
> - *Clostridium difficile* infection should be excluded with appropriate stool testing.

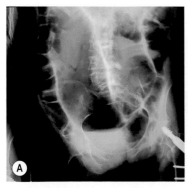

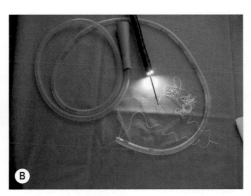

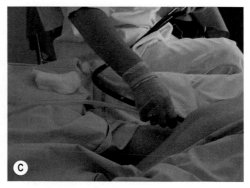

Figure 8 Acute colonic pseudo-obstruction. (A) A plain abdominal film with evidence of large bowel dilation due to pseudo-obstruction. (B) A rectal decompression tube. (C) Insertion of the tube parallel to the colonoscope.

> **Box 1** Treatment of acute colonic pseudo-obstruction: conservative measures
>
> - Patients should be kept nothing by mouth.
> - Nasogastric decompression should be initiated.
> - Test for and correct any electrolyte imbalance (in particular potassium, magnesium, calcium, and phosphorus).
> - Test for and treat thyroid dysfunction.
> - Discontinue or minimize offending drugs, such as narcotics and anticholinergics, if possible.
> - Mobilize patients out of bed if feasible.
> - Manage concurrent illnesses.
> - Obtain abdominal radiographs once every 12–24 h to follow cecal diameter.
> - Serial abdominal examinations should be performed to assess for tenderness, worsening abdominal distension and signs of peritonitis.
> - Water-soluble contrast enemas may be tried to liquefy the stool and stimulate colon motility.

Therapy of acute colonic pseudo-obstruction can be divided into conservative treatment and active interventions. Conservative measures should be tried for 24–48 h, after which the condition usually resolves in most patients (at least in 75% of cases). Active interventions should be implemented if the disease progresses or does not respond to conservative measures.

Active interventions, including treatment with neostigmine and/or colonoscopic decompression, should be considered in patients who do not respond to a maximum of 48 h of conservative therapy, those with extreme abdominal pain, and those with cecal diameter >12 cm.

Neostigmine, an anticholinesterase parasympathomimetic agent, is usually the first medical agent tried in patients who do not have any contraindications to its use.

> **Box 2** Facts about neostigmine
>
> - Three placebo-controlled double-bind randomized trials have documented the effectiveness of neostigmine.
> - The majority of patients (80–90%) will respond to neostigmine with prompt evacuation of flatus and/or stool and a reduction in abdominal distension.
> - It is given as a 2 mg intravenous dose. The dose may be repeated every 3 (or more) hours in case of recurrence.
> - It has a low side-effect profile but potential serious side-effects, such as bronchospasm, bradycardia, hypotension, and seizures may occur. Side-effects are usually short lasting because of the short half-life of neostigmine.
> - Neostigmine should only be given under close cardiac monitoring (continuous EKG monitoring and intermittent blood pressure measurements for 30 min after the dose is given). Atropine should be immediately available and should be given only for severe, prolonged, or symptomatic bradycardia.
> - Other side-effects include salivation, nausea, vomiting, abdominal pain, restlessness, tremor, miosis, and sweating.
> - The elimination half-life is prolonged in patients with renal insufficiency.
> - Absolute contraindications to the use of neostigmine include the following: known hypersensitivity and mechanical urinary or intestinal obstruction. Relative contraindications include recent myocardial infarction, acidosis, asthma, bradycardia, peptic ulcer disease, and therapy with beta-blockers.

> **Box 3** Facts about colonoscopic decompression in patients with acute colonic pseudo-obstruction
>
> - Colonoscopic examination aids in ruling out mechanical obstruction and signs of colonic ischemia or necrosis.
> - Decompression colonoscopy reduces colonic distension and prevents ischemia and perforation.
> - Air insufflation should be kept to a minimum and the use of carbon dioxide, if available, for insufflation is advisable.
> - Initial colonoscopic decompression is successful in about 70% of patients. In up to 40% of cases, the distension recurs requiring repeat colonoscopy.
> - After repeat colonoscopy, the overall clinical success rate increases to 73–85%.
> - Placement of a decompression tube in the right colon (proximal to the splenic flexure) increases the success rate to >90%.
> - Decompression colonoscopy, although technically demanding, can be preformed safely with a reported mortality rate of 1% and a morbidity rate of 3% (mainly perforation risk).
> - It is debatable if colonoscopy should be aborted if signs of colonic ischemia are present.
> - Placement of a decompression tube has been shown to decrease recurrence rate.
> - Colon preps/enemas are not needed because the stool remaining in the colon is usually liquefied and the colonic lumen is distended.
> - Each colonic segment should be decompressed as soon as it is entered with the colonoscope.
> - Cecal intubation is desired (if possible) for cecal examination and complete decompression.
> - A guidewire is placed through the working channel of the colonoscope and advanced to the cecum (or the most proximal point reached by the colonoscope). The endoscope is then withdrawn and the decompression tube is placed over the wire.
> - Fluoroscopy is needed for optimal tube placement to avoid the common problems of coiling of the tube and distal guidewire migration (which usually results in distal placement of the tube in the left colon).
> - The tube should be taped securely to the buttocks, placed on low intermittent suction, and flushed with water or saline every 6 hours to prevent clogging.
> - Daily abdominal radiographs should be obtained to follow colonic diameter and exclude pneumoperitoneum.

Colonoscopic decompression with placement of decompression tube should be performed in patients who fail neostigmine treatment.

Patients who fail medical and endoscopic treatment and those with signs of colonic perforation/necrosis should be treated surgically with cecostomy or colectomy. Figure 9 illustrates an algorithm suggested by the ASGE for treating patients with ACPO.

> **Warning!**
>
> - Conservative treatment alone should only be implemented when pain and abdominal distension are not extreme, and cecal diameter is <12 cm.
> - Conservative treatment alone should be tried for a maximum of 48 hours in patients with tolerable symptoms because perforation risk increases significantly after 4–5 days.

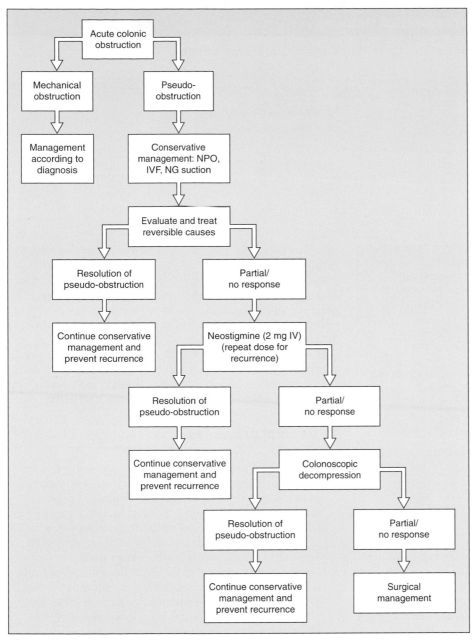

Figure 9 ASGE algorithm for managing patients with ACPO.

Further Reading

Eisen GM, Baron TH, Dominitz JA, et al: Acute colonic pseudo-obstruction, *Gastrointest Endosc* 56:789–792, 2002.

Godshall D, Mossallam U, Rosenbaum R: Gastric volvulus: case report and review of the literature, *J Emerg Med* 17:837–840, 1999.

Loftus CG, Harewood GC, Baron TH: Assessment of predictors of response to neostigmine for acute colonic pseudo-obstruction, *Am J Gastroenterol* 97:3118–3122, 2002.

Madiba TE, Thomson SR: The management of cecal volvulus, *Dis Colon Rectum* 45:264–267, 2002.

Ponec RJ, Saunders MD, Kimmey MB: Neostigmine for the treatment of acute colonic pseudo-obstruction, *N Engl J Med* 341:137–141, 1999.

Renzulli P, Maurer CA, Netzer P, Buchler MW: Preoperative colonoscopic derotation is beneficial in acute colonic volvulus, *Dig Surg* 19:223–229, 2002.

Tejler G, Jiborn H: Volvulus of the cecum. Report of 26 cases and review of the literature, *Dis Colon Rectum* 31:445–449, 1988.

Tsang TK, Walker R, Yu DJ: Endoscopic reduction of gastric volvulus: the alpha-loop maneuver, *Gastrointest Endosc* 42:244–248, 1995.

7.3 Esophageal, duodenal and colorectal stenting

Mouen Khashab, Jean-Christophe Létard, Jean Marc Canard, Sanjay Jagannath

Key Points

- Covered self-expandable metal stents (SEMS) resist tumor ingrowth, may be removable, and have a higher incidence of migration. Uncovered SEMS are non-removable, migrate less often, but tumor ingrowth occurs frequently.
- The various esophageal SEMS are equivalent in technical success, efficacy, and complication rates when used for malignant strictures.
- Patients with malignant gastric outlet obstruction and short life expectancy are best treated with endoscopic stenting.
- Main indications for colonic stenting are bridge to surgery in patients with colorectal cancer who present with colonic obstruction and palliation of inoperable malignant colorectal obstruction.

Introduction

Advances in interventional endoscopy over the last two decades have made an immense impact on clinical care. One such advance is the endoscopic placement of stents for the treatment and palliation of benign and malignant strictures involving the esophagus, duodenum, and colorectal regions of the gastrointestinal tract.

Esophageal cancer is one of the most lethal malignancies in the Western world. The incidence of esophageal cancer is rising at a faster rate as compared to any other GI cancer, and fewer than 50% of cases are curable and the 5-year survival rate is only 5–10%. For these reasons, palliative treatment of esophageal cancer remains an essential part of its management. Palliative esophageal surgery is associated with unacceptably high morbidity and mortality; it has largely been replaced by chemoradiation, brachytherapy, and/or endoscopic therapy. Among the available endoscopic techniques, endoluminal stenting is the most commonly employed because of its efficacy and wide availability.

Tumors involving the gastric outlet or the duodenum cause symptoms and signs of gastric outlet obstruction. Neoplasms that most commonly result in gastric outlet obstruction include pancreatic cancer, gastric cancer, carcinoid tumor, and metastases from other primary malignancies. Multiple studies have shown that palliative stent placement for unresectable tumors, as compared with palliative surgery, is more efficacious, cost-effective, and is associated with less morbidity and mortality.

Colorectal cancer, the third leading cause of new cancer diagnoses in the USA, often presents with partial or complete colon obstruction. Colorectal stenting has been used effectively for both palliation of malignant obstruction and as a bridge to curative surgery.

This aim of this chapter is to describe the general principles of GI luminal stenting and to focus on the use of endoscopically placed stents to treat benign and malignant obstruction of the esophagus, duodenum, and colon.

1. General principles

- Two broad categories of stents exist currently: self-expandable metal stents (SEMS), and self-expandable plastic stents (SEPS). In the past, semi-rigid plastic stents were used, but were associated with a higher complication rate, longer hospital stay, and worse clinical outcome when compared to SEMS and SEPS. Semi-rigid plastic stents are no longer used.
- Several manufacturers retail SEMS designed specifically for esophageal, duodenal, biliary, or colonic placement. These products differ in their physical properties and characteristics (length, diameter, flared endings, shortening during expansion, rigidity, material, radial expansive force, removability, and delivery systems).
- Covered and uncovered SEMS are available. Covered SEMS are designed to resist tumor ingrowth, while uncovered SEMS embed into the stricture and surrounding tissue. Fully covered SEMS (Fig. 1) may be removable, but have a higher incidence of migration. Uncovered SEMS are non-removable, migrate less often, but tumor ingrowth occurs frequently.
- Covered stents offer better long-term palliation for malignant disease than uncovered stents.
- One self-expandable plastic stent (Polyflex, Boston Scientific, Natick, MA) is available for esophageal use. This stent does not embed into the tissue and is approved by the US Food and Drug Administration (FDA) for benign disease and removability.
- All self-expandable stents may be placed with high rates of technical success with fluoroscopic guidance.

Table 1 FDA-approved expandable esophageal stents

Stent type	Manufacturer	Material	Covering	Deployment diameter (mm)	Release system	Degree of shortening	Features
Ultraflex	Boston Scientific	Nitinol	Partial or uncovered	18, 22	Proximal or distal	30–40%	Proximal flared end, no bare metal ends
Wallstent II	Boston Scientific	Cobalt-based alloy	Partial	20	Distal	20–30%	Flared ends, bare metal ends, reconstrainable
Z-stent	Cook Endoscopy	Stainless steel	Full or partial	18	Distal	None	Flared ends
Z-stent with Dua Antireflux Valve	Cook Endoscopy	Stainless steel	Full	18	Distal	None	Windsock on distal end to prevent gastroesophageal reflux when placed across gastroesophageal junction
Alimaxx-E	Alveolus	Nitinol	Full (internally lined)	18, 22	Distal	None	Internally lined
Polyflex	Boston Scientific	Polyester/silicone	Full	16, 18, 21	Distal	30–40%	Proximal flared end, approved for removability

2. Esophageal stenting

2.1. General concepts

- Of patients with esophageal cancer, 50–60% present with surgically unresectable disease
- Dysphagia is the most distressing symptom
- Dilation only transiently improves dysphagia and carries a significant risk of perforation
- Dilation is primarily used as an adjunct treatment for stenting
- Stenting provides rapid relief of dysphagia
- All esophageal SEMS are covered
- The three most commonly studied SEMS are: Ultraflex, Wallstent, and Z-stent. Other stents exist
- The Polyflex stent is FDA-approved for the palliation of malignant diseases and for the treatment of benign diseases of the esophagus
- Currently available esophageal stents are not placed through the scope.

2.2. FDA-approved expandable esophageal stents (Table 1)

2.2.1. Ultraflex stent

- Ultraflex stent is partially coated (with a polyurethane membrane lining the middle of the stent while the proximal and distal 1.5 cm is uncovered).
- It has an easy-to-use delivery system which is 5.3 mm in diameter and can be deployed from the proximal to the distal end or vice-versa.
- The flared proximal end reduces the risk of food pocket formation between the stent and the wall and anchors the stent to the esophageal wall.

- The stent can theoretically be repositioned, if necessary, by means of a wire at its upper end.
- It is slow to expand (encouraging the patient to start eating again cautiously and gradually).
- Expansion is occasionally incomplete, requiring balloon dilation, which is not always effective. Perforation is rare.
- The Ultraflex stent has no bare metal edges and is less traumatic to the mucosa compared to the Wallstent.

 Clinical Tips

Among all SEMS, the Ultraflex stent produces the least radial expansive force which, in theory, may be clinically relevant:
- Decreased risk of fistula formation
- Decreased risk of perforation
- Diminished efficacy (less relief from dysphagia).

2.2.2. Wallstent II

- This stent is partially coated with bare proximal and distal ends (2 cm on each end).
- It is easy to place and can be repositioned during the procedure. The stent can be recaptured as long as <50% of the stent has been deployed.
- The stent may foreshorten after deployment.
- The stent exerts a high radial force which may translate into better dysphagia relief, but increased post-procedural pain.
- It appears ideal for patients with advanced lesions.

2.2.3. Z-stent

- This stent is available as fully coated or partially coated with exposed flanges.

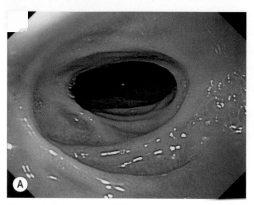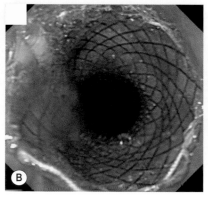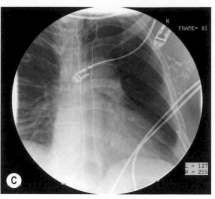

Figure 1 Fully covered SEMS. (A) Patient with multiple esophageal strictures, which were resistant to repeat dilation. (B) Fully covered esophageal stent inserted across the stricture. (C) Fluoroscopic image.

- The delivery system is rigid, and stent assembly is more complicated than other commercially available SEMS.
- A Z-stent with a 'Dua' antireflux valve is available for lesions that extend across the gastroesophageal junction (GEJ). The antireflux valve is an 8 cm extension of the polyurethane coating beyond the distal stent border. This polyurethane 'windsock' creates a one-way valve that shuts, with a rise in intragastric pressure, by collapsing on itself. With further increase in intragastric pressure, the valve can invert to allow vomiting or belching and returns, following a sip of water, to the intragastric position.

2.2.4. Alimaxx-E stent

- This is a relatively new stent and data are limited.
- The delivery system (7.4 mm in diameter) is easy to use.
- It is the only SEMS that is completely covered with a biocompatible membrane.
- The Alimaxx-E stent is the only SEMS in which removability is included in the guidelines for use (not FDA-approved yet).
- To remove the stent, grasp with suture, which is located at the proximal end of the stent, with a rat-tooth forceps. Then, apply firm, continuous traction by pulling on the endoscope in order to 'peel' the stent off the esophageal wall, and thus facilitate relatively atraumatic repositioning or removal.

2.2.5. Polyflex stent

- This is the only available SEPS (Fig. 2).
- The delivery system (diameter of 13 mm) is cumbersome. As such, Polyflex deployment frequently requires predeployment stricture dilation to 12–14 mm.
- It is the only stent approved for treatment of benign diseases of the esophagus and for removability (up to 9 months after placement).

2.3. Technique of stent placement

- The Ultraflex, Alimaxx-E, and Polyflex stents may be placed endoscopically without fluoroscopic guidance; however, fluoroscopic guidance is commonly used.

- The proximal and distal borders of the tumor are marked by endoscopic clips, injection of contrast material using sclerotherapy needle, or placement of external radio-opaque markers (Fig. 3).

> **☑ Clinical Tips**
>
> - If a stricture is not traversable with a standard endoscope, a pediatric endoscope (6 mm diameter) may be used, if available.
> - If the stricture is not traversable with the endoscope, stent placement must be performed under fluoroscopic guidance.
> - The stricture needs to be dilated to allow passage of the delivery system (usually to a diameter of 9–10 mm and not exceeding 12–14 mm).
> - If an endoscope cannot be passed beyond the stricture, the length and geometry of the stricture can be defined using a balloon and water insoluble contrast.

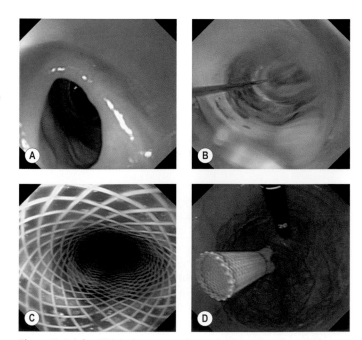

Figure 2 Polyflex. This is the same patient as in Figure 1, with multiple esophageal strictures (A). The strictures were dilated (B) and a Polyflex stent inserted (C). However, this migrated into the stomach (D) necessitating removal and insertion of an fully covered removable SEMS.

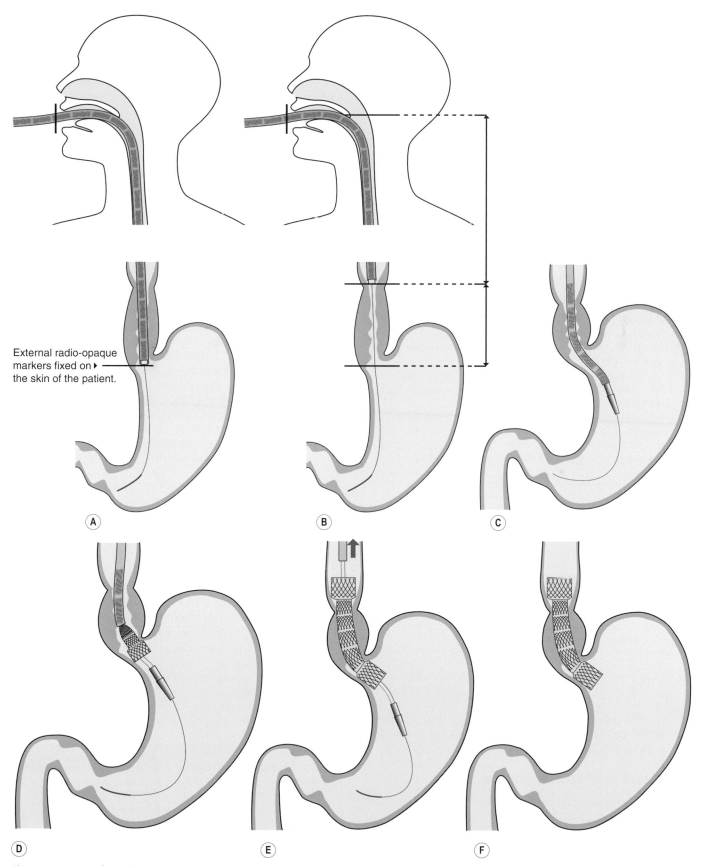

External radio-opaque markers fixed on ▸ the skin of the patient.

(A) (B) (C)

(D) (E) (F)

Figure 3 Insertion of esophageal stent. (A) Placement of radio-opaque marker and guide wire. (B) Measure distance of proximal and distal tumor margins from the teeth. (C) Delivery system through the stenosis. (D) Distal stent deployment. (E) The system is withdrawn. (F) Stent deployed.

Clinical Tip

It is best to have the patient in supine position when external markers are placed, for optimal fluoroscopic visualization. Keep patient in same position during stent deployment.

- A stiff guidewire is positioned in the stomach through the stenosis.
- The scope is withdrawn.
- The delivery system with the stent is passed to the stomach over a stiff guidewire. The system is then withdrawn and the stent deployed with the assistance of fluoroscopy, so that the markings on the stent indicate that placement will be with at least a 2 cm margin proximal and distal to the marked tumor margins.
- Repeat endoscopic examination may be done to confirm the proximal end of the stent is above the proximal tumor margin.

Clinical Tips

- Avoid traversing the stent after deploying it because of migration risk, as the stent has not fully expanded. Full stent expansion takes about 48 h.
- It is crucial to choose the proper stent length that will bridge the entire tumor. This may be accomplished by measuring the tumor length endoscopically or fluoroscopically.
- Remember that the chosen stent should be 2–4 cm longer than the stricture to allow for a 1–2 cm margin above and below the stricture proximal and distal margins. This allows for the covered portion of the stent to cover the stricture, thus reducing tumor ingrowth.

- More than one stent may be needed to cover long strictures. The second stent is placed in the same manner and positioned such that the two stents overlap for a distance of about 1–2 cm.

Clinical Tip

Do not leave an excessive length of stent in the stomach because of the risk of gastric ulceration and bleeding when the stent rubs against the opposite gastric wall.

- If deployment is suboptimal based on fluoroscopic appearance, the stent may be dilated using a TTS balloon.
- Prescribe pain medications and proton pump inhibitor therapy before patient is discharged. Patients should also be advised on specific nutritional guidelines (Box 1).

2.4. Stent retrieval techniques

- The most commonly used method for retrieving stents is to grasp the proximal end of the stent with forceps or endoscopic snares, and then to pull out the endoscope, stent, and forceps/snare as one unit. Injury to the gastric or esophageal mucosa may occur and an overtube or a retrieval hood can be used to minimize this.
- The stent may be removed using a regular upper endoscope. Some endoscopists prefer using the double-channel therapeutic endoscope with two rat-tooth

Box 1 Nutritional guidelines following esophageal stent placement

- Have liquids for the first 24 h as the stent has not fully expanded.
- Chew all food properly and avoid dense and fibrous foods.
- Eat 5–6 small meals per day if needed.
- Eat slowly and take small bites.
- Sit upright while eating.
- Drink fluids in between meals if one feels 'full' with meals.
- Remain in an upright position at least 30–60 min after eating.
- If food ever feels 'stuck' in your throat, take sips of Coca-Cola. One may repeat this throughout the day, especially before and after meals.

forceps or a rat-tooth forceps and a snare for stent removal.

2.5. Outcome data (efficacy)

- Technical success rates for placement of esophageal SEMS is close to 100%. Placement of SEPS (Polyflex) is more cumbersome and the technical success rate is reportedly lower than that of SEMS (approximately 85%).
- Rapid and prolonged improvement of dysphagia occurs in the majority of patients.
- Polyflex has higher migration rates compared to SEMS, especially when placed across the GE junction.
- Migration rates are higher with benign disease (30–70%) and efficacy is significantly lower. Some studies report long-term improvement in as few as 6% of patients.
- Although the Alimaxx-E stent is not FDA-approved for removability, it is the only SEMS that has an indication for removability. It is currently being widely used to treat both malignant and benign diseases of the esophagus. The stent appears easier to remove if it has been in place for a shorter period of time (e.g. 4–6 weeks).

2.5.1. Fistula formation

- This typically occurs between the esophagus and the respiratory tract. Most common etiologies include esophageal carcinoma, bronchogenic carcinoma, radiation therapy, laser therapy, and esophageal stents. This latter occurrence is due to pressure necrosis at the edge of a previously placed SEMS (due to high radial expansive force).
- Endoscopic placement of a covered SEMS is currently the primary and preferred form of therapy of malignant

Box 2 Take home points

- Newer stents (SEMS and SEPS) are superior to the obsolete semi-rigid plastic stents.
- The various SEMS are equivalent in technical success, efficacy, and complication rates when used for malignant strictures.
- The choice of a particular SEMS depends on device availability, familiarity and personal preference.
- SEPS is approved for removability.
- Benign strictures of the esophagus may be treated with either the Polyflex or the Alimaxx-E stents.
- Migration rates are higher when treating benign strictures.

esophagorespiratory fistula with clinical success rates of 80–100%.

- Patients with persistent ERF may benefit from parallel stent placement: placement of a stent in the esophagus in combination with another stent in the trachea and/or bronchi.

2.5.2. Parallel stent placement

- As mentioned above, this may be performed for non-healing esophagorespiratory fistula.
- Esophageal cancer may invade/encroach the trachea causing dyspnea. In addition, mediastinal tumors causing extrinsic esophageal compression may also cause tracheal/bronchial compression. These patients are best treated with parallel stent placement because of risk of respiratory compromise. Place the tracheal or bronchial stent first.
- Proximal esophageal stents may compress the trachea. A low index of suspicion for tracheal compression is advocated in these patients, especially if they develop dyspnea.
- Complications, including fatal complications, occur more commonly with parallel stent placement because of tissue necrosis caused by the radial expansive force of both stents.

2.5.3. Proximal esophageal carcinoma

- Several small studies have shown that placing esophageal stents very close to the upper esophageal sphincter is feasible. The rate of efficacy is decreased, and there is a greater incidence of foreign body and globus sensation (8%) compared to more distal stents.
- If one chooses to place a stent in the cervical esophagus, close to the upper esophageal sphincter, choose a stent with the following favourable characteristics:
  - Minimal to no foreshortening and a proximal release system to ensure precise deployment
  - Small body diameter of 18 mm or less to minimize globus sensation
  - Compliant characteristics in order to conform to the proximal esophageal anatomy
  - 1–2 mm should be left between the upper esophageal sphincter and the proximal margin of the stent.

2.5.4. Extrinsic compression

- Esophageal stents have been used for palliation of malignant esophageal obstruction due to extrinsic lesions with favorable results.
- The degree of clinical improvement in such is significantly less than that in patients with malignant esophageal obstruction due to intrinsic lesions.

2.6. Complications

Early (or procedure-related) complications of esophageal stent placement occur in 10% of procedures and consist of chest pain, aspiration pneumonia, stent misplacement (can be minimized by choosing a stent 4 cm longer than the length of the stricture) and perforation. Late complications occur in 35–45% of patients and consist of gastrointestinal bleeding, development of ERF, stent migration, food bolus impaction, gastroesophageal reflux, and tumor overgrowth at either end of the stent. Stents placed across the gastroesophageal junction have higher complication rates when compared to stents placed in the mid-esophagus. In like manner, there is a statistically significant increased rate of life-threatening complications and associated increased mortality rate when placing stents in patients with a prior history of chemotherapy or radiotherapy. It appears that tissue integrity is compromised with administration of chemotherapy or radiation therapy, and this predisposes SEMS patients to a higher risk of life-threatening complications. Tumor ingrowth is a late complication that has been reduced with the advent of silicone or polyurethane covering, but unfortunately at the risk of increased stent migration (16% migration rate for covered SEMS vs 4% for uncovered SEMS). Treatment options for management of tumor ingrowth include laser therapy, injection therapy, electrocoagulation, photodynamic therapy, argon plasma coagulator, and placement of an overlapping second SEMS.

Clinical Tips

- When placing a stent across the gastroesophageal junction, choose a large diameter stent to decrease migration risk.
- An antireflux stent may be useful.

3. Duodenal stenting

3.1. General concepts

- Patients with gastric outlet obstruction were historically treated with gastrojejunostomy with or without choledochojejunostomy.
- A recent systematic review of palliative stent placement versus open or laparoscopic gastrojejunostomy for the treatment of patients with malignant gastric outlet obstruction suggested that endoscopic treatment is the preferred modality in patients with short life expectancy (<6 months).
- The two FDA-approved duodenal stents are uncovered and can be placed through the working channel of a therapeutic endoscope (need a working channel ≥3.8 mm).
- It is frequently not possible to traverse the stricture with the endoscope since a therapeutic endoscope is usually warranted.
- Duodenal stents are best placed under fluoroscopic guidance.
- There is usually no need to aggressively dilate the stricture in order to minimize risk of perforation.
- Duodenal stents are not used for benign disease.
- Patients with malignant duodenal obstruction often have or are at risk for biliary obstruction. Consider placing a biliary SEMS prophylactically before placing a duodenal SEMS.
- Duodenal strictures are dilated (18–22 mm) only if biliary drainage is to be performed, since access to the papilla requires the use of a large diameter therapeutic duodenoscope.

3.2. FDA-approved expandable duodenal stents

See Table 2.

3.3. Technique of stent placement

- The insertion procedure of a duodenal stent is similar to that of an esophageal stent (Figs 4, 5).
- Patients with gastric outlet obstruction have high gastric residuals and suction of gastric contents should be performed if possible, to minimize aspiration risk and optimize visualization.
- Patients should be in supine or prone position to optimize fluoroscopic visualization.
- If a patient is deemed high risk for aspiration, consider endotracheal intubation prior to stent placement.

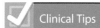

> **Clinical Tips**
> - The status of the biliary tree should be assessed before gastroduodenal stent placement.
> - Placement of SEMS across the papilla will render endoscopic biliary access difficult, if not impossible.

- If the tumor is located in the proximal duodenum without involvement of the papilla, a stent that is long enough to cross the lesion should be chosen, but not excessively long which will prevent access to the papilla. Therefore, accurate assessment of the length and location of the malignant stricture is important.

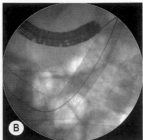
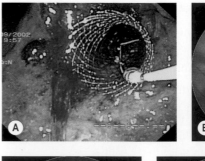
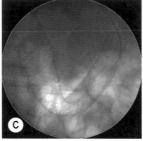
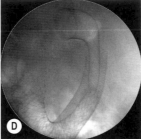

Figure 5 Duodenal stenting. Tumor ingrowth in a previously placed duodenal stent. A wire is placed across the stent under (A) endoscopic and (B) fluoroscopic guidance. A second, followed by a third stent is deployed (C). (D) The final radiographic image with three duodenal stents. (Courtesy of Dr Ian Penman.)

> **Clinical Tips**
> - An expandable metal biliary stent should be placed before the duodenal stent is placed if there is known or impending biliary obstruction.
> - To treat biliary obstruction after placement of a duodenal stent, a percutaneous transhepatic approach is usually required.
> - Stenting of both the duodenum and the bile duct is the non-surgical equivalent of a traditional double surgical bypass (gastrojejunostomy and choledochojejunostomy).

- The stricture may then be accessed with a standard biliary balloon catheter over a guidewire under fluoroscopic guidance. Injecting dye through the stricture may help delineate the length, geometry, and extension of the stricture.
- The selected stent should be about 4 cm longer than the stricture.
- Prior to discharge, patients should be advised to advance from liquids to solids as tolerated and to avoid leafy vegetables, which may result in stent occlusion.

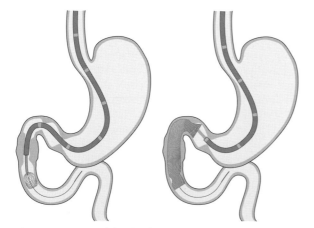

Figure 4 Insertion of duodenal stent.

Table 2 FDA-approved expandable duodenal stents

Stent type	Manufacturer	Material	Covering	Deployment diameter (mm)	Degree of shortening	Features
Wallstent Enteral	Boston Scientific	Cobalt-based alloy	Uncovered	20, 22	40–50%	TTS delivery, reconstrainable
Wallflex Enteral duodenal	Boston Scientific	Nitinol	Uncovered	22	30–40%	Proximal flaring, TTS delivery, reconstrainable

3.4. Outcome data (efficacy) and complications

One systematic review that included 606 patients summarized the published evidence of the effectiveness and safety of gastroduodenal stenting. Technical success and clinical success were achieved in 97% and 89% of patients, respectively. There was no procedure-related mortality and serious complications (bleeding and perforation) were observed in 1.2% of patients. In addition, migration and obstruction (primarily due to tumor ingrowth) occurred in 5% and 18% of patients, respectively.

Jejunal stents may also be placed. These can sometimes be placed with a pediatric colonoscope; however, augmented enteroscopy with double balloon, single balloon or spiral enteroscope (Fig. 6) provide a stable platform for stent insertion.

4. Colonic stenting

4.1. General concepts

- All four FDA-approved colonic stents are SEMS.
- All colonic stents currently in use are uncovered because the use of covered stents in the colon is associated with an unacceptably high migration rate.
- Two SEMS can be placed through the scope (TTS) and the other two are non-TTS.
- Few data exist on the use of colonic stents for the treatment of benign diseases of the colon.
- Main indications for colonic stenting are:
  - Bridge to surgery in patients with colorectal cancer (CRC) who present with total or subtotal colonic obstruction.

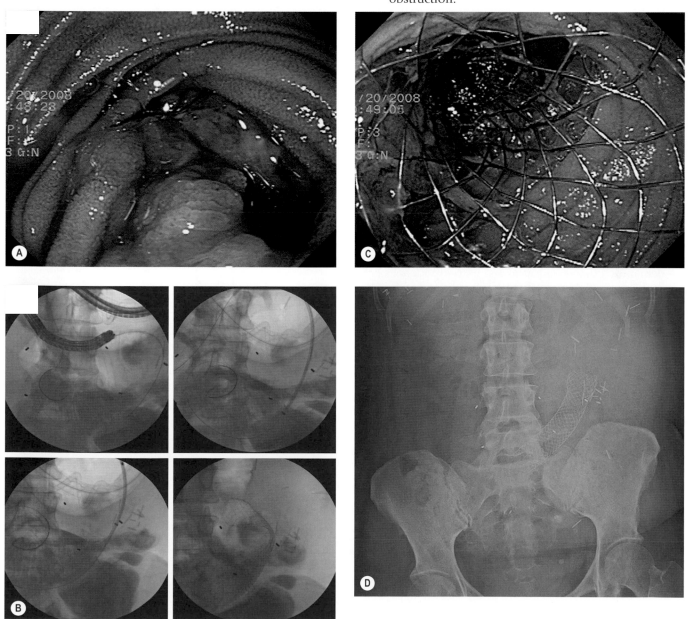

Figure 6 Jejunal stent insertion using spiral enteroscopy. (A) Small-bowel obstruction with tumor. (B) Deployment of SEMS using Endo-Ease Discovery overtube. (C) Endoscopic image of deployed SEMS. (D) Radiographic image of deployed SEMS. (Courtesy of Dr Anne Marie Lennon, from Lennon AM, Chandrasekhara V, Shin EJ, Okolo PI. Spiral-enteroscopy-assisted enteral stent placement for palliation of malignant small-bowel obstruction. Gastrointestinal Endoscopy 2010; 71(2): 422-425.)

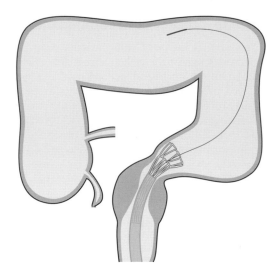

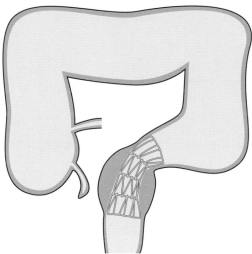

Figure 7 Insertion of colonic stent.

- Palliation of inoperable malignant colorectal obstruction.
- Smaller diameter stents are appropriate for proximal colonic stenting because the stool is still liquefied and smaller diameter stents may carry a lower perforation risk. Larger diameter stents are more appropriate for distal colonic strictures to prevent solid stool impaction within the stent lumen
- Enema preps suffice for patients with total colonic obstruction or distal colonic obstruction. All other patients require standard colonoscopy preparation.

4.2. FDA-approved expandable colonic stents

Table 3.

4.3. Technique of stent placement (Figs 7, 8)

- Placement of colonic stents is more technically demanding than esophageal and gastroduodenal stents. Endoscopic placement alone can be performed for traversable strictures. Because of the frequent complexity of colonic strictures, colonic angulations, and the presence of stool, the use of fluoroscopic guidance is advocated.
- For endoscopic placement alone, a small calibre endoscope is used to traverse the stricture. The stricture can be carefully dilated to 12–14 mm if needed. The geometry and length of the stricture are then determined with the endoscope. Subsequently, the guidewire is placed through the stricture and the scope is withdrawn. Only non-TTS stents may be used since TTS stents do

not fit into the therapeutic channel of a small calibre endoscope. The stent is then placed over the guidewire, the endoscope is positioned just distal to the lesion, and the stent is deployed under endoscopic guidance.
- Combined endoscopic and fluoroscopic placement obviates passage of the endoscope across the stricture. A therapeutic channel endoscope and a TTS-stent may be used. A biliary balloon catheter is passed through the stricture over a stiff guidewire and water-soluble

Table 3 FDA-approved expandable colonic stents

Stent type	Manufacturer	Material	Covering	Deployment diameter (mm)	Degree of shortening	Features
Ultraflex Precision Colonic	Boston Scientific	Nitinol	Uncovered	25	25%	Non-TTS, non-reconstrainable, proximal flaring
Wallstent Enteral	Boston Scientific	Cobalt-based alloy	Uncovered	20, 22	40–50%	TTS delivery, reconstrainable
Wallflex Enteral Colonic	Boston Scientific	Nitinol	Uncovered	22, 25	30–40%	TTS delivery, reconstrainable, proximal flaring
Colonic Z-Stent	Cook Endoscopy	Stainless steel	Uncovered	25	None	Non-TTS

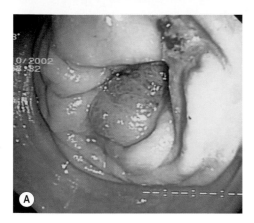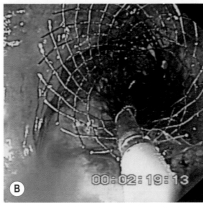

Figure 8 Colonic stent insertion. (A) Malignant colonic obstruction (B) that was palliated with placement of a self-expandable metal stent.

dye is injected to delineate the geometry and length of the stricture. The stent is then placed under endoscopic and fluoroscopic guidance as described previously.
- The stent chosen should be 4 cm longer than the stricture.

4.4. Outcome data (efficacy) and complications

- Table 4 summarizes pooled analysis from a 14-year data collection that included 1198 patients.

- SEMS may be used effectively to treat patients with malignant rectal obstruction within 5 cm from the anal verge (anal pain occurs in 62% of patients).
- SEMS may be used effectively to treat patients with malignant proximal colonic obstruction (technical success 95%, clinical success 85%).
- Colonic stents are generally less effective for palliation of colorectal obstruction due to extrinsic malignant obstruction.

Table 4 Pooled analysis of technical and clinical success rates

	Group	Patients (*n*)	Cumulative (%)
Technical success	Overall	1198	93.2
	Bridge to surgery	407	91.9
	Palliative	791	93.3
Clinical success	Overall	1198	88.6
	Bridge to surgery	407	71.7
	Palliative	791	91

Table 5 Preoperative and palliative colorectal stents complications (n = 826)

Mortality	0.3%
Morbidity	5–10%
Perforation	3%
Migration	9%
Bleeding/pain/tenesmus	10%
Re-obstruction	9% (tumor ingrowth/overgrowth 74%, fecal impaction 20%, migration 6%)

Further Reading

Baerlocher MO, Asch MR, Dixon P, et al: Interdisciplinary Canadian guidelines on the use of metal stents in the gastrointestinal tract for oncological indications, *Can Assoc Radiol J* 59:107–122, 2008.

Baron TH: Expandable gastrointestinal stents, *Gastroenterology* 133:1407–1411, 2007.

Baron TH: Expandable metal stents for the treatment of cancerous obstruction of the gastrointestinal tract, *N Engl J Med* 344:1681–1687, 2001.

Dormann A, Meisner S, Verin N, et al: Self-expanding metal stents for gastroduodenal malignancies: systematic review of their clinical effectiveness, *Endoscopy* 36:543–550, 2004.

Eloubeidi MA, Lopes TL: Novel removable internally fully covered self-expanding metal esophageal stent: feasibility, technique of removal, and tissue response in humans, *Am J Gastroenterol* 104:1374–1381, 2009.

Mougey A, Adler DG: Esophageal stenting for the palliation of malignant dysphagia, *J Support Oncol* 6:267–273, 2008.

Nathwani RA, Kowalski T: Endoscopic stenting of esophageal cancer: the clinical impact, *Curr Opin Gastroenterol* 23:535–538, 2007.

Sebastian S, Johnston S, Geoghegan T, et al: Pooled analysis of the efficacy and safety of self-expanding metal stenting in malignant colorectal obstruction, *Am J Gastroenterol* 99:2051–2057, 2004.

Tierney W, Chuttani R, Croffie J, et al: Enteral stents, *Gastrointest Endosc* 63:920–926, 2006.

7.4 Argon plasma coagulation

Vikesh K. Singh, Jean Marc Canard

Summary

1. General principles 179
2. Equipment 179
3. Technique 179

4. Clinical applications 181
5. Complications 183

Key Points

- Argon plasma coagulation (APC) is a non-contact monopolar electrocoagulation technique.
- APC probes can direct high frequency current towards tissue in a parallel or perpendicular fashion.
- The depth of coagulation is dependent on the properties of the target tissue, the generator power setting, the distance between the probe and tissue, and duration of current application.
- Power settings of 40–60 W and gas flow rates of 1 L/min are used for superficial hemostasis and ablation of vascular ectasias. Power settings of 70–90 W are used for tissue ablation.
- APC is used for the treatment of gastric antral vascular ectasia, angiodysplasia, radiation proctopathy, and residual adenomatous tissue seen after piecemeal colonic polypectomy.

1. General principles

Argon plasma coagulation (APC) is a non-contact monopolar electrocoagulation technique, initially used for endoscopic applications in the digestive tract in 1994 by Grund and Farin. APC is used primarily for superficial hemostasis and tissue ablation.

The probe of the delivery catheter contains a tungsten electrode through which a high frequency electric current is delivered to the target tissue using ionized argon gas (argon plasma). This results in the coagulation of the target tissue. The depth of coagulation is dependent on the power of the electrosurgical generator, the distance between the probe and the target tissue, and the duration of application. The physical properties of the treated tissue also affects the depth of tissue injury. Treated tissue demonstrates three zones of effect. The outermost zone, closest to the probe, is the dessication zone followed by the coagulation and devitalization zone (Fig. 1).

2. Equipment

APC requires a monopolar electrosurgical generator, argon gas source, gas flow meter, flexible delivery catheter, foot activation pedal, and grounding pads.

There are two manufacturers of APC generators (Conmed, Utica, NY and ERBE Electromedizen, Tubingen, Germany). Power can be adjusted between 0 and 150 W and gas flow rates between 0.5 and 7.0 L/min. The flexible delivery catheters are disposable and are available in a 1.5 mm, 2.3 mm, and 3.2 mm diameters with lengths of 220 cm and 300 cm. The most commonly used is the 2.3 mm diameter, 220 cm long catheter. The wider diameter catheters are used if a larger treatment area is required. The 300 cm catheters are used for treatment of lesions in the small bowel during push enteroscopy. Catheters can direct current in a parallel or 'forward firing' versus perpendicular or 'side firing' manner, in relation to the longitudinal axis of the catheter. The 'side firing' probe can be used for lesions which are difficult to access, such as those located behind a fold or around a sharply-angled corner (Fig. 2). The foot activation pedal synchronizes delivery of the current and argon gas which ionizes the argon gas and allows current to be delivered to the target tissue.

Grounding pads are required as APC is a monopolar coagulation technique necessitating that the current circuit is completed via a return electrode.

3. Technique

- Patients requiring colonic APC should be given a full bowel preparation prior to the procedure, even if therapy is to only be directed to the rectum because there is a risk of explosion. It is also imperative to aspirate the gas that is released in the colon during an APC procedure as failure to do so can result in colonic distension.
- Apply the grounding pad. Care must be taken in patients with cardiac pacemakers and defibrillators when using APC. The grounding pad should always be placed away from these devices.
- Check the generator and gas flow settings are appropriate for the desired indication prior to administering APC (Table 1).
- Flush the probe before firing. This should be followed by test firing the probe before inserting the probe into the operating channel of the endoscope.
- Insert the probe until it protrudes slightly from the operating channel with at least one black mark on the probe visible to prevent injury to the tip of the endoscope.
- The probe should be kept 1–2 mm from the target tissue. If the probe is at a distance greater than this, ionization of the argon gas will not occur. Probe

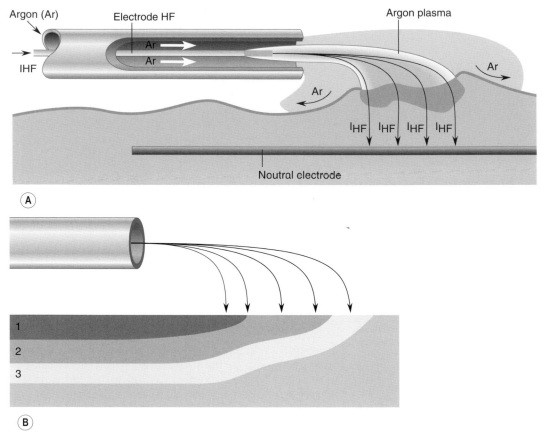

Figure 1 (A) The argon beam follows the path of least electrical resistance and; therefore, will direct itself away from treated tissue to adjacent areas of untreated tissue. This property allows administration of current in both a perpendicular and parallel manner from the tip of the catheter probe. (B) Three zones of effect: (1) dessication (2) coagulation (3) devitalization.

should initially touch the target tissue and then withdrawn prior to firing to ensure the proper distance.

- Take care to make sure that an actively firing probe does not touch the mucosa, as this increases the risk of perforation and allows for the passage of non-ionized gas into open blood vessels.

- Avoid repeatedly firing in the same area as this increases the risk of perforation.
- If an increased distance is required between the probe and the target lesion, increasing the power, as opposed to the gas flow rate, will increase the length of ionized argon gas arc. Alternatively, a 'side-firing' probe can be

Table 1 APC setting

Indication	Power setting (W)	Flow rate (L/min)	Tips
Radiation proctopathy	40–60	1–1.5	If there is extensive hemorrhage, set power to 60 W and wash/ suction blood before therapy
GAVE	40–100	2.0	
Angiodysplasia	40–60	2.0	For cecal angiodysplasias, consider submucosal injection of 2–3 cc of saline and/or dilute epinephrine (1:200000) with a power setting of 50 W and gas flow rate of 2 L/min prior to APC treatment. Application of pulses should be 1 s in duration
Post polypectomy	40–65	0.8–2.0	Use 50 W with short application duration (1–2 s) for right colon and 60–65 W for left colon
Tumor palliation[a]	70–90	2.0	Limit to those patients who are not good candidates for other palliative modalities

[a]For example, in the treatment of occluded esophageal stent, palliation of obstruction in inoperable esophageal cancer or palliation of inoperable gastric cancer. Also when it is impossible to put a stent when the cancer is developed near or on the sphincter superior of the esophagus because the upper part of the stent can 'avoid deglutition'.

used, particularly if the target lesion is located lateral to the probe or is behind a fold.

- Avoid contact with the mesh from a metal stent as the wire may melt.
- Avoid contact with a clip, as conduction of current can cause secondary perforation (particularly in the duodenum).

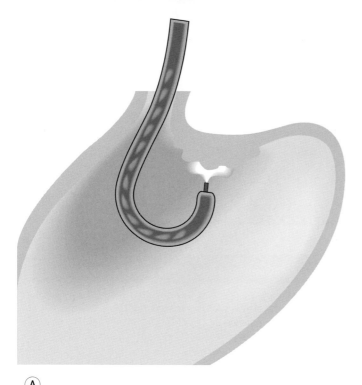

Clinical Tips

How to decrease risk of perforation

- Always apply APC under direct visual control.
- Start with multiple, short activations before using long activations.
- Direct contact of the probe with the mucosa increases the risk of perforation and should be avoided.
- Avoid repeated treatment of the same area.
- Avoid excessive insufflation by asking the nurse to monitor for abdominal distension and suctioning regularly.
- Limit the power of the generator to the level required for adequate coagulation of the target tissue.
- Patients undergoing APC in the colon, even on the rectum, MUST have a full bowel preparation.
- Avoid contact with clips to avoid secondary perforation.

4. Clinical applications

4.1. Radiation proctopathy

APC has been shown to be an effective treatment for gastrointestinal bleeding associated with radiation proctopathy in several case series studies (Fig. 3).

- Patients must have a full bowel preparation, even if only treating the rectum, as there is an increased risk of explosion in an unprepared colon.
- Care should be taken to avoid treatment close to the dentate line.
- Power settings of 40–60 W and gas flow rates of 1–1.5 L/min have been evaluated.
- Treatments are repeated every 1–2 months, with between 1 and 3 sessions usually required.

Complications include post procedure pain, particularly when treatment is administered close to the dentate line. Rare complications which have been reported include transient urinary retention, rectovaginal fistula, and rectal strictures. There are currently no randomized prospective trials comparing APC with laser and medical therapies.

4.2. Vascular lesions

APC is an effective treatment for gastric antral vascular ectasia (GAVE) (Fig. 4) and angiodysplasia (Fig. 5), and prevents recurrent bleeding associated with these lesions.

GAVE (Fig. 4) is an uncommon cause for upper gastrointestinal blood loss associated with cirrhosis and other chronic diseases (Box 1). Involvement of the antrum can be patchy or diffuse. Patients often present with iron deficiency anemia. Improvements in hemoglobin levels and a decrease in transfusion requirements are seen in most patients. However, recurrence can be seen in 30–40% of patients

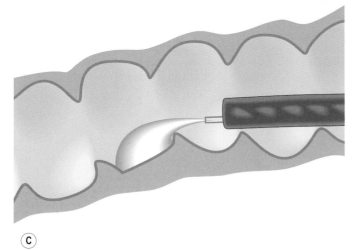

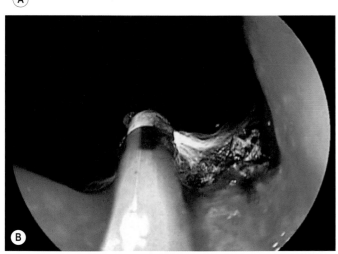

Figure 2 Role of APC in areas which are difficult to access. (A) APC is very useful for treating areas in the retroflexed position. It has the advantage over other modalities of not damaging the endoscope. (B) APC of the cardia. (C) APC is useful for inaccessible blind areas, e.g. behind a fold.

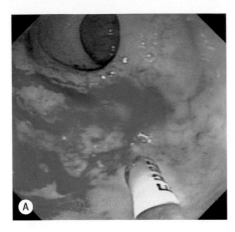

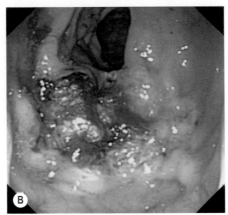

Figure 3 Radiation proctopathy. (A) Rectum with active bleeding from radiation proctopathy. (B) Following APC.

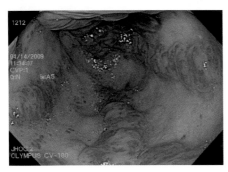

Figure 4 Classic appearance of gastric antral vascular ectasia.

Box 1	Conditions associated with GAVE

- Cirrhosis.
- Collagen vascular disease (e.g. scleroderma).
- Ischemic heart disease.
- Chronic renal failure.
- Pernicious anemia.
- Bone marrow transplant recipients.

between 20 and 30 months after therapy, which often requires further APC treatment.

- Power settings between 40 and 100 W have been used.
- Treatments are repeated every 1–2 months, with between 2 and 3 sessions usually required.

Angiodysplasias (Fig. 5) can be found throughout the gastrointestinal tract and are effectively treated with APC. Angiodysplasias can be found throughout the gastrointestinal tract and are effectively treated with APC.

- The 300 cm probes will often be required to ablate angiodysplasias of the mid and distal small bowel during push enteroscopy.
- Successful ablation of angiodysplasia(s) is indicated by the presence of a white coagulum after treatment.
- APC treatment of diffuse angiodysplasias require moving a probe in an side-by-side and up-and-down arc which is commonly referred to as 'painting' the lesion with short, 1–2 s applications.
- For cecal angiodysplasias, consider submucosal injection with saline and/or dilute epinephrine prior to treatment to reduce the risk of perforation.
- APC therapy significantly improves hemoglobin values and is associated with lower rates of overt bleeding in about 85–90% of patients.

4.3. Treatment of remnant polypoid tissue after piecemeal resection of large colonic polyps

APC has been shown to be effective in devitalizing any remnant polypoid tissue at the rim and base of a piecemeal polypectomy site. Polyps which are large (>1.5 cm), flat, extended, and/or located behind a fold or an angulated area of the colon often require piecemeal resection techniques. Patients undergoing APC have been shown to have significantly fewer recurrences. Treatment should be focused along the rim of the polypectomy site but short applications at the base can also be used. However, there has only been one small randomized study demonstrating these results.

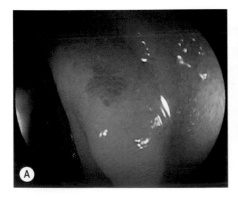

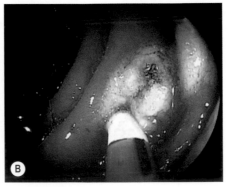

Figure 5 APC treatment of angiodysplasia. (A) Small angiodysplastic lesion before coagulation. (B) Following APC.

4.4. Other applications

APC has been used for palliative debulking of obstructive tumors of the esophagus (Figs 6, 7), stomach, ampulla, and rectum (Figs 8, 9). While symptomatic improvement is seen in >90% of patients, multiple treatment sessions are often required. While there have been few randomized studies, a large series of patients with obstructive esophageal and cardia tumors underwent APC with maintenance of luminal patency in 64% of patients until death.

APC has also been studied as therapy for bleeding peptic ulcers but concerns center on its inability to seal a bleeding vessel and the risk of precipitating further bleeding, especially from arteries >1 mm. Another potential role for APC in the future may be for shortening or trimming metal stents which have become displaced over time to prevent perforation or bleeding.

5. Complications

- Perforation can occur with APC (0.2% in one large study), particularly when treating lesions in the right colon. It is associated with increased power setting, long duration of application, and short probe to tissue distance.

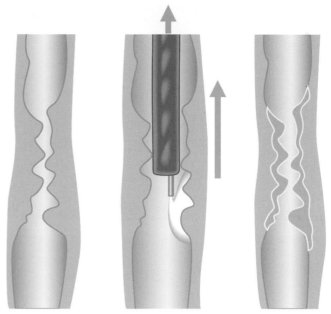

Figure 6 APC for the palliative treatment of an esophageal tumor. Start at the most distal extent of the tumor and work proximally.

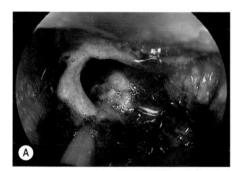 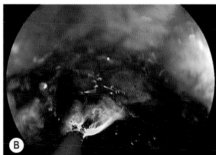 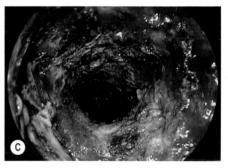

Figure 7 (A) Esophageal cancer pre-treatment. (B) APC treatment of the tumor. (C) Esophageal cancer following treatment.

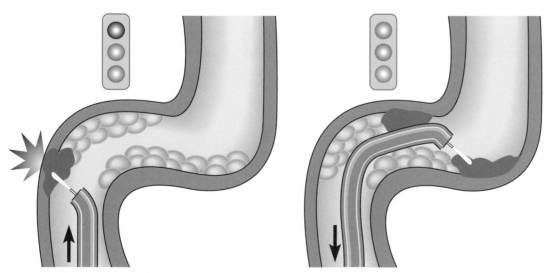

Figure 8 Palliative treatment of a tumor in the sigmoid colon. Start at the most distal extent of the tumor to avoid coagulation in the wrong direction.

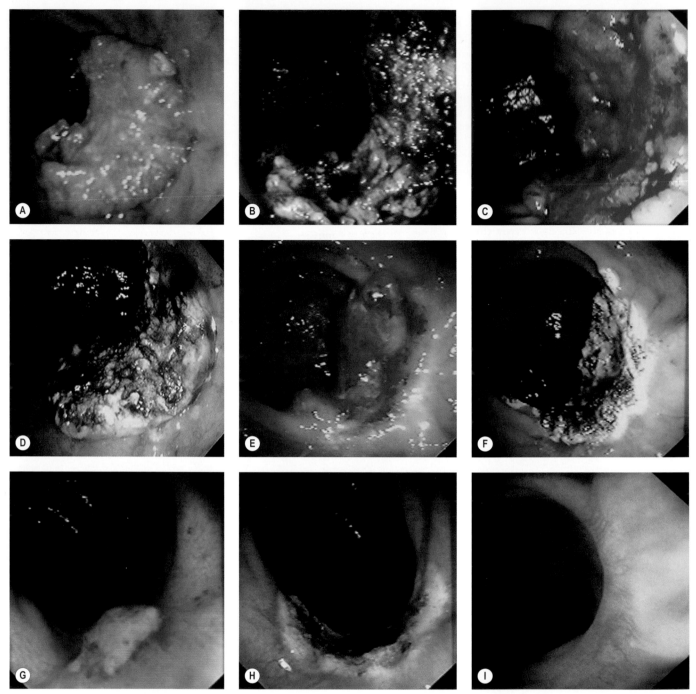

Figure 9 APC treatment for palliation of rectal cancer. (A) Rectal cancer pre treatment. (B) After the first session of APC. (C) Prior to commencing second session of APC. (D) Following second session. (E) Appearance during treatment. (F) Appearance after the session. (G) Appearance before the last session. (H) Last session of APC. (I) Scar with complete destruction. As a result of this example, YAG laser has been replaced with APC.

- Abdominal distension is not uncommon as even a few minutes of application can lead to significant quantities of argon gas release.
- Colonic explosion has been described in patients who had not undergone a full bowel preparation or if a fermentable, sugar-containing laxative is used prior to the procedure.

- APC can also cause a neuromuscular stimulation which can sometimes be painful.
- Rare complications include transient urinary retention, rectovaginal fistula, rectal strictures and subcutaneous empyema.

Further Reading

Canard JM, Fontaine H, Vedrenne B: Electrocoagulation par plasma d'Argon: première expérience française rapportée [Argon plasma electrocoagulation: first French experience reported], *Gastroenterol Clin Biol* 21:A36, 1997.

Canard JM, Vedrenne B: Clinical applications of Argon plasma coagulation in gastro-intestinal endoscopy: has the time come to replace the laser? *Endoscopy* 33(4):353–357, 2001.

Canard JM, Vedrenne B, Bors G. et al: Résultats à long terme du traitement des rectites radiques hémorragiques par la coagulation au plasma d'Argon [Long-term results of the treatment of hemorrhagic radiation proctitis by argon plasma coagulation], *Gastroenterol Clin Biol* 27:455–459, 2003.

Farin G, Grund KE: Technology of argon plasma coagulation with particular regard to endoscopic applications, *Endosc Surg Allied Technol* 2:71–77, 1994.

Dumot JA, Greenwald BD: Argon plasma coagulation, bipolar cautery, and cryotherapy: ABCs of ablative techniques, *Endoscopy* 40:1026–1032, 2008.

Ginsberg GG, Barkun AN, Bosco JJ, et al: The argon plasma coagulator, *Gastrointest Endosc* 55:807–810, 2002.

Manner H: Argon plasma coagulation therapy, *Curr Opin Gastroenterol* 24:612–616, 2008.

Morris ML, Tucker RD, Baron TH, et al: Electrosurgery in gastrointestinal endoscopy: principles to practice, *Am J Gastroenterol* 104:1563–1574, 2009.

Postgate A, Saunders B, Tjandra J, et al: Argon plasma coagulation in chronic radiation proctitis, *Endoscopy* 39:361–365, 2007.

Selinger CP, Ang YS: Gastric antral vascular ectasias (GAVE): an update on clinical presentation, pathophysiology, and treatment, *Digestion* 77:131–137, 2008.

Suzuki N, Arebi N, Saunders BP: A novel method of treating colonic angiodysplasias, *Gastrointest Endosc* 64:424–427, 2006.

Vargo JJ: Clinical applications of the argon plasma coagulator, *Gastrointest Endosc* 54:81–88, 2004.

Jean-Christophe Létard, Marcel Happi Nono

Key Points

- 80–90% of foreign bodies and food bolus impactions pass spontaneously.
- Always assess for perforation.
- Drug packets should never be removed by endoscopy.
- Have a low threshold for seeking anesthetic input to protect the airway.
- Test the instrument you are going to use to remove the foreign body before performing endoscopy.

Introduction

Removal of foreign bodies is a common procedure for gastroenterologists. In the majority of cases the type of foreign body ingested can be determined by a careful history or by speaking to relatives or friends.

The majority (80%) of foreign bodies are ingested by children, with a peak between the ages of 6 months to 3 years. Prisoners, psychiatric patients, alcoholics, patients with a history of digestive surgery or malformations (rings or webs) and edentulous elderly patients are at risk of foreign body ingestion.

The commonest sites for obstruction are the glottis, valleculae, larynx, cricopharyngeal muscle, aortic arch, lower esophageal sphincter, pylorus, ileocecal valve or anus or at areas associated with pathology (i.e. esophageal stricture).

Once in the stomach, most foreign bodies pass through the GI tract without complication within 1–2 weeks (Box 1). Exceptions to this rule are objects longer than 5 cm or wider than 2 cm, which may not pass through the pylorus or duodenum.

If endoscopy is required it is successful in greater than 95% of cases. The majority of series report morbidity rates of less than 5% and usually 0%.

1. Clinical assessment

1.1. Foreign body lodged in the respiratory tract

This should be suspected if the patient has difficulty breathing or has wheezing.

1.2. Foreign body in the upper gastrointestinal tract

The ingestion of a foreign body can cause retrosternal pain, odynophagia, dysphagia, hypersialorrhea and sometimes vomiting in the case of large, obstructive objects. Subcutaneous emphysema can occur with esophageal perforation, while peritonitis suggests small or large bowel perforation. Sharp objects, such as toothpicks, meat or fish bones, razors, lapel badges, dentures or needles, can cause bleeding or perforation.

A high degree of suspicion is required in children or mentally impaired adults as 20–38% of children are asymptomatic, while up to 40% of children or non-communicative adults have no history of foreign body ingestion.

2. Imaging

Plain radiographs in two planes should be performed promptly. Anteroposterior and lateral radiographs of the chest and abdomen should be performed. This allows for localization of the foreign body and will also detect the presence of pneumomediastinum, pleural effusion or subcutaneous air, which are associated with perforation. Anteroposterior and lateral films of the neck and chest should be performed if there is a suspicion of a foreign body in the esophagus versus the trachea (Fig. 1).

Box 1 Outcome of ingested foreign bodies

- 80–90% pass spontaneously.
- 10–20% require endoscopy.
- <1% require surgery.

Clinical Tip

Respiratory tract or esophagus?

A coin with a round face on AP film is usually in the esophagus; if it has a linear surface, it is most likely the trachea owing to the orientation of the vocal cords (see Fig. 1).

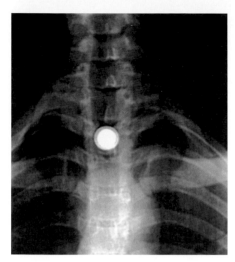

Figure 1 Anteroposterior CXR with characteristic image of a battery in the esophagus. Note the 'Halo' sign which is seen because the two sides have a different diameter. If the battery is in the trachea, it would be seen in profile.

Not all foreign bodies are visible on a plain radiograph. Radio-opaque objects are visible; however, non-radio-opaque objects will not be seen (Table 1). Thus, plain radiographs will miss 50–80% of swallowed bones later identified on endoscopy. Computerized tomography is superior to plain radiographs, and will identify the location of 80–100% of foreign bodies. Barium studies should not be performed due to risk of acute pulmonary edema if aspiration occurs.

3. Timing of endoscopy

Most foreign bodies pass spontaneously and do not require endoscopic intervention. Patients who are symptomatic usually require endoscopy.

Table 1 Radiolucency of foreign bodies

Radiolucency	Foreign body
Radio-opaque	Metal (such as coins), batteries, needles and pins
Not always visualised	Cartilage, meat or fish bones, pieces of plastic and occasionally glass or alloy are not always visualized on plain films
Radiolucent	Food

Foreign bodies obstructing the hypopharynx, sharp or pointed foreign bodies and batteries located in the esophagus should be removed as an emergency.

The majority of foreign bodies which reach the stomach can be watched. Exceptions to this rule are:

- Foreign bodies >2 cm thick or >5 cm long, as they are unlikely to pass through the pylorus and ileocecal valve, and will require endoscopic removal.
- Sharp objects.

4. Equipment

- Diagnostic and therapeutic upper endoscopes should be available
- Rat-tooth or crocodile type forceps (Fig. 2)
- Tripod forceps (Fig. 2)
- Biopsy forceps (Fig. 3)
- Polypectomy snare
- Dormia and Roth baskets
- Overtubes (Fig. 4)
  - Standard (extend past the upper esophageal sphincter)
  - 45–60 cm (extend past the lower esophageal sphincter)
- Rubber hood (Fig. 5).

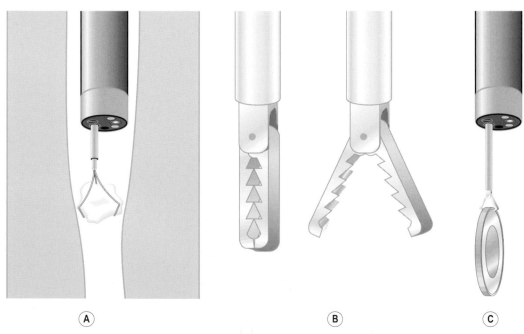

(A)   (B)   (C)

Figure 2 Instruments used for removal of foreign bodies. (A) Removal of an esophageal foreign body using tripod forceps. (B) Crocodile forceps. (C) Removal of a coin using rat-tooth forceps.

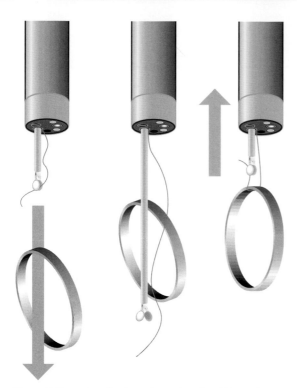

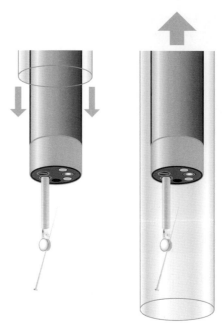

Figure 4 Removal of a sharp foreign body. An overtube should be used to withdraw a sharp foreign body.

Figure 3 Extraction of a ring using a thread and biopsy forceps passed through the ring.

5. Endoscopy technique

General anesthesia is required in pediatric patients or in those with complex or multiple foreign bodies.

Endoscopic strategy depends on the size of the foreign body ingested, its shape, the material it is made of, the anatomical location of the obstruction, the experience of the endoscopist and the technical resources available. Foreign bodies located above the cricopharyngeal muscle should be removed by laryngoscopy. Foreign bodies below this level should be removed with endoscopy.

✓ **Clinical Tip**

Endoscopic 'dry run'
Simulate foreign body removal outside the body prior to endoscopy with the object to determine what technique and equipment work best.

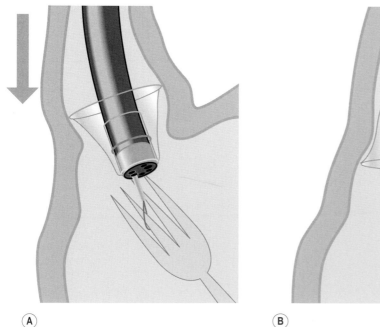

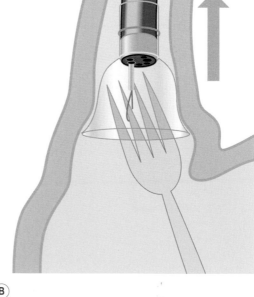

Ⓐ   Ⓑ

Figure 5 Removal of long foreign body. A rubber hood or overtube should be used to remove objects which are longer than 45 cm.

Overtubes can be used to extract foreign bodies whose removal could cause bleeding or perforation, such as pointed, sharp or long foreign bodies (Fig. 4). Standard overtubes extend past the upper esophageal sphincter, while longer overtubes (45–60 cm) pass the lower esophageal sphincter and are used to remove sharp objects from the stomach. Overtubes are also useful where there is a risk of aspiration or where multiple attempts will be made to remove a foreign body (i.e. food bezoars in non-intubated patient). Overtubes are rarely used in children, given their diameters.

5.1. Food bolus obstruction

Food impaction occurs in patients with anatomical anomalies such as web, ring or stricture or in patients with esophageal cancer. In the absence of esophageal obstruction, an endoscopy should be performed within 24 h. Endoscopy is successful in 95–99% of cases. An attempt should be made to pass the endoscope between the esophageal wall and the food bolus and into the stomach. The angle of the gastroesophageal junction and the cause of the obstruction should be noted. The food bolus will sometimes pass into the stomach with this maneuver. If this fails, the endoscope can be repositioned and the food gently pushed into the stomach. This should not be attempted if there are bones within the food bolus, as these can perforate if pushed into the mucosa. If this is unsuccessful, the food bolus can be broken into smaller pieces. These smaller pieces can sometimes be gently pushed into the stomach or can be removed using a Roth net.

5.2. Bezoars

These are usually encountered in adults without teeth or with anatomical anomalies such as atresia, stenosis, diverticulum or cancer of the esophagus, hiatus hernia or Schatzki ring. They may cause nausea, vomiting or loss of appetite. There are three types of bezoars. Trichobezoars are concretions of hair found in women aged 10–19 years who practice trichophilia or trichophagy. Phytobezoars consist of vegetable matter. Lactobezoars occur in premature, low-birthweight babies or infants fed for the first week of life with concentrated milk.

In the absence of bowel obstruction, wait 24 h before performing endoscopy. Fizzy drinks can be tried. Intravenous glucagon causes relaxation of the lower esophageal sphincter, and is effective in 30–50% of cases.

When endoscopy is required, an attempt should be made to pass the endoscope between the esophageal wall and the bezoars and into the stomach. The bezoar will often follow the endoscope into the stomach (Fig. 6). If this fails, or if the bezoar is large, it should be broken into smaller fragments, which can then be extracted with a basket or Roth net.

5.3. Round blunt foreign bodies

These are commonly swallowed in children aged between 6 and 12. Ingestion is asymptomatic in 16% of cases. In the remaining cases, the object will lodge at the level of the cricopharyngeal muscle (60–80% of cases), at the aortic arch (10–20%), or at the lower esophageal sphincter (5–20%).

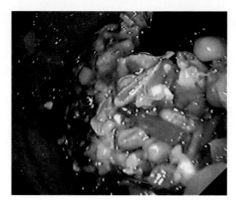

Figure 6 Bezoar in the stomach.

The management of round, blunt foreign bodies (i.e. coins) depends on their size, the patient's symptoms and the location. Objects which measure 2.5 cm or less will pass through the pylorus and may be watched (Table 2). If they are located in the esophagus, they should be removed if they have not passed within 24 h. If they are located in the stomach, they should be removed if they have failed to pass after 4–6 days. If the foreign body has passed through the pylorus, patients may be placed on a regular diet, with plain radiographs every week to confirm passage through the gut. Prokinetic medication has not been proved to be effective.

If endoscopy is required, most round, blunt objects can be removed using a Dormia basket, a Roth net, a polyp snare or forceps (Fig. 7). It is essential to ensure that the airway is protected from aspiration or inadvertent loss of the foreign body into the upper airways (i.e. coin).

5.4. Batteries

Batteries are blunt objects which yield a 'halo' image on standard radiographs (Fig. 1), because they have two sides with different diameters. Their ingestion requires emergency treatment, as there is a high risk of perforation. Mucosal

Table 2 Classification of lesions seen up to 24 h after caustic burn

Stage	Endoscopic findings	Management and outcome
0	Normal mucosa	Excellent
I	Mucosal erythema and edema	Spontaneous recovery in 1–3 days
IIa	Ulceration of the mucous membrane with exudates and bleeding	Commence liquid diet and progress to solid after 48 h
		No endoscopic follow-up necessary
IIb	Circumferential or deep ulceration	Major risk of stricture formation
		Initiate nasoenteric feeding after 24 h with liquid at 48 h if clinically well
III	Extensive necrosis	High risk of perforation
		Monitor carefully for 10 days
		Surgery indicated

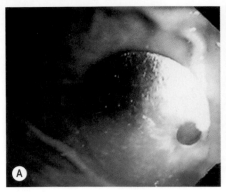
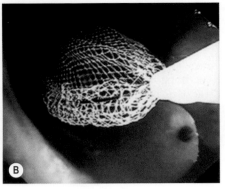
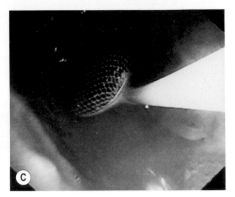

Figure 7 Removal of a round metal object located in the stomach using a Roth net.

damage can occur in the esophagus in 1 h, muscular damage in 2–4 h, with perforation occurring in 8–12 h.

Batteries can be removed in a similar manner to round objects described in section 5.3. The airway should be protected by intubation or by using an overtube. The battery itself can be removed with a Roth net or basket. Graspers and forceps should be avoided to avoid puncturing the battery. Once they have passed into the stomach, approximately 85% pass spontaneously. In these cases, passage should be confirmed with serial radiographs. Surgery is indicated if the battery fails to pass within 3 days, or the patient develops severe abdominal pain.

5.5. Sharp foreign bodies

Sharp objects require emergency treatment if they are impacted in the esophagus, owing to the risk of perforation (15–35%) and hemorrhage. If they have passed through the pylorus, daily radiographs should be performed. Surgery is indicated if the sharp object has remained in the same place for more than 3 days.

To extract a sharp object, ensure that the blunt end of the object is closest to the endoscope, with the sharp end following. This is done to avoid damaging or perforating the mucosa while extracting the foreign body. These objects can usually be removed using a forceps, polypectomy snare, Dormia basket or Roth net. If there is significant risk of trauma, an overtube or rubber hood should be used (Fig. 4). An alternative that has been described uses a simple latex glove: the tip is cut off and secured with a thread to the distal end of the endoscope. The foreign body is grasped and the latex glove inverts around the foreign body as it comes through the lower esophageal sphincter.

> Clinical Tip
>
> Always remove sharp objects blunt end first to avoid perforation.

5.6. Long foreign bodies

Long objects (>5 cm) need urgent endoscopy if they are in the esophagus or stomach. They are usually pens, spoons or toothbrushes. These should be maneuvered using a polypectomy snare so that the widest part is adjacent to the endoscope. The endoscope and the long foreign body should then be withdrawn. This should be done in combination with either an overtube or a rubber hood. An overtube is recommended if the object is >45 cm long (Fig. 5).

5.7. Body packages containing drugs

Body-packing involves the use of condoms filled with drugs such as cocaine or heroin. *No attempt should be made to extract these drug packets* since they may burst, causing a fatal overdose. Radiographs should be obtained daily, and surgery considered if perforation is suspected or if the packets remain for >48 h in the intestine.

5.8. Parasitic foreign bodies

Parasitic foreign bodies can occur, e.g. *Ascaris lumbricoides* trapped in the bile ducts or *Anisakis* impacted in the stomach wall. Endoscopic extraction is performed using forceps, a basket or occlusion balloon. It is important to ensure that the worm is completely extracted from the bile duct as remnants can lead to stone formation.

6. Complications

- Perforation
  - Fever, pain, distension, crepitus in the neck or chest, swelling, guarding or rebound on abdominal examination should prompt investigation for perforation.
  - Risk increases if objects are left in the esophagus for >24 hour.
  - In patients with symptoms, the perforation rate is up to 5%, increasing to 35% for sharp foreign bodies.
- GI bleeding
- Fistulae
- Aspiration
- Abscess formation.

7. Ingestion of toxins

7.1. Ingestion of caustic toxins

Take a detailed history and examine the patient to assess:

- The type of product ingested, quantity, contact time and whether it is a recent acute event.

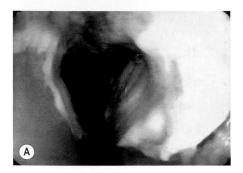 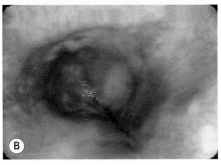

Figure 8 Caustic injury to the esophagus. (A) Caustic injury to the esophagus after ingestion of tetracycline. (B) Repeat endoscopy 3 weeks later.

- Examine the patient to assess for laryngeal damage (hoarseness or dyspnea with stridor) or severe esophageal damage (odynophagia, hypersialorrhea or refusal of food) or perforation.
- Patients should be managed in an intensive or high dependency unit.
- Patients should be kept fasting and have serial chest and abdominal films.
- Proton pump inhibitors should be prescribed.

Basic (caustic cleaners, dishwasher products or hair conditioner), acidic products or bleaching agents are caustic to the pharynx, larynx, esophagus and also the stomach and duodenum (Fig. 8).

7.2. Timing of endoscopy following ingestion of caustic substances

Upper endoscopy should be performed as soon as possible, and within 24 h of ingestion of a caustic substance. If upper endoscopy has not been performed within 48 h after ingestion, endoscopy should be deferred for 2 weeks due to the increased risk of perforation.

7.3. Contraindications and requirement for upper endoscopy

- Upper endoscopy is contraindicated if a perforation is suspected.
- In the absence of burns to the lips, buccal mucous membrane or oropharynx, caustic ingestion is rarely responsible for severe esophageal or gastric lesions and upper endoscopy is therefore unnecessary.
- The ingestion of certain metals (antimony, arsenic, barium, cadmium, chromium salts, copper salts and thallium) is not associated with caustic lesions and upper endoscopy is not indicated.

 Clinical Tip

Nasogastric intubation and emetics are contraindicated due to the risk of re-exposing the esophagus to caustic substance.

7.4. Endoscopy

- Endoscopy provides information on the early risk of perforation and on the late risk of stenosis.
- There is no requirement for antibiotic prophylaxis for endoscopy.

- There is currently no role for prophylactic esophageal stenting.
- Steroid injection is not recommended.
- Introduction of the endoscope should only be performed under visual control to minimize the risk of perforation.
- Note the appearance, location, extent and depth of caustic lesions (Table 2).

7.5. Post-endoscopy

- Prescribe proton pump inhibitors.
- Corticosteroid therapy at 2 mg/kg per day for 21 days seems effective for stage 2 burns and is believed to reduce the risk of stenosis due to scarring.
- Penicillamine or N-acetylcysteine may reduce collagen formation.

7.6. Special cases

7.6.1. Dilute bleach

Ingestion of dilute bleach (5–6% sodium hypochlorite) has a good prognosis. Endoscopy is performed only if there are ENT symptoms.

7.6.2. Formaldehyde

Formaldehyde does not destroy tissue; it acts as a fixative but the architecture of the tissues is preserved. Motility disappears and the mucous membrane gradually becomes grayish, discolored, rigid, and atonic. The examination needs to be repeated to assess the lesions.

7.6.3. Paraquat

The appearance of esophageal and gastric lesions after ingesting Paraquat (weed killer) indicates a poor prognosis and may precede sometimes fatal pulmonary fibrosis.

7.6.4. Meprobamate

The formation of gastric masses of meprobamate may cause prolonged poisoning, and even recurrences. They can be broken up endoscopically and removed via the upper route.

7.6.5. Potassium permanganate

The ingestion of potassium permanganate tablets involves a high risk of perforation for several hours afterwards.

An emergency plain abdominal X-ray is useful as the tablets are radio-opaque. The mucous membrane is colored dark purplish-black, which may erroneously suggest digestive necrosis and in this case endoscopy will not allow correct evaluation of the lesions which are usually localized.

7.7. Complications from ingestion of caustic toxins

The ingestion of caustic substances can be complicated by perforation, mediastinitis or peritonitis. One of the commonest complications dealt with by an endoscopist is stricture formation.

- Stenosis appears in 10–15% of cases.
- Dilation should be deferred until 3–6 weeks after ingestion of caustic substance due to the risk of perforation.
- Treatment with temporary plastic stent insertion has been described.
- Pyloric stenosis with gastric outlet can develop months to years later.
- Surgery is necessary in some cases with replacement of the esophagus with colonic or jejunal interposition, or gastroplasty.
- There is a 1000-fold increase in the risk of squamous esophageal cancer in these patients.

Surveillance, commencing 15–20 years after caustic ingestion, and repeated every 1–3 years, is recommended.

Further Reading

Cotton PB: Overtubes (sleeves) for upper gastrointestinal endoscopy, *Gut* 24(9):863–866, 1983.

Kay M, Wyllie R: Pediatric foreign bodies and their management, *Curr Gastroenterol Rep* 7:212–218, 2005.

Webb WA: Management of foreign bodies of the upper gastrointestinal tract: update, *Gastrointest Endosc* 41:39–51, 1995.

Wells CD, Fleischer DE: Overtubes in gastrointestinal endoscopy, *Am J Gastroenterol* 103(3):745–752, 2008.

7.6 Endoscopy in obesity

Jean-Christophe Létard, Pierre-Adrien Dalbies, Ian Penman

Key Points

- Endoscopic or surgical management of obesity is only indicated after medical therapy has failed for patients with a BMI ≥40 (or 35 with co-morbidity).
- All patients with upper GI symptoms should undergo preoperative upper endoscopy.
- Endoscopy should also be performed in all patients in whom gastric bypass is planned irrespective of symptoms.
- A large hiatal hernia is a relative contraindication to gastric banding.
- Endoscopists should understand the different types of bariatric procedures, the resulting anatomy and the different complications that may arise from these.
- ERCP is technically difficult following Roux-en-Y gastric bypass and alternative means of diagnosis (MRCP) or treatment (percutaneous transhepatic cholangiography) should be considered. ERCP should be undertaken selectively and in specialist centers.

 Clinical Tip

Endoscopic or surgical therapy may be indicated when medical management has failed in patients with a BMI of ≥40, or over 35 when there is major co-morbidity. Careful patient selection is vital.

1. Endoscopy and bariatric surgery

Two types of surgical procedures are performed:

- Restrictive procedures aiming to reduce gastric capacity (vertical banded gastroplasty (VBG) and laparoscopic adjustable gastric banding (LAGB)).
- Procedures combining a reduction in gastric capacity with maldigestion/malabsorption (Roux-en-Y gastrojejunal bypass, RYGB) or duodenal switch and biliopancreatic diversion (DS/BPD).

It is important for endoscopists to understand the different types of operation, the resulting anatomical alterations and the different complications that can arise following these procedures (Fig. 1).

2. Preoperative endoscopy

All patients with upper GI symptoms should undergo endoscopy to detect and treat underlying conditions such as gastritis and gastric or duodenal ulceration. This may be impossible postoperatively, as the distal stomach and duodenum may be excluded and impossible to visualize endoscopically following RYGB or DS/BPD. A large hiatus hernia is also a relative contraindication to LAGB because of an increased risk of band slippage. Detection and eradication of *Helicobacter pylori* infection is also important as infection may increase the risk of anastomotic marginal ulcers. In contrast, there is less evidence to justify routine upper endoscopy in asymptomatic patients prior to bariatric surgery but it is still commonly performed.

3. Postoperative endoscopy

Clear understanding of the exact operation that has been performed is essential and personal discussion with the surgeon involved is often useful as the length of the Roux limb or afferent limb may vary from 50 to 150 cm in RYGB procedures and the size of the gastric pouch and the diameter of its outlet may also vary following VBG or LAGB.

Introduction

Obesity is excess body fat and has a harmful effect on health resulting from an increased risk of cardiovascular disease (hypertension and cerebrovascular accidents), hyperlipidemia and type 2 diabetes. All cause mortality is also significantly higher in obese people. It is defined in clinical practice by the body mass index (BMI) which is calculated as weight/height^2 (kg/m^2). The WHO classification of obesity is shown in Table 1.

In the USA, 32% of the population are obese and 5% are morbidly obese. The treatment of obesity requires multidisciplinary management (nutritionist, endocrinologist, and psychiatrist) and it is only after dietary, pharmacological and behavioral therapy have been unsuccessful that endoscopic or surgical treatment should be offered.

Table 1 WHO definitions of obesity

BMI	Description	Obesity grade
<18.5	Thin	
18.5–24.9	Normal	
25–29.9	Overweight	
30–39.9	Obese	I (30–34.9), II (35–39.9)
≥40	Morbidly obese	III

Warning!

Endoscopy should be undertaken with care in the early postoperative period, as excess air insufflation may disrupt newly created anastomoses. Contrast radiology studies may better delineate postoperative anatomy and are preferred when a leak or fistula is suspected.

When undertaking endoscopy, the size of any gastric pouch should be carefully documented, suture lines and anastomoses should be inspected for evidence of fistulation, stenosis or marginal ulceration, the latter occurring most commonly on the intestinal side. Stomas are generally 10–12 mm in diameter and stenosis is defined as a diameter <10 mm. The possibility of band slippage or erosion following LAGB should always be considered and looked for as these occur in 5–10% of patients. Anastomotic stenoses can be safely and gradually dilated without difficulty, either by

bougienage or using balloon dilators. Dilatation should probably not be performed to >15 mm, as this may be associated with future weight gain.

 Warning!

Following RYGB the Roux limb may be tunnelled through the transverse mesocolon and can stricture at this point. Dilatation here is associated with a high risk of perforation and should be avoided.

4. Gallstone disease and ERCP following bariatric surgery

Both obesity and rapid weight loss are independent risk factors for cholelithiasis. After LAGB, ERCP can be performed normally but after gastric bypass procedures, it can be technically difficult or impossible. The likelihood of success is

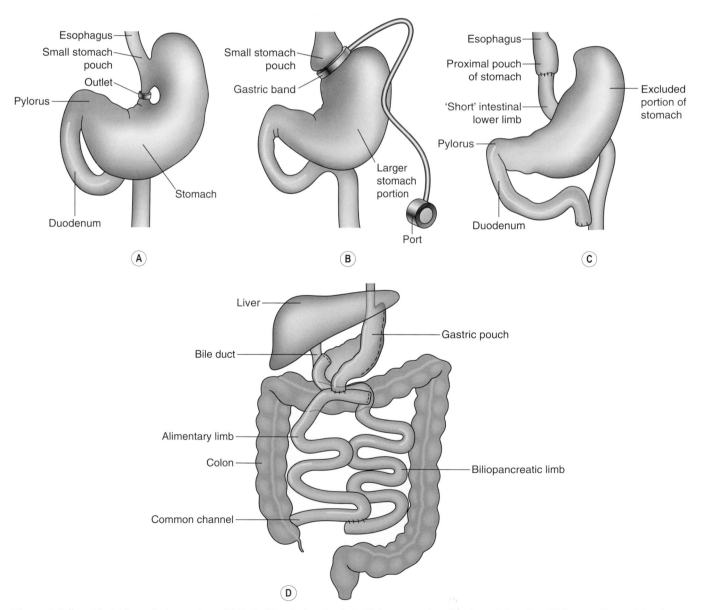

Figure 1 Different bariatric surgical procedures. (A) Vertical banded gastroplasty. (B) Laparoscopic assisted gastric banding. (C) Roux-en-Y gastrojejunal bypass. (D) Duodenal switch and biliopancreatic diversion.

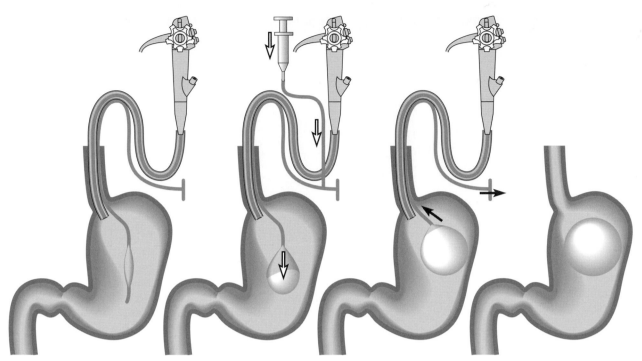

Figure 2 Insertion of an intragastric balloon.

lower if the Roux and/or afferent limbs are long. Highly skilled endoscopists can achieve success in up to two-thirds of patients with experience, time and using a range of equipment including side-viewing duodenoscopes, forward-viewing gastroscopes or colonoscopes or even a double balloon enteroscope. A variety of specifically designed ERCP accessories is often also necessary to achieve cannulation, sphincterotomy and/or stent placement. Alternatives should be considered in patients with suspected biliary tract disease following bariatric surgery including the use of MRCP or percutaneous transhepatic cholangiography (PTC).

5. Endoscopic placement of intragastric balloons

This is undertaken in some countries as an alternative to bariatric surgery but has become less popular in recent years as bariatric surgery has developed. They have not been shown to be a convincing means of achieving major weight loss but offer prospects to non-morbidly obese patients not being considered for surgery, those unwilling to undergo an operation and those awaiting surgery.

Endoscopic insertion of intragastric balloons was introduced in 1985 by Garren-Edwards and Taylor. The balloons were round or oval, made of polyurethane, and filled with 300–600 cc of air or water. The first balloons were a source of numerous complications including migration, gastric perforation or ulceration. The criteria for balloon design were subsequently refined and the 'ideal' balloon should be effective as regards weight loss, smooth, radio-opaque, strong and water-filled, its volume should be adjustable and it should be easy to insert and remove. Progress has been made with the water-filled balloon (Bioenterics Intragastric Balloon, BIB, Inamed Health, Santa Barbara, USA); however, its volume is no longer adjustable.

5.1. Equipment and technique

The water-filled balloon is made of silicone, equipped with an antireflux valve, and is round so it is easily positioned after an endoscopic examination of the digestive tract under anaesthesia (Fig. 2). It is released into the stomach after filling with 500–600 mL of physiological saline containing methylene blue (Figs 3, 4). The IGB is released by traction, against the gastric cardia. The covering membrane frees itself gradually, releasing the balloon from its constraint.

5.2. Indications

The use of an IGB depends on the patient's history of obesity, associated co-morbidity and careful dietary assessment. Endocrinological and psychiatric consultations are not legally required but are recommended. Balloons can also be recommended for very obese patients waiting for surgery. In this setting, evidence of efficacy may influence the decision to operate because patients who have clearly lost weight over 6 months would potentially respond well to surgical treatment (the 'IGB test').

5.3. Contraindications

There is no consensus about contraindications (Box 1), but the presence of a large hiatus hernia, malignancy or active

Box 1 Contraindications to use of intragastric balloons
• Severe/untreated psychiatric disease.
• Alcohol or drug addiction.
• Coagulopathy/anticoagulation.
• Pregnancy.
• Varices.
• Hiatal hernia >3 cm.
• Grade C or D esophagitis.

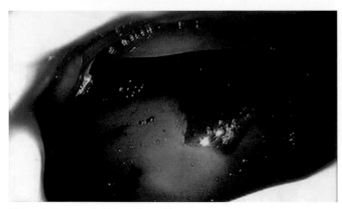

Figure 3 Intragastric balloon in position.

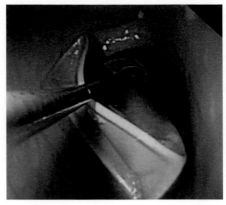

Figure 5 Extraction of an IGB with grasping forceps after removal of its contents by suction.

gastric or duodenal ulceration, may postpone the procedure or alter the approach. General anesthesia and intubation of the patient is advisable when balloons are inserted, because of the risk of aspiration. Given current knowledge of IGB, their use in adolescents is not recommended at present.

5.4. Monitoring

Patients should undergo clinical monitoring weekly or monthly after insertion of an IGB (laboratory tests in the event of vomiting, X-ray or ultrasound if fracture or migration is suspected), and regular consultations with a dietitian are an essential supplement of therapy for the duration of treatment. A mean weight loss of 10–12% over 6 months can be expected. According to the manufacturer's recommendations, the IGB is left in position for 6 months and removed by puncture and suction of the physiological saline using a removable trocar mounted in a plastic catheter. Once flattened, the IGB is extracted using tripod forceps or a polypectomy snare (Figs 5, 6). As few perforations as possible should be made in the IGB because this may cause it to empty partially like a watering-can rose, forming pockets of fluid, which make it more difficult to remove.

5.5. Complications

Expected immediate complications after insertion of an IGB are functional, such as vomiting (90% in the first week). This requires readmission to hospital in 5% of cases, because of hypokalemia and dehydration. Vomiting may last 1 week but

can persist for more than 3 weeks in 20% of patients. Heartburn is present in up to 15% of patients, with or without esophagitis, and erosive gastritis an also occur. Colicky abdominal pain with diarrhea responds to antispasmodic and antidiarrheal agents. It is only rarely necessary (2–3%) to remove the IGB early because of persistent vomiting or pain. Spontaneous elimination of the balloon may occur in 2.5% of patients, usually without the patient's awareness, despite the methylene blue. Cases of mechanical obstruction have been reported as a result of this.

5.6. Future developments

Air-filled balloons are still under investigation. Their insertion system is more rigid and removal more difficult because of the size of the valve. In contrast with water-filled balloons, the removal of air-filled balloons requires multiple puncture holes. Other devices including implantable intragastric prostheses, semi-stationary antral balloons and an implantable endoscopic duodenal-jejunal bypass sleeve are under development. In summary, the intragastric balloon is one of a number of methods available to doctors treating obesity and it should be offered only after the medical therapy has failed and a multidisciplinary medical decision has been taken, as in the case for surgery. There are no data on long-term efficacy, outcomes or quality of life and more studies are needed. They do not achieve the degree of durable weight loss that occurs following surgery but may be useful in selected patients, although more evidence of efficacy and safety are required.

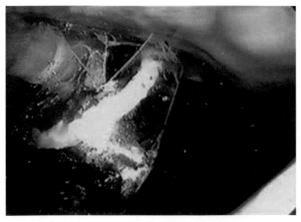

Figure 4 Release of a water-filled balloon (unfolding the covering membrane).

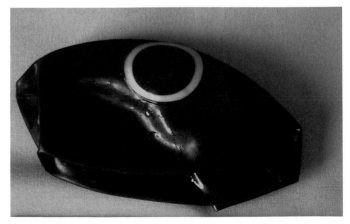

Figure 6 Water-filled balloon after removal.

Further Reading

ASGE standards of practice committee: Guideline. Role of endoscopy in the bariatric surgery patient, *Gastroinest Endosc* 68:1–9, 2008.

Coté GA, Edmundowicz SA: Emerging technology: endoluminal treatment of obesity, *Gastrointest Endosc* 70(5):991–999, 2009.

Feitoza AB, Baron TH: Endoscopy and ERCP in the setting of previous upper GI tract surgery. Part I: Reconstruction without alteration of pancreaticobiliary anatomy, *Gastroinest Endosc* 54:743–749, 2001.

Feitoza AB, Baron TH: Endoscopy and ERCP in the setting of previous upper GI tract surgery. Part II: postsurgical anatomy with alteration of the pancreaticobiliary tree, *Gastrointest Endosc* 55(1):75–79, 2002.

Sauerland S, Angrisani L, Belachew M, et al: European Association for Endoscopic Surgery. Obesity surgery: evidence-based guidelines of the European Association for Endoscopic Surgery (EAES), *Surg Endosc* 19:200–221, 2005.

Tsesmeli N, Coumaros D: Review of endoscopic devices for weight reduction: old and new balloons and implantable prostheses, *Endoscopy* 41(12):1082–1089, 2009.

Wright BE, Cass OW, Freeman ML: ERCP in patients with long-limb Roux-en-Y gastrojejunostomy and intact papilla, *Gastrointest Endosc* 56:225–232, 2002.

7.7 Polypectomy

Mouen Khashab, Jean Marc Canard, Anthony N. Kalloo

Key Points

- Optical enhancement techniques, such as narrow-band imaging, FICE, or staining with 0.2% indigo carmine, may be used to predict polyp histology.
- Forceps polypectomy is best suited for diminutive polyps. Pedunculated polyps ≤5 mm and sessile polyps ≤7 mm may be resected with cold snaring.
- Polyps that exhibit the non-lifting sign and polyps that are ulcerated may harbor carcinoma. These polyps should be biopsied to exclude cancer prior to resection.
- Large sessile polyps resected in piecemeal fashion should be followed-up with repeat examination in 2–6 months to exclude residual or recurrent adenoma.
- Management of antithrombotic agents in the peri-endoscopic period depends on the bleeding risk from polypectomy and the thromboembolic risk associated with interruption of medications.
- Colonoscopy should be performed urgently in patients with active post-polypectomy hemorrhage.

Introduction

Colorectal cancer (CRC) is one of the leading causes of cancer death worldwide. The lifetime risk of developing CRC is 6%, with the majority of cancers occurring in people older than 50 years. CRC is believed to arise from adenomas through the adenoma to carcinoma sequence. Interruption of this progression through polypectomy is one of the most effective cancer prevention means in medicine. The National Polyp study showed that colonoscopy with removal of adenomas decreased the incidence of CRC by 76–90%. More recent studies showed that colonoscopy with polypectomy is associated with a relative reduction in CRC death of 65%. However, colonoscopy is imperfect and incident cancers after clearing colonoscopies continue to occur. Up to one-third of incident cancers are believed to be due to ineffective polypectomy. All endoscopists should therefore be familiar with effective and safe polypectomy techniques.

The aim of this chapter is to discuss techniques of removal of small polyps, large pedunculated polyps, and large sessile polyps. In addition, the chapter discusses the management of antithrombotic agents during the peri-endoscopic period, the treatment of malignant colorectal polyps, and the management of complications of polypectomy.

1. Optical enhancement techniques

Optical enhancement techniques, such as narrow-band imaging (NBI), chromoendoscopy (CE), autofluorescence (AF), Fuji Intelligent Chromo Endoscopy (FICE), and I-Scan, may be used to improve polyp detection and/or predict polyp histology in real time (Fig. 1) (see Ch. 6.2). The discussion of the former use is beyond the scope of this chapter. However, understanding the use of such techniques to predict polyp histology may assist in determining the need for polypectomy.

NBI and CE are the most studied optical enhancing technologies. CE involves spraying of dye, and is cumbersome and time-consuming. NBI has been called digital

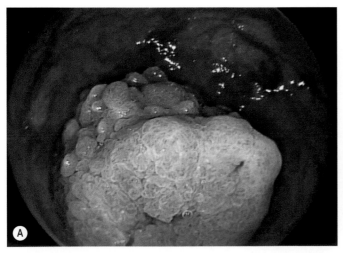
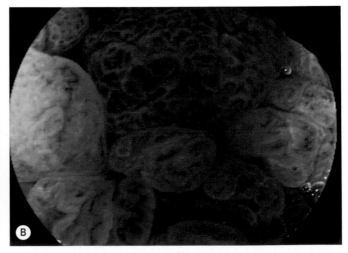

Figure 1 Sessile polyp. (A) This polyp in the transverse colon was identified as a sessile polyp using FICE and optical zoom. (B) Note the tubular pit patterns with no sign of adenocarcinoma.

Table 1 Endoscopic features predictive of polyp histology when viewed by NBI

Adenomatous polyps	Hyperplastic polyps
Short thick blood vessels	Thin blood vessels crossing polyp surface and not surrounding pits
Overall brown color	Bland, featureless appearance
Tubular or oval pits	Pattern of black dots surrounded by white
Central brown depression	

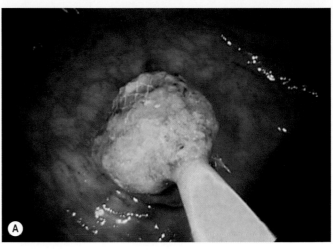

chromoendoscopy, does not involve spraying of dye, and is an efficient means of predicting colon polyp histology. Table 1 depicts the endoscopic features that are predictive of adenomatous and hyperplastic histology when viewed by NBI. Experienced endoscopists can correctly predict adenomatous and hyperplastic histology of diminutive polyps (≤5 mm) in 90–95% of cases. NBI may, thus, identify small distal hyperplastic polyps that need not be resected (or resected and discarded). All proximal hyperplastic polyps, however, should be resected as they may represent serrated adenomas, which are now recognized as precancerous lesions.

Another potential use of optical enhancement techniques is examination of polypectomy sites to assess the adequacy of polypectomy and the presence of residual or recurrent adenomatous tissue at the index or follow-up colonoscopic examinations, respectively.

2. Equipment

Box 1   Equipment
• Polypectomy snares[a].
• Cold and hot biopsy forceps.
• Tripod grasper forceps.
• Injection needle.
• Endoscopic clips.
• Detachable loops.
• Polyp retrieval 'Roth' nets (Fig. 2).
• Polyp trap (Fig. 2).
• Tattoo (Sterile carbon suspension rather than India Ink).
• Epinephrine.
[a]Snares come in a variety of shapes and sizes. We usually use hexagonal snares, as they can be half opened to remove small polyps, and fully opened to remove large polyps.

3. Small polyp removal

3.1. General concepts

- Small polyps have a maximum diameter of <10 mm and diminutive polyps have a maximum diameter of ≤5 mm.
- Most colon polyps are diminutive (80%) or small (90%).
- The optimal technique for resection of small polyps has not been established.
- The benefit of removal of all diminutive adenomas is not known.
- Most polypectomy complications result from small polyp removal because of their prevalence.

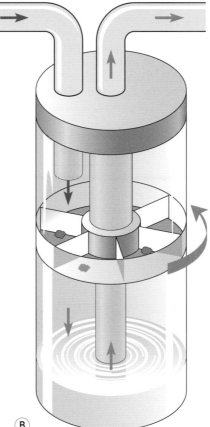

Figure 2 Polyp retrieval devices. (A) Polyp retrieval net (Roth). (B) A polyp trap is useful for small polyps which can be suctioned and then captured in the trap.

- Most polypectomy complications are electrocautery-related.
- Electrocautery is not needed in the resection of many small polyps.

3.2. Cold biopsy forceps

- Cold forceps are appropriate for the resection of smallest polyps (1–3 mm in size).
- Hot forceps are best suited for resection of diminutive flat polyps that are harder to grasp with a snare.

- Resection of larger polyps using a biopsy forceps in piecemeal fashion is inefficient and may result in residual adenomatous tissue.

Clinical Tips

- Polyps >3 mm are usually resected in piecemeal fashion when forceps are used for resection. The endoscopic field may become bloodied, which may obscure the margins of the residual polyp. It is better to use hot biopsy forceps.
- Cold forceps are not associated with increased complication risks and can be used safely in anticoagulated patients and patients on anti-platelet agents.

3.3. Hot biopsy forceps

- The tip of the polyp should be grasped and tented away from the colonic wall to create a pseudo-stalk. Lumen should be first deflated and electrocautery is then applied. Since the electric current density concentrates at the narrowest point, the pseudo-stalk is cauterized.
- Hot forceps are also best suited for resection of diminutive polyps. Resection of larger polyps with hot forceps involves piecemeal resection and risks incomplete polyp removal.
- Hot forceps are associated with an increased risk of delayed post-polypectomy bleeding and transmural thermal injury.
- Hot forceps biopsies are associated with a 8–16% risk of residual polyp.

Clinical Tips

- The right colon is particularly susceptible to transmural injury and perforation. Great care must be taken when using hot biopsies in the right colon.
- The American Society for Gastrointestinal Endoscopy (ASGE) recommends that hot forceps should be used only for polyps ≤5 mm.

3.4. Cold snare

- The V of the open snare should be positioned at the point the endoscopist wants the snare to close. This is usually at the junction between the polyp and the adjacent normal tissue (Figs 3, 4). Be careful to check that the colon wall is not caught in the snare before cutting (Fig. 5).
- In general, snaring techniques are more effective than forceps techniques for efficient and complete eradication of polyps.
- Cold snares are effective for resecting sessile polyps up to 7 mm in size and pedunculated polyps up to 5 mm in size.

Clinical Tips

- Hot snaring should be used for resection of larger (>5 mm) pedunculated polyps because their stalk may enclose large blood vessels; electrocautery coagulates blood vessels and helps avoid bleeding complications.
- There is no need to lift or tent the polyp away from the colonic wall when using cold snare technique. Avoiding tenting may help keep the resected polyp in the endoscopic field.

Clinical Tip

Some authorities recommend resecting 1–2 mm rim of normal tissue around the polyp edge along with polyp to ensure complete resection. This should be avoided when using hot snaring because it increases the size of the cautery burn.

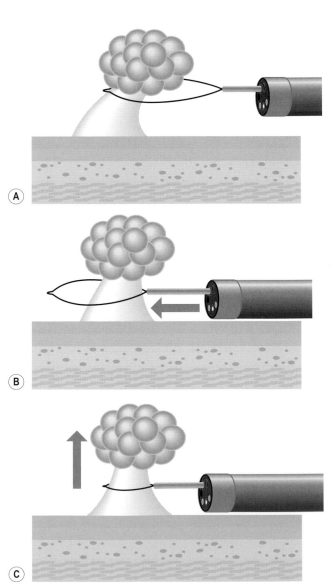

Figure 3 How to place a diathermy snare around the stalk of the polyp. (A) Position the polyp in the 6 o'clock position. Open the snare beyond the polyp and then place it over polyp. (B) Push the snare forward slightly to advance it onto the stalk of the polyp. (C) Once it is around the stalk, close the snare slowly, withdrawing the polyp slightly.

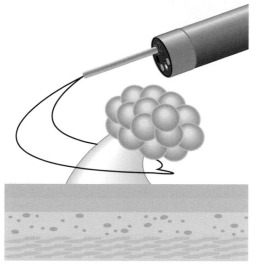

Figure 4 An alternative technique is to place the snare over the front of the polyp and then close the snare behind the polyp. This technique is used when the polyp is difficult to snare using the classic technique.

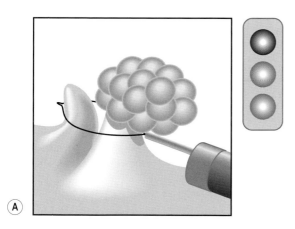

(A)

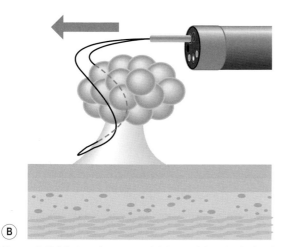

(B)

Figure 5 Pitfalls in polypectomy. (A) Be careful to check that the colon wall is not caught in the snare before cutting. (B) This can be avoided by first advancing the snare over the polyp under direct vision before closing.

Table 2 Types of currents used for polypectomies

Current type	Early bleeding risk	Delayed bleeding risk
Coagulation	↓	↑
Cutting	↑	↓
Blended	↑	↓

The type of current affects the risk of early or late bleeding. Thus coagulation is associated with an increased risk of delayed bleeding, while using a cutting current is associated with a decreased risk of delayed bleeding but an increased risk of early bleeding.

3.5. Hot snare

- Different types of currents may be used for hot snare polypectomies (Table 2). There is currently no consensus for the optimal type of current that should be used. The intensity of the heat delivered per mm of contact depends on the contact area (Fig. 6).
- We usually use endo-cut mode as this setting has a low risk of bleeding while having sufficient cutting current to resect a polyp.
- The ensnared polyp should be lifted away from the colonic wall and the lumen deflated prior to the application of electrocautery to minimize the risk of transmural injury.
- Pedunculated polyps >5 mm are best resected with a hot snare.

4. Large pedunculated polyp removal

- Large pedunculated polyps are most commonly found in the sigmoid colon.

> **! Warning!**
>
> Caution needs to be exercised not to mistake a pedunculated mucosal prolapse or a large lipoma for an adenoma. Mucosal prolapse has a normal pit pattern. Lipomas exhibit a positive pillow sign.

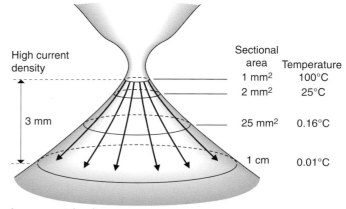

High current density

3 mm

Sectional area   Temperature
1 mm² 100°C
2 mm² 25°C
25 mm² 0.16°C
1 cm 0.01°C

Low current density

Figure 6 The intensity of the heat delivered per millimeter of contact depends on the contact area.

- A pedunculated polyp of any size should be able to be removed by a single transection. Piecemeal resection of the head may be performed if the polyp cannot be ensnared, until the residual polyp can be encircled with the snare.

Clinical Tip

If a pedunculated polyp is resected in piecemeal fashion, then the portion of polyp nearest to the pedicle should be submitted to pathology in a separate jar, because this section will determine the need for further therapy if cancer is found.

- Epinephrine injection of the stalk prior to polyp resection decreases immediate, but not delayed, post-polypectomy bleeding risk. This is particularly important in polyps with a large (>1 cm) stalk that may contain a large artery (Fig. 7).
- Epinephrine injection into the stalk may also result in shrinking of the polyp. For this purpose, injection is best performed during scope insertion so that the delayed effect of shrinkage is appreciated during scope withdrawal.
- Placement of a detachable loop around the pedicle of large pedunculated polyps decreases the risk of immediate and delayed post-polypectomy bleeding (Figs 8–10). This should be avoided in polyps with short stalks, as it may render snare resection more cumbersome and may slip off and result in massive hemorrhage. A detachable loop should be closed gently, as excessive tightening of the loop can transect the polyp stalk.

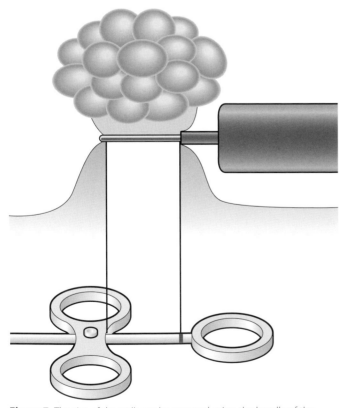

Figure 7 The size of the stalk can be assessed using the handle of the closed loop.

Box 2 Non-lifting sign

- Polyps that do not lift after submucosal saline injection display the non-lifting sign.
- Such polyps should be biopsied with cold forceps, and resected if biopsies fail to reveal carcinoma.
- Prior failed attempts at polyp resection with snaring produce a false non-lifting sign due to submucosal fibrosis.
- The positive predictive value of the non-lifting sign for invasive carcinoma is 83%.

- The snare should be placed over the pedicle such that half or upper third of the pedicle will be resected (Figs 3, 11). This is crucial to ensure R0 resection if cancer is found in the polyp head. In addition, this leaves adequate residual pedicle to grasp and treat if bleeding occurs.
- Larger snares should be used for giant pedunculated polyps. The colonoscope should be advanced proximal to the polyp, the snare opened widely, and then the polyp ensnared during colonoscope withdrawal.

5. Large sessile polyp removal

- Large sessile colon polyps are those ≥2 cm in size, and 'giant' polyps refer to those ≥3 cm. These lesions have a propensity to harbor or transform to cancer.
- These polyps must be biopsied to exclude the presence of carcinoma. If carcinoma is present, the polyp should be resected surgically.
- Polyps that exhibit the non-lifting sign and polyps that are ulcerated may harbor carcinoma.
- Most large sessile polyps are removed using piecemeal technique (Fig. 12). Submucosal injection, although non-mandatory, facilitates the safe resection of such polyps (Figs 13, 14).
- Initial snaring of the polyp is usually performed using large snares, removing large pieces if possible (Fig. 12). Smaller residual polypoid tissue is then resected using

Warning!

When to use submucosal injection

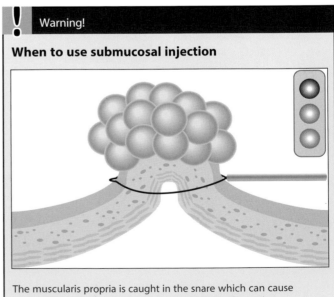

The muscularis propria is caught in the snare which can cause perforation. Submucosal injection should be performed.

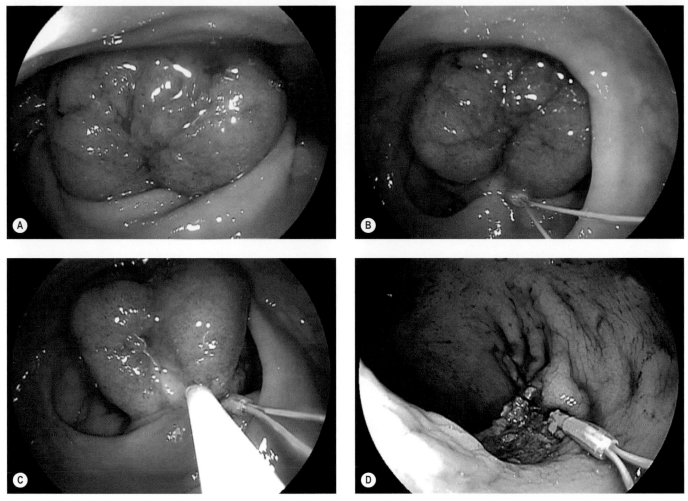

Figure 8 (A–D) Non effective use of a detachable loop in a patient with a large and short pedunculated polyp.

smaller snares. All remaining flat adenomatous tissue can then be ablated using argon plasma coagulation (see Ch. 7.4) when it is not possible to resect with a snare.

- Spiral snares can be used to grasp residual small areas of very flat adenomatous tissue.
- The use of APC to ablate the edges of the polypectomy site and any visible residual adenomatous tissue has been shown in randomized controlled trials to decrease the incidence of polyp recurrence.
- Large polyps outside the cecum should be tattooed to facilitate endoscopic localization during follow-up examinations. Tattoos should be placed to the right and

left of the polyps. If surgical localization is required, tattoos should be placed in three or four quadrants around the polyp. Transmural injection of the tattoo should be avoided as it may render subsequent surgery more difficult.

- Small pieces of resected tissue can be suctioned through the scope into the retrieval trap (Fig. 2B). A single remaining large piece can be grasped with the snare. Multiple larger pieces can be grasped with a Roth retrieval basket (Fig. 2A). The catheter can be advanced few centimeters beyond the colonoscope tip, which allows colonic examination during withdrawal.

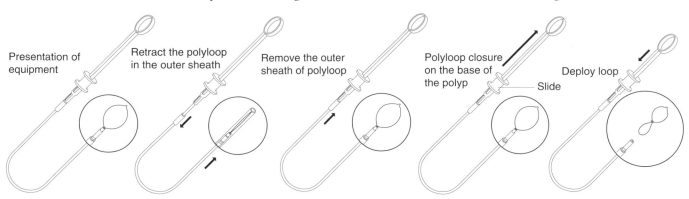

Presentation of equipment | Retract the polyloop in the outer sheath | Remove the outer sheath of polyloop | Polyloop closure on the base of the polyp — Slide | Deploy loop

Figure 9 Use of detachable loops.

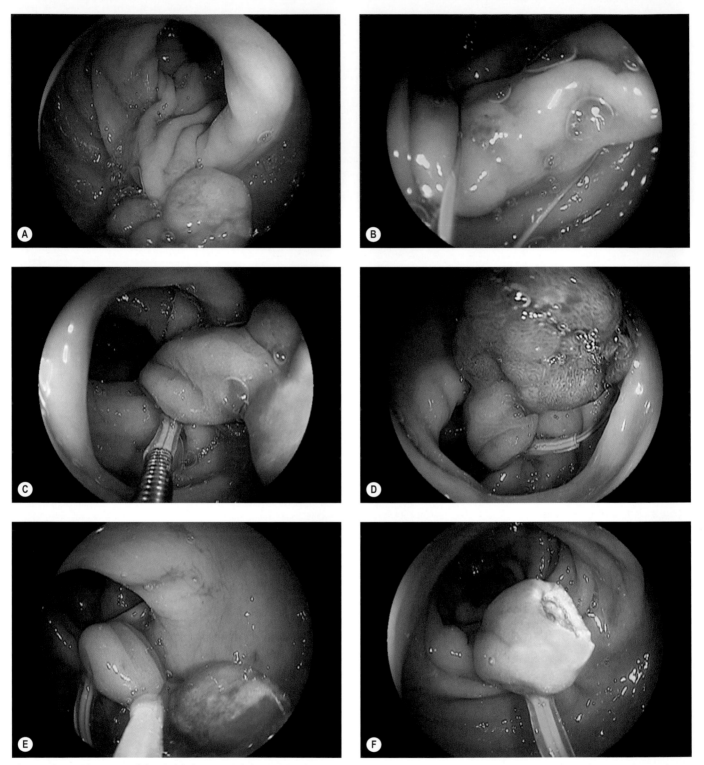

Figure 10 A–F Placement of detachable loop around the pedicle of a large pedunculated polyp.

- Guidelines recommend inspection of the polypectomy site 2–6 months after resection, followed by a second examination 1 year later. The polypectomy scar should be biopsied at follow-up even if macroscopic recurrence is not present. Negative scar biopsy specimen at the first follow-up is predictive of long-term eradication.

6. Special clinical situations

6.1. Malignant polyps

- In general, all malignant colon polyps are best treated surgically.

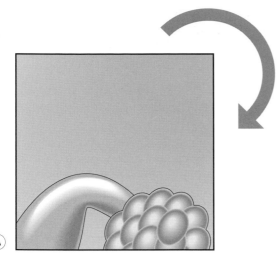
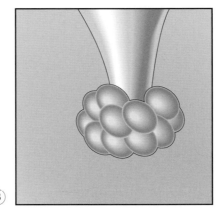

Figure 11 Snaring a large pedunculated polyp. (A) The orientation of the polyp is poor. (B) The patient is repositioned, which improves the orientation of the polyp.

- Some malignant pedunculated polyps with favorable histology can be treated endoscopically.
  - Favorable histology: well-differentiated and moderately-differentiated adenocarcinoma
  - Unfavorable histology: poorly-differentiated adenocarcinoma, mucinous adenocarcinoma, and signet-ring cell carcinoma
  - Carcinoma involving the head of the polyp (above the junction between the adenoma and its stalk), the neck of the polyp (junction between adenoma and its stalk), or the proximal part of the stalk (given that the lower resection margin of the stalk is free of cancer), may be treated with endoscopic resection
  - Carcinoma invading into the submucosa of the bowel wall below the stalk should be surgically resected
  - No surgery is required for cases where the tumor infiltration extends <1000 μm into submucosal and is well- or moderately-differentiated adenocarcinoma with no lymphatic involvement.

Warning!

Great care must be taken when performing a polypectomy when a clip has been placed. It is important to ensure that the diathermy loop does not touch the clip, as if this occurs, the current will be transmitted through the clip and may cause perforation.

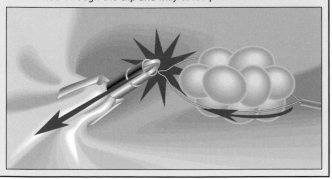

7. Complications

7.1. Hemorrhage

- This is the most common complication of polypectomy and can be immediate or delayed. Immediate bleeding is more common with cutting or blended current while

---

Box 3 Submucosal injection: technique and advantages

- The ideal solution, which will result in substantial bulge and will not dissipate quickly, has not been defined. Most experts in the USA use saline.
- Other solutions used for submucosal injection include hypertonic saline, 50% dextrose sodium hyaluronate, hydroxypropyl methylcellulose (artificial tears), fibrinogen and blood.
- Methylene blue or indigo carmine can be added to the injection solution to delineate the injected mound and to demarcate the edges of the polyp.
- Inclusion of epinephrine in the submucosal injection solution decreases the risk of immediate post-polypectomy bleeding but increases the risk of delayed bleeding.
- Although submucosal injection has been shown to decrease injury to the muscularis propria in an animal model, there is no controlled evidence that it decreases perforation rate in humans.
- The only contraindication for submucosal injection is presence of surface ulceration because of the theoretical risk of tumor seeding if carcinoma is present. Tumor seeding has only been reported in one patient.
- The easiest way to locate the submucosal space is to start injecting before puncturing the mucosal surface. The polyp will lift when the needle enters the submucosal space, which is the only compartment that will accommodate fluid due to the presence of areolar tissue.
- In most cases, injection should begin through the polyp. Injection into the distal (close to the scope) should be avoided, because a large bleb may render the polyp hard to visualize.
- When most of the polyp is hidden from view behind a fold or wrapped around a fold in clamshell fashion, fluid should be injected into the normal mucosa at the proximal (far) edge of the polyp.

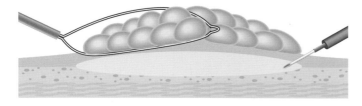

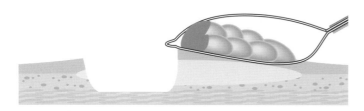

Figure 12 Piecemeal resection of a sessile polyp. Submucosal injection is performed to raise the polyp. The polyp is then removed piece by piece until fully resected.

delayed bleeding is more common with coagulation current. Delayed bleeding can occur up to 1 month after polypectomy.

- The overall risk is about 1–2% for snare polypectomy.
- Risk factors for bleeding include coagulopathy, large polyp size, and proximal polyp location.
- Immediate hemorrhage can be treated with epinephrine injection, bipolar electrocautery, and/or clip placement (Fig. 15, Table 3).
- Approximately 70% of patients with delayed hemorrhage stop bleeding spontaneously, as evidenced by decreasing frequency or cessation of stooling, and can be managed conservatively.
- Colonoscopy should be performed urgently in patients with active hemorrhage. Since the location (s) of polypectomy site(s) are known a priori, colonoscopy

Table 3 Treatment of immediate post-polypectomy bleeding

Methods	Comments
Grasp the stalk with the snare	Hold for stalk for few minutes Do not transect the remaining stalk
Inject the stalk with epinephrine	Therapeutic effect is by vasoconstriction and tamponade
Apply coaptive coagulation with bipolar electrocautery	Bleeding vessel is tamponaded and sealed by a protein coagulum
Place detachable snare around stalk	This method may be cumbersome and impractical in the case of vigorous bleeding
Place hemoclips over the bleeding vessel	Efficient method for treating post-polypectomy hemorrhage

may be performed without bowel purging. Bleeding is best treated with epinephrine injection and clip placement, since thermal therapy can potentially extend tissue injury.

7.2. Post-polypectomy syndrome and perforation

- Post-polypectomy syndrome, also known as transmural burn syndrome, results from transmural burn due to electrocautery but without free perforation. Patients present with abdominal pain (often with rebound

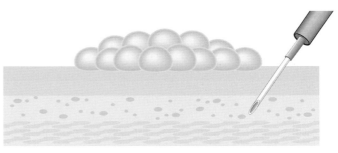

(A)

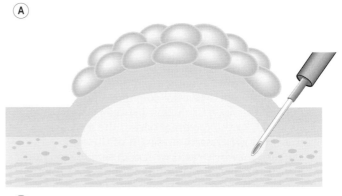

(B)

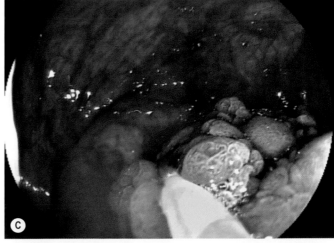

(C)

Figure 13 How to perform submucosal injection. (A) Injection should begin through the polyp. Injection into the distal (close to the scope) should be avoided, because a large bleb may render the polyp hard to visualize. When most of the polyp is hidden from view behind a fold or wrapped around a fold in clamshell fashion, fluid should be injected into the normal mucosa at the proximal (far) edge of the polyp. (B) Continue injection until the polyp has been raised. This indicates that there is no invasion of the muscularis propria. (C) Submucosal injection of a polyp.

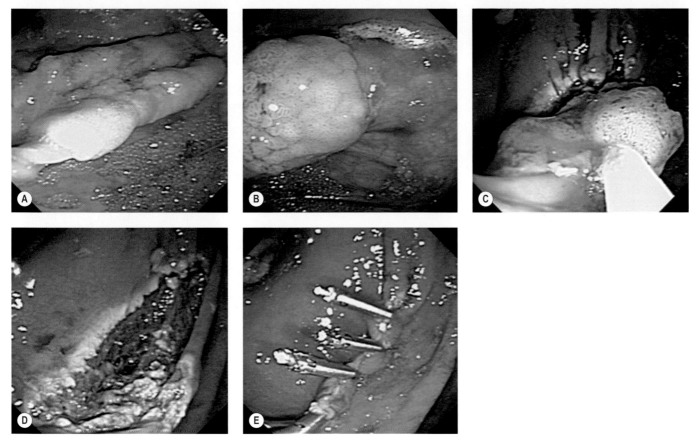

Figure 14 Piecemeal resection of a 35 mm sessile cecal polyp. (A) Large sessile cecal polyp; (B) after submucosal injection; (C) during piecemeal resection; (D) after resection and treatment with APC and (E) after polypectomy site closure with clips.

tenderness), fever, and leukocytosis. Abdominal imaging may reveal air in the bowel wall but not free air in the abdomen, as seen with free perforations.
- Abdominal computed tomography (CT) should be obtained in patients with high suspicion for perforation even if abdominal radiographs are non-revealing.
- Management of post-polypectomy syndrome includes nil per os, antibiotics, and surgical consultation. In properly managed patients, the risk of evolution to frank perforation is low.

- Endoscopic clipping may be useful in closing small perforations that are recognized immediately.

Most patients with colon perforations are treated surgically, although successful conservative management has been reported.

Patients with polyps require surveillance colonoscopy. Guidelines can be found in Table 4.

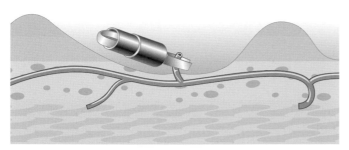

Figure 15 Clip placement. A clip has been placed across a bleeding vessel following polypectomy.

Table 4 Guidelines for surveillance of small adenomas

	Surveillance period
Patients with 1 or 2 small adenomas	5 years after initial polypectomy
Patients with 3–10 small adenomas	3 years after initial polypectomy
Patients with >10 small adenomas	<3 years after initial polypectomy
Patients with any adenoma with villous features or with high-grade dysplasia	3 years after initial polypectomy
Patients with adenomas that are removed piecemeal	2–6 months to verify complete removal

Further reading

Anderson MA, Ben-Menachem T, Gan SI, et al: Management of antithrombotic agents for endoscopic procedures, *Gastrointest Endosc* 70:1060–1070, 2009.

Fatima H, Rex DK: Minimizing endoscopic complications: colonoscopic polypectomy, *Gastrointest Endosc Clin N Am* 17:145–156, viii, 2007.

Haggitt RC, Glotzbach RE, Soffer EE, et al: Prognostic factors in colorectal carcinomas arising in adenomas: implications for lesions removed by endoscopic polypectomy, *Gastroenterology* 89:328–336, 1985.

Herrera S, Bordas JM, Llach J, et al: The beneficial effects of argon plasma coagulation in the management of different types of gastric vascular ectasia lesions in patients admitted for GI hemorrhage, *Gastrointest Endosc* 68:440–446, 2008.

Khashab M, Eid E, Rusche M, et al: Incidence and predictors of 'late' recurrences after endoscopic piecemeal resection of large sessile adenomas, *Gastrointest Endosc* 70:344–349, 2009.

Levin TR, Zhao W, Conell C, et al: Complications of colonoscopy in an integrated health care delivery system, *Ann Intern Med* 145:880–886, 2006.

Norton ID, Wang L, Levine SA, et al: Efficacy of colonic submucosal saline solution injection for the reduction of iatrogenic thermal injury, *Gastrointest Endosc* 56:95–99, 2002.

Rex DK: Narrow-band imaging without optical magnification for histologic analysis of colorectal polyps, *Gastroenterology* 136:1174–1181, 2009.

Uno Y, Munakata A: The non-lifting sign of invasive colon cancer, *Gastrointest Endosc* 40:485–489, 1994.

Winawer SJ, Zauber AG, Ho MN, et al: Prevention of colorectal cancer by colonoscopic polypectomy. The National Polyp Study Workgroup, *N Engl J Med* 329:1977–1981, 1993.

7.8 Endoscopic treatment of upper gastrointestinal hemorrhage in patients with peptic ulcer

Nicholas I. Church, Jean-Christophe Létard

Key Points

- Some 80% of ulcers stop bleeding spontaneously; therapy is required for the remainder with stigmata of recent hemorrhage.
- Clinical and endoscopic scoring systems can be used to stratify patients at risk of a poor outcome.
- Only ulcers with Forrest I, IIA and IIB stigmata of hemorrhage require endoscopic intervention.
- Prompt resuscitation and close attention to co-morbid conditions is vital prior to endoscopy.
- Endoscopy should be performed within 24 h of the initial bleed.
- Best outcomes are achieved with combination therapy (injection plus either thermal ablation or mechanical clipping).
- *Helicobacter pylori* status should be determined in patients presenting with peptic ulcer bleeding.
- Intravenous proton pump inhibitors reduce re-bleeding after endoscopic therapy for peptic ulcer.

Box 1   Factors associated with poor prognosis

- Presence of shock.
- Passage of fresh red blood.
- Age >60 years.
- Hemoglobin <10 g/dL.
- Presence of significant co-morbid disease.
- Bleed from varices or large peptic ulcer.
- Onset in hospital.
- Recurrent bleeding.

Introduction

Gastroduodenal ulcers are the cause of non-variceal upper gastrointestinal bleeding (NVUGIB) in approximately 35% of cases. Ulcers are usually associated with *Helicobacter pylori* infection or the use of antiplatelet or NSAID therapy. Bleeding may be exacerbated by concurrent steroid or anticoagulant therapy. In 80% of cases, bleeding stops spontaneously and endoscopic therapy is only required in the 20% of ulcers with endoscopic stigmata of hemorrhage. Re-bleeding rates of ulcers treated by endoscopic therapy are 5–20%. Despite advances in endoscopic intervention, the overall mortality rate from peptic ulcer bleeding remains 10%, largely as a result of the increasing age and co-morbidity of the patients. Endoscopy in this situation is often the most challenging that endoscopists undertake and careful assessment, resuscitation and preparation of patients for endoscopy is vital, to ensure a safe and successful outcome.

1. Risk assessment

Clinical factors associated with a poor prognosis after an upper GI bleed are shown in Box 1. A number of risk scoring systems have been developed to stratify risk of poor outcome and of these the Rockall and the Glasgow Blatchford systems have been most widely studied (Tables 1, 2). The Rockall score can be used to predict mortality but not re-bleeding. The advantage of the Glasgow Blatchford score is that it may be used before endoscopy to predict the need for intervention to treat bleeding. Low scores (≤ 2) have been shown to be associated with a very low risk of adverse outcome.

Endoscopic factors predicting a high risk of ulcer re-bleeding are shown in Box 2. Stigmata of recent hemorrhage are described by the Forrest classification (Box 3, Fig. 1A–C). Only ulcers with Forrest I, IIA, and IIB stigmata require endoscopic intervention.

2. Initial management

Patients with signs of major bleeding and hemodynamic instability should be managed in a high dependency or intensive care unit. Prompt resuscitation and close attention to co-morbid conditions is vital prior to endoscopy. Patients should have two large bore intravenous cannulae and cross-match of at least four units of red cell concentrate. Aim to transfuse to a hemoglobin of 10 g/dL (hematocrit 30%) prior to endoscopy to minimize cardiorespiratory compromise. Correct coagulopathy to INR <1.5 and platelet count to $>50 \times 10^9/L$ if required and feasible (see Chapter 2.1). This should not delay endoscopy in an emergency. Stop NSAID and antiplatelet therapy. The prokinetic effects of intravenous erythromyicn (1 g) or metoclopramide (10–20 mg) 1 hour before endoscopy may improve views but is not routinely necessary.

Warning!

Adequate resuscitation and stabilization of the patient is essential before undertaking urgent endoscopy in patients with severe upper gastrointestinal bleeding. Obtunded patients may require intubation and ventilation to facilitate endoscopy and prevent aspiration.

Table 1   Blatchford score

Admission risk marker	Score component value
Blood urea (mmol/L)	
≥6.5, <8.0	2
≥8.0, <10.0	3
≥10.0, <25.0	4
≥25	6
Hemoglobin (g/L) for men	
≥12.0, <13.0	1
≥10.0, <12.0	3
<10.0	6
Hemoglobin (g/L) for women	
≥10.0, <12.0	1
<10.0	6
Systolic blood pressure (mmHg)	
100–109	1
90–99	2
<90	3
Other markers	
Pulse ≥100 (per min)	1
Presentation with melena	1
Presentation with syncope	2
Hepatic disease	2
Cardiac failure	2

Score is equal to '0' if the following are all present:
1. Hemoglobin level >12.9 g/dL (men) or >11.9 g/dL (women)
2. Systolic blood pressure >109 mmHg
3. Pulse <100/min
4. Blood urea nitrogen level <6.5 mmol/L
5. No melena or syncope
6. No past or present liver disease or heart failure.

3. Endoscopy

Endoscopy should be performed after adequate resuscitation and within 24 h of the initial bleed. The majority of patients may be endoscoped on the next available list. However, when hemodynamic instability recurs after initial resuscitation or the patient fails to respond to resuscitation, emergency endoscopy is required. If the patient has a reduced consciousness level, significant respiratory disease or large volume hematemesis, anaesthetic support to protect the

---

> **Box 2**   Endoscopic predictors of re-bleeding
>
> - Ulcer with active bleeding.
> - Ulcer with stigmata of recent hemorrhage.
> - Ulcer size >20 mm.
> - Posterior duodenal ulcer (gastroduodenal artery involvement).

> **Box 3**   Forrest classification of stigmata of hemorrhage
>
> - Forrest 1a: spurting hemorrhage.
> - Forrest 1b: oozing hemorrhage.
> - Forrest 2a: non-bleeding visible vessel.
> - Forrest 2b: tightly adherent clot.
> - Forrest 2c: hematin in ulcer base.
> - Forrest 3: clean based ulcer.

airway should be sought. Endoscopy should be performed in a clinical area with access to full resuscitation facilities, videoendoscopy equipment, and with the support of staff familiar with endoscopic hemostatic procedures. Endoscopic injection and at least one thermal or mechanical therapeutic modality should be available (Box 4).

4. Endoscopic technique

In many patients, endoscopy may be safely performed under anesthesia, topical pharyngeal local anesthetic or intravenous (IV) sedation. Buscopan 10–20 mg IV in patients without glaucoma or glucagon 1 mg IV reduces spasm and significantly improves visualization, particularly of the pylorus and duodenal cap.

In patients with signs of major bleeding, use of a therapeutic endoscope with a large bore channel (GIF-1T160 or 1T260) or a twin channel (Olympus 2T160 or 2T260; Fujinon EG 450D) and with a water pump is advantageous to facilitate suction of blood and clot, while simultaneously deploying therapeutic accessories.

The bleeding point may be obvious, but if this is not the case, careful and systematic inspection of the gastroesophageal junction, fundus, high lesser curve, incisura, pyloric channel, duodenal cap, D1/D2 junction and second part should reveal the source of bleeding. Washing devices such as the 'Waterpik' or Heater probe (Olympus HPU 20) facilitate visualization of bleeding lesions by clearing blood and clot.

> **Box 4**   Conditions and equipment needed when undertaking endoscopy for upper GI bleeding
>
> ### General
>
> - Properly resuscitated patient: correct hypovolemia, hypotension, coagulopathy, hypoxia.
> - Skilled endoscopist and nursing assistants: trainees must be adequately supervised.
> - High dependency or intensive care facilities and anesthetic support for unstable patients.
> - Standard and large channel 'therapeutic' gastroscopes.
> - Water pump for irrigation and washing.
>
> ### Specific equipment
>
> - 23 G injection sclerotherapy needles.
> - 1:10 000 epinephrine.
> - Endoscopic clips.
> - Heater probe or BICAP probe.
> - Argon plasma coagulation (APC) generator and catheters.
> - Do not forget intravenous proton pump inhibitor for appropriate cases.

Table 2 Rockall score

Variable	Score 0	Score 1	Score 2	Score 3	Score
Age	<60	60–79	>80		
Shock	No shock	Pulse >100	Systolic BP <100		
Co-morbidity	Nil major		CCF, IHD, major morbidity	Renal/liver failure, metastatic cancer	
Diagnosis	Mallory–Weiss tear or normal	All other diagnoses	GI malignancy[a]		
Evidence of bleeding	None		Blood in stomach, adherent clot, visible or spurting vessel[b]		
				Final score (range 0–11)	

[a]Malignancy and varices have the worst prognosis.
[b]These features are associated with a high risk of re-bleeding. Re-bleeding (fresh hematemesis or melena associated with shock or a fall of Hb >20 g/L over 24 h) is associated with a 10-fold increased risk of death.

5. Endoscopic hemostasis

Accurate identification of the bleeding source is essential for effective therapy. Tightly adherent blood clot (Forrest 2B) should be vigorously washed. Some experts recommend removal of such clots with snares to reveal the underlying stigmata. Prior injection of epinephrine around the clot before removal reduces the risk of torrential bleeding.

The best outcomes are achieved with combination therapy. This involves the delivery of injection therapy, followed by either thermal ablation or the application of mechanical clips. Selection of the therapeutic method depends upon the location and type of ulcer, availability of equipment and endoscopist expertise. Use of a single hemostatic method is better than no therapy. Very recent studies have highlighted the efficacy and safety of a nanopowder ('Hemospray') that can be sprayed onto bleeding ulcers with rapid cessation of bleeding. Trials of this new treatment are awaited.

5.1. Injection

Injection therapy is straightforward, accessible, portable, and cheap. Injection is applicable to ulcers in any location. Numerous agents have been investigated, but none has proven superior to dilute epinephrine. Sclerosants such as polidocanol are associated with perforation and are not recommended. The mechanism of action of injected epinephrine includes tamponade, vasoconstriction, and stimulation of platelet aggregation. Injected volumes of 13–20 mL are associated with reduced re-bleeding rates compared with smaller volumes.

Injection therapy is delivered via a standard 23 G endoscopic injection needle in a 7 F catheter sheath (Fig. 2). Injection of 1:10 000 epinephrine should be delivered in 1–2 mL aliquots into the fibrous base of the ulcer circumferentially around the bleeding point or visible vessel (Fig. 3). Injection should continue until active bleeding has ceased and the surrounding mucosa demonstrates a blanching effect. It is common for injection sites to ooze small amounts of blood. It is not necessary to inject oozing edges of ulcers.

> ### ✓ Clinical Tip
>
> Inject dilute epinephrine circumferentially around a visible or bleeding vessel before targeting the vessel itself. The same applies to application of thermal therapy.

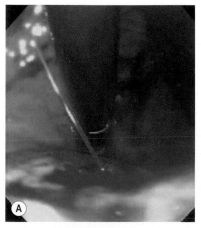
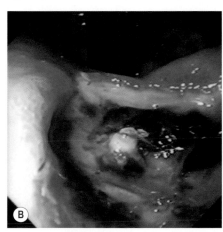
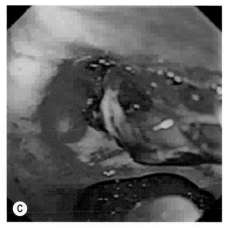

Figure 1 Examples of stigmata of hemorrhage. (A) Forrest IA: spurting hemorrhage from an ulcer in gastric cardia. (B) Forrest IIA: non-bleeding visible vessel. (C) Forrest IIB: tightly adherent clot in ulcer base.

5.2. Thermal therapy

The most widely used thermal probes are the heater probe and the BICAP. Monopolar coagulation is associated with perforation, and laser therapy is no longer used for peptic ulcer treatment. Argon plasma coagulation has a superficial effect which is generally unsuitable for arterial bleeding caused by peptic ulceration.

The heater probe (Fig. 4) has a Teflon coated tip which delivers preset amounts of direct heat energy according to the probe settings. It has the advantage of a powerful water jet which facilitates location of the bleeding source. Settings of 20–30 J should be used according to tissue effect.

The BICAP is a bipolar probe requiring an electrosurgical plate to be applied to the patient, usually on the posterior thigh; 20–30 W settings should be used. A particular version of the BICAP is the Gold probe (Boston Scientific) which combines a BICAP probe with an injection needle, this allowing for complete therapy using a single accessory.

Thermal probes use the technique of coaptive coagulation. The vessel is compressed, opposing the vessel walls before heat is applied to minimize therapy-induced bleeding (Fig. 5). Probes may be applied tangentially, which may be a particular advantage in awkwardly placed ulcers in the duodenum. Pulses should be delivered circumferentially around the bleeding point before therapy to the vessel itself. The desired end result is cavitation and blackening of the vessel, usually requiring at least 8–10 pulses of therapy.

5.3. Mechanical clips

There are three types of clip in general use (Fig. 6). The Olympus QuickClip 2, the Cook TriClip and the Boston

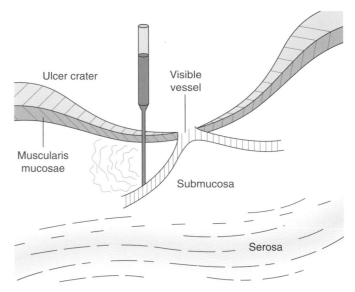

Figure 3 Injection therapy. Injection should be into the fibrous ulcer base around the vessel. In the case of epinephrine this will result in vasoconstriction and a tamponade effect, both resulting in clotting within the vessel.

Scientific Resolution clip. All have been shown to be effective, although the QuickClip 2 (Fig. 7) has the best trial evidence of efficacy. Clips produce mechanical compression of the bleeding point, but are problematic to apply tangentially, rendering posterior duodenal and high lesser curve ulcers difficult to treat. In addition, the tough fibrous base of a chronic ulcer may be impossible to clip adequately. All types of clip are delivered singly and are deployed from a delivery sheath. The control handle may be used to rotate the clips to the desired alignment.

Once the bleeding lesion is located, the clip is advanced from the sheath. If the endoscope is retroflexed to visualize the ulcer, it may be necessary to straighten the scope before clip advancement and then reposition with the clip ready to apply. In the case of the QuickClip, the clip must be primed before application to the lesion in order to achieve correct placement. The advantage of the Resolution clip is that it may be opened and closed numerous times before final deployment, thus facilitating correct positioning. The clip is

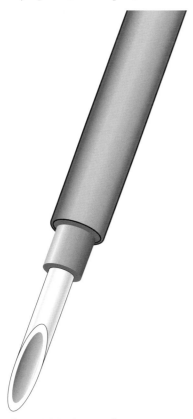

Figure 2 Injection needle.

> **⚠ Warning!**
>
> Clips may be difficult to apply when the ulcer is awkwardly placed (posterior duodenal bulb, high lesser curve) or in chronic ulcers with fibrotic bases.

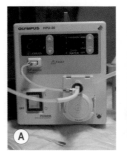 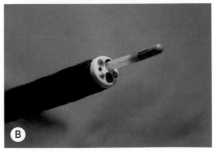

Figure 4 Heater probe unit (A) with 3.2 mm heater probe in a therapeutic channel gastroscope (B).

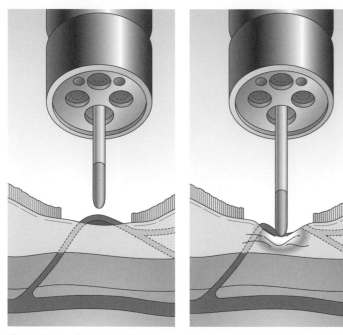

Figure 5 Coaptive coagulation.

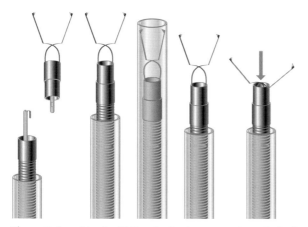

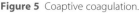

Figure 6 Reusable clip. (1) The clip (hook, compression cylinder, jaws) and the transmission system (cable for anchoring the clip with lug, spiral sheath for advancing the closing cylinder and a protective sheath). (2) The clip fixed by its hooking system is locked onto the spiral sheath. (3) The clip and the spiral sheath are covered with the protective sheath. (4) The clip is pushed out of the protective sheath over the lesion to be clipped. (5) Maximum opening of the clip achieved when the assistant begins to close the clip: it is only from this point that the clip is ready to be deployed onto the lesion.

advanced to the lesion and then pressed onto the ulcer at the base of the lesion. Back pressure on the control handle deploys the clip which then detaches from the sheath. Two to three clips should be applied for maximum efficacy (Figs 8–10).

5.4. Second-look endoscopy

Evidence that an early 'second-look' endoscopy improves outcomes in ulcer bleeding is controversial but this should be considered in selected cases – for example, when complete views of the source of bleeding have been obscured by blood or there is doubt about the adequacy of endoscopic therapy in patients regarded as high risk for surgery should they rebleed.

6. *Helicobacter* testing

Patients in whom an ulcer is found should have biopsies taken for *H. pylori* testing at the index endoscopy. Blood in the stomach may buffer the reagent in a rapid urease test and so this should be combined with antral biopsies sent to pathology to maximize the diagnostic yield. Eradication of *H. pylori* facilitates ulcer healing and has been shown to reduce re-bleeding.

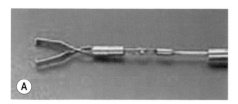
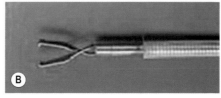

Figure 7 (A,B) Reusable clip.

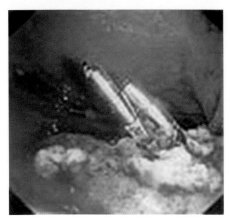

Figure 8 Clips in position after hemorrhage.

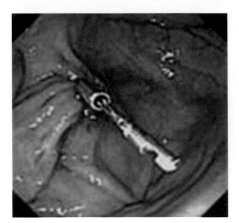

Figure 9 Triclip released.

7. Proton pump inhibitor therapy

Intravenous proton pump inhibitors (IV PPI) reduce re-bleeding after endoscopic therapy for peptic ulcer. The trial evidence suggests that an IV bolus of 80 mg of Omeprazole or Pantoprazole followed by a continuous infusion of 8 mg/h for 72 h will reduce both re-bleeding and surgery rates. There is no evidence that IV PPIs are required in other groups, and no robust evidence to support their use before endoscopy.

Clinical Tips

- Resuscitate prior to endoscopy.
- Buscopan facilitates adequate visualization.
- Combination therapy improves outcome.
- Inject into the ulcer base around vessels.
- 13–20 mL epinephrine injection gives optimum results.
- Apply heater probe circumferentially around vessel before application to vessel.
- Prime QuickClip before application to vessel.

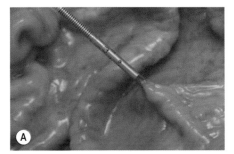

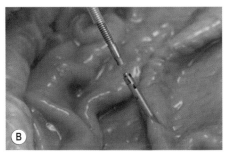

(A)

(B)

Figure 10 (A) Disposable clip which can be repositioned. (B) Clip released in pig stomach.

Further Reading

ASGE Committee: Guideline: the role of endoscopy in acute non-variceal upper-GI hemorrhage, *Gastrointest Endosc* 60(4):497–504, 2004.

ASGE Technology status evaluation report: Endoscopic hemostatic devices, *Gastrointest Endosc* 69(6):987–996, 2009.

Barkun AN, Bardou M, Kuipers EJ, et al: International Consensus Upper Gastrointestinal Bleeding Conference Group. International consensus recommendations on the management of patients with nonvariceal upper gastrointestinal bleeding, *Ann Intern Med* 152(2):101–113, 2010.

BSGE Committee: Non-variceal upper gastrointestinal hemorrhage: guidelines. British Society of Gastroenterology Endoscopy Committee, *Gut* 51(Suppl IV):iv1–iv6, 2002.

Blatchford O, Murray WR, Blatchford M: A risk score to predict need for treatment for upper-gastrointestinal hemorrhage, *Lancet* 356:1318–1321, 2000.

Church NI, Palmer KR: Acute non-variceal gastrointestinal hemorrhage: treatment. In McDonald JW, Burroughs AK, Feagan BG, et al, editors: *Evidence-based gastroenterology and hepatology*, ed 3, London, 2010, BMJ Books, pp 165–189.

Scottish Intercollegiate Guidelines Network: *Management of acute upper and lower gastrointestinal bleeding*. A national clinical guideline. Guideline No. 105. 2008. www.sign.ac.uk/pdf/sign105.pdf

Stanley AJ, Ashley D, Dalton HR, et al: Outpatient management of patients with low-risk upper-gastrointestinal haemorrhage: multicentre validation and prospective evaluation, *Lancet* 373(9657): 42–47, 2009.

7.9 Endoscopic treatment of upper gastrointestinal hemorrhage secondary to portal hypertension

Nicholas I. Church, Jean-Christophe Létard

Summary

Key Points

- Variceal bleeding occurs in 30% of cirrhotic patients during the course of their disease.
- Mortality of variceal bleeding is determined by the severity of the underlying liver disease.
- Endoscopy should be undertaken as soon as possible after resuscitation.
- Endoscopic band ligation is superior to injection sclerotherapy for esophageal varices.
- Gastric varices may be treated by endoscopic injection of thrombin or cyanoacrylate tissue glue.
- TIPSS insertion is an effective rescue therapy when endoscopic therapy fails.
- Antibiotic therapy reduces mortality in variceal bleeding.

Introduction

Variceal bleeding occurs in 30% of cirrhotic patients at some stage in their life. Risk factors for bleeding include variceal size, portal pressure, wall tension, and severity of underlying liver disease. Endoscopic therapy is effective for variceal bleeding but re-bleeding rates may be 20–50%. Bleeding is associated with a significant risk of death, which is largely determined by the severity of liver disease. For a patient with Child's cirrhosis (Child's A), the mortality risk of a first variceal bleed is 5% but this rises to 50% in Child's C disease. Overall mortality in all patients presenting with variceal bleeding is 14%. Mortality may be reduced by the administration of antibiotics for 5 days after a bleed.

1. General management

The general principles of risk assessment, resuscitation, and management of co-morbid conditions apply to patients with variceal bleeding in the same way as to those with bleeding ulcer (see Ch. 7.8). Factors suggestive of variceal rather than ulcer bleeding include a previous history of variceal bleeding, known liver disease or clinical signs of cirrhosis and portal hypertension. Excessive blood transfusion should be avoided, as this may increase portal pressure and exacerbate coagulopathy: aim for Hb 8–10 g/dL (hematocrit 0.30). In patients with a high suspicion of variceal bleeding, terlipressin 2 mg IV 4 times daily. should be commenced in addition to antibiotic therapy with quinolones or third generation cephalosporins. Patients may be agitated or obtunded secondary to encephalopathy, resulting in a high risk of aspiration, particularly during endoscopy or insertion of a balloon tamponade device. In such cases, anesthetic support should be sought early.

2. Endoscopy

As with a bleeding peptic ulcer, patients should be adequately resuscitated prior to endoscopy. However, endoscopy should be undertaken as soon as resuscitation is achieved rather than waiting until the next available list. The procedure should be undertaken in a high dependency area with full resuscitation facilities, videoendoscopic equipment and staff familiar with endoscopic hemostatic procedures. Light sedation may be adequate, but in agitated or obtunded patients, deeper sedation and endotracheal intubation is often required. Band ligation devices, injection needles, sclerosants and ideally thrombin or tissue glue should be available in addition to the equipment required for ulcer hemostasis (Box 1). A Sengstaken or Minnesota tube should also be readily available.

3. Endoscopic technique

It is preferable to start with a regular diagnostic endoscope as a standard diameter banding cap will not fit the large channel therapeutic scope. The other principles are similar to those for peptic ulcer bleeding.

Esophageal varices may be graded endoscopically as in Box 2. Esophageal varices occur mainly in the palisade zone, which extends from the gastroesophageal junction for 4–5 cm towards the mid-esophagus (Fig. 1). Active bleeding is usually obvious (Fig. 2), although the exact site of the bleeding may be difficult to identify. Signs of recent bleeding include fibrin plugs or red spots (the 'red wale' sign). In general, if varices are present and the patient has signs of a significant bleed in the absence of other causative lesions, it is reasonable to assume that the varices were the source of bleeding.

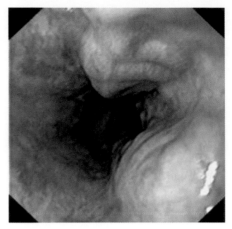

General

The same considerations apply as for peptic ulcer bleeding (Ch. 7.8).

Specific equipment

- Variceal ligation devices.
- 5% ethanolamine (if variceal ligation devices not available).
- Thrombin (fibrin tissue sealant, Tisseel, Baxter International, Deerfield, IL, USA).
- Tissue adhesive glue (n-butyl cyanoacrylate or 2-octyl cyanoacrylate).
- Sengstaken/Minnesota tube.
- Do not forget intravenous antibiotics (cephalosporin or quinolone or piperacillin with tazobactam).

Figure 1 Grade 2 esophageal varices.

4. Endoscopic therapy for esophageal varices

4.1. Variceal band ligation (EVL)

Band ligation has become the therapy of first choice, as it is effective and associated with fewer complications than sclerotherapy. The treatment involves placing an elastic band onto the variceal column. This results in initial thrombosis and hemostasis. Ischemia of the mucosa and submucosa develops during the days following ligation, followed by the formation of granulation tissue and re-epithelialization after 14–21 days.

4.1.1. Method

Two banding devices are currently in widespread use. These are the Cook 4,6,10 Shooter Saeed Multi-Band Ligator and the SpeedBand SuperView Super 7 Multiple Band Ligator from Boston Scientific. These devices allow the placement of 4–10 elastic bands during the same session. The steps required to set up an endoscopic variceal ligator are shown in Figure 3. Following the initial diagnostic endoscopy, the scope is withdrawn and the banding device attached. Re-intubation with the banding cap *in situ* is slightly more difficult than usual, but if the scope is inserted in the midline and directed posterior to the cricoarytenoid cartilage, gentle forward pressure will usually result in successful passage into the esophagus. The transparent end cap is positioned over a varix which is aspirated into the operating channel. Optimum placement occurs when a 'red-out' is seen, indicating that sufficient tissue has been aspirated into the cap (Fig. 4). The ligating band is then released by turning the wheel of the banding device clockwise (Fig. 5). If not enough mucosa is aspirated, the band will tend to slide off after deployment,

which may exacerbate bleeding. Banding should commence close to the gastroesophageal junction, continuing upwards in a spiral fashion until there is at least one band on each variceal column (Fig. 6). Aim to band in the distal 5 cm of the esophagus. Usually 4–8 bands are required, although the placement of more than six has not been shown to improve outcome. Ligation sessions should then be performed at intervals of 7–14 days, until the varices have been completely eradicated, which may need 2–4 sessions on average but sometimes more than this.

4.1.2. Complications

Minor complications such as short-lived dysphagia and thoracic discomfort are common. In contrast to sclerotherapy, esophageal stricturing, mediastinitis and perforation are rare. Post-ligation ulcers occasionally bleed, but in cases of significant bleeding standard hemostatic methods such as injection of epinephrine are effective.

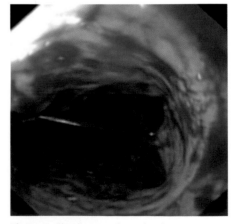

Figure 2 Bleeding esophageal varix.

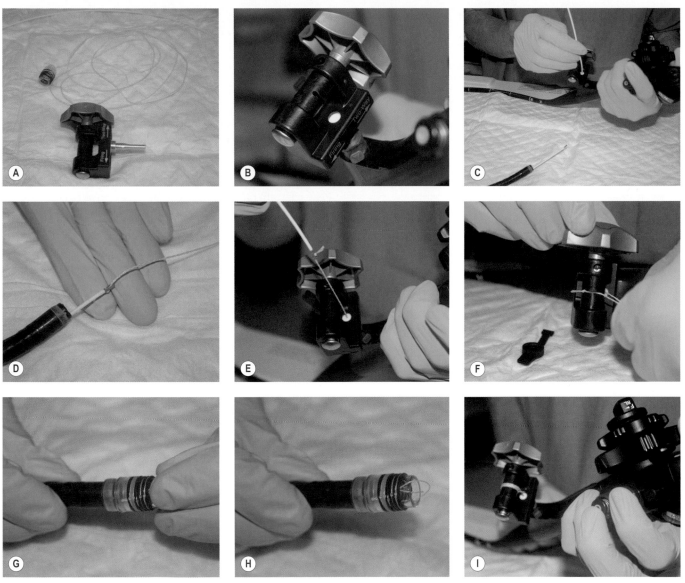

Figure 3 Setting up an endoscopic variceal ligator. (A) The kit consists of a handle, cap with bands and thread, and an introducer. (B) The handle is securely fitted into the endoscope instrument channel. (C) The plastic introducer is passed down through the rubber slit in the ligator handle until exits the distal tip of the endoscope. (D) The knot on the thread is attached to the hook at the end of the introducer. (E) The thread is drawn up the instrument channel until it appears through the ligator handle. (F) The thread is slotted into the groove on the ligator handle. (G) The cap is fitted snugly onto the endoscope tip. (H,I) Any slack in the thread is taken up by slowly turning the wheel on the handle. The cap is rotated so that the threads lie at 7–9 o'clock on the endoscopic image so they do not interfere with the view (see Figure 6).

4.2. Endoscopic sclerotherapy (EST)

Injecting a sclerosing agent into and around a variceal lumen results in inflammation, necrosis, and thrombosis. During an active hemorrhage, the aim of treatment is to stop bleeding, either directly by achieving rapid thrombosis of the bleeding vessel, or indirectly by compression of the vessel by tissue oedema. Prophylactic sclerotherapy results in inflammation of the variceal wall and surrounding tissues, leading to fibrosis and thus obstruction of the vessel. EST is now second-line therapy after EVL, in view of its propensity to cause complications (see below). The most commonly used agents are 1–3% polidocanol and 5% ethanolamine oleate in Europe; 1–2% sodium tetradecyl sulphate and 5% sodium morrhuate in the USA. No one agent is superior to the others.

4.2.1. Method

Standard disposable 23-gauge injection needles are used. Commence injection at the gastroesophageal junction and proceed around the circumference (Fig. 7). 1–2 mL of sclerosant is injected at each site, up to a maximum of 12–20 mL per session. Injection should be avoided in the proximal or mid-esophagus since a leak of sclerosant could enter the azygos vein and pulmonary circulation, causing serious harmful effects. After successful initial control of bleeding, the patient should commence an eradication program as described above.

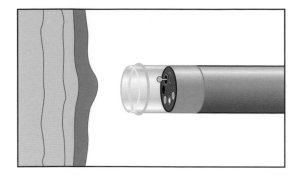

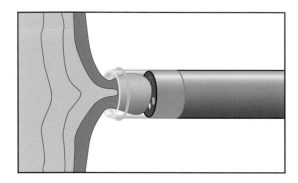

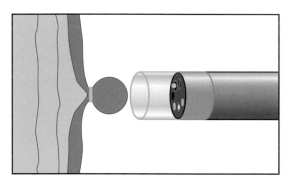

Figure 4 Esophageal varices banded.

 Warning!

Do not inject sclerosant into the mid- or proximal esophagus as sclerosant may enter the azygous vein and pulmonary circulation.

4.2.2. Complications

Minor complications (slight fever, retrosternal pain or temporary dysphagia) occur within 24–48 h and do not usually need any treatment. Deep ulceration of the esophageal mucosa and submucosa is the commonest major complication, appearing within 24 h in more than 90% of patients. Ulceration may cause recurrent hemorrhage in 20% of cases. Post-sclerotherapy esophageal stenoses have been reported in 2–10% of cases. They respond to dilation but this procedure may be hazardous in the context of esophageal varices. Esophageal perforation is rare but serious, since the mortality rate is >50%. Rare regional complications may also occur after sclerotherapy. These include respiratory distress syndrome, bronchoesophageal fistula, pneumothorax, chylothorax or mediastinitis.

5. Endoscopic therapy for gastric varices

Gastric varices may be classified endoscopically as in Box 3. They differ from esophageal varices, in that they lie more deeply in the submucosa and tend to have a greater vessel

Box 3 Endoscopic grading of gastric varices
• Gastroesophageal varices type 1 (GOV1): esophageal varices which extend onto the lesser curve of stomach.
• Gastroesophageal varices type 2 (GOV2): esophageal varices which extend into the fundus.
• Isolated gastric varices type 1 (IGV1): isolated gastric varices in the fundus.
• Isolated gastric varices type 2 (IGV2): isolated gastric varices at ectopic sites in the stomach or in the first part of duodenum.

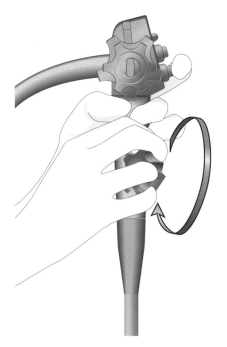

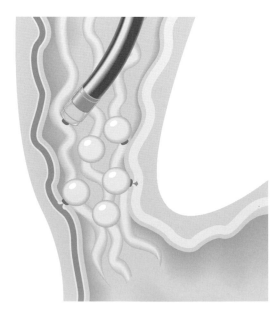

Figure 5 Technique of elastic ligation of esophageal varices.

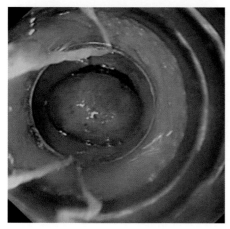

Figure 6 Application of several elastic bands.

diameter. The incidence of bleeding from gastric varices is half that of esophageal varices, but when gastric variceal bleeding does occur, it is more severe, and endoscopic therapy is more difficult. Band ligation and sclerosant injection are ineffective and the two therapeutic options are injection of either thrombin or cyanoacrylate tissue adhesive. Neither of these agents has been subjected to adequately powered randomized clinical trials.

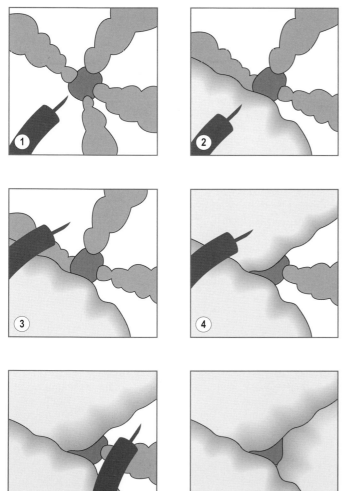

Figure 7 Sclerotherapy technic for esophageal varices (paravariceal injection).

5.1. Thrombin injection

5.1.1. Method

Initial case series reported the injection of bovine thrombin to be effective. This agent is no longer available due to the risk of transmission of vCJD. Human thrombin is now available and small studies have shown efficacy in terms of initial hemostasis and reduction of re-bleeding.

Thrombin is presented as a freeze dried powder which is reconstituted with 5 mL of normal saline to produce a thrombin solution containing 1000 IU/mL. The injection is performed using a standard sclerotherapy needle and requires no special preparation. 1 mL aliquots are injected into the gastric varix until hemostasis is secure. It is common for the puncture site to bleed transiently after removal of the needle, but clotting occurs rapidly. The total volume of injection required depends on the size and number of varices, but is usually 2–10 mL. No major complications of thrombin injection have been reported.

> ✓ **Clinical Tip**
>
> To minimize bleeding from gastric varices after each thrombin injection, withdraw the needle but keep the catheter sheath firmly pressed against the vessel for 30 s.

5.2. Cyanoacrylate tissue glue injection

5.2.1. Method

Tissue glue is a liquid monomer, which rapidly polymerizes on contact with living tissues to form a hard acrylic plastic. Two forms are available in Europe: n-butyl-2-cyanoacrylate (Histoacryl) and isobutyl-2-cyanoacrylate (Bucrylate). In the USA, 2-octyl cyanoacrylate (SurgiSeal) has been used for treatment of gastric varices. The evidence for efficacy is from small, generally non-randomized case series. Glue injection is potentially hazardous for staff and equipment due to the rapidity of hardening of the glue, and close attention to the correct technique is required.

Eye protection should be worn by the patient, operators and assistants. Injection is performed with a standard 23-gauge sclerotherapy needle. A 'dry run' before filling the needle with glue may be beneficial to confirm that the needle will operate successfully in the retroflexed position. Several needles should be available as they may become inoperable due to glue polymerization. The volume of dead space in the needle is determined by prior injection with sterile water (saline would cause polymerization of the glue). A 2 mL syringe containing 0.5 mL glue and 0.5 mL Lipiodol is then prepared and a volume equivalent to two-thirds of the dead space is used to prime the needle. The biopsy port is coated and the channel flushed with Lipiodol and the primed needle inserted. The needle sheath is placed close to the varix and the needle advanced and placed into the varix. The remainder of the glue/Lipiodol mix is then injected, followed by a flush of either water or Lipiodol equivalent in volume to the dead space of the needle, thus flushing the glue out of the needle. The needle is then removed from the varix without retracting it into the sheath and a continuous flush of water is used to prevent the needle from becoming jammed. The needle should be removed immediately to prevent it sticking to the varix. A short-lived rush of blood and glue from the injection site is common. Contamination of the tip of the endoscope with glue may be minimized by prior coating of the tip with Lipiodol, maintaining a safe distance of the scope from the injection site and continuous air insufflation during the injection procedure. If the needle can then be retracted following injection, the sheath may be used to compress and assess the varix. If it is soft, further injections are needed and the process is repeated by re-priming the needle with glue. If the needle cannot be retracted a new needle is required. Injection volumes of >1 mL of glue should not be used to minimize the risk of embolization.

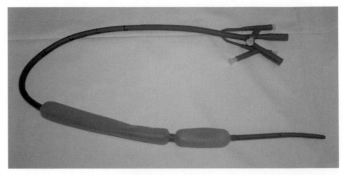

Figure 8 Minnesota tube.

 Warning!

Use of tissue glue

- Eye protection is essential for patient and staff.
- Take care to avoid glue polymerization in the scope channel.
- The needle needs to be flushed after every injection.
- The needle should be removed immediately after injection but not retracted into its sheath to avoid sticking.

5.2.2. Complications

Complications of tissue glue injection have been reported. These include portal and splenic vein thrombosis, pulmonary embolism and emboli to heart and brain. Ulceration and perforation at the injection site may also occur.

6. Rescue therapy

For cases in which endoscopic hemostasis is unsuccessful or unavailable, balloon tamponade may be life-saving, although this is only a temporary measure to stabilize the situation before definitive therapy. A Sengstaken–Blakemore or Minnesota tube is used (Fig. 8). Tips for insertion are given in Box 4.

Transjugular intrahepatic portosystemic shunt (TIPSS) insertion is the mainstay of definitive therapy when

---

Box 4 Tips for insertion of tamponade balloon

- Protect the airway – aspiration is a major risk.
- Pass the tube through the mouth – passage through the nose risks damage to the nasal turbinates and soft palate.
- Inserting a guidewire into the tube before tube insertion may help to prevent the tube kinking in the esophagus reducing the risk of esophageal perforation.
- Once in the stomach, blow up the gastric balloon with 200–250 mL of air – there is no need to fill the balloon with water and water will render the balloon difficult to locate on check X-ray.
- If the tube is difficult to pass, insertion over an endoscopically placed guidewire may be helpful.
- Inflation of the esophageal balloon is rarely necessary and risks ischemic necrosis of the esophagus and perforation.
- Once the gastric balloon is inflated, apply gentle traction and fix the tube by clamping it between two tongue depressors placed above and below it, with their ends taped together under tension, resting against a gauze pad at the lips.
- Check tube position with X-ray.

---

endoscopic methods are ineffective. A correctly placed TIPSS will stop bleeding in the majority of cases, although its use is limited by the availability of equipment and expertise and a significant proportion of patients become encephalopathic following insertion.

Surgery is now rarely employed as rescue therapy, except in the situation of isolated gastric varices due to splenic vein thrombosis, in which case splenectomy may be required.

Further Reading

ASGE Committee: Guideline: the role of endoscopy in the management of variceal hemorrhage (updated July 2005), *Gastrointest Endosc* 62(5):651–655, 2005.

Samonakis DN, Triantos CK, Thalheimer U, et al: Management of portal hypertension, *Postgrad Med J* 80:634–641, 2004.

Scottish Intercollegiate Guidelines Network: *Management of acute upper and lower gastrointestinal bleeding*. A national clinical guideline. Guideline No. 105. 2008. www.sign.ac.uk/pdf/sign105.pdf

Tripathi D, Hayes PC: Endoscopic therapy for bleeding gastric varices: to clot or glue? *Gastrointest Endosc* 68(5):883–886,2008.

7.10 Endoscopic treatment of non-variceal non-ulcer gastrointestinal hemorrhage

Nicholas I. Church, Jean-Christophe Létard

Summary

1. Upper GI tract   221

2. Lower GI tract   222

Key Points

- Upper GI tract lesions, which may be result in arterial bleeding, include esophagitis, Mallory–Weiss tear, and Dieulafoy lesions.
- Arterial bleeding in the lower GI tract may be caused by diverticulosis or following polypectomy.
- Endoscopic techniques for the treatment of arterial bleeding are similar to those for bleeding peptic ulcer.
- Non-arterial bleeding is best treated with argon plasma coagulation, but lesions may not require therapy.

1. Upper GI tract

1.1. Esophagitis

Severe esophagitis may be a cause of hematemesis in some patients. Usually no treatment is required other than proton pump inhibitor therapy. However, erosion into submucosal vessels may result in more significant hemorrhage. Such lesions may be seen as actively bleeding lesions, non-bleeding visible vessels or have adherent clot. They respond well to injection of epinephrine 1 : 10 000, thermal probes, and mechanical clips. The techniques of therapy are as described in section 7.8. Care should be taken to differentiate such lesions from bleeding esophageal varices, which are treated by banding as described in section 7.9.

1.2. Mallory–Weiss syndrome

Typically presenting with hematemesis after an episode of vomiting, Mallory-Weiss tears (Fig. 1) are longitudinal tears around the gastroesophageal junction. They may be best visualized with the endoscope retroflexed in the fundus. Severe bleeding is unusual, but when present is treated with injection, thermal probes or clips as above. Re-bleeding after therapy is rare.

1.3. Dieulafoy's lesion

This uncommon lesion is a developmental malformation of a submucosal artery, which results in the vessel retaining a caliber 10 times that of normal submucosal vessels. Bleeding results when a superficial mucosal defect occurs over the vessel, possibly due to the progressive mechanical effect on the mucosa of the pulsation of the underlying artery. The majority of Dieulafoy lesions are found within 6 cm of the gastroesophageal junction, usually on the high lesser curve of the stomach, but they may occur anywhere in the gut.

A presentation with recurrent, severe hemorrhage in a young patient, in whom blood is found in the upper GI tract without an obvious cause endoscopically, should alert the endoscopist to the possibility of a Dieulafoy lesion. This lesion appears as a protruding vessel, without significant surrounding ulceration, which may be actively bleeding, or may be seen as a small area of adherent clot (Fig. 2). Endoscopic hemostasis with epinephrine injection and clips produces the best results, although thermal probes may be used also (Fig. 3). Some operators have reported good outcomes following the application of bands. Endoscopic therapy is effective in the majority of cases.

Clinical Tip

The site of a Dieulafoy's lesion can be difficult to identify especially when bleeding is brisk. Once identified and treated, the site can be marked with a tattoo in case repeat endoscopy is required.

1.4. Angiodysplasia

Angiodysplasias are vascular lesions composed of ectatic, thin walled mucosal and submucosal vessels, often with arteriovenous malformations. Lesions are frequently found in the fundus and upper body of the stomach, the second part of duodenum and the small bowel but the colon is the most common site. Angiodysplasias usually cause recurrent occult blood loss, although bleeding may sometimes be overt. Lesions may be masked by blood or considered an artefact associated with suctioning, but with careful inspection, their frond-like appearance around a central vessel is characteristic.

The most effective endoscopic treatment is superficial ablation using the argon plasma coagulator (APC, see Ch. 7.4). Coagulation depth is limited to around 3 mm which is advantageous when treating lesions in the colon. Straight and side firing versions of the catheter are available and choice depends on endoscopist preference and the orientation of the lesion. The power should be set to 40–60 W in the upper GI tract, but may be reduced according to tissue effect. The catheter is advanced until close to the lesion and the pedal is activated to deliver short pulses of coagulation until the lesion is desiccated and appears white. APC generates irritant gasses, which should be regularly suctioned to minimize patient discomfort. Angiodysplasias may also be treated with conventional thermal probes such as the BICAP.

Warning!

Low-power (20–30 W) argon plasma coagulation is adequate for treating superficial angiodysplastic lesions in the upper GI tract. Lower power (15–20 W) should be used in the thinner right colon. Contact of the probe tip with the mucosa may force gas into the submucosa, risking perforation, and should be avoided.

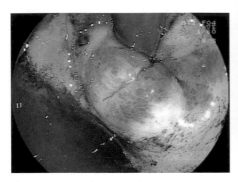

Figure 1 Linear ulcer at esophagogastric junction secondary to Mallory–Weiss tear.

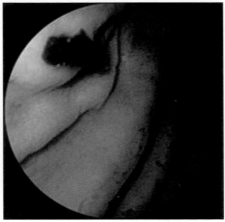

Figure 2 Dieulafoy's lesion with a characteristic clot confirming the diagnosis.

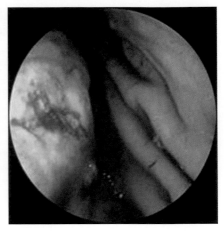

Figure 3 Dieulafoy's lesion after argon plasma coagulation (APC).

1.5. Gastric antral vascular ectasia (GAVE)

This condition usually presents with occult GI hemorrhage or iron deficiency anemia, but may present with hematemesis. Numerous thin-walled ectatic vessels develop in the antrum of the stomach, radiating out from the pylorus in lines, leading the condition to be commonly named watermelon stomach.

Endoscopic treatment is with the APC as above (see Ch. 7.4). To coagulate the lines of vessels, the APC may be activated and the scope pulled back along the line. Prolonged and repeated sessions of therapy may be required before all vessels are ablated.

1.6. Malignant lesions

Malignant lesions in the esophagus and stomach may cause significant bleeding. Superficial coagulation with the APC is the most effective endoscopic therapy. It is possible to coagulate large lesions, although this may be time consuming. Re-bleeding is common.

1.7. Other lesions

'Cameron lesions' are linear ulcers occurring in the neck of a hiatal hernia sac and thought to result from trauma from repeated herniation (Fig. 4). Portal hypertensive gastropathy (Fig. 5) causes diffuse minor bleeding. It does not respond to endoscopic therapy. Mucosal erosions may be responsible for minor bleeding. Treatment involves PPI therapy and discontinuation of irritant medications or treatment of *H. pylori*. Esophageal microerosions occasionally cause upper GI bleeding (Fig. 6) Aortoduodenal fistula may present with a herald bleed. The endoscopic appearance is of a red/purple bulge in the second part of duodenum, usually in a patient with a history of aortic aneurysm. Urgent vascular surgical repair is the treatment.

2. Lower GI tract

2.1. Diverticulosis

Diverticular bleeding may be profuse but in 75% of cases bleeding stops spontaneously. Submucosal arteries become stretched around the neck of the diverticulum and bleeding may occur from the neck or the base. Urgent colonoscopy most commonly reveals non-bleeding diverticulae (Fig. 7), but occasionally active bleeding or a non-bleeding visible vessel is seen in one particular diverticulum. Epinephrine 1:10 000 injection in 1 mL aliquots in four quadrants around the bleeding site is effective. The BICAP thermal probe used on low-power (10–15 W) settings may also be

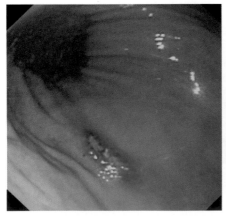

Figure 4 Linear ('Cameron') erosion in a hiatus hernia sac.

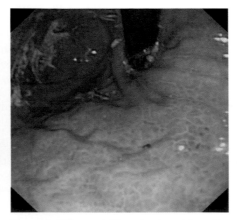

Figure 5 Diffuse portal hypertensive gastropathy with small petechiae.

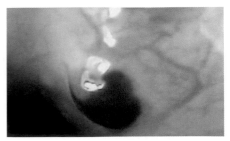

Figure 6 Bleeding esophageal microlesion.

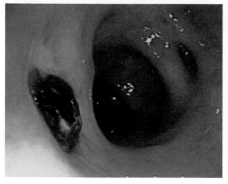

Figure 7 Blood clot in a colonic diverticulum.

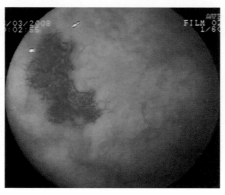

Figure 8 Colonic angiodysplasia.

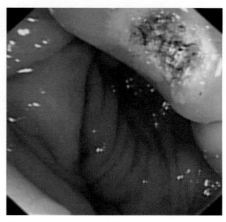

Figure 9 Colonic angiodysplasia after APC therapy.

used. Thermal energy is delivered in single short pulses around and then onto the bleeding vessel using coaptive coagulation (see below). The bleeding site should be marked with a tattoo to facilitate visualization in cases of re-bleeding.

2.2. Post-polypectomy bleeding

Bleeding following polypectomy (see Ch. 7.7) is usually self-limiting, occurring up to 7–10 days after the procedure. If there is torrential or persistent bleeding, epinephrine injection, thermal coagulation, clip application, and the application of endoloops are all effective.

2.3. Angiodysplasia

Angiodysplasias are most commonly found in the colon (Figs 8, 9). They are treated with APC set at 40–60 or the BICAP set at 10–15 W.

2.4. Malignancy

Bleeding from colonic tumors may be treated with APC as above.

2.5. Other lesions (Figs 10–12)

Ulcerative colitis, thermometer-related ulceration, solitary rectal ulcer syndrome (SRUS) and radiation proctitis generally cause diffuse mild bleeding. Endoscopic therapy is not required. Hemorrhoids generally respond to medical therapy or proctoscopy and banding. Rectal varices can be ligated as for esophageal varices but are best treated by insertion of a TIPSS shunt.

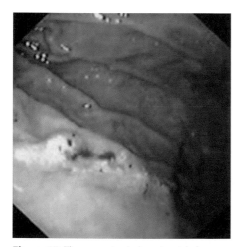

Figure 10 Thermometer-induced rectal ulcer.

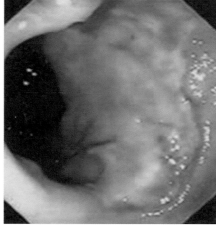

Figure 11 Solitary rectal ulcer.

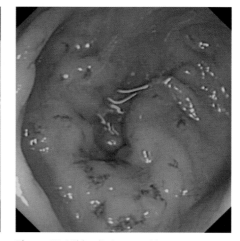

Figure 12 Mild radiation proctitis.

Further Reading

ASGE Committee: Guideline: the role of endoscopy in acute non-variceal upper-GI hemorrhage, *Gastrointest Endosc* 60(4):497–504, 2004.

BSGE Committee: Non-variceal upper gastrointestinal hemorrhage: guidelines. British Society of Gastroenterology Endoscopy Committee, *Gut* 51(suppl IV):iv1–iv6, 2002.

Chung SC, Lau JY, Rutgeerts P, et al: Thermal coagulation for non-variceal bleeding, *Endoscopy* 34:89–92, 2002.

No authors listed: Les anti-ulcéreux: indications chez l'adulte (recommandations de bonne pratique) [Antiulcer agents: indications in adults (good practice recommendations)], *Gastroenterol Clin Biol* 24(4):447–460, 2000.

Park CH, Sohn YH, Lee WS, et al: The usefulness of endoscopic hemoclipping for bleeding Dieulafoy lesions, *Endoscopy* 35(5):388–392, 2003.

7.11 Percutaneous endoscopic gastrostomy

Anne Le Sidaner

Key Points

- Percutaneous endoscopic gastrostomy is the most commonly performed therapeutic upper GI endoscopic procedure.
- The appropriateness of PEG feeding must be carefully considered before proceeding.
- The pull-type technique is the most widely used.
- The commonest indication is for prolonged enteral nutrition in patients who are unable to swallow adequately or safely.
- Antibiotic prophylaxis is recommended for all PEG procedures.
- Major complications occur in 3% and minor complications in up to 43% of patients.

Introduction

Percutaneous endoscopic gastrostomy (PEG) is the standard technique for long-term enteral nutritional support (>4 weeks). It is the commonest therapeutic procedure performed during upper digestive endoscopy. The decision to insert a PEG is often ethically challenging and the indication for the procedure must be carefully considered. Careful discussion with the patient and/or carers is essential and informed consent must be obtained. The procedure can be performed at the bedside or in the endoscopy room, provided that strict asepsis is followed. It can be performed under conscious sedation but general anesthesia is preferable in uncooperative patients and the procedure takes, on average, 30 min. An abdominal surgical field must be prepared, and oral disinfection carried out (povidone iodine mouthwash), especially when there is oral or ENT disease. The patient must fast for at least 8 hours.

 Clinical Tip

Antibiotic prophylaxis is necessary because the procedure carries a 4.3–16% risk of local, soft tissue infection. A single dose of cephazolin 2 g or cefuroxime 750 mg is given pre-procedure. If allergic, teicoplanin 400 mg can be used.

1. PEG equipment

Several disposable sterile PEG kits are available. Contents and exact tube design vary but all include a puncture trocar,

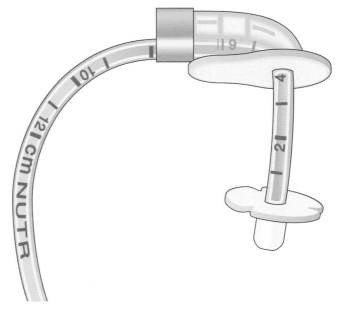

Figure 1 Non-extractable tube.

a double-stranded wire, gastrostomy tube, external securing collar and adaptor. Tube diameter varies from 9 to 24 F. Tubes are made of silicone or polyurethane, both inert and well-tolerated materials. Silicone tubes may deteriorate more quickly, but dysfunction and complications are similar in the long term.

- Non-extractable tubes with a rigid internal collar are available (Fig. 1). These may be preferable in agitated patients or those with cognitive impairment who might unintentionally dislodge their tube. Replacing the tube requires cutting it close to the skin and pushing the device into the stomach, to be recovered endoscopically. Allowing the device to pass naturally risks obstruction or perforation in 1% of cases.

- Extractable tubes have a flexible internal collar (Fig. 2) or a deflatable balloon retention system (Fig. 3), so they can be removed through the skin by traction on the tube. These tubes may migrate spontaneously and become incarcerated in the gastric wall or abdominal cavity (3 weeks to 2 months after insertion) with blockage to feeding and 'buried bumper syndrome', requiring surgical or endoscopic treatment.

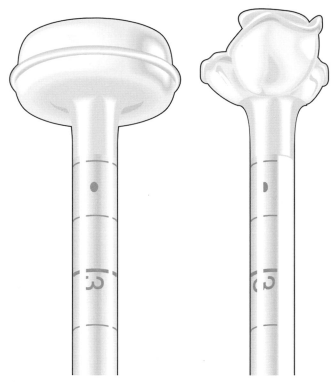

Figure 2 Inflatable retention dome tube.

- Some devices have an option to extend the PEG tube with a jejunostomy tube (J-PEG or JET-PEG) (Fig. 4), but this is only necessary in a minority of patients and the procedure can be difficult.

The lifespan of a PEG tube is approximately 730 days (range 180–1305). Replacement may be necessary if the tube deteriorates, leaks or is blocked. After insertion, it is preferable to wait 2–3 months for a mature fistula to be established before replacing the tube. Various replacement systems are available, e.g. a tube with a flexible internal obturator-type collar requiring a rigid stylet for introduction (Fig. 5). The majority of replacement devices are silicone balloon tubes that can be inflated with water (Fig. 6) but they have a short lifespan (3–4 months). Skin level devices ('buttons') have the advantage of an aesthetic appearance (Fig. 7). They are indicated in young children and outpatients.

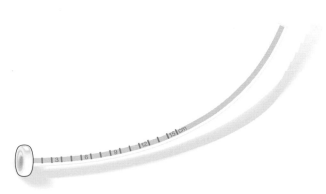

Figure 3 Flexible dome extractable tube.

After final removal of the PEG, the tract closes within a few (24–48) hours. Very rarely, a gastrocutaneous fistula persists and requires surgical closure.

2. Techniques

PEG is performed by two endoscopists, one performing endoscopy, and the other performing the abdominal aspects of the procedure. Upper endoscopy is first carried out as far as the second part of the duodenum to identify any contraindications or abnormalities requiring specific treatment (e.g. ulcer or esophagitis).

2.1. Pull-type technique (Fig. 8)

This technique was described by Gauderer and Ponsky in 1980 and is the most widely used (see Box 1).

2.2. Push-type technique

This was described by Sacks-Vine (Fig. 19). It is less widely used and does not differ greatly from the technique described above. The guidewire is tensioned by pulling simultaneously on the abdominal and buccal ends. Outside the mouth, the lubricated feeding tube is pushed onto the guidewire then positioned so the tapered end exits through the abdomen. By exerting traction on this tapered end, the collar of the tube can be applied to the stomach wall.

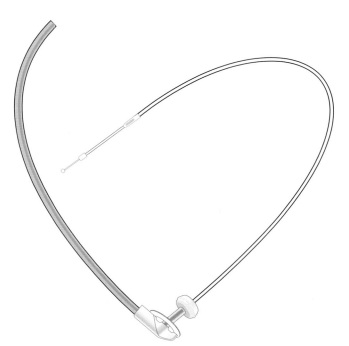

Figure 4 Jejunostomy tube for PEG.

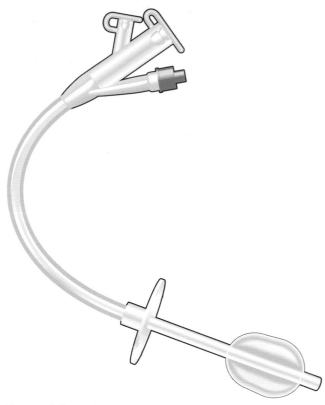

Figure 5 Balloon tube.

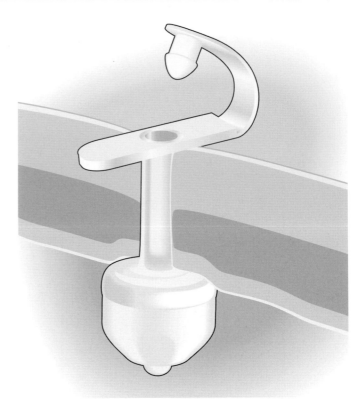

Figure 7 Gastrostomy button with a flexible obturator-type dome.

2.3. Introducer-type technique

This technique (Fig. 20) was described by Russell in 1984 and is similar to radiological gastrostomy ('RIG'). Introduction of the tube into the stomach occurs by direct puncture from outside, under endoscopic control and with air insufflation. Securing the tube requires using a special peelable catheter.

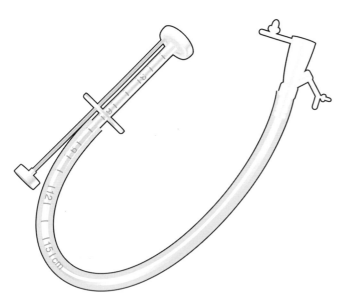

Figure 6 Flexible dome replacement tube with stylet.

Box 1   Steps for pull-type PEG insertion

- Patient lies supine.
- Stomach is insufflated so that it lies close to the abdominal wall.
- Puncture site is located (Figs 9, 10) by transillumination (switch off room lights).
- Optimum position for puncture is confirmed (anterior surface of distal gastric body) by finger indentation on the abdominal wall. Failure to transilluminate is a contraindication to proceeding (Fig. 11).
- Disinfection of the skin.
- Local anesthesia of the path through the wall using syringe and needle. This confirms the correct needle path and that gastric and abdominal walls are apposed (Fig. 12).
- Short incision of the skin with a scalpel (>1 cm or diameter of the tube) (Fig. 13).
- Puncture with trocar, perpendicular to the wall, until endoscopist sees it appear in the stomach (Fig. 14).
- Stylet introducer is withdrawn and guidewire is passed into stomach (Fig. 15).
- Guidewire is grasped (rat-tooth or foreign body forceps or polypectomy snare) and brought out patient's mouth by withdrawing the endoscope.
- PEG tube, which has a loop at its tapered end, is secured at oral end of guidewire and lubricated.
- By exerting gentle traction on the abdominal end of the wire, tube is pulled into stomach until the internal retaining collar gently abuts gastric wall (Fig. 16).
- External fixing device is attached, checking it is neither too tight (pain and wall necrosis) nor too loose (peristomal leak) (Fig. 17).
- Tube is cut to desired length (approx. 15 cm) and adaptor fitted (Fig. 18).
- Correct positioning of the tube is confirmed endoscopically (Fig. 21).

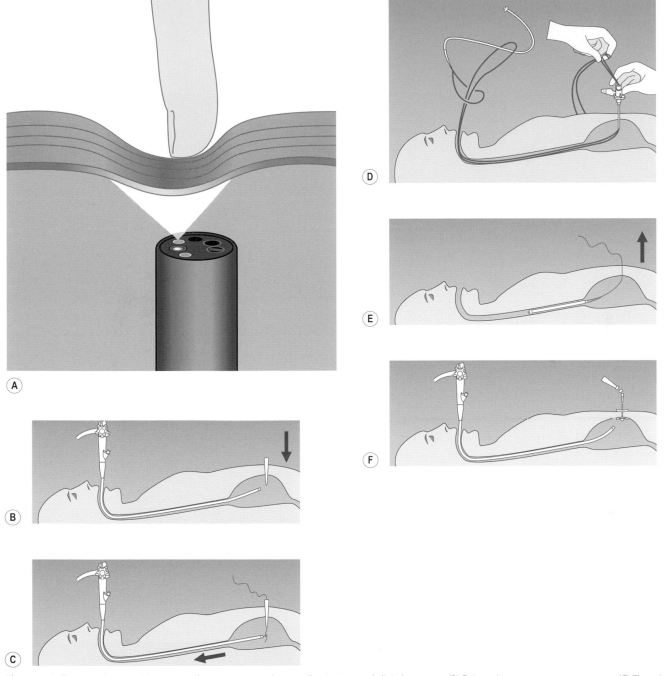

Figure 8 Pull-type technique. (A) Locating the puncture site by transillumination and digital pressure. (B) Epigastric transcutaneous puncture. (C) The wire is introduced into the trocar and grasped using endoscopic forceps. (D) The wire is pulled out of the mouth and the gastrostomy tube is secured. (E) The wire is pulled in the opposite direction towards the epigastric region and the tube traverses the gastric wall from internal to the external. (F) The gastrostomy tube is secured and the procedure checked endoscopically.

2.4. Aftercare following PEG insertion

- Antiseptic cleaning with application of a sterile dressing daily for 8 days
- Thereafter the area should be washed daily with soap and water
- The tube can be used early (within 3–6 h) by flushing it with sterile physiological saline (this also allows detection of a peristomal leak).

3. Indications

The main indications are:

- Prolonged enteral nutrition in patients who cannot swallow adequately or safely as a result of:
  - Neurological disorders: cerebrovascular accident, Parkinson's disease, prolonged coma, anoxic or traumatic brain injury, multiple sclerosis, amyotrophic lateral sclerosis, brain tumor

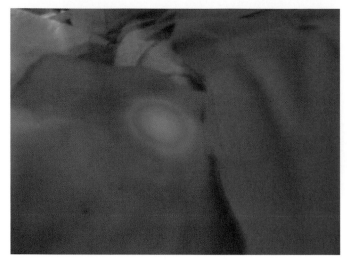

Figure 9 Transillumination of the abdominal wall.

- ■ Tumors of the head and neck or esophagus and their sequelae
- ■ Severe craniofacial trauma
- ■ Malignant dysphagia not controlled by laser or stenting
- ■ Congenital ENT malformations
- ■ Prior to radical therapy for head and neck cancer.
- • Severe nutritional deficiency in patients with anorexia, inflammatory gut disorders (e.g. Crohn's disease), cancer, cardiorespiratory failure or HIV-AIDS
- • Elderly patients who refuse food (depression, senile dementia), choking on food, deficiency due to inadequate intake

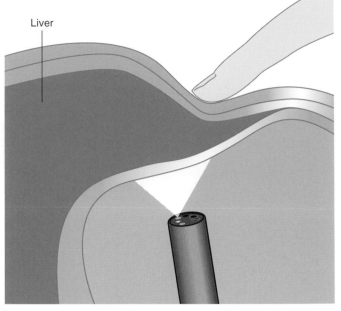

Figure 11 Absence of transillumination owing to the interposition of the liver. Puncture is contraindicated. at this point.

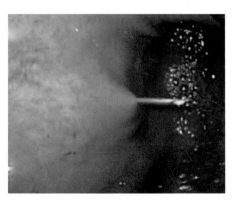

Figure 12 Local anesthesia and location of the correct puncture path.

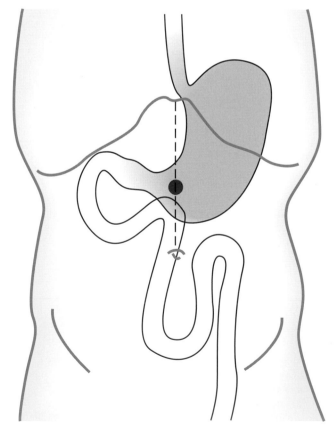

Figure 10 Puncture site for insertion of a PEG.

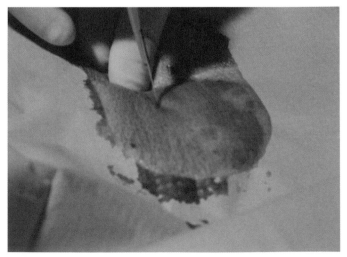

Figure 13 Skin incision with a scalpel.

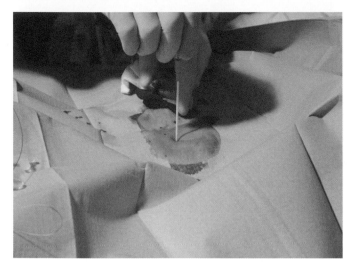

Figure 14 Trocar puncture under endoscopic control.

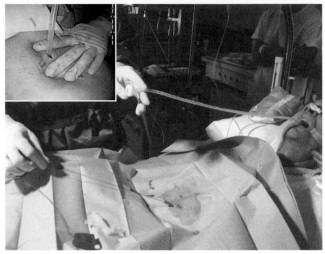

Figure 16 Gentle traction on the abdominal part of the guidewire and extraction of the tube.

- In children, sequelae of cerebral anoxia, congenital neuromuscular disorders, encephalopathy, cystic fibrosis
- To provide gastric aspiration ('venting' gastrostomy)
  - Peritoneal carcinomatosis or intestinal obstruction
  - Esophageal perforation.

4. Contraindications

- Absolute contraindications are few:
  - Severe coagulopathy
  - Inflammation, infection or neoplasia affecting the gastric wall or abdominal skin
  - Significant ascites, major obesity, organ interposition (left lobe of liver, transverse colon), absence of

transillumination. In these cases, the alternative is a laparoscopically-assisted PEG
  - Anticipated prognosis <1 month
  - intestinal failure due to short bowel syndrome: parenteral nutrition is indicated
  - Patients undergoing peritoneal dialysis
  - Fistula of the proximal small intestine
- Relative contraindications (these should be discussed on an individual basis):
  - Portal hypertension (esophageal or gastric varices)
  - Large hiatus hernia
  - Active gastric ulcer.

PEG is also possible in patients with a ventriculoperitoneal or peritoneovenous shunt if it is located fluoroscopically and the tube is kept well away from the shunt.

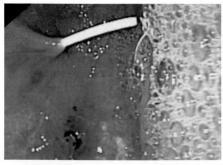

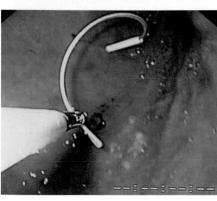

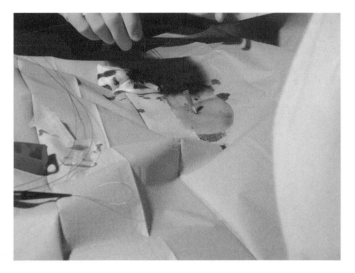

Figure 15 Guidewire passing into the trocar, grasped by forceps in the gastric lumen.

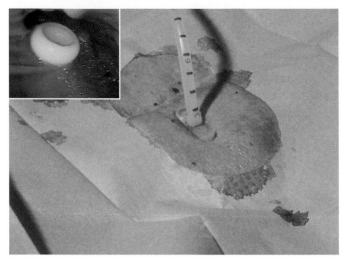

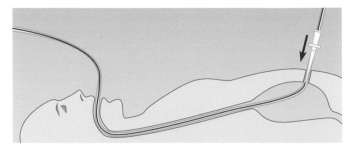

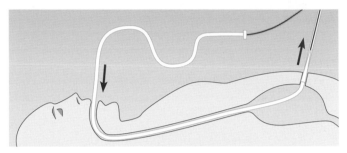

Figure 17 External collar in position and endoscopic check on the correct position of the tube.

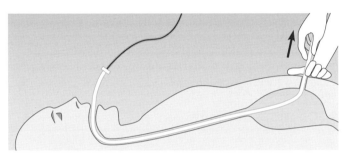

Note

Total or partial gastrectomy is not a contraindication. The tube should be placed in the gastric stump away from the anastomosis or in the jejunum (in this case use a small-diameter tube as there is a risk of the internal bumper causing jejunal obstruction). If there is an abdominal scar, obtain good transillumination away from the scar and choose the puncture site with care.

5. Complications

The procedure has a low mortality rate of 0.1–3%, due to cardiorespiratory problems, laryngospasm and massive pulmonary aspiration.

- Minor complications: frequent (1.4–43%)
  - Peristomal soft tissue infection (3–30%) associated with inflammatory granuloma, prevented by antibiotic prophylaxis
  - Bowel obstruction or abdominal pain with fever, resolving with antibiotics

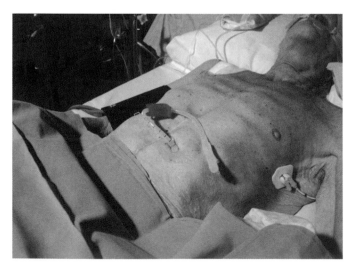

Figure 18 Gastrostomy tube in position.

Figure 19 Push-type technique.

  - Gastroesophageal reflux; not always prevented by a jejunostomy extension tube
  - Abdominal wall hematoma, peristomal gastric ulcer
  - Obstruction, displacement or expulsion of the tube, incarceration of the collar in the wall, localized pain caused by excessive traction requiring repositioning of the tube
  - Benign pneumoperitoneum, resolving spontaneously
  - Reflex ileus, resolving spontaneously in 48 h
  - Leakage of contents at the abdominal opening (caused by manipulating the tube too early or an excessively wide skin incision)
- Major complications: rare (3%)
  - Gastrocolic fistula, gastric perforation or esophageal tear
  - Gastric hemorrhage or gastric ulcer
  - Peritonitis (0.8–2%)
  - Wall necrosis (necrotizing fasciitis)
  - Migration of the tube with risk of perforation and small intestinal obstruction, requiring surgery.

Clinical Tip

Radiologically inserted gastrostomy ('RIG') is indicated:
- If the patient cannot open his/her mouth sufficiently
- If undilatable esophageal or pharyngeal stricturing is present prior to radical therapy for head and neck cancer. Passage of a PEG tube through the tumor using the pull method can rarely result in tumor seeding of the gastric wall or abdominal tract.

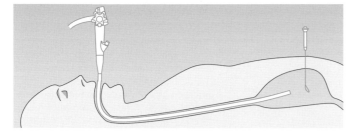

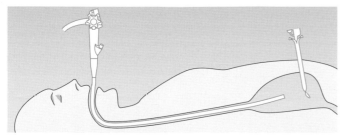

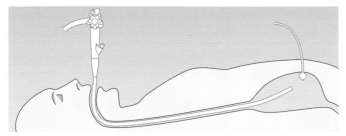

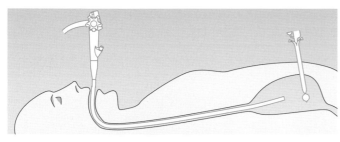

Figure 20 Introducer technique.

6. Nutrition and local treatment

6.1. Enteral nutrition

The administration of nutrient preparations through the tube may begin within 24 h of the procedure. Iso-osmolar mixtures are used, providing 1 kcal/mL, with an infusion rate of <2 mL/min (1 L over 3–4 h), increasing progressively as tolerated. The mixtures are administered by gravity or using a pump. Do not inject drugs at the same time as nutrition; instead they should be administered in liquid form or finely crushed with water. The tube should be flushed well with 60–100 mL of water before and after each use. If the tube becomes obstructed, try to unblock it by injecting pressurized warm water at 40°C, using a small syringe (10–20 mL).

6.2. Local aftercare

This should be explained to the patient, his/her carers, and the nursing team.

- Wash the peristomal skin daily with warm water and simple soap and dry carefully; a daily shower is permitted after a few days
- Clean the mouth 2–3 times daily
- Apply povidone iodine if there is any peristomal redness or inflammation
- Treat granulation tissue with silver nitrate
- Check daily that the tube is in the correct position by rotating it, moving it gently backwards and forwards, checking the distance markings and the application of the external collar to the skin.

> ✓ **Clinical Tip**
>
> Polymeric feeds are generally used unless absorption capacity is greatly reduced, in which case semi-elemental mixtures are preferred.

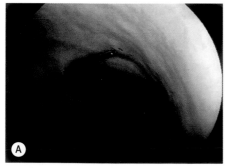
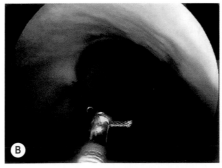

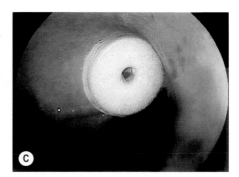

Figure 21 (A) Trocar. (B) Grasping the guidewire. (C) Internal collar of the gastrostomy tube in position.

Further Reading

Arpurt JP, Barthet M, Boustière C, et al: Recommendation sheets: antibiotic prophylaxis and digestive endoscopy, *Acta Endosc* 34(1), 2004.

Beau P: Complications tardives de la gastrostomie percutanée endoscopique (GPE) [Late complications of percutaneous endoscopic gastrostomy (PEG)], *Nutr Clin Metab* 14:153–156, 2000.

Gauderer MW, Ponsky JL, Izant RJ: Gastrostomy without laparoscopy: a percutaneous endoscopic technique, *J Pediatr Surg* 15:872–875, 1980.

Le Sidaner A: Gastrostomie percutanée endoscopique [Percutaneous endoscopic gastrostomy], *Acta Endosc* 32:739–754, 2002.

Loser C, Aschl G, Hebuterne X, et al: ESPEN guidelines on artificial enteral nutrition – percutaneous endoscopic gastrostomy (PEG), *Clin Nutr* 24:848–861, 2005.

Mellinger JD, Ponsky JL: Percutaneous endoscopic gastrostomy: state of the art, *Endoscopy* 30:126–132, 1998.

Verdon R, Dargere S: Complications infectieuses de la gastrostomie percutanée endoscopique [Infectious complications of percutaneous endoscopic gastrostomy], *Nutr Clin Metab* 14:149–152, 2000.

Westaby D, Young A, O'Toole P, et al: The provision of a percutaneously placed enteral tube feeding service, *Gut* 59:1592–1605, 2010.

7.12 Endoscopic mucosal resection

Jean Marc Canard, Ian Penman

Key Points

- Endoscopic mucosal resection (EMR) is the most accurate staging modality for assessing depth of invasion of superficial cancers.
- EMR is also a curative therapy for selected superficial cancers.
- The decision to proceed to EMR should be discussed carefully with the patient and the appropriate multidisciplinary team.
- Familiarity with different EMR techniques and equipment is vital.
- Paris type 0–III lesions and those that fail to lift following submucosal injection are not suitable for EMR.
- The risk of lymph node invasion is <5% for T1m(1–3) lesions and these are considered cured by EMR when margins are clear.
- Submucosal involvement (T1sm), discovered at EMR, carries a risk of lymph node involvement of 19–44% and is an indication for surgery in fit patients.
- With experience, perforation rates are low (1–5%).

Introduction

Endoscopic mucosal resection (EMR), also known as mucosectomy, has become an accepted curative treatment for superficial tumors of the digestive tract: benign flat or sessile lesions, high-grade intraepithelial neoplasia and superficial cancers with little or no risk of lymph node involvement in the esophagus, cardia, stomach, duodenum, ampulla of Vater, colon or rectum.

EMR allows resection of the mucosa, the muscularis mucosae and part or even all of the submucosa. It allows histological analysis of the entire lesion unlike ablative therapies such as laser or argon plasma coagulation. It also allows further treatment (surgery or radiochemotherapy) to be considered should the pathology reveal high risk features for lymphatic invasion (see below) or incomplete resection.

EMR techniques were developed originally in Japan, for the treatment of superficial cancers of the stomach and squamous esophagus. These are common in Japan and all Japanese people are offered screening endoscopy from the age of 40. As such, many superficial cancers are diagnosed and this led to the development of EMR.

These lesions are less common in Western countries but advances in endoscopic imaging and the fortuitous discovery of dysplastic lesions or superficial cancers have resulted in the adoption of these techniques. EMR has also been used for many years for colonic lesions, especially flat, sessile polyps and those larger than 2 cm.

1. Indications and limitations

The feasibility of EMR throughout the upper and lower gastrointestinal tract has been clearly demonstrated in recent years, although every lesion must be assessed on its individual merits and site-specific caveats apply in different parts of the gut (see below).

1.1. Benign lesions

For benign lesions, the limitations are essentially technical, related to difficulties in resecting very large lesions, which require piecemeal resection. Neither size nor location is a factor in the decision to consider EMR: very large lesions may be entirely benign and, conversely, small lesions may be malignant and endoscopically unresectable as a result of infiltration of the deep submucosa or muscularis propria.

1.2. Cancers

For cancers, the indications for EMR are determined by the risk of lymph node involvement which varies depending on:

- Site
- Size
- The degree of differentiation (well, moderate or poor) and
- Vertical depth of invasion.

According to the original Japanese classification and the modified 'Paris Classification', T1 lesions are considered resectable by EMR and may be divided into six subgroups, according to the level of invasion (Fig. 1).

- **T1m1** corresponds to disease confined to the epithelium. This represents *in situ* cancer which does not invade the basement membrane and thus carries no risk of lymph node involvement.
- **T1m2** corresponds to infiltration of the lamina propria, not involving the muscularis mucosae and with a low lymph node risk (0–2%).
- **T1m3** corresponds to invasion into but not beyond the muscularis mucosae (lymph node risk up to approximately 9%).

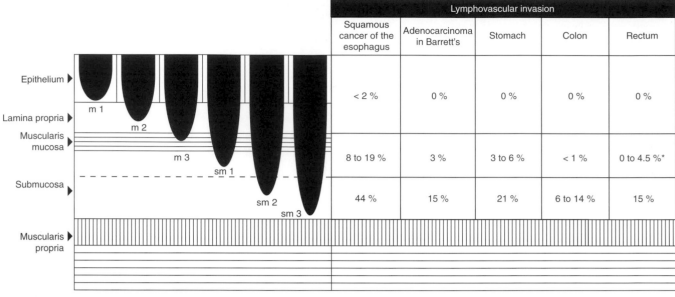

	Lymphovascular invasion				
	Squamous cancer of the esophagus	Adenocarcinoma in Barrett's	Stomach	Colon	Rectum
	< 2 %	0 %	0 %	0 %	0 %
	8 to 19 %	3 %	3 to 6 %	< 1 %	0 to 4.5 %*
	44 %	15 %	21 %	6 to 14 %	15 %

Epithelium ▶
m 1
Lamina propria ▶
m 2
Muscularis mucosa ▶
m 3
sm 1
Submucosa ▶
sm 2
sm 3
Muscularis propria ▶

Figure 1 Japanese classification of superficial malignant lesions of the digestive tract (T1) – *0% without lymphovascular invasion – 4.5% with lymphovascular injection.

- **T1sm1** corresponds to superficial invasion of the submucosa (upper third). These cancers are invasive and the risk of lymph node invasion is 0–19%.
- **T1sm2** corresponds to invasion of the middle third of the submucosa.
- **T1sm3** corresponds to invasion of the deep submucosa. The risk of lymph node invasion is 6–44% for T1sm2 and T1sm3 lesions.
- **T2** corresponds to invasion of the muscularis propria. These cancers are advanced and not suitable for EMR, which would not be curative and also risks removing the muscularis propria and causing a perforation.

 Clinical Tip

Patients with T1m1, T1m2 or T1m3 lesions may be regarded as cured by successful EMR. T1sm1, sm2 and sm3 lesions may require surgical resection or chemoradiotherapy depending on the risk of surgery which may be very high, particularly for esophageal resection.

2. Conditions for performing EMR

Careful consultation is essential prior to EMR so that patients understand their condition, the rationale for EMR, its risks and the alternatives including minimally invasive surgery. Arrangements can be made for patients taking antiplatelet or anticoagulant therapy. Anesthetic assessment is also important in high-risk patients because it is a high-risk procedure. In many centres, EMR is performed under general anesthesia, allowing the endoscopist to concentrate solely on the complex task in hand.

 Warning!

Aspirin therapy can continue but warfarin (3–5 days) and clopidogrel (7–10 days) must be stopped prior to EMR.

Local practices will determine whether EMR is performed under conscious sedation or general anesthesia. The latter should be considered if a long procedure is anticipated, e.g. a large lesion of the cardia, stomach or duodenum, or if an overtube is being used for multiple esophageal intubations.

Relatively simple EMR procedures can be performed as a day case but more complex cases require at least overnight stay afterwards and may be best admitted the day beforehand. The patient needs to be prepared because of the risks of serious complications, although these are uncommon.

3. Evaluation prior to EMR

Careful endoscopic evaluation is necessary to predict the risk of deep invasion into the submucosa or beyond as this would contraindicate EMR. The decision to proceed to EMR is based on the morphological appearances, results of endosonography and, in appropriate cases, the response to submucosal injection.

3.1. Appearance on endoscopy

Size and the Paris endoscopic classification will determine with reasonable precision the risk of submucosal invasion for cancers, particularly in the stomach. The risk is virtually zero for tumors measuring less than a centimeter and low for those measuring 1–2 cm. The Paris classification (Ch. 3, Fig. 25) distinguishes between polypoid (type I), flat (type II) and ulcerated (type III) lesion types. Flat lesions may be slightly elevated (IIa), truly flat (IIb) or slightly depressed (IIc). Any combination of forms may exist, e.g. type IIa+IIc.

EMR is not technically possible for type III lesions. Type I lesions are usually resectable without difficulty but site-specific factors must be considered: e.g. squamous esophageal type I lesions are associated with submucosal involvement in >90% of cases. This is not true in Barrett's cancers, the stomach or colon. Generally the best indications for EMR are type IIa, IIb or IIc lesions, in which the risk of submucosal invasion is <10%.

3.2. Endosonography

Conventional endosonography at 7.5 and 12 MHz can differentiate between T1 and T2 stages with a diagnostic accuracy of 90%. 30 MHz catheter miniprobes can distinguish between T1 and T2 stages in almost 100% of cases in expert hands. Some studies suggest that EUS can differentiate between T1m and T1sm stages with 90% accuracy. There is a problem with overstaging as a result of peri-tumoral fibrosis and inflammation and because of this, lesions classified as T1sm by endosonography should not be automatically rejected for possible EMR.

The diagnostic accuracy of miniprobes in intramucosal tumors has been reported as approximately 95% but recent data suggests that accuracy may only be around 80%. As a result, and because EMR techniques have become easier in recent years, a 'diagnostic' EMR is often performed to allow more accurate and definitive pathological staging of the depth of invasion.

3.3. Submucosal injection

The response to submucosal injection ('lifting sign') was described by Kato and predicts deep infiltration that precludes EMR (Figs 2–4).

4. Equipment

This varies depending on whether EMR is being performed 'freehand' or whether cap-based methods are used (see below). Units performing EMR should have available a full range of necessary endoscopes, electrosurgical equipment and accessories and be familiar with their use (Box 1).

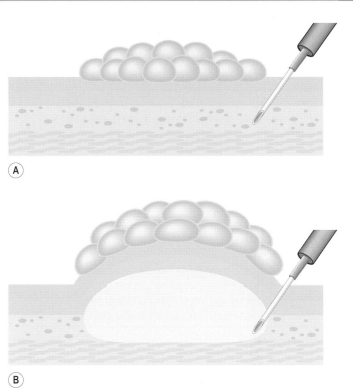

Figure 3 Inject and cut. (A) Needle in the submucosa. (B) Submucosal injection: elevation indicates absence of invasion of the muscularis propria.

Warning!
Do not attempt EMR for type 0–III (ulcerated) lesions, those that fail to lift on submucosal injection or if EUS suggests T2 disease or nodal involvement.

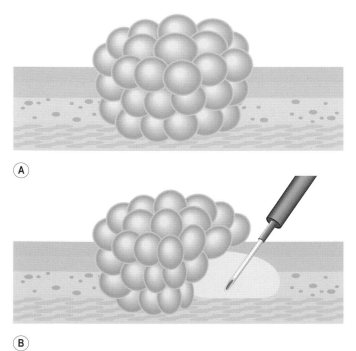

Figure 2 (A) Invasion of the muscularis propria. (B) Absence of elevation on submucosal injection ('non-lifting sign').

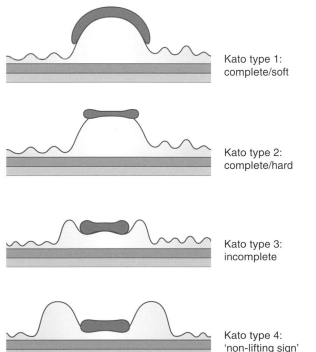

Kato type 1: complete/soft

Kato type 2: complete/hard

Kato type 3: incomplete

Kato type 4: 'non-lifting sign'

Figure 4 The 'lifting sign' following submucosal injection. EMR is contraindicated for type 4 and should be undertaken with care in type 3.

235

Box 1 Equipment for EMR

- High definition videoendoscopes.
- Twin channel videoendoscopes.
- Videocolonoscope with optical zoom facility.
- Videocolonoscope with two operating channels for retreatment of lesions previously subjected to incomplete resection.
- Electrosurgical diathermy equipment with 'endo-cut' mode and argon plasma coagulation.
- Stains for chromoendoscopy:
  - 1% Lugol's iodine solution
  - 0.2% indigo carmine
  - 1% acetic acid (Barrett's).
- Spray catheters.
- Diathermy snares (hexagonal, crescentic, and barbed).
- Injection needles.
- Clips for hemostasis and to attempt closure of perforations.
- Oblique transparent caps (standard = 16 mm).
- 50 mL syringes for washing and chromoendoscopy.
- Tissue retrieval devices: Roth nets, tripod grasping forceps, baskets.

---

5. Techniques

5.1. Locating the lesion

Assessing the horizontal extent of a lesion is made easier by chromoendoscopy and is essential for flat lesions. Lugol's iodine solution 1% (squamous esophageal lesions) and 0.2–0.4% indigo carmine (glandular mucosa) are mostly used. The margins of the lesion can be marked with electrocoagulation points using the tip of a snare or APC. This is useful only in the stomach and duodenum where staining sometimes may fail to delineate the margins for long enough, risking incomplete resection and the need for repeated sessions to clear residual neoplastic tissue.

5.2. Submucosal injection

This confirms that the lesion lifts away from the deep layers and, importantly, creates an insulating cushion that reduces the risk of perforation.

Physiological saline without epinephrine is most commonly used. Injection of epinephrine may temporarily prevent bleeding from a vessel which may subsequently begin to bleed and require repeat endoscopy for hemostasis. It is therefore preferable to detect immediate bleeding and to use clipping or thermal methods to achieve durable hemostasis. Saline is absorbed quickly and repeated injections may be necessary but there is no limit to the volume that can be used. Hyaluronic acid, 10% dextrose, 2% hydroxypropylmethylcellulose (HPMC) or other solutions have been used to allow a longer lasting injection but are generally reserved for submucosal dissection procedures (ESD).

5.3. Excision procedure

Several procedures for EMR have been described and these can be roughly divided into four types: inject and cut, pull and cut, suck and cut, simplified aspirate and cut.

5.3.1. Inject and cut (Fig. 3)

Elevation of the lesion by submucosal injection is the first step and resection removes a portion of the wall containing mucosa, muscularis mucosae, and part or all of the submucosa. To reduce the risk of perforation, it is vital to maintain sufficient lifting of the lesion throughout the procedure. This may require the injection of 10–20 mL (or up to 50 mL in some cases). Injection is undertaken at several points around the previously marked area. If there is no elevation of the lesion ('non-lifting'), this is strong evidence of deeper than expected invasion and the procedure must be stopped. The elevated lesion is grasped in a polypectomy snare. An 'endocut' current or blended or pure cutting current may be used (see Ch. 1.4). The risk of perforation from deep electrocoagulation of the wall is reduced by keeping the resulting cutting plane away from the submucosal injection. This method is used mainly in the colon or rectum where it is the standard technique for small lesions, but can also be used at other sites.

5.3.2. Pull and cut

This technique requires a twin-channel endoscope. A snare passed through one channel is placed around the lesion and biopsy or grasping forceps of different size close around the apex of the lesion via the second channel. The lesion can then be pulled towards the endoscope tip before the snare is closed and resection by diathermy occurs.

5.3.3. Aspirate and cut

Several techniques have aspiration of the lesion before resection in common. Aspiration can be achieved using a plastic hood ('cap method', Olympus) or a band ligation device (multiband mucosectomy, 'Duette', Cook Medical). Some Japanese experts use an overtube in the esophagus.

Cap method

A transparent oblique plastic cap (Fig. 5) is mounted on the endoscope. The cap has a notch that should be aligned with the instrument channel of the endoscope. The snare (a miniloop specially designed to open on contact with the inner rim of the distal end of the cap) is inserted into the cap, the lesion is aspirated into the hood and the loop is then closed, grasping the tumor. Suction is released and the loop and the tumor are pushed out of the hood. Resection is then carried out using Endo-cut mode (ERBE ICC 200 generator setting 120 W, effect 2, for 2–3 s or ERBE VIO generator endocut Q, effect 2). This technique is recommended in the esophagus and cardia. The fragile snare deforms easily and for piecemeal resections a new snare should be used for each resection.

Band ligation

The same technique may be used with a band ligation device (multiband mucosectomy, MBM, Fig. 6) or a diathermy snare outside the distal hood (Fig. 7). After aspirating the lesion and applying the band, resection of the pseudopolyp is carried out using a 5–7F hexagonal monofilament snare supplied with the kit. The snare should be placed *below* the band. This technique can be used in the stomach or esophagus and is comparable with the cap method in ease of use, outcomes and complication rates. Submucosal injection is unnecessary. The size of the resected tissue correlates with

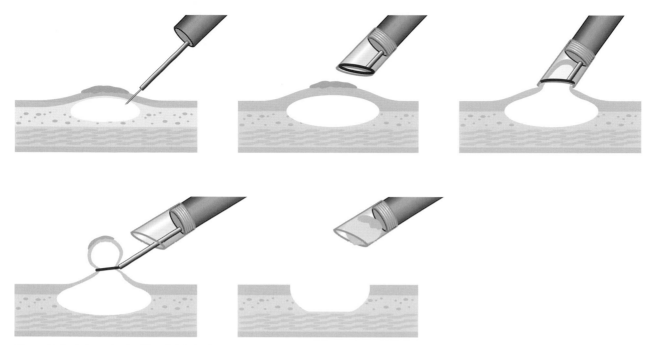

Figure 5 Aspirate and cut with a distal plastic cap.

the amount of suction into the hood – a 'red-out' is needed for large lesions while less vigorous suction is necessary for small lesions.

Transparent plastic overtube

The use of a transparent plastic overtube (Fig. 8) specially designed for esophageal endotherapy has been proposed by Japanese teams and seems particularly useful for dysplasia or flat superficial cancers extending over large surface areas. It is currently unavailable in many Western countries and insertion-related perforations have been reported.

> **! Warning!**
>
> Submucosal injection is essential before each resection when using the Olympus cap method to avoid perforation. Injection is unnecessary in the esophagus when using multiband mucosectomy as the risk of perforation is extremely low but the risk of a complete resection is lower.

5.3.4. Simplified aspirate and cut

The use of a monofilament pediatric snare through an endoscope with a large operating channel has been suggested as

an alternative to submucosal injection or suction with a cap. By using a large operating channel, there is still sufficiently powerful aspiration despite the introduction of the snare, which is progressively closed around the lesion during aspiration. This technique, which has been validated for small cancers of the esophagus, can also be considered for benign sessile colonic tumors.

> **! Warning!**
>
> Whichever technique is used, the electrosurgical current power settings should be adapted to the type of snare used (monofilament or braided).

> **✓ Clinical Tip**
>
> **Handling and preparation of resected specimens**
>
> A key component of the procedure is providing the pathologist with well-oriented specimens so that accurate assessment of lateral and, more importantly, vertical depth of invasion can be performed. Tissue should be fixed on a flat cork board or wax slab using pins and placed face down in fixative.

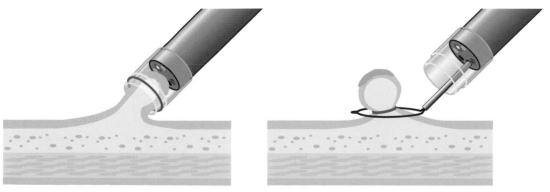

Figure 6 EMR using a band ligation device (Duette, Cook Medical).

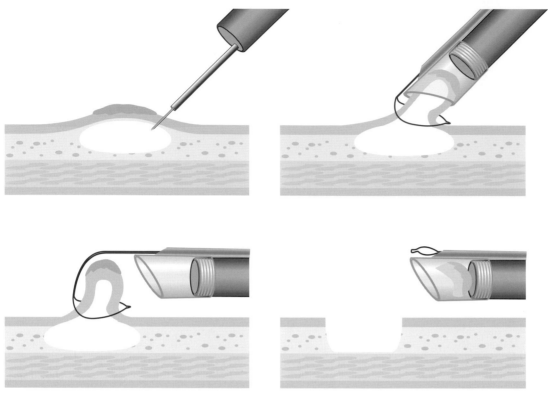

Figure 7 Cap-assisted EMR with a diathermy snare outside the endoscope.

Box 2	Practical considerations for EMR

- Extensive training is necessary for successful EMR: training courses, simulators, and animal tissue models are all available. Practice on these before undertaking cases.
- Two experienced nurses are needed to assist with EMR.
- General anesthesia is recommended so that the patient is perfectly still.
- Inject beneath all lesions, regardless of their location in the digestive tract, except when using MBM in the esophagus.
- Stain the esophagus with Lugol's solution and the stomach and colon with indigo carmine.
- Mark the margins of gastric and duodenal lesions with the tip of a diathermy snare (20–40 W).
- Use the cap method for the esophagus and cardia.
- Have all equipment ready before starting an EMR, including epinephrine, clips and coagrasper forceps.
- Aim to resect lesions completely in a single session and preferably en-bloc.

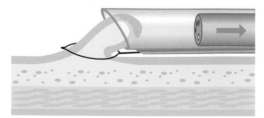

Figure 8 EMR with an overtube.

6. Complications

Immediate bleeding is common and is part of the procedure. It should be treated during the same session, usually by clipping or coagulation with diathermy forceps ('Coagraspers', Fig. 9). Perforations (Fig. 10) occur in <5% and, if small and detected immediately, attempts should be made to close these with clips (Fig. 11). Perforation and haemorrhage may also be delayed (by up to 10 days for hemorrhage). Surgery is rarely required.

Very wide and particularly circumferential mucosectomies may be complicated by stenosis in up to 50% (rectum and esophagus). Dilatation is usually easy and is performed until a normal lumen has been restored. Stenoses can be avoided by performing large EMRs in two or more sessions.

7. Results

The success rate of EMR is 90–94%. Results are determined by how complete the excision is. For superficial cancers, survival rates of more than 80% have been reported, with disease-specific mortality of 2–3%. These results are equivalent to those of surgery. The recurrence rate after resection with negative margins is approximately 2% for superficial cancers of the stomach and less than 10% in the colon. Many of these recurrences are small and endoscopically treatable.

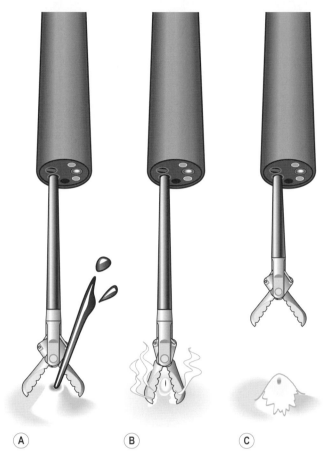

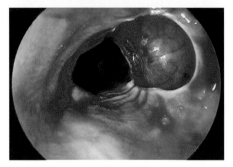

Figure 10 'Pseuodperforation' (i.e. only adventitia remains) treated successfully with parenteral nutrition, antibiotics and antisecretory agents for 15 days.

Figure 9 Coagrasper forceps for coagulating a vessel during EMR (80 W, soft coag setting). (A) Grasping the vessel in the Coagrasper jaws. (B) Coagulation by gentle tenting of the grasped vessel. (C) Opening the forceps before retraction.

8. Future developments

The development of surveillance and screening endoscopy targeted at patients at risk of GI cancers, advances in imaging techniques (high resolution) and education of endoscopists about the appearances of subtle abnormalities and their significance should help to increase the proportion of superficial cancers detected. It is vital that endoscopists appreciate what to look for and allow enough time for a thorough examination. New equipment will allow the resection of circumferential lesions of the esophagus, particularly dysplasia in Barrett's esophagus, as well as extensive superficial gastric and colonic cancers. Known as endoscopic submucosal dissection (ESD) (Figs 12–14), this technique may replace some of the EMR currently performed. It has been widely adopted in Asia and is slowly emerging in other parts of the world. ESD has the advantages of complete en bloc resection of very large lesions with low recurrence rates. The procedure is at present technically challenging and time-consuming with a long learning curve. In Western countries the number of patients suitable for ESD is far smaller than in Asia and expertise should be concentrated in a small number of specialist centers.

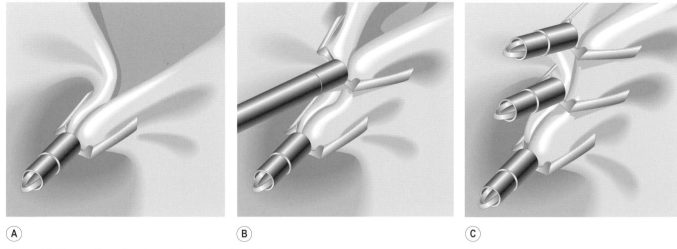

Figure 11 Closure of a perforation starting at lateral margin.

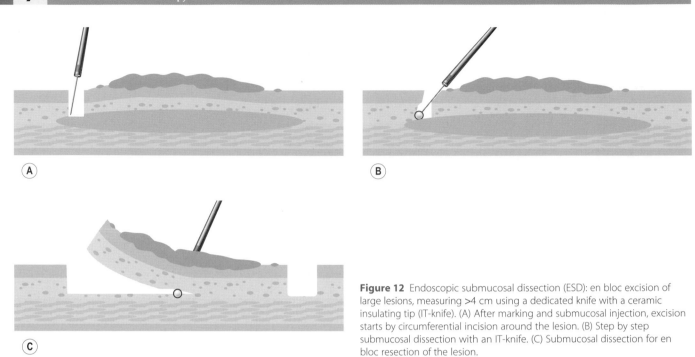

(A)

(B)

(C)

Figure 12 Endoscopic submucosal dissection (ESD): en bloc excision of large lesions, measuring >4 cm using a dedicated knife with a ceramic insulating tip (IT-knife). (A) After marking and submucosal injection, excision starts by circumferential incision around the lesion. (B) Step by step submucosal dissection with an IT-knife. (C) Submucosal dissection for en bloc resection of the lesion.

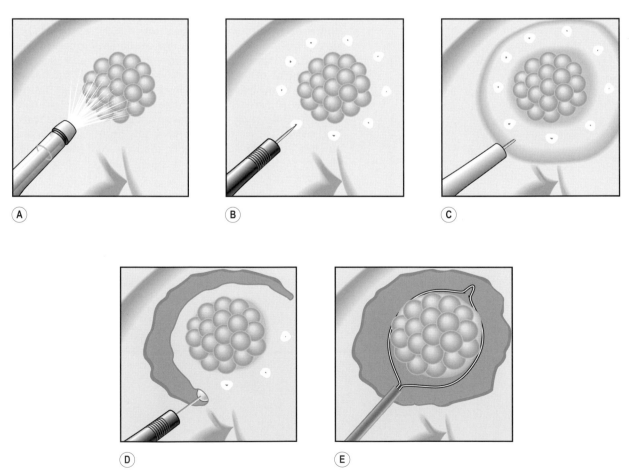

(A)

(B)

(C)

(D)

(E)

Figure 13 Endoscopic submucosal dissection: inject and cut. (A) Staining in the esophagus and colon. (B) Marking in the stomach and duodenum only. (C) Submucosal injection. (D) Dissection using a ceramic-tipped knife. (E) Removal of the lesion as a single piece, grasped in a large snare.

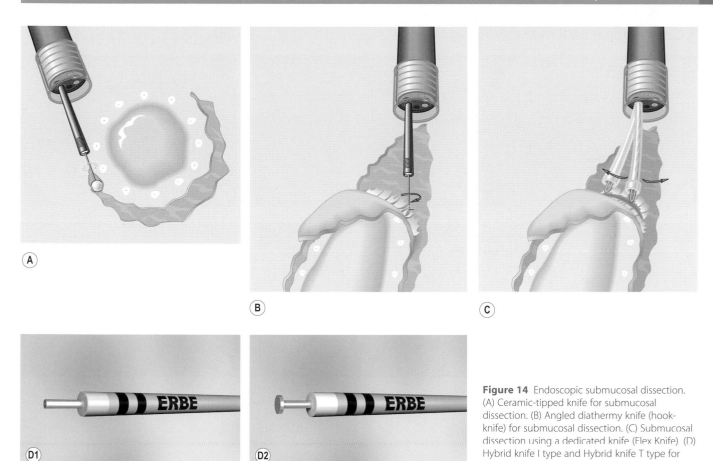

Figure 14 Endoscopic submucosal dissection. (A) Ceramic-tipped knife for submucosal dissection. (B) Angled diathermy knife (hook-knife) for submucosal dissection. (C) Submucosal dissection using a dedicated knife (Flex Knife) (D) Hybrid knife I type and Hybrid knife T type for injection and dissection with the same device.

9. Images

9.1. EMR of the esophagus: aspirate and cut in a single piece

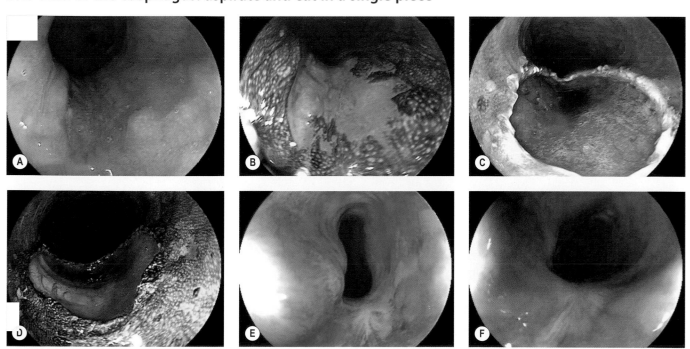

Figure 15 EMR of the esophagus: aspirate and cut in a single piece. (A) Small squamous cancer of the esophagus. (B) After 1% Lugol's solution. (C) After cap-assisted resection. (D) Follow-up image with 1% Lugol's solution showing complete resection in a single session. (E) EMR scar at 6 months after 1% Lugol's solution. (F) EMR scar using the FICE system (Fujinon).

9.2. Additional EMR of the esophagus

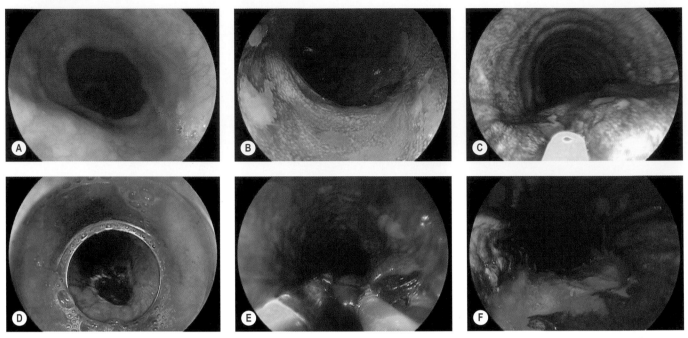

Figure 16 Additional EMR of the esophagus. (A) Follow-up of EMR at 3 months. (B) Staining with 1% Lugol's solution with residual fragment. (C) Effective submucosal injection. (D) Difficult, limited resection (cap method). (E) Resection with a twin-channel endoscope. (F) Follow-up and further staining with Lugol's solution.

9.3. Semi-circumferential cancer of the esophagus resected in a single session

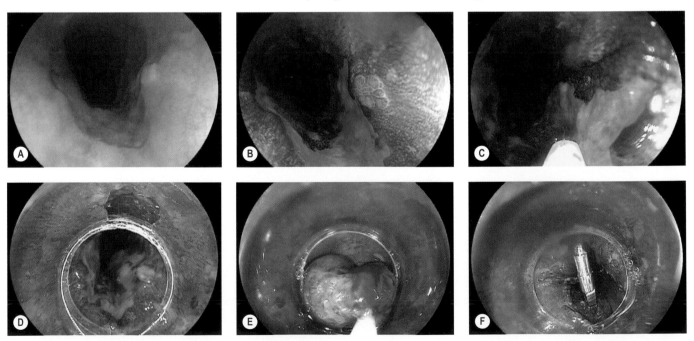

Figure 17 Semi-circumferential cancer of the esophagus resected in a single session. (A) Semi-circumferential squamous cancer of the esophagus. (B) After 1% Lugol's solution. (C) Submucosal injection. (D) Cap. (E) Lesion in the cap (resection in a single piece). (F) Clip to control bleeding.

9.4. EMR of the esophagus combining two techniques: aspirate and cut then pull and cut

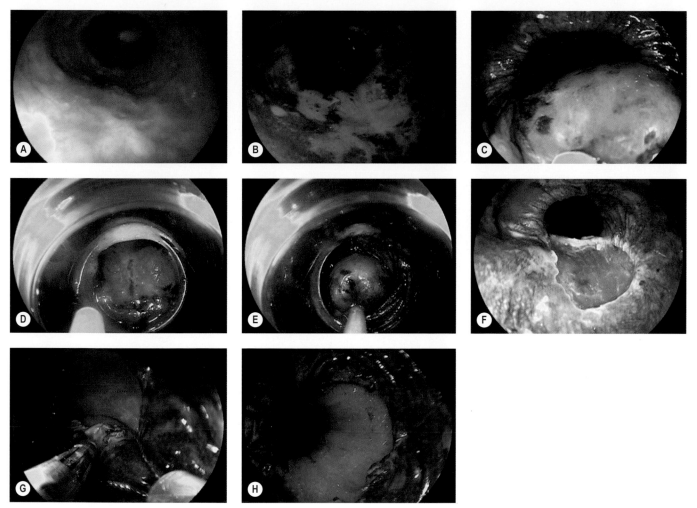

Figure 18 EMR of the esophagus combining two techniques: aspirate and cut then pull and cut. (A) Long squamous cancer. (B) Squamous cancer after 1% Lugol's solution. (C) Submucosal injection. (D) Resection cap + EMR snare. (E) Lesion in the snare. (F) After resection. (G) Residual fragment needing resection with an endoscope with two operating channels. (H) Follow-up with 1% Lugol's solution; lesion resected whole in a single session.

9.5. Resection of extensive superficial cancer of the esophagus

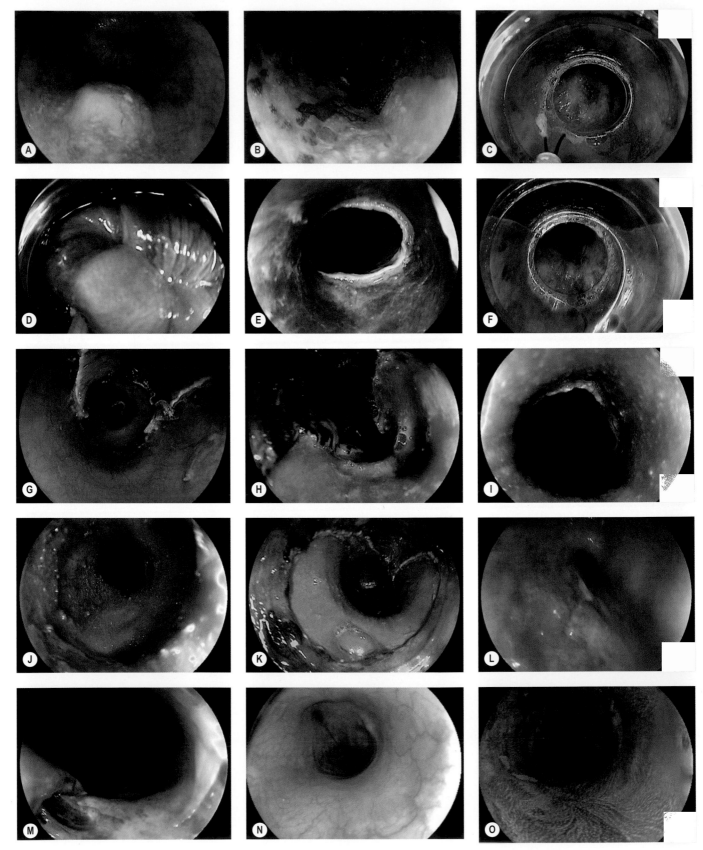

Figure 19 Resection of extensive superficial cancer of the esophagus. (A) Superficial esophageal cancer. (B) After staining with Lugol's solution, the lesion appears to be very extensive. (C) Centring the upper part of the lesion in the cap. (D) Aspiration. (E) Circumferential resection. (F) Continuing the resection of the lower part of the lesion. (G) After cap resection. (H) Residual tumor tissue bridge between two resection zones – resected with a twin channel endoscope. (I) Lower end of the resection zone. (J) Middle part. (K) Upper part – resection in a single session, in total 10 cm long and 7 cm in circumference: normal. (L) Stenosis due to scarring at 4 weeks. (M) After dilation. (N) EMR scar at 6 months. (O) Scar after 1% Lugol's solution: no residual or recurrent lesion. Follow up at 5 years normal.

9.6. EMR of the cardia

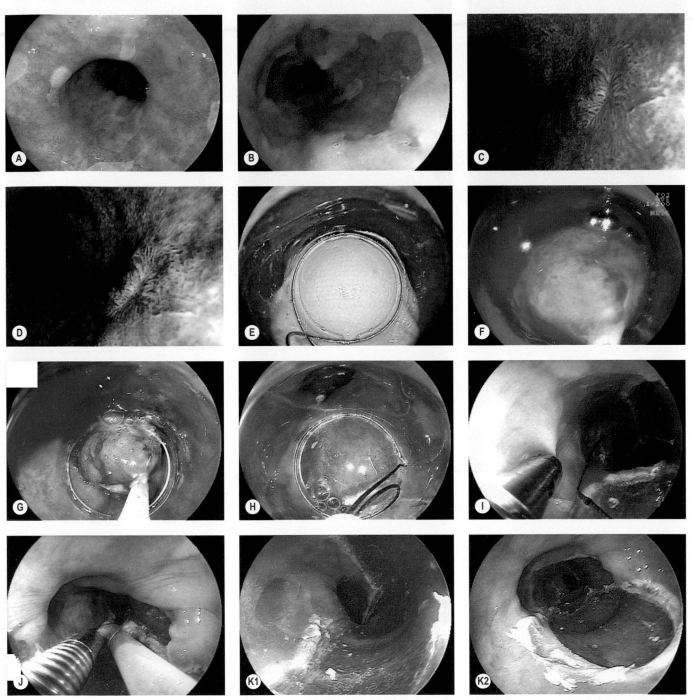

Figure 20 EMR of the cardia. (A) Circumferential Barrett's esophagus. (B) High-grade dysplasia on a proximal tongue of Barrett's epithelium. (C) 1% acetic acid + electronic zoom ×1.5 in the dysplastic zone. (D) 1% acetic acid + electronic zoom (×1.5) + FICE in the dysplastic zone. (E) Oblique transparent cap + special EMR snare with aspiration test on the endoscopist's glove. (F) Aspiration of the lesion into the cap and closure of the snare. (G) Lesion outside the cap. (H) Second resection close to the first one. (I) Continued resection with an endoscope with two operating channels, the snare on the right, the forceps on the left to remove a residual fragment between two resected areas. (J) Closed snare. (K) Resection of two-thirds of circumferential Barrett's esophagus and the tongue-like projection with the lesion. A second session will take place in 3 months for resection of the remaining Barrett's epithelium. Treatment in two sessions to minimize the risk of stenosis.

9.7. EMR of high-grade dysplasia in Barrett's esophagus using a band ligation device

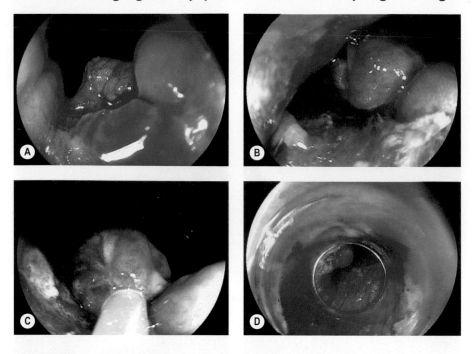

Figure 21 EMR of high-grade dysplasia in Barrett's esophagus using a band ligation device. (A) High-grade dysplasia in Barrett's esophagus. (B) 1 band placed on the edge of a previously treated area. (C) Resection by snare. (D) Resection of two-thirds of the Barrett's segment with the lesion.

9.8A. Gastric EMR

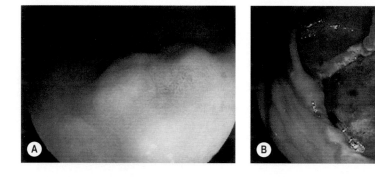

Figure 22 Gastric EMR. (A) Antral adenoma with high grade dysplasia. (B) After resection.

9.8B. Gastric ESD

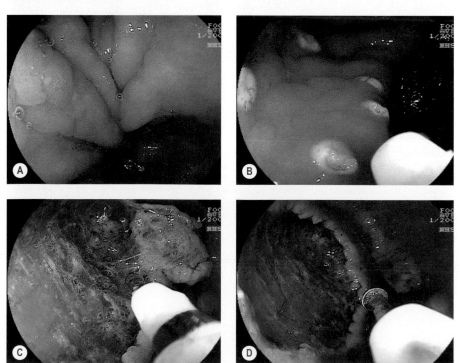

Figure 23 Gastric ESD. (A) Superficial gastric cancer T1m1. (B) Marking the limit of the resection. (C) ESD with Hybrid Knife T type. (D) After resection.

9.9. Duodenal EMR

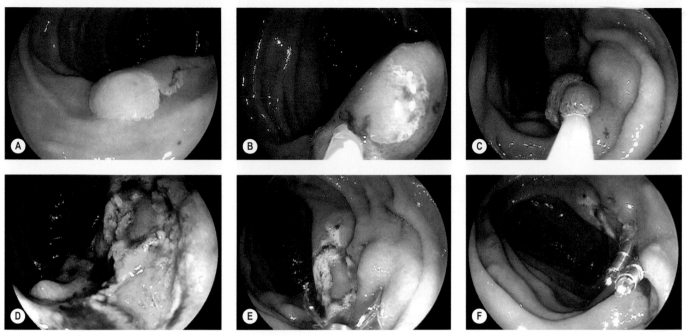

Figure 24 Duodenal EMR. (A) Small duodenal polyp. (B) Injection under the polyp. (C) Resection with the snare. (D) Confirmation of complete resection with 0.2% indigo carmine. (E) Closing with a clip to prevent secondary bleeding. (F) 2nd clip in position.

9.10. EMR of a large duodenal polyp

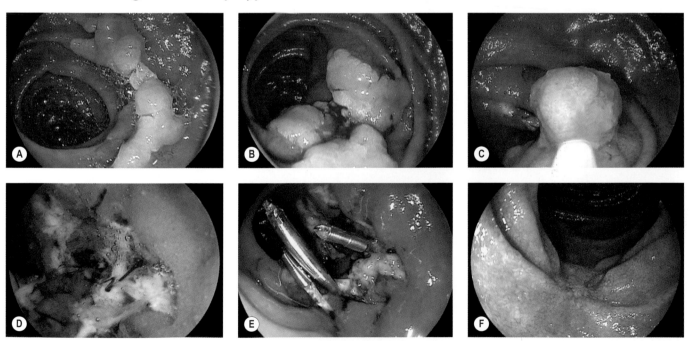

Figure 25 EMR of a large duodenal polyp. (A) Large duodenal polyp. (B) Submucosal injection. (C) Partial resection. (D) Oozing seen after immersion of D2 under water. (E) Clips to close the resection zone to prevent secondary bleeding. (F) Duodenal EMR scar at 3 months.

9.11. Colonic EMR: sessile lesion in the caecum

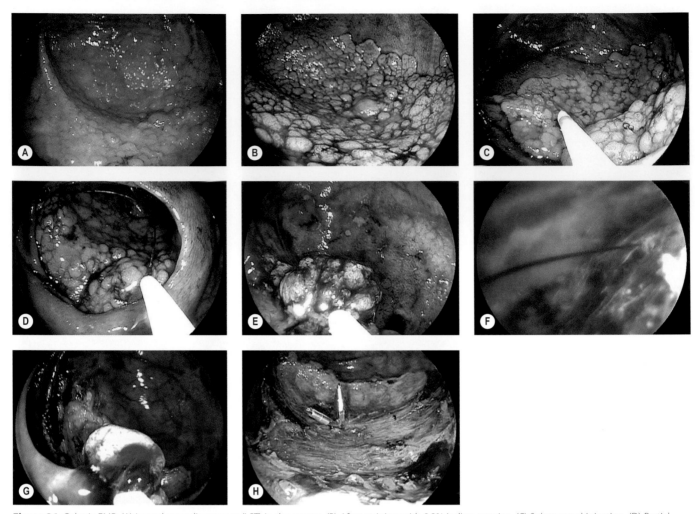

Figure 26 Colonic EMR: (A) Lateral spreading tumor (LST) in the cecum. (B) After staining with 0.2% indigo carmine. (C) Submucosal injection. (D) Partial resection with snare. (E) Resection of another fragment. (F) Active bleeding from a small vessel requiring clipping in order to continue. (G) Continuing the procedure. (H) End of the procedure.

9.12. EMR of a serrated adenoma: the only situation where marking is necessary in the colon

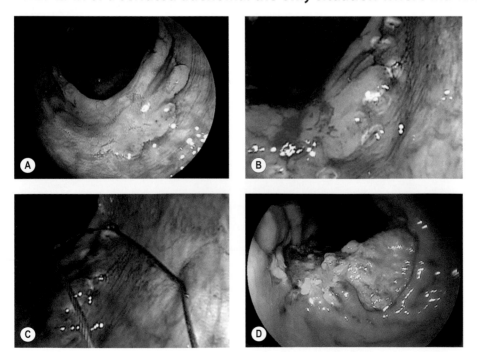

Figure 27 EMR of a serrated adenoma: the only situation where marking is necessary in the colon. (A) Serrated adenoma. (B) Marking necessary before resection. (C) A snare and a colonoscope with two operating channels may be useful for this type of lesion. (D) Complete resection in a single session.

9.13. EMR of a sessile rectal polyp

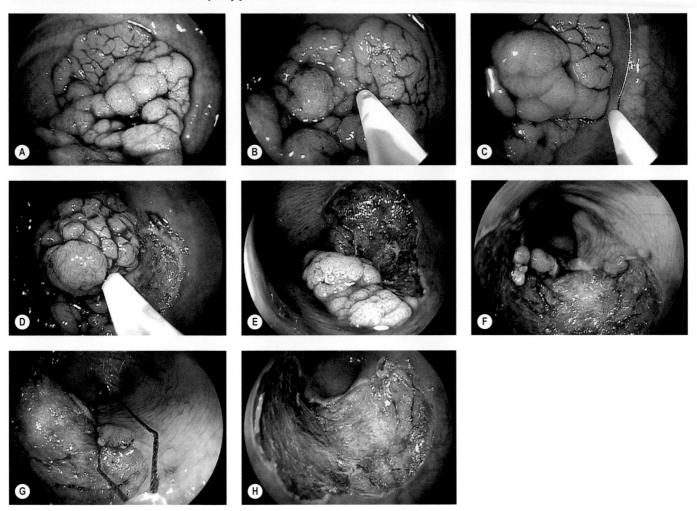

Figure 28 EMR of a sessile rectal polyp. (A) Staining with 0.2% indigo carmine. (B) Submucosal injection. (C) Piecemeal resection. (D) Resection of successive fragments. (E) Partial resection. (F) Follow-up showing residual adenoma at the resection margin. By using a colonoscope with optical zoom, the adenoma with elongated crypts can be clearly distinguished from normal mucosa with rounded crypts. (G) Resection of the final fragment. (H) Complete resection in a single session.

9.14. Perforation treated by clipping

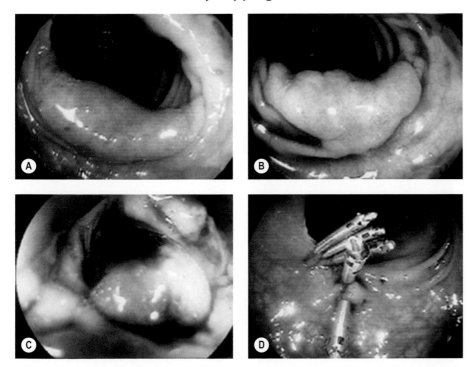

Figure 29 Perforation treated by clipping. (A) Recurrence of an incompletely resected sessile polyp. (B) After staining. (C) Intraperitoneal fatty tissue emerging through the site of perforation. (D) Closing the perforation: additional treatment with antibiotics and a fiber-free diet for 7 days before discharge.

Further Reading

ASGE Committee: Technology status evaluation report. Endoscopic mucosal resection and endoscopic submucosal dissection, *Gastrointest Endosc* 68:11–18; 2008.

Canard JM, De Leusse A, Palazzo L, et al: Traitement endoscopique du carcinome épidermoïde superficiel et de la dysplasie de haut grade de l'oesphage [Endoscopic treatment of superficial squamous carcinoma and high-grade dysplasia of the esophagus], *Gastroenterol Clin Biol* 28:A2, 2004.

Canard JM, Rahmi G, Manière T, et al: Long term outcome of endoscopic mucosal resection of high grade dysplasia and squamous cell carcinoma of the esophagus, *Acta Endosc* In press, 2010.

Cao Y, Liao C, Tan A, et al: Meta-analysis of endoscopic submucosal dissection versus endoscopic mucosal resection for tumors of the gastrointestinal tract, *Endoscopy* 41:751–757, 2009.

Fujischiro M, Yahagi N, Kashimura Y, et al: Comparison of various submucosal injection solutions for maintaining mucosal elevation during endoscopic mucosal resection, *Endoscopy* 36:579–589, 2004.

Murata Y, Napoleon B, Odegaard SY: High frequency endoscopic ultrasonography in the evaluation of superficial esophageal cancer, *Endoscopy* 35:429–436, 2003.

Ono H, Kondo H, Gotoda T, et al: Endoscopic mucosal resection for treatment of early gastric cancer, *Gut* 33:568–573, 2001.

Paris Workshop Participants: The Paris Endoscopic Classification of superficial neoplastic lesions: esophagus, stomach and colon, *Gastrointest Endosc* 58:S3–S27, 2003.

Pech O, May A, Rabenstein C, Ell C: Endoscopic resection of early oesophageal cancer, *Gut* 56:1625–1634, 2007.

Soetikno RM, Gotoda T, Nakanishi Y, et al: Endoscopic mucosal resection, *Gastrointest Endosc* 57:567–579, 2003.

7.13　Endoscopic pH monitoring in gastro-esophageal reflux disease

Jean-Christophe Létard, Jean Marc Canard

Key Points

- Gastroesophageal reflux disease (GERD) is a common disorder, affecting approximately 20% of adults, requiring long-term treatment.
- The implantable pH meter (Bravo probe) provides similar results compared with conventional pH meter.
- Good technique is essential to ensure adequate attachment to the esophageal mucosa.
- Chest pain is common, with 1% of patients requiring removal of the capsule due to pain.

Introduction

Gastroesophageal reflux disease (GERD) occurs when the gastroesophageal pressure gradient falls below 3 mmHg or if intra-abdominal pressure exceeds lower esophageal sphincter resistance. Medical treatment with proton pump inhibitors (PPI) controls the symptoms of GERD in 85–95% of patients. Surgical treatment (Nissen's fundoplication) relieves the symptoms of GERD in 80–90% of cases. Several endoscopic devices were developed with the hope of providing an alternative to surgery; however, the majority have since been withdrawn from the market and are no longer used.

In patients with refractory GERD, it is important to document the presence of ongoing acid reflux. This can be performed either by placing a probe transnasally or alternatively a capsule (Bravo capsule) can be placed endoscopically. This consists of a pH-meter capsule which is attached endoscopically 5 cm above the gastroesophageal junction. The probe records acidity over a 48-hour period and then spontaneously falls off the esophageal wall and passes out in the stools. Concordance for the diagnosis of gastroesophageal reflux disease (GERD) is excellent during the first 24 hours when the telemetry capsule is compared with conventional pH-meter. Patients often prefer placement of a capsule rather than the conventional pH meter.

1. Indications

Bravo probe placement is indicated to confirm the diagnosis of GERD.

2. Equipment

- Upper endoscope
- Bravo pH capsule with delivery system
- pH receiver.

3. Technique

- Remove the plastic covering protecting the capsule inserted over the implantation kit. Take care to hold the capsule on either side so that it does not become detached from its insertion. Avoid bending the implantation kit (Fig. 1).
- Remove the magnet white rigid plastic to start the batteries (Fig. 2).
- Calibrate the capsule by inserting it into the Bravo pH system for 10 minutes in the pH 7 medium (Fig. 3). Take care to ensure that the whole capsule is immersed. This procedure should be performed at room temperature.
- Switch on the Bravo receiver, check that the time and date are correct, then use the '*Set up*' menu to set the various user options.
- Use the '*Calibrate*' menu to start calibration (follow the prompts displayed on the device).
- Once calibrated, use the '*pH study*' menu to start recording, check that the implantation device number matches that shown on the receiver.

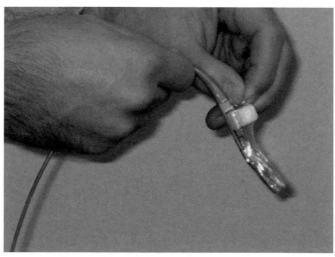

Figure 1 Removal of the protective plastic covering.

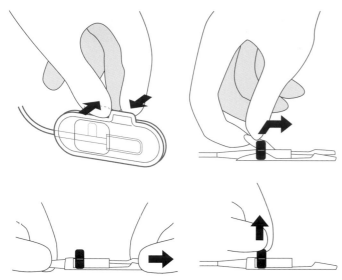

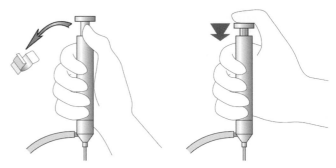

Figure 2 Remove the capsule from its protective case and remove the magnet (white rigid plastic) to start the batteries.

> **Warning!**
>
> The Bravo probe is delicate and must be treated with care. It is important to follow the directions carefully.

- An upper endoscopy is performed. The level of the gastroesophageal junction (GEJ) should be noted. The endoscope is withdrawn and the capsule and delivery system is introduced through the mouth or nose, with the capsule facing downwards
- Position the capsule 5 cm above the GEJ using the graduations marked on the delivery system
- Once in position, make sure that the delivery device does not move by holding it firmly at the nostrils or

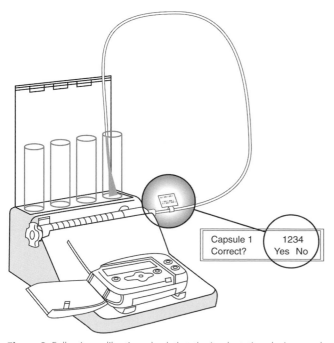

Figure 3 Following calibration, check that the implantation device number (highlighted in figure) matches that shown on the receiver.

Figure 4 Remove the clip which prevents deployment. Depress the button and turn it one quarter turn clockwise. Then allow the button to return automatically to its original position.

mouth. Connect the vacuum tube to the kit handle, switch on the pump and maintain pressure of 500 mmHg (see pump dial) for at least 30 seconds.

> **Warning!**
>
> - Effective suction is essential for successful placement of the pH probe.
> - Ensure that the suction channel is clear.
> - Do not use gel or biopsy the esophagus before introducing the capsule and delivery system, as these may block the suction channel.
> - If there is blood, withdraw the system and place it in sterile water, blowing air through the channel provided.
> - Avoid bending the delivery system as this can damage the catheter.
> - Avoid any movement once the pH probe is in position.
> - Ensure that the vacuum is maintained at 500 mmHg for at least 30 seconds.
> - Check that the probe is in a stable position after deployment.

- To deploy the capsule, remove the clip which prevents deployment (Fig. 4), depress the button and turn it one quarter turn clockwise. Then allow it to return to its original position. The capsule is deployed after the vacuum has been stopped. This can be performed with or without endoscopic monitoring. If performed without endoscopic monitoring, the endoscope is usually reinserted to confirm that the capsule is appropriately attached (Fig. 5).
- Before discharging the patient, check that recording has started properly.

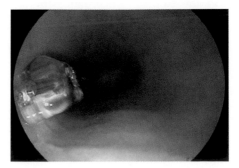

Figure 5 Bravo probe after deployment.

4. Complications

Chest pain and foreign body sensation are the commonest side-effects. Other side-effects include nausea and dysphagia. Rarer complications include mucosal tear, and one report of esophageal perforation. Known endoscopy-related complications include attachment failure, failure to transmit from the capsule to the receiver. 1% of patients require the capsule removal due to severe, intractable chest pain.

Further Reading

Ayazi S, Lipham JC, Portale G, et al: Bravo catheter-free pH monitoring: normal values, concordance, optimal diagnostic thresholds, and accuracy, *Clin Gastroenterol Hepatol* 7(1):60–67, 2009.

Chotiprashidi P, Liu J, Carpenter S, et al: Technology Assessment Committee, American Society for Gastrointestinal Endoscopy, *Gastrointest Endosc* 62(4):485–487, 2005 Oct.

Håkanson BS, Berggren P, Granqvist S, et al: Comparison of wireless 48-h (Bravo) versus traditional ambulatory 24-h esophageal pH monitoring, *Scand J Gastroenterol* 44(3):276–283, 2009.

Hirano I, Richter JE: Practice Parameters Committee of the American College of Gastroenterology, *Am J Gastroenterol* 102(3):668–685, 2007 Mar.

Kahrilas PJ, Shaheen NJ, Vaezi MF; American Gastroenterological Association Institute; Clinical Practice and Quality Management Committee: American Gastroenterological Association Institute technical review on the management of gastroesophageal reflux disease, *Gastroenterology* 135(4):1392–1413, 2008.

Lacy BE, Edwards S, Paquette L, et al: Tolerability and clinical utility of the Bravo pH capsule in children, *J Clin Gastroenterol* 43(6):514–519, 2009.

National Institute for Health and Clinical Excellence. IPG187 Catheterless oesophageal pH monitoring – guidance. www.nice.org.uk.

Yamaguchi T, Seza A, Odaka T, et al: Placement of the Bravo wireless pH monitoring capsule onto the gastric wall under endoscopic guidance, *Gastrointest Endosc* 63(7):1046–1050, 2006.

7.14 Ablative therapies for esophageal neoplasia

Jacques Etienne, Ian Penman

Key Points

- Photodynamic therapy (PDT) and radiofrequency ablation (RFA) are different ablative therapies for early esophageal neoplasia.
- Each can eradicate Barrett's high-grade dysplasia in approximately 80–90% of patients and delay progression to cancer.
- Porfimer sodium is more efficacious than 5-ALA at treating intramucosal cancer but has greater toxicity.
- Strictures can occur in patients who undergo PDT with porfimer sodium.
- All photosensitizers cause cutaneous phototoxicity after therapy.
- RFA can eradicate high-grade dysplasia in 80% of patients and reduce progression to cancer.
- 360° balloon-based catheters and 90° focal ablation electrodes are available.
- Care must be taken in selecting the correct size of the RFA balloon catheter, especially in patients with strictures or previous EMR.
- Major complications such as perforation are very rare with RFA.
- Careful follow-up with biopsies is essential after treatment with either PDT or RFA.

Introduction

This chapter discusses ablative therapies for early esophageal neoplasia. In this context, early neoplasia refers to high-grade dysplasia (HGD) or intramucosal carcinoma (IMC). While PDT has been used for palliation of advanced cancer, its role as a curative modality for early neoplasia is discussed here. The newer technique of radiofrequency ablation (RFA, Halo, BARRX, Sunnyvale, USA) is also applicable to early neoplasia. Both techniques are currently used in practice and so will be described here. At present, there are no studies directly comparing the efficacy, safety or cost-effectiveness of these two modalities. PDT is also used in conjunction with biliary stenting for the palliation of non-resectable cholangiocarcinoma and this is considered separately in Chapter 10 (ERCP).

1. Photodynamic therapy (PDT)

PDT utilizes the non-thermal photochemical effects of lasers that result from interactions between a photosensitizer and laser light in the presence of molecular oxygen (Fig. 1).

1.1. Principle of photochemical effects of lasers

Different photosensitizers are administered intravenously, orally, or topically and are retained for longer in neoplastic compared with normal cells, thus requiring a delay between administration and light irradiation. The optimal time delay is determined by the maximum concentration of the photosensitizer in tissue and this varies among photosensitizers. Illumination by laser light at an appropriate wavelength (red or green light) induces absorption of photons by the photosensitizer with release of phototoxic products, ultimately causing direct tumor cell necrosis (Figs 2, 3). Other mechanisms of action include vascular endothelial cell death with hypoxia and activation of the immune system and inflammatory responses.

1.2. Photosensitizers

1.2.1. Three most commonly used photosenstizers

Originally hematoporphyrin derivatives (an insoluble mixture of active products) were used for PDT. Sodium porfimer (Photofrin II), a more stable and defined mixture, is used now instead. The agent localizes in the mucosa and submucosa but also reaches the muscularis propria, explaining both the high efficacy and the significant risk of strictures (30–50%). These are major drawbacks, as is skin phototoxicity, which can persist for up to 6 weeks. Other agents such as 5-aminolaevulinic acid (5-ALA) localize in the mucosa and are effective in the treatment of high-grade dysplasia but less so for intramucosal carcinoma as a result of the limited depth of tissue destruction achieved. A newer agent, meta-tetrahydroxyphenylchlorine (m-THPC, Foscan) has two absorption wavelength peaks in the red (630 nm) and green light (514 nm) ranges. The penetration depth of green light is 1.25 mm, while red light penetrates to an approximate depth of 4.16 mm, hence the stricture rate is reduced with green light. Table 1 summarizes the properties of the three most commonly used photosensitizers.

New photosensitizers are under development and include Pd-bacteriopheophorbide (Tookad).

1.2.2. Afamelanotide

Skin phototoxicity is an important side-effect of PDT, requiring protection against exposure to spot light, daylight and direct sunlight. Afamelanotide, an agonist for

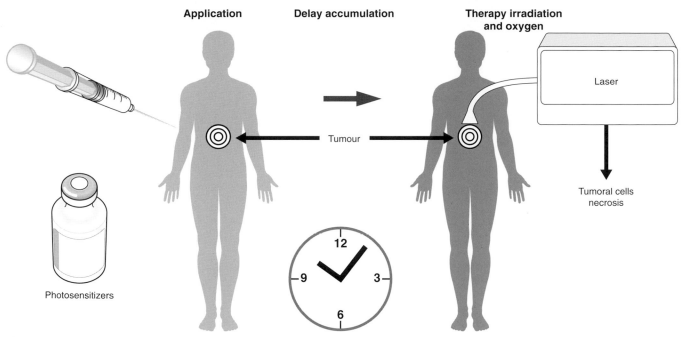

Figure 1 Basic principle of photodynamic therapy.

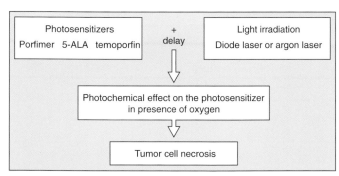

Figure 2 Photodynamic therapy: basic mechanism.

melanogenesis, provides dermal photoprotection and is being evaluated to determine whether it can reduce the period of skin phototoxicity in patients undergoing Photofrin PDT. The drug is a potent and long-acting analogue of α-MSH. It causes the production of eumelanin and consequently increases melanin levels within epidermal melanocytes. Eumelanin acts as a neutral density filter and unlike most sunscreens reduces penetration of all wavelengths of light equally so that photoprotection is essentially independent of wavelength. A clinical case shows progressive skin tanning observed over a period of a month after implant administration (Fig. 4). Afamelanotide is supplied as a 16 mg implant for subcutaneous injection. A phase II, multicenter, double-blind, placebo-controlled pilot study has been undertaken in 2009, to examine its ability to mitigate phototoxicity in Photofrin PDT and improve postoperative quality of life in oncology patients.

1.3. Dosimetry

The parameters of light illumination must be precise for each PDT session. They include:

- Fluence = total light energy = dose (J/cm^2)
- Irradiance (mW/cm^2)
- Irradiation time (s).

Fluence = irradiance × irradiation time. Precise calculation of these requires close collaboration between endoscopists and medical physicists. Dosimetry remains a major issue for PDT treatment and must be adapted according to the lesion and its localization. The appropriate dosimetry for Barrett's HGD using a semi-circular windowed diffuser is given in Table 2.

1.4. Equipment for PDT

Different types of lasers and diffusers are required in PDT practice to activate photosensitizers.

1.4.1. Light sources

For some time, lasers have been considered as the best light sources for PDT (Table 2). They effectively emit coherent directional and monochromatic light corresponding to the different absorption peaks of photosensitizers. Diode lasers, developed in the last 10 years, are small, portable, and easy to use (Fig. 5). Furthermore, they do not require any specific installation (air cooling, standard voltage outlet), are compatible with all optical fibers, and durable with low maintenance.

1.4.2. Light diffusing devices

Two types of *diffusers* are available: semicircular windowed diffusers (Figs 6, 7) and circular balloon diffusers. Diffusing balloon catheters serve two main purposes: to stretch the wall of the esophagus and smooth out esophageal folds; and to ensure uniform distribution of light emitted by the cylindrical light diffuser positioned within the balloon. The

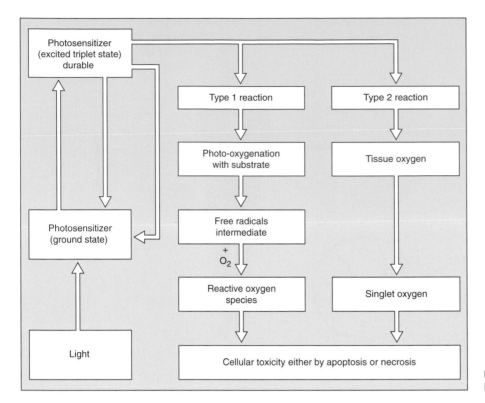

Figure 3 Mechanisms of tumour cell death with PDT.

Table 1 Comparison of the three main photosensitizers

Characteristics	Porfimer sodium (Photofrin)	m-THPC (Foscan)	5-ALA
Dose mg/kg	2	0.15	60
Route	IV	IV	Oral
Delay before irradiation	2 days	4 days	4–5 h
Wavelength (nm)	630	514	635
Localization	m, sm, mp	m	m, sm
Light source	Diode laser	Diode laser	Diode laser
Fluence J/cm^2	25	75	150
Irradiance mW/cm^2	48	100	10O
Irradiation time	15 min	8 min	15 min
Diffuser	Balloon or sectorial windowed diffuser	Sectorial windowed diffuser	Balloon
Efficacy	++	++ (HGD)	++ HGD; ± carcinoma
Strictures	++ (30–50%)	±	−
Phototoxicity	6 weeks	3 weeks	Brief

HGD, high-grade dysplasia; m, mucosa; sm, submucosa; mp, muscularis propria.

Table 2 Suppliers of PDT diode lasers

Manufacturer	Reference	Power (W)	Wavelength (nm)
Biolitec/CeramOptec	PDT630	2–4	630
Diomed	630PDT	2	630

Table 3 Dosimetry for Barrett's HGD using a semicircular windowed diffuser

Parameters	Green light (514 nm)	Red light (630 nm)
Fluence	75 J/cm^2	25 J/cm^2
Irradiance	100 mW/cm^2	28 mW/cm^2
Irradiation time	12 min, 30 s	15 min

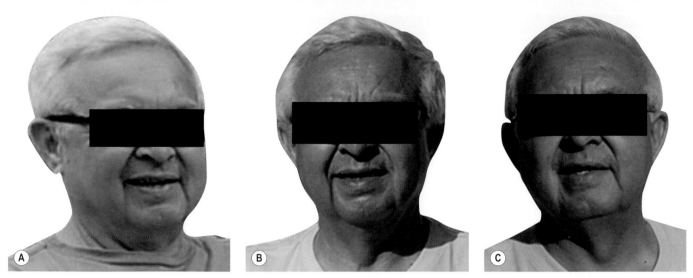

Figure 4 Skin tanning progression over a month following afamelanotide implant. (A) Before implant. (B) Day 7. (C) Day 30.

balloon catheter (Medlight, Ecublens, Switzerland) is 17 mm in diameter with radio-opaque markers at each end of the diffuser. Introduction of the fiber into the balloon catheter allows a radial illumination length varying from 1 to 7 cm. The light dose applied is a fluence of 130 J/cm of diffuser length. Use of a bare diffuser fiber is not recommended for Barrett's HGD as, eccentric placement can lead to uneven light distribution and significant under- or overdosing effects.

1.4.3. Fibers

Two different *optical fibers* are available: plastic and silica. The former are more flexible, while the latter are more transparent, transmitting about 95% of laser light power. The core sizes vary from 400 to 600 μm (0.4–0.6 mm).

1.5. Technique of PDT

It is essential that all staff must be well trained and understand the procedures and the need to protect patients from phototoxicity. All patients are photosensitive and precautions to protect patients are vital (Box 1). Porfimer should be administered as a single slow intravenous injection over 3–5 min at 2 mg/kg body weight. Care should be taken to prevent extravasation at the injection site. If this does occur, the area should be protected from light for a minimum of 90 days. After the appropriate dosing delay, the segment to be treated is carefully measured and mapped out. The appropriate balloon length is chosen (1–7 cm) and the deflated balloon is inserted into the esophagus over a guidewire (Fig. 7). A pediatric endoscope is usually placed alongside the balloon to allow direct visualization of the procedure. The diffuser is inserted into the centring balloon and treatment is performed according to the calculated dosimetry settings (Table 3). Atropine (0.4 mg) or glucagon (1 mg) IV may be helpful if there is excessive esophageal peristalsis. Treatment can be repeated if areas of dysplastic mucosa persist.

> **! Warning!**
>
> Using the aiming beam facility of the laser, the integrity of the fiber should be checked prior to calibration. If red light leakage is apparent, the fiber must be rejected.

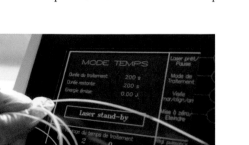

Figure 5 Diode laser (Biolitec) transmitting red light via a fiber introduced through a non-inflated balloon catheter.

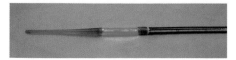

Figure 6 Green light illuminating the half-windowed diffuser.

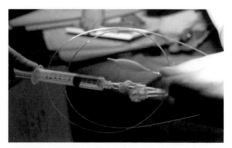

Figure 7 Balloon diffuser (medlight) being inflated before treating total circumference of esophagus.

> **Warning!**
>
> Patients may experience temporary worsening of dysphagia after PDT and should follow a pureed/liquid diet for the first few days post-treatment.

1.6. Role of PDT versus other local therapies

The different techniques available for mucosal destruction represent a real advance in the management of early neoplasia in the esophagus allowing prevention of the development of invasive carcinoma. All procedures, i.e. thermal destruction (e.g. laser, APC), EMR and PDT differ in efficacy and appropriateness in different settings. EMR is currently routine for visible lesions but cannot be undertaken when there is non-visible or multifocal disease. PDT techniques represent the most widely studied treatments (Table 4) but the recent development of radiofrequency ablation may offer similar benefits in future (see below). A problem reported for all ablative techniques is the possibility of small remnants of Barrett's tissue underneath the neosquamous epithelium (so-called 'buried glands'), which may or may not harbor future neoplastic potential.

1.7. Results, side-effects and complications

1–3 sessions of PDT with porfimer can achieve complete eradication of HGD or intramucosal carcinoma in 77–90% of patients. When using 5-ALA, successful ablation of HGD occurs in around 90% of patients (Fig. 8) but success rates for intramucosal carcinoma (Fig. 9) are only approximately 50%. Only small scale studies using m-THPC have been reported with promising results but further trials are awaited. Results of ablation with porfimer or m-THPC are better in early Barrett's neoplasia (80–90%) compared to squamous dysplasia, where success occurs in about 70%.

After PDT with m-THPC or porfimer for early esophageal lesions most side-effects are mild. Chest pain, odynophagia and, less frequently, temporary loss of weight, dysphagia and bouts of hiccups occur. Asymptomatic pleural effusions and arrhythmias have been reported rarely. *Strictures* and *cutaneous phototoxicity* are the two major adverse events that may occur. After treatment the diameter of the esophageal lumen is narrowed but normal eating is possible if it remains >12 mm. Risk factors for the development of strictures are circumferential illumination and previous endoscopic mucosal resection, strictures or radiotherapy. Measures to minimize the risk of phototoxicity are outlined in Box 1.

Box 1   Protecting patients from phototoxicity

- Careful patient counseling about the procedure and precautions afterwards.
- Masks, gloves and sunglasses to be provided.
- Curtains drawn in procedure room and recovery area.
- Patient should be transported rapidly to the procedure room.
- Patient lies facing away from light and is covered with a protective sheet.
- Sunblock creams are not protective and protective clothing is essential (hat, long-sleeved shirts, gloves).
- Remaining in shaded areas (200 lux evaluated by a lightmeter) helps but gentle exposure to ambient light is also beneficial ('photobleaching') and may shorten the period of photosensitivity.

Table 4 Comparison of three different methods of destruction of early neoplasia

	Endoscopic mucosal resection (EMR)	Thermal ablation	Photodynamic therapy
Advantages	Visible lesions only Histologic sample obtained	Visible lesions only	Relatively selective destruction of malignant cells Multifocal lesions Invisible lesions
Disadvantages	Resection extent limited Risk of stricture if circumferential resection Low risk of stricture if resection <50% circumference	No tissue sample Recurrence in remaining mucosa Risk of stricture if circumferential treatment	No tissue sample
			Porfimer Phototoxicity: 6 weeks Low risk of stricture if sectorial illumination at 3-month interval Recurrence in remaining mucosa
			ALA Phototoxicity: 2 days Frequent recurrences in buried glands and remaining mucosa
			m-THPC Phototoxicity: 3 weeks Low risk of stricture if sectorial illumination at 3-month interval Recurrence in remaining mucosa

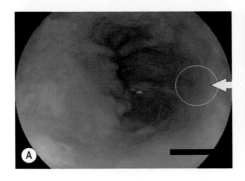
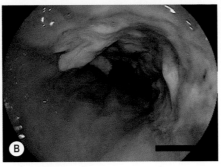

Figure 8 (A) Non-visible high-grade dysplasia detected by random four-quadrant biopsies in short Barrett's (arrow). (B) Necrosis 7 days post-PDT with a 180° windowed diffuser.

1.8. Follow-up

After treatment, endoscopic follow-up is very important especially for patients with risk factors for residual or recurrent HGD and/or IMC, such as:

- Piecemeal EMR
- Long-segment Barrett's esophagus
- Multifocal neoplastic lesions
- Persisting non-dysplastic Barrett's mucosa after complete response of abnormal areas.

Follow-up intervals vary but 3, 6, and 12 months is practical and then yearly thereafter for 5 years. Treatment sessions can be repeated for residual disease.

2. Radiofrequency ablation (RFA)

2.1. Introduction

Barrett's esophagus is an increasing public health issue and represents the only known risk factor for development of esophageal adenocarcinoma. Approximately 4% of Barrett's patients will progress to low-grade dysplasia annually while 0.9% will develop high-grade dysplasia each year and cancer develops annually in 0.5%. Regular surveillance with systematic four-quadrant biopsy protocols and the use of advanced imaging techniques have led to more patients with Barrett's being diagnosed with high-grade dysplasia or early intramucosal carcinoma. While endoscopic mucosal resection of focal visible lesions is highly effective, it leaves behind a premalignant background Barrett's mucosa on which further neoplasia may develop over time.

Recently, a radiofrequency ablation (RFA) system has been developed for treating dysplastic Barrett's esophagus (Halo,

BÂRRX Medical, Sunnyvale, CA, USA). The RF generator delivers a fixed amount of radiofrequency energy density with fixed power in an automated fashion via a bipolar electrode array. This allows uniform, controlled ablation of the mucosa to a depth of 0.5–1 mm. This is deep enough to destroy all Barrett's glands but does not involve the muscularis mucosae or submucosa thereby minimizing subsequent stricturing.

2.2. Equipment

The Halo system (Figs 10–13) comprises:

- Radiofrequency (RF) energy generators (separate for 360° and 90° systems)
- Sizing balloon catheters for measuring the inner esophageal diameter
- 360° balloon ablation catheters (ranging from 18 mm to 31 mm in diameter)
- 90° focal ablation catheters (20 × 13 mm)
- Footswitch.

Halo 360° RF energy generator This delivers 300 W of energy to the 360° balloon catheter electrode via an output cable connected to the catheter and activated by a footswit Settings can be adjusted.

Sizing catheters These are transparent, 4 cm long non-compliant balloons mounted on a catheter. The generator automatically inflates these to 4 psi (0.28 atm) to calculate the mean internal diameter of the esophagus.

360° electrode ablation catheters Similar to the sizing catheter, this consists of a 4 cm balloon containing a 3 cm 360° bipolar electrode comprising 60 electrode rings that alternate in polarity. They are available in outer diameters of 18, 22, 25, 28 and 31 mm. Energy is delivered in <1 s.

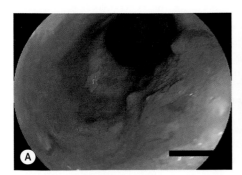
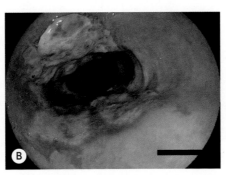

Figure 9 (A) Intramucosal carcinoma at 3 o'clock in long segment Barrett's. (B) Homogenous necrotic area 7 days after PDT with a 240° windowed diffuser.

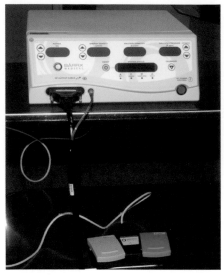

Figure 10 360° radiofrequency generator and footswitch (Halo, BARRX, Sunnyvale, CA, USA).

Halo 90° ablation catheter This consists of a 20 × 13 mm bipolar electrode plate on a 160 cm long, 4 mm wide catheter which can be mounted on a tip of a standard gastroscope. It connects to a dedicated energy generator. Short tongues of Barrett's can be treated with this device as can residual islands of intestinal metaplasia that persist after Halo 360° treatment. It can also be used to treat the Z-line so that one can be confident that all Barrett's mucosa has been ablated.

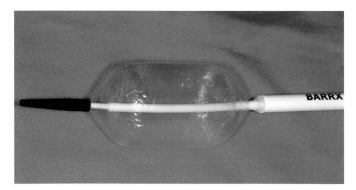

Figure 11 Sizing balloon catheter and markings for measuring esophageal diameter prior to 360° RFA.

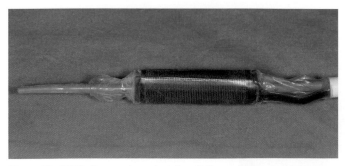

Figure 12 360° balloon catheter (uninflated). The multiple electrode rings can be clearly seen.

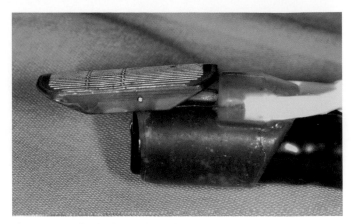

Figure 13 90° focal ablation electrode.

Footswitch This has two pedals. The left (gray) pedal activates automatic inflation of the balloon to the specified diameter while the right (blue) pedal triggers automated delivery of RF energy from the generator.

Other non-proprietary accessories are required for performing RFA procedures and these are listed in Box 2.

2.3. Technique

The procedure is performed under either conscious sedation or general anesthesia with the patient in the left lateral position. The esophagus is carefully inspected and, using the Prague criteria, the Barrett's esophagus is carefully mapped out, also noting the position of the Z line and the extent of any hiatus hernia present. The site of any previous EMR should be carefully inspected and its position measured (in cm from the incisors). Similarly the presence of any stricturing must be noted.

> **! Warning!**
>
> 360° RFA should not be performed until the site of a recent EMR has completely healed as there is a risk of laceration with bleeding or perforation. This usually takes 6–8 weeks.

Excess surface mucus is removed by washing with 1% acetylcysteine, which is then flushed away with water. The guidewire is then placed endoscopically in the stomach and the endoscope removed.

Box 2 Additional accessories for RFA procedures

- Stiff 0.035″ guidewire.
- Soft endoscope attachment cap.
- Dye spraying catheter.
- Esophageal balloon dilator inflation handle, e.g. Alliance/Boston Scientific.
- 20 mL 1% acetylcysteine (dilute 5 mL of 20% NAC in 100 mL of saline).
- 60 mL syringe for washing.
- Cotton gauze swabs.
- 50–70% alcohol solution.

2.3.1. Calculating the inner esophageal diameter

The next step is to measure the inner esophageal diameter. A sizing catheter is connected to the generator and will calibrate automatically. It is passed over the guidewire into the esophagus without using lubricant gel as this impedes contact and delivery of RF energy to the mucosa. The sizing catheter is positioned 5 cm above the proximal extent of the Barrett's esophagus and the esophageal diameter is measured by pressing the gray foot pedal which inflates the balloon. The digital display on the generator shows the calculated diameter and this should be noted down. Using the centimeter markings on the catheter shaft, the balloon is advanced in 1 cm intervals with measurements taken each time. The catheter must be grasped firmly to prevent it moving in or out during balloon inflation. This process is repeated every 1 cm until there is a sudden rise in calculated diameter, indicating that the balloon is in either a hiatus hernia sac or the stomach.

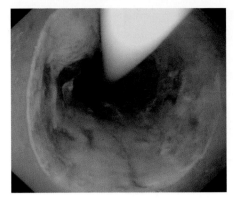

Figure 14 Appearances immediately after one application of 360° ablation.

 Clinical Tip

Lubricant gel impedes delivery of RF energy to the mucosa and should not be used to lubricate the endoscope or balloon catheters – use water instead.

2.3.2. Selecting the appropriate ablation catheter

This is done by reviewing the list of measured esophageal diameters. An ablation catheter one size smaller than the smallest measured diameter should be chosen. If there has been a previous EMR a catheter one *further* size smaller should be chosen because of the small but significant risk of perforation at the EMR site (the esophageal wall here is scarred and lacks the normal distensibility).

! Warning!

There may be eccentric narrowing at the site of a previous EMR. This fibrotic area lacks the normal compliance seen elsewhere in the esophagus and there is a risk of laceration or perforation upon inflation of the balloon. A balloon two sizes smaller than the smallest measured esophageal diameter should be chosen in such cases.

2.3.3. Performing the ablation

The sizing catheter is removed and replaced over the guidewire by the selected ablation catheter. This is connected to the generator with settings of 300 W power and an energy setting of 12 J/cm^2. The endoscope is introduced alongside the catheter and the proximal margin of the ablation electrode on the balloon is positioned visually 1 cm proximal to the proximal extent of the Barrett's segment. Pressing the gray pedal inflates the balloon, and when the generator beeps, the blue pedal is then pressed to deliver the RF energy. The mucosa of the treated segment will appear whitened and the balloon is advanced forward to treat the next portion of the Barrett's mucosa, leaving about 10 mm of overlap with the previously treated segment (Fig. 14). The procedure is repeated in steps until the entire segment has been treated once.

 Clinical Tip

Gentle suction immediately prior to delivery of RF energy will deflate the esophagus slightly and maximize contact of the mucosa with the surface of the balloon.

2.3.4. Cleaning between first and second passes

The catheter and endoscope are removed together, alcohol and swabs are used to clean any coagulum or debris from the electrode and while this is being done the endoscope is reintroduced with a soft distal cap mounted on its end. This is used to scrape very gently any slough off the esophagus. Vigorous spraying of the mucosa using a CRE balloon inflation handle and a 60 mL syringe of water attached to a spray catheter will also physically remove slough. This is an essential step as the presence of adherent coagulum (Figs 14–16) reduces the quality of contact with the electrode for the second pass. Once this is done the entire Barrett's segment is re-treated for a second time. Adequately treated areas have a yellow-brown hue (Fig. 17).

2.3.5. Aftercare

The procedure is generally well tolerated and patients are usually discharged home the same day. Cold drinks and a sloppy diet are advised for a few days and simple analgesia may be necessary for mild retrosternal discomfort or sore

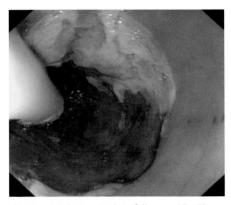

Figure 15 White coagulum following RFA. This must be removed before the second RFA pass.

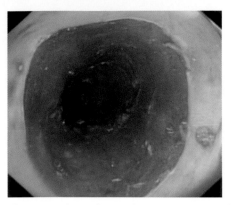

Figure 16 After washing with water via a spray catheter and gentle scraping with a soft distal attachment cap on the end of a gastroscope.

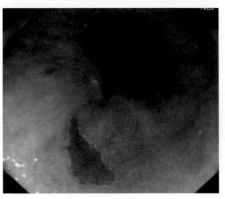

Figure 18 Residual islands of Barrett's mucosa seen with narrow band imaging after one session of 360° RFA.

throat. To encourage regeneration with a neosquamous epithelium and to minimize the risk of stricturing, it is important that the patients take potent acid suppression therapy with a high dose proton pump inhibitor, e.g. Omeprazole 40 mg twice daily or equivalent. Some experts also recommend the addition of Ranitidine 300 mg at night and Sucralfate 1 g 4 times daily to maximize acid suppression and promote healing. Patients should be given written information at discharge and instructed to seek medical advice urgently if they experience dysphagia, severe chest pain, fever, hematemesis, melena or vomiting. The procedure may require to be repeated and a further endoscopic evaluation with a view to further treatment should be scheduled for 8–12 weeks.

2.4. Results of RFA

A number of studies have demonstrated the efficacy and safety of RFA in both non-dysplastic and dysplastic Barrett's esophagus. Complete resolution of all Barrett's esophagus occurs in approximately 77% of patient after 1–3 sessions of treatment. Low-grade dysplasia can be eradicated in 90% and complete eradication of high-grade dysplasia in approximately 80%. Available data have also shown a significant reduction in any progression of Barrett's to a higher grade and notably a reduction in progression to cancer, at least in the short to medium term. One concern about RFA treatment is the possibility of residual submucosal 'buried'

glands, which may be undetectable beneath a new squamous epithelium. Studies of RFA therapy involving thousands of follow-up biopsies have failed to demonstrate that this occurs. RFA is currently expensive, catheters costing €1000–1500 each – a course of three sessions of RFA is therefore costly and in many countries an appropriate reimbursement code and tariff have not been agreed. This is currently limiting widespread uptake of the procedure in these countries.

2.5. Complications

A mild sore throat, chest discomfort and nausea are relatively common for a few days post-procedure but major complications are rare. A mucosal tear with bleeding can be avoided by using a smaller balloon and taking care. Perforations have been recorded but are rare (<0.5%).

2.6. Focal ablation with the Halo 90 RFA system

The Halo 90° system is ideal for very short segments of Barrett's esophagus (≤2 cm), islands of residual Barrett's after previous treatment (Fig. 18) and for treating the Z-line effectively. The Halo 90° electrode comes attached to a transparent rubber cap on the tip of the catheter sheath. It is mounted onto the tip of an endoscope and rotated until the electrode is visible at the 12 o'clock position on the endoscopy image. It is dampened with water to ease intubation but, like the 360° catheter, lubricant gel should be avoided. Introducing the endoscope with the mounted catheter can be tricky and must be performed gently to avoid trauma to the pharynx or larynx. As the endoscope is advanced over the tongue the endoscope tip and electrode are deflected upwards using the large wheel on the endoscope and this is then relaxed into a more neutral position when the larynx is seen. The electrode is hinged and should deflect easily.

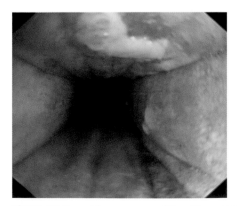

Figure 17 Brownish appearance of Barrett's mucosa after two applications of 360° RFA.

 Clinical Tip

If there are difficulties achieving intubation a 10–12 mm through-the-scope dilator balloon can be passed and gently inflated at the level of the upper esophageal sphincter to act as a bougie and facilitate gentle introduction of the endoscope into the esophagus.

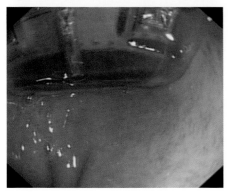

Figure 19 Endoscopic image with 90° focal ablation electrode mounted in the correct position.

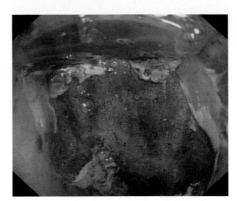

Figure 20 Appearances after 90° focal ablation of residual Barrett's mucosa.

Once in the esophagus any area of residual Barrett's should be carefully identified and marked out (Fig. 19). This is often easier using enhanced imaging techniques such as narrow band imaging. The endoscope should be rotated until the area to be treated is positioned at the 12 o'clock position. The electrode is gently pressed against the mucosa until there is good contact and energy delivered by activating the foot pedal as above. Without removing the electrode a second pulse of energy is delivered. The electrode is then gently removed and the area treated should reveal a rectangular whitish area of coagulum (Fig. 20). The endoscope is rotated and adjacent areas treated with slight overlap of a few millimeters. Once all Barrett's areas have been treated with two pulses of energy, the coagulum is gently scraped away using the distal lip of the electrode and gentle to and fro movements of the endoscope in a 'snow plough' fashion. Vigorous washing as described for the 360° system can also be used. The endoscope is removed, coagulum that is adherent to the electrode surface is removed and the procedure is then repeated, i.e. areas of Barrett's are treated four times (2 × 2). Care should be taken to make sure that the Z-line is treated circumferentially. The generator will allow a maximum of 80 pulses of energy to be delivered by a single electrode before a new one must be used. Aftercare is identical to that described above and patients should be endoscopically evaluated and, if necessary, retreated after an interval of approximately 8 weeks. Further endoscopies should then be scheduled at 6 and 12 months and annually thereafter. High resolution endoscopes, preferably with NBI, FICE or iSCAN should be used to allow detection of residual Barrett's mucosa. A rigorous and systematic biopsy protocol should be followed at all follow-up endoscopic procedures to confirm eradication of dysplasia and intestinal metaplasia and to exclude the presence of buried glands.

Conclusion

Both PDT and RFA can effectively and safely eradicate high-grade dysplasia in Barrett's and delay or prevent progression to cancer. Both offer a non-invasive alternative to surgery for selected patients but the decision to proceed should be carefully discussed beforehand in a multidisciplinary environment. It is not possible at present to say whether one technique is superior to the other but RFA is perhaps simpler and is not associated with either stricturing or phototoxicity. In many centers RFA is replacing PDT as the first choice ablative therapy for HGD in Barrett's esophagus.

Further Reading

Dunn J, Lovat L: Photodynamic therapy using 5-aminolaevulinic acid for the treatment of dysplasia in Barrett's esophagus, *Expert Opin Pharmacother* 9:851–858, 2008.

Etienne J, Dorme N, Bourg-Heckly G, et al: Photodynamic therapy with green light and m-tetrahydroxyphenyl chlorin for intramucosal adenocarcinoma and high grade dysplasia in Barrett's esophagus, *Gastrointest Endosc* 59:880–889, 2004.

Fleischer DE, Overholt BF, Sharma VK, et al: Endoscopic radiofrequency ablation for Barrett's esophagus: 5-year outcomes from a prospective multicenter trial, *Endoscopy* 42(10):781–789, 2010.

Overholt BF, Lightdale CJ, Wang KK, et al: Photodynamic therapy with porfimer sodium for ablation of high-grade dysplasia in Barrett's esophagus: international, partially blinded, randomized phase III trial, *Gastrointest Endosc* 62:488–498, 2005.

Peters FP, Kara MA, Rosmolen WD, et al: Poor results of 5-aminolevulinic acid-photodynamic therapy for residual high-grade dysplasia and early cancer in Barrett's esophagus after endoscopic resection, *Endoscopy* 37:418–424, 2005.

Pouw RE, Sharma VK, Bergman JJ, et al: Radiofrequency ablation for total Barrett's eradication: a description of the endoscopic technique, its clinical results and future prospects, *Endoscopy* 40:1033–1040, 2008.

Shaheen NJ, Sharma P, Overholt BF, et al: Radiofrequency ablation in Barrett's esophagus with dysplasia, *N Engl J Med* 360:2277–2288, 2009.

Sharma VK, Wang KK, Overholt BF, et al: Balloon-based, circumferential, endoscopic radiofrequency ablation of Barrett's esophagus: 1-year follow-up of 100 patients, *Gastrointest Endosc* 65:185–195, 2007.

Zhang YM, Bergman JJ, Weusten B, et al: Radiofrequency ablation for early esophageal squamous cell neoplasia, *Endoscopy* 42(4):327–323, 2010.

Complications of gastrointestinal endoscopy

Mouen Khashab, Jean Marc Canard

Summary

Introduction   264

1. Complications of upper gastrointestinal endoscopy   264

2. Complications related to specific upper gastrointestinal procedures   268

3. Complications of endoscopic ultrasonography (EUS)   270

4. Complications of device-assisted enteroscopy and capsule endoscopy   272

Key Points

- Endoscopists need to implement strategies to minimize complications of endoscopy and be able to recognize and treat them efficiently and effectively.
- There are currently no data to prove a causal link between endoscopic procedures and infective endocarditis. In like manner, there are no data to demonstrate that antibiotic prophylaxis in the peri-endoscopic period decreases the risk of infective endocarditis.
- Immediate endoscopic closure of perforation and in case of failure, early treatment is key to successful conservative management. Delay in the diagnosis is associated with a poor outcome.
- Drainage of infection and fluid collections is paramount for successful endoscopic closure of a perforation.
- Complications of endoscopic ultrasound include FNA-related and non-FNA-related complications.
- Complications that appear to be increased after double-balloon enteroscopy include acute pancreatitis, gastrointestinal hemorrhage, and perforation. Perforation risk is increased in patients with altered surgical anatomy.
- Capsule retention, perforation, aspiration, and small bowel obstruction are reported complications of capsule endoscopy. Among these, capsule retention is the most common complication and occurs in 1.2–2.6% of cases.

Introduction

Complications are inherent to gastrointestinal endoscopy and do not signify negligence by the endoscopist. Due to the technical and invasive nature of endoscopic procedures and the recent trend towards aggressive therapeutic interventions, post-procedural complications may occur, ranging from minor (requiring brief hospitalization) to severe, with permanent disability or death. Endoscopists need to be cognizant of complications that may occur with any endoscopic procedure and those that are specific to the procedure being performed. In addition, endoscopists need to implement strategies to minimize these untoward occurrences and be able to recognize and treat them efficiently and effectively.

This chapter summarizes the complications that are associated with various upper endoscopic procedures, including endoscopic ultrasonography (EUS), with emphasis on strategies aimed at minimizing and treating these complications. Complications related to sedation and those related to the performance of colonoscopy, percutaneous endoscopic gastrostomy (PEG) tube placement, and endoscopic retrograde cholangiopancreatography (ERCP) are discussed elsewhere (see Chapter 8).

1. Complications of upper gastrointestinal endoscopy

1.1. Infection complications

Endoscopy related infection may occur under the following circumstances:

- Exogenous infections: microorganisms may be spread from patient to patient by contaminated equipment.
- Endogenous infections: microorganisms may spread from the GI tract through the bloodstream during an endoscopy to susceptible organs or prostheses, or may spread to adjacent tissues that are breached as a result of the endoscopic procedure.
- Microorganisms may be transmitted from patients to endoscopy personnel and perhaps from endoscopy personnel to patients.

Recently, the American Society for Gastrointestinal Endoscopy (ASGE) published guidelines on infection control in gastrointestinal endoscopy (Box 1).

DOI: 10.1016/B978-0-7020-3128-1.00008-0

Transmission of infection as a result of endoscopes is extremely rare, and reported cases are invariably attributable to lapses in currently accepted endoscope reprocessing protocols or to defective equipment.
- Endoscopes should undergo high-level disinfection as recommended by governmental agencies and all pertinent professional organizations for the reprocessing of GI endoscopes.
- Extensive training of staff involved in endoscopic reprocessing is obligatory for effective infection control.
- General infection control principles should be adhered to at the endoscopy unit.
- Transmission of infection from patients to endoscopy personnel can be avoided by application of standard precautions.

1.1.1. Endogenous complications

Bacteremia can occur after any endoscopic procedure due to bacterial translocation as a result of mucosal trauma that occurs during endoscopy. Bacteremia is thought of as a surrogate marker for infective endocarditis (IE) risk. However, there are currently no data to prove a causal link between endoscopic procedures and IE. In like manner, there are no data to demonstrate that antibiotic prophylaxis in the peri-endoscopic period decreases the risk of IE (see Ch. 2.2). Although previous recommendations have been to administer antibiotic prophylaxis prior to procedures with high risk of bacteremia, namely esophageal dilation and sclerotherapy, the most recent ASGE guidelines stated that this policy to prevent IE is no longer recommended before endoscopic procedures. Notable exceptions to this guideline are detailed in Box 2.

1.2. Perforation

- Perforation related to diagnostic upper endoscopy is rare and occurs at a rate of 0.03%, with a mortality rate of 0.001%.
- Box 3 lists known factors that increase perforation risk during upper endoscopy.
- Signs and symptoms of perforation include pain, pleuritic chest pain, fever, crepitans, leukocytosis and/or pleural effusion
- Early recognition of the perforation is key to successful conservative (least-invasive) management. Delay in the diagnosis is associated with a poor outcome
- Water-soluble esophagogram is the initial test of choice for the localization of suspected perforations. If the site

of perforation is not recognized, endoscopy or computed tomography may be used.

Clinical Tip

Endoscopy is safe to diagnose esophageal perforations and should be undertaken, if necessary, after a negative CT scan or esophagogram, to exclude the diagnosis.

- Stable patients may be managed conservatively with nothing per os, placement of a nasogastric tube, administration of broad-spectrum antibiotics, and with parenteral hyperalimentation.

Clinical Tips

Management
- Surgical consultation should be implemented early even if conservative management is undertaken.
- Surgical management is usually required for larger perforations, when the pleural space is involved, and in patients who fail to respond to conservative therapy.

1.2.1. Endoscopic management of perforations

Although interest in endoscopic closure began in the early 1990s with the first description of clip closure of gastric perforation, Natural Orifice Transluminal Endoscopic Surgery (NOTES) has provided the momentum for development of this field. NOTES has opened the realm for new endoscopic techniques, innovative endoscopic instruments, and pioneering treatment modalities, which made endoscopic closure of perforations possible.

Clinical Tip

Management

Tension pneumoperitoneum or pneumothorax may complicate GI perforations, should be checked for, and if present, should be managed with immediate decompression with a wide-bore needle puncture.

- ERCP with anticipated incomplete drainage (e.g. primary sclerosing cholangitis, hilar strictures).
- ERCP in the setting of a communicating pseudocyst.
- Transmural drainage of pancreatic fluid collection.
- EUS-guided fine-needle aspiration (EUS-FNA) of cystic lesions.
- PEG tube placement.
- Cirrhosis with acute GI bleeding (required regardless of endoscopic procedures).

- Anterior cervical osteophytes.
- Zenker's diverticulum (Fig. 1).
- Malignant esophageal obstruction.
- Complex esophageal strictures (defined as strictures with at least one of the following features: asymmetry, diameter ≤12 mm, or inability to pass the endoscope).
- Radiation-induced strictures.
- Eosinophilic esophagitis.
- Inexperienced endoscopist.

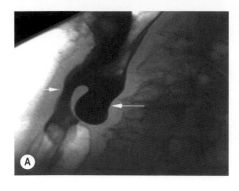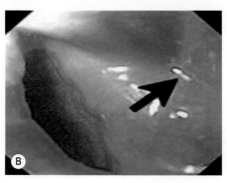

Figure 1 (A) Zenker's diverticulum: barium esophagogram showing a large diverticulum arising from the posterior wall of the upper esophagus (long arrow) producing extrinsic narrowing of the anterior esophageal lumen (short arrow). (B) Endoscopic picture showing a large Zenker's diverticulum. The black arrow points at the lumen. Zenker's diverticulum is a risk factor for perforation of the cervical esophagus during EUS.

- Currently, endoscopic clips are the only devices available in the market for closure of perforations, whereas suturing and stapling devices are not available for clinical use. Clips can be used to close perforations that are <2 cm in size. Five different designs of clips are currently available:
  1. *Resolution Clip* (Boston Scientific, Natick, MA) has the ability to reopen up to five times before final deployment, thus maximizing the chance to realign the clip for better tissue approximation.
  2. *TRICLIP* (Cook Medical Inc, Winston-Salem, NC) is a tri-pronged single-use clip device with a flushing mechanism designed to orient on the target site without the need for rotation of the prongs.
  3. *QuickClip2* (Olympus Corp, Melville, NY) is a rotatable clip device that is ready for use immediately after taking out of the package, unlike its predecessor that required loading of clips on a reusable applicator.
  4. *InScope Multiclip Applier* (Ethicon Endosurgical Inc, Cincinnati, OH) has the ability to deliver four clips, 1:1 rotation to align the jaw openings across the defect and reopening of the clip if necessary.
  5. *Over-the-scope clip* (Ovesco Endoscopy, Tuebingen, Germany) is a nitinol clip loaded at the tip of the endoscope that can capture small perforations.
- Clip closure of perforations should not be performed by endoscopists with no prior experience with the use of clips. It is critical for both the endoscopist and his assistant to be conversant with the use of clips before undertaking endoscopic closure of perforations. Attention to the details as outlined below is critical for successful clip closure of perforations. Technique of clip closure of perforations is detailed in Box 4.

Box 4   Technique of closure of perforations with clips (Figs 2–5)

- The most critical component of closure of perforations is the placement of the first clip.
- Keep the clip close to the end of the endoscope with the clip and the endoscope acting as a single unit.
- Place the wide-open clip across the defect at 90° to the defect.
- Gently push the clip-endoscope unit as one unit while applying gentle suction to collapse the lumen so that as much tissue away from the edge of perforation as possible could be grasped while slowly closing the clip.
- Be patient and confirm satisfactory clip closure of the perforation with approximation of the edges before deployment of the clip. A misplaced clip might render placement of additional clips technically difficult.
- Place additional clips from top-to-bottom in linear perforations or left-to-right in circular perforations after satisfactory application of the first clip.
- Over inflating the lumen with air can widen the defect: avoid over inflation and decompress the lumen before withdrawal of the endoscope.
- Use carbon dioxide (CO_2) rather than air for insufflation.

- Large perforations (>2 cm in diameter) cannot be approximated effectively with clips because all current available clips have a wingspan <2 cm. In addition, the edges of a malignant perforation may not be effectively approximated with clips, which tend to tear through cancerous tissue rather than grip the edges of the perforation.
- Covered self-expandable metal stents (SEMS) can be used to seal esophageal perforations, especially larger perforations that are not amenable to closure by clips (Fig. 6). To prevent mechanical complications, including stent embedment into the esophageal wall, the stent should be removed preferably within 8 weeks after placement.
- Although a covered self-expanding plastic stent (SEPS) (Polyflex, Boston Scientific, Natick, MA) is commercially available, it is not the stent of choice in the setting of a perforation because its delivery system is cumbersome.
- The different FDA-approved SEMS and the technique of stent placement are discussed in detail in Chapter 7.3.

1.3. Bleeding

- Significant bleeding occurs only rarely after diagnostic upper endoscopy.

Clinical Tips

- Drainage of infection and fluid collections is paramount for successful endoscopic closure of perforations.
- If an *en-face* approach to the perforation is unsuccessful, the use of a rotatable clip may be helpful. In addition, the use of a cap-fitted endoscope may render tissue approximation feasible in these instances. It is often possible to bring the defect *en-face* by drawing it into the cap even when it is situated tangential to the endoscope. Moreover, the transparent cap maintains a certain distance between the endoscope lens and the defect, enabling a more effective clip placement.

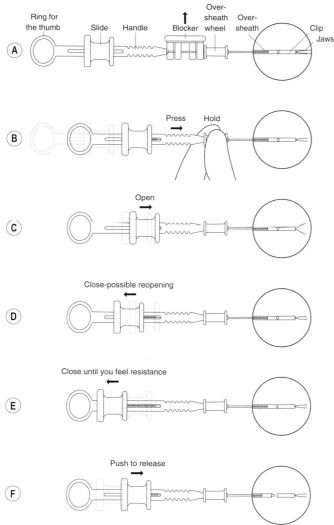

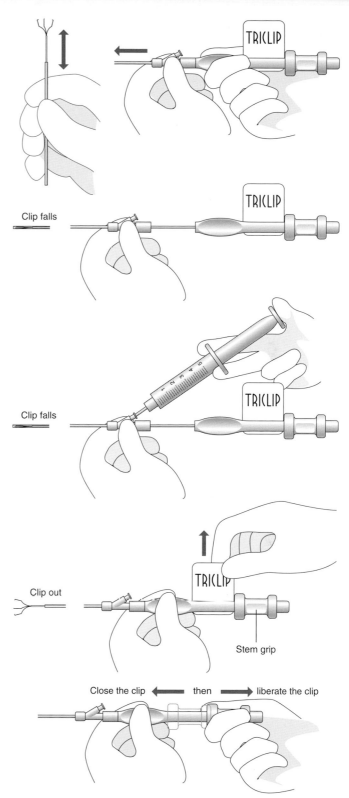

Figure 2 Boston Scientific hemostatic clip. (A) When the endoscopist is in the correct position, remove the safety stopper located between the over-sheath grip and the handle. (B) To release the jaws of the clip, hold the sheath grip firmly and push the handle towards the grip until they come into contact. (C) Open the jaws of the clip by sliding the slider over the handle towards the over-sheath grip. (D) To close the clip without releasing it, bring the slider towards you until feel slight resistance. If the clip is incorrectly positioned, it can be re-opened by sliding the slider towards the over-sheath grip. (The clip may be opened or closed five times at most.) (E) When the clip is correctly positioned, close it until you feel resistance. After hearing the first click, continue to close it until you hear the second click. The slider should reach the ring on the handle. Never try to re-open a clip after the second click. (F) To release the clip, push the slider back towards the over-sheath. Once separation has occurred, release the slider and advance the over-sheath so that the safety stopper can be replaced. Never try to withdraw the endoscopic device until this maneuver has been completed, otherwise the endoscope may be seriously damaged if the distal over-sheath does not cover the material for anchoring the clip entirely.

Figure 3 Cook TRICLIP. (A) Hold the handle firmly with one hand and advance the sheath with the other until the clip is completely covered by the sheath. (B) When the lesion has been located, introduce the TRICLIP, when instructed by the endoscopist, into the operating channel until it emerges from the distal end of the endoscope. If necessary, flush the lesion using a suitable syringe for the injection site. (C) When instructed by the endoscopist, deploy the TRICLIP by bringing the sheath device towards you. Immediately before releasing the clip, when instructed by the endoscopist, remove the cardboard tab from the handle. (D) To clip the lesion and close the clip, advance the stem grip towards the sheath. To release the clip, pull the stem grip towards you.

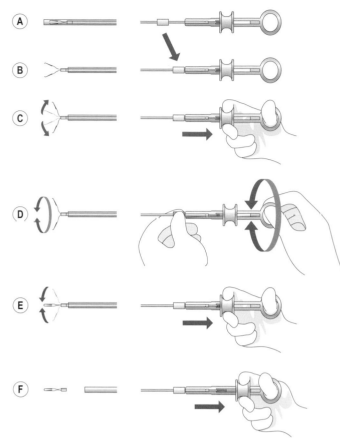

Figure 4 Olympus hemostatic clip. (A) Introduce the clip into the biopsy channel. (B) When the device is correctly positioned, remove the stopper when instructed by the endoscopist. (C) Release the clip by bringing the yellow ring towards the handle. The opening width of the clip can be increased by moving the handle very slightly in the same direction as for closing. (D) If necessary, improve the position of the clip by rotation: to do this, hold the device by the yellow ring in the left hand and rotate the handle with the right hand. (E) When instructed by the endoscopist, close the clip by closing the handle. (F) After the device has been completely closed, the clip is automatically released.

- Risk factors for bleeding include coagulopathy and/or severe thrombocytopenia (platelet count <20 000).
- Mucosal biopsies should be performed with caution in patients with severe thrombocytopenia and platelet transfusion prior to endoscopy should be strongly considered.
- Diagnostic upper endoscopy can be performed safely in anticoagulated patients, as long as the anticoagulant levels are within therapeutic range.

1.3.1. Management of antithrombotic agents in patients undergoing upper endoscopic procedures

- Management of antiplatelet agents (e.g. aspirin, NSAIDs, thienopyridines, e.g. clopidogrel and ticlopidine) and anticoagulants (e.g. warfarin, heparin, and LMWH) in patients undergoing endoscopy requires the endoscopist to be cognizant of bleeding risk associated with endoscopy and thromboembolic risk associated with interruption of antithrombotic agents (Box 5) (see also Ch. 2.1).
- Aspirin and other NSAIDs can be continued in the peri-endoscopic period, even after high-risk endoscopic procedures
- Current guidelines recommend withholding clopidogrel for at least 7 days prior to high-risk procedures. This often requires consultation with patients' cardiologist
- For anticoagulated patients undergoing high-risk procedures and who are at low risk of thromboembolic events, warfarin is withheld 3–5 days prior to the procedure. For patients who are at high risk for thromboembolism, bridging therapy (Box 6) with heparin or LMWH is required.

2. Complications related to specific upper gastrointestinal procedures

2.1. Dilation and enteral stenting

Complications related to dilation of benign and malignant strictures of the gastrointestinal tract and of pneumatic dilation in achalasia patients are detailed in Chapter 7.1.

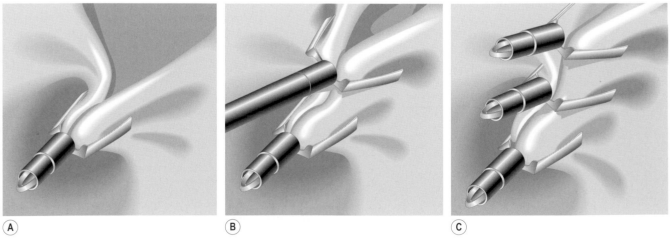

Figure 5 (A–C) Closing a perforation starting from one side.

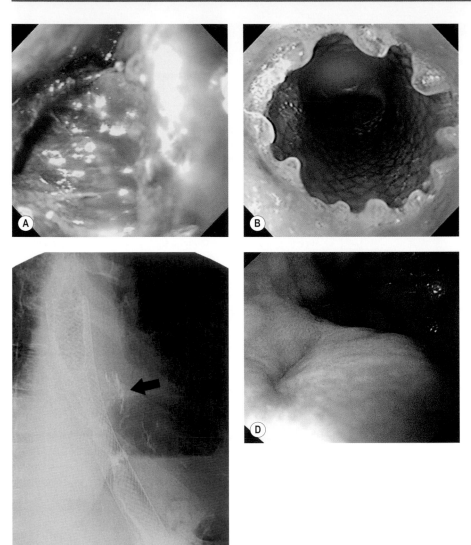

Figure 6 (A) Endoscopic view showing perforation in distal esophagus through which mediastinal cavity is visible. (B) Endoscopic view of distal esophagus immediately after placement of metallic stent showing stent to be fully expanded and perforation sealed. (C) Esophagogram after placement of metallic stent showing no leakage of contrast. Note contrast medium injected into wall of esophagus (arrow) to mark area approximately 4 cm proximal to perforation. (D) Endoscopic view of distal esophagus 3.5 weeks after complicated stent removal showing residual scar at site of original perforation. (From Siersema et al. Use of large-diameter metallic stents to seal traumatic nonmalignant perforations of the esophagus. Gastrointestinal Endoscopy 2003; 58: 356–361.)

Complications of enteral stenting are discussed in Chapter 7.3.

2.2. Hemostatic technique

2.2.1. Endoscopic non-variceal hemostasis

- Tissue necrosis and ulceration, but not perforation, can occur due to epinephrine injection.
- The reported perforation rate after bipolar or multipolar electrocoagulation is 0–2%.
- Bleeding is common after electrocoagulation and occurs in up to 5% of cases. Usually, bleeding is immediate and can be controlled during the same endoscopic session.
- The use of clips for the control of GI bleeding is being increasingly used and appears to be safe and well tolerated. The main risk is misplacement of the clip, which can render further attempts at hemostasis more difficult.

2.2.2. Endoscopic variceal hemostasis

- Endoscopic variceal band ligation (EVBL) is a safe procedure with low rate of serious complications (mortality and perforation risk <1%).
- Superficial ulcerations occur commonly (5–15%) after EVBL. Treatment with proton pump inhibitors after EVBL may decrease the risk of bleeding from resulting esophageal ulcerations.
- Superficial ulceration is more common with sclerotherapy (90%). Deep ulceration may also occur and results in re-bleeding in 5% of cases.
- Stricture formation occurs in 2–20% of sclerotherapy cases.
- Other less frequent but serious complications include perforation, mediastinitis, pleural effusion, and portal vein thrombosis.
- The techniques and complications of gastric variceal treatment with adhesives are discussed in Chapter 4.

Box 5 Risk of upper endoscopic procedures for bleeding and risk of cardiovascular conditions for thromboembolism

Low risk procedures for bleeding

- Diagnostic EGD (including biopsy).
- Diagnostic coloscopy (including biopsy).
- Enteroscopy and diagnostic balloon-assisted enteroscopy.
- Capsule endoscopy.
- Enteral stent placement (without dilation).
- ERCP without sphincterotomy.
- EUS without FNA.

High-risk procedures for bleeding

- Polypectomy and endoscopic mucosal resection.
- Ampullectomy.
- Pneumatic or bougie dilation.
- Endoscopic hemostasis.
- Treatment of varices.
- PEG placement.
- Tumor ablation.
- Therapeutic balloon-assisted enteroscopy.
- ERCP with sphincterotomy.
- EUS with FNA.

Low-risk conditions for thromboembolism

- Uncomplicated or paroxysmal nonvalvular atrial fibrillation.
- Bioprosthetic valve.
- Mechanical valve in the aortic position.
- Deep venous thrombosis.

High-risk conditions for thromboembolism

- Atrial fibrillation associated with valvular heart disease.
- Mechanical valve in the mitral position.
- Mechanical valve in any position and previous thromboembolic event.
- Recently (<1 year) placed coronary stent.
- Acute coronary syndrome.
- Non-stented percutaneous coronary intervention after myocardial infarction.

EGD, upper endoscopy; ERCP, endoscopic retrograde cholangiopancreatogram; EUS, endoscopic ultrasound; FNA, fine needle aspiration.

2.3. Polypectomy and endoscopic mucosal resection

- Gastric polyps are detected in up to 3% of upper endoscopic evaluations.
- The ASGE has published its recommendations on management of gastric polyps (Box 7).

Box 6 Bridging therapy

- Warfarin is withheld 3–5 days prior to high risk procedures.
- Heparin or LMWH is started when INR approaches lower limit of normal.
- LMWH is more convenient than heparin because it can be administered subcutaneously on an outpatient basis.
- Heparin should be stopped 4–6 h before the procedure while LMWH should be stopped 8–12 h prior.
- Warfarin is typically restarted on the evening of the procedure and heparin/LMWH is restarted the same evening.
- Discontinue heparin or LMWH 1 or 2 days later when INR is between 2 and 3.

Box 7 ASGE recommendations for the management of gastric polyps

- Polyps causing symptoms, such as obstruction and bleeding, should be removed, preferably endoscopically.
- Polyps >2 cm in size should be endoscopically excised wherever feasible.
- Asymptomatic polyps that are non-adenomatous and are <2 cm in size can be managed expectantly.
- When multiple gastric polyps are encountered, the largest polyps should be biopsied or excised, and representative sample biopsies taken from some others. Further management should be based on histologic results.
- Surveillance endoscopy 1 year after removal of an adenomatous polyp is reasonable. If this examination is negative, repeat surveillance endoscopy should be repeated no more frequently than 3- to 5-year intervals.
- No surveillance endoscopy is needed after removal of non-adenomatous gastric polyps.

- The incidence of hemorrhage from gastric polypectomy is about 2%.
- Complications after endoscopic resection of duodenal adenomas are similar in nature to complications of colonoscopic polypectomy and include perforation, bleeding, and complications related to sedation.
- Submucosal injection of saline or epinephrine and the application of loops and clips have been used during resection of large gastroduodenal polyps.
- Placing clips after EMR can avoid delayed bleeding, particularly in the duodenum.

2.3.1. Endoscopic mucosal resection (EMR)

- EMR involves the lifting of a lesion from the muscularis propria of the gut wall, either by injection or by suction of the lesion into a cap fitted to the tip of the endoscope, followed by snare removal of the lesion. Several EMR techniques have been described:
  - Inject and cut technique
  - Inject, lift, and cut technique
  - EMR with ligation
  - Cap-assisted EMR
- Complications of EMR include bleeding, perforation, and luminal stenosis (Table 1).

2.4. Ablative techniques

Complications associated with various ablative techniques are described in Table 2.

2.5. Removal of foreign bodies

Management and complications of endoscopic removal of ingested foreign bodies are detailed in Ch. 7.5.

3. Complications of endoscopic ultrasonography (EUS)

3.1. Non-FNA related complications

3.1.1. Perforation

- Duodenal perforations have been reported to occur in 0.03% of upper EUS procedures.

Table 1 Complications of endoscopic mucosal resection (EMR)

Bleeding	Most common complication of EMR (up to 17% of cases). Most bleeding is immediate, but can be delayed (>24 h). Most important risk factor for delayed bleeding is immediate bleeding. Size >1–2 cm has been reported to be another risk factor for bleeding. No association has been found between risk of bleeding and EMR technique, lesion morphology (flat, raised, or depressed), type of electrocautery current used, amount of saline injected, and location of lesion except in duodenum. Bleeding is best managed with epinephrine injection and clip placement, because this method eliminates the risk of additional cautery injury to the EMR site.
Perforation	Gastric EMR perforation rate is high (1–5%). Avoid performing EMR in patients who had prior attempts at endoscopic resection. Scar tissue may prevent adequate lifting of the lesion and, thus, may increase risk of perforation. Small perforations that are recognized early in stable patients can be managed conservatively with clip placement (Fig. 7). Patients should be placed nil per os and treated with broad spectrum antibiotics.
Luminal stenosis	It has been described after extensive luminal resections, mainly when more than three-fourths of the luminal circumference has been excised in one endoscopic session. Luminal stenosis occurs most commonly after EMR of esophageal lesions. Incremental resections in multiple treatment sessions may decrease the risk of post-EMR strictures. Post-EMR strictures can be treated successfully with serial dilations and/or temporary stent placement.

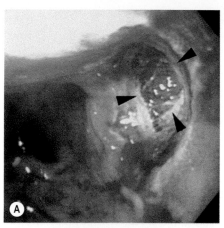

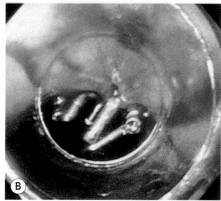

Figure 7 (A) Endoscopic view of perforation (arrowheads) that occurred during EMR. (B) Closure of perforation by application of six clips. (From Tsunada S et al. Endoscopic closure of perforations caused by EMR in the stomach by application of metallic clips Gastrointestinal Endoscopy 2003; 57(7): 948-951.)

- Since these perforations are typically retroperitoneal and are difficult to recognize, a low threshold of suspicion should be maintained in cases of difficult duodenal intubation.
- Perforation during cervical esophageal intubation is rare but has been associated with difficult intubation during prior upper endoscopy, older age, presence of large cervical osteophytes, and operator inexperience.

Table 2 Complications associated with different ablative techniques

Laser light	Mortality 1% Perforation rate: 1–9% Major bleeding: up to 12% Others: Stricture and fistula formation
Photodynamic therapy (PDT)	Strictures: up to 30% Prolonged skin sensitivity Perforation and fistula formation Others: dysphagia, odynophagia, chest pain, fever, nausea (all occur commonly)
Argon plasma coagulation (APC)	Serious complications are very uncommon Abdominal distention is common Strictures are uncommon but can occur as a late complication

3.2. FNA-related complications

3.2.1. Infectious complications

- The incidence of EUS-FNA related bacteremia is approximately 5%, which is comparable with that of diagnostic upper endoscopy.
- Prophylactic antibiotics are not recommended for EUS-FNA of solid pancreatic lesions.

 Clinical Tip

During EUS-FNA of cystic lesions, complete aspiration of cystic fluid content and limiting the number of passes may help decrease the risk of infection.

- In contrary, there is evidence supporting the routine administration of prophylactic antibiotics during EUS-FNA of cystic lesions. The ASGE recommends that prophylaxis with antibiotics, such as a fluoroquinolone, be administered before or during EUS-FNA of cystic lesions, and may be continued for 3–5 days after the procedure.

Clinical Tip

Avoiding the main pancreatic duct during puncture may decrease the risk of pancreatitis.

3.2.2. Pancreatitis

- EUS-FNA induced pancreatitis is relatively uncommon with reported incidence rates of 0% to 2%.

3.2.3. Hemorrhage

- Mild intraluminal bleeding post-FNA is not uncommon and is usually self-limited.
- Clinically significant bleeding occurs in just under 1% of EUS-FNA procedures.
- EUS-FNA-induced intracystic bleeding is usually self-limited and recognition of this complication and cessation of further FNA attempts appear to be adequate management. Prophylactic antibiotics are recommended since the intracystic hematoma can serve as a nidus for bacterial infection.
- Cessation of anticoagulants and antiplatelet medications for at least 5 days prior to the procedure is generally recommended prior to EUS procedures with anticipated FNA. Limiting the number of passes, use of Doppler mode to identify and avoid large vascular structures, and use of smaller gauge needles may decrease the risk and limit the severity of bleeding.

3.2.4. Celiac plexus blockade and neurolysis

- EUS-guided celiac plexus blockade (using corticosteroids) and neurolysis (using absolute alcohol) are used as a means of achieving analgesia in patients with chronic pancreatitis and pancreatic cancer, respectively.
- Both procedures appear to be generally safe and associated with fewer complications compared to the percutaneous approach.
- Transient diarrhea has been reported in 9–15%, transient orthostasis in 1%, and transient increase in pain in 9%.
- Prophylactic antibiotics and adequate intravenous fluid hydration prior to and during the procedure should be administered to reduce the incidence of infection and orthostasis, respectively.

4. Complications of device-assisted enteroscopy and capsule endoscopy

4.1. Device-assisted enteroscopy

Device-assisted enteroscopy techniques, including double-balloon enteroscopy (DBE), single balloon enteroscopy (SBE), and spiral enteroscopy (SE), have both diagnostic and therapeutic capabilities. DBE is the most studied and established deep enteroscopy (DE) technique to date.

- Complications that can be associated with DE comprise complications common to all endoscopic procedures including sedation-related adverse events, infection, and aspiration pneumonia.

 Clinical Tip

The use of carbon dioxide (CO_2) rather than air for insufflation during DE has been shown to decrease post-procedural cramping. In addition, it improves intubation depth in DBE.

- The most reported adverse symptom after DE has been abdominal pain, which occurs in 2–20% of procedures.
- Complications that appear to be increased after DBE include acute pancreatitis (0.2%), gastrointestinal hemorrhage, and perforation (0.2%). Perforation risk is increased in patients with altered surgical anatomy.

 Clinical Tip

Advanced age, poor general condition with dehydration or myopathy, dysphagia, poor dentition, alcohol or drug use, and underlying neurologic disease are risk factors for capsule aspiration and indications for endoscopic placement of the capsule.

4.2. Capsule endoscopy

- Since its introduction at the turn of the century, capsule endoscopy (CE) has gained worldwide acceptance.
- CE has proven to be a useful tool for evaluating patients with suspected small bowel disorders, and has made it possible to view the entire small bowel in about 83% of patients.
- Although capsule endoscopy can visualize the entire small intestine, a main disadvantage is the inability to obtain biopsies, navigate altered anatomy or perform therapeutic maneuvers.
- CE has an extraordinarily safety profile which is partly due to its purely diagnostic ability.
- Capsule retention, perforation, aspiration (Fig. 8), and small bowel obstruction are reported complications of CE. Among these, capsule retention is the most common complication and occurs in 1.2–2.6% of cases.
- Although retained capsules can eventually pass spontaneously or by drug promotion in a few patients, surgical intervention is needed in most cases due to obstructing lesions, such as malignant or Crohn's strictures. Crohn's disease accounts for 37% of capsule retention cases. Box 8 lists factors associated with increases capsule retention risk.
- A rare complication of CE is capsule aspiration which occurs in 0.13% of cases.

Box 8 Factors associated with increased capsule retention risk (Fig. 9)

- Prolonged non-steroidal anti-inflammatory drug use.
- Abdominal radiation injury.
- Extensive Crohn's disease.
- Prior major abdominal surgery.
- Prior small bowel resection.

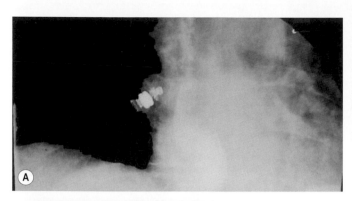

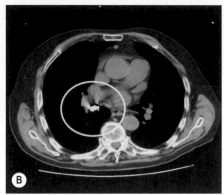

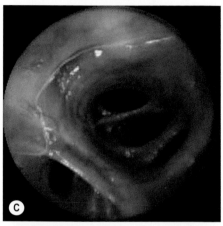

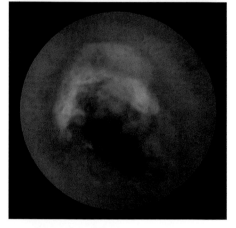

Figure 8 (A) Plain radiograph showing capsule endoscope at right border of mediastinum. (B) Chest CT showing capsule in right lower lobe bronchus. (C) Capsule endoscope image showing right lower lobe bronchus. (From Tabib S, Fuller C, Daniels J, Lo SK. Asymptomatic aspiration of a capsule endoscope. Gastrointestinal Endoscopy 2004; 60(5): 845-848.)

Figure 9 CE of a retained capsule shows NSAID enteropathy (diaphragm disease) – associated ulcer and stricture. (From Li F et al. Retention of the capsule endoscope: a single-center experience of 1000 capsule endoscopy procedures. Gastrointestinal Endoscopy 2008; 68(1): 174-180.)

Further Reading

Anderson MA, Ben-Menachem T, Gan SI, et al: Management of antithrombotic agents for endoscopic procedures, *Gastrointest Endosc* 70:1060–1070, 2009.

Banerjee S, Shen B, Baron TH, et al: Antibiotic prophylaxis for GI endoscopy, *Gastrointest Endosc* 67:791–798, 2008.

Banerjee S, Shen B, Nelson DB, et al: Infection control during GI endoscopy, *Gastrointest Endosc* 67:781–790, 2008.

Barkay O, Khashab M, Al-Haddad M, et al: Minimizing complications in pancreaticobiliary endoscopy, *Curr Gastroenterol Rep* 11:134–141, 2009.

Eisen GM, Baron TH, Dominitz JA, et al: Complications of upper GI endoscopy, *Gastrointest Endosc* 55:784–793, 2002.

Gerson LB, Tokar J, Chiorean M, et al: Complications associated with double balloon enteroscopy at nine US centers, *Clin Gastroenterol Hepatol* 7:1177–1182, 2009.

Guidelines on Complications of Gastrointestinal Endoscopy: See 'Guidelines Index'. 2006. www.bsg.org.uk Accessed January 5, 2010.

Li F, Gurudu SR, De Petris G, et al: Retention of the capsule endoscope: a single-center experience of 1000 capsule endoscopy procedures, *Gastrointest Endosc* 68(1): 174–180, 2008.

Liao Z, Gao R, Xu C, et al: Indications and detection, completion, and retention rates of small-bowel capsule endoscopy: a systematic review, *Gastrointest Endosc* 71:280–286, 2010.

Raju GS: Endoscopic closure of gastrointestinal leaks, *Am J Gastroenterol* 104:1315–1320, 2009.

Siersema PD, Homs MY, Haringsma J, et al: Use of large-diameter metallic stents to seal traumatic nonmalignant perforations of the esophagus, *Gastrointest Endosc* 58:356–361, 2003.

Tabib S, Fuller C, Daniels J, et al: Asymptomatic aspiration of a capsule endoscope, *Gastrointest Endosc* 60:845–848, 2004.

Tsunada S, Ogata S, Ohyama T, et al: Endoscopic closure of perforations caused by EMR in the stomach by application of metallic clips, *Gastrointest Endosc* 57(7):948–951, 2003.

CHAPTER 9

Endosonography

Laurent Palazzo, Anne Marie Lennon, Ian Penman

Summary

Key Points

- Endoscopic ultrasound (EUS) is firmly established in the locoregional staging of cancers of the esophagus, stomach, pancreas, extrahepatic bile duct, anal canal, and rectum.
- EUS is complementary to cross-sectional imaging, e.g. CT, MRI, PET in the evaluation of GI cancers and benign pancreaticobiliary disease.
- It also has a major role in the diagnosis and management of submucosal lesions of the GI tract, choledocholithiasis, chronic pancreatitis, and cystic pancreatic lesions.
- A thorough understanding of anatomy and experience are key to accurate EUS performance.
- Radial and linear EUS are complementary: for many indications, radial examination is easier to learn and quicker to perform; linear EUS is necessary for performing FNA biopsy.
- Interventional EUS is a key component of modern EUS.

- EUS-FNA is safe with a major complication rate of <1%.
- EUS-FNA will yield a diagnosis in >80% of solid masses.
- Optimum handling and preparation of cytology samples is critical for diagnosis.
- EUS is the preferred method for performing celiac plexus neurolysis.
- EUS-guided drainage of pancreatic pseudocysts offers many potential advantages over other methods.
- Therapeutic EUS relies on a combination of EUS imaging and other endoscopic procedures, e.g. guidewire exchanges and stent insertion.
- Further new roles for therapeutic EUS are likely to be developed soon, but will require new accessories and devices and possibly modified echoendoscopes.

Introduction

By introducing a miniature ultrasound probe into the gastrointestinal tract, bringing the structure to be examined close to the transducer, high frequencies can be used, achieving a satisfactory compromise between excellent image resolution and the resulting poor depth of field that can be assessed. Endoscopic ultrasound (EUS) is a particular aspect of gastrointestinal ultrasonography, since the miniature transducer is placed at the tip of an endoscope equipped with video optics. Gastrointestinal endosonography began in the mid-1970s, was developed in the mid-1980s, and is now used in current practice in gastrointestinal oncology, but also in the diagnosis of biliary

DOI: 10.1016/B978-0-7020-3128-1.00009-2

obstruction and in assessing neoplastic and inflammatory disorders of the pancreas. Several other less common indications have been developed, for example submucosal tumors of the gut wall, portal hypertension, esophageal motor disorders and assessment of various anorectal and gynecological disorders, in particular deep subperitoneal endometriosis.

1. Principles

This imaging technique, which has the highest resolving power currently available for evaluating the digestive tract wall and the organs in contact with it, has undergone a rapid evolution in the last decade with the development of EUS-guided histology, the development of EUS-guided therapeutic techniques and the advent of technological refinements such as elastography and contrast-enhanced EUS.

It is important to bear in mind that this imaging technique, in which the quality of the results depends directly on operator experience, requires considerable investment in terms of diverse, expensive equipment, long specific training (except for therapeutic endoscopic ultrasound which is easy for an interventional endoscopist to learn) and finally the recruitment of many types of personnel. Its use is therefore justified only at referral centers where all these conditions are met.

Although therapeutic endoscopic ultrasound is the most exciting part of the technique, it is not currently in widespread use because of the limited indications and small number of patients who may benefit from it.

Diagnostic EUS and EUS-guided FNA thus remain more than ever the main applications of the technique and are its future in the short and medium term.

2. Technical aspects

2.1. Introduction

The resolving power of an ultrasound probe is directly proportional to the frequency emitted: with a frequency of 7.5 MHz, widely used in EUS, the spatial resolution is in the order of 1 mm. On the other hand, the depth of field that can be analyzed is inversely proportional to the frequency used (Table 1).

In recent years, equipment manufacturers have increased the range of frequencies that can be used on the same endoscope by adding relatively low frequencies (5 and 6 MHz), which allow accurate analysis to a depth of 6–8 cm, thus achieving better management of some pancreatic disorders.

2.2. Equipment

Two types of ultrasound technique are used in endoscopic ultrasound.

2.2.1. Radial imaging

Radial imaging provides 360° ultrasound images perpendicular to the axis of the endoscope.

This technique has many advantages, namely:

- Excellent image quality, allowing real-time study of the circumference of the digestive tract through 360° (Fig. 1), making the examination easier overall for all types of gut pathology, particularly for assessing locoregional involvement of cancers and their surveillance or other indications related to diseases of the gastrointestinal wall
- The ability to visualize constantly the major vascular landmarks, facilitating localization of pathology regardless of the oblique optics of the ultrasound image obtained, thus allowing precise evaluation of the structures and organs around the intestinal lumen, particularly the pancreaticobiliary region.

Its main drawback is that it is impossible to carry out EUS-FNA as the path of the needle passes through the plane of the ultrasound image and cannot therefore be monitored in real-time.

Because radial imaging is long-established and relatively easy to perform, it currently remains the most widely used EUS technique. Three types of apparatus have been developed as a result:

Table 1 EUS transducer frequency and depth of field

Frequency (MHz)	Depth of field (cm)
7.5	5–6
12	3
20	1.5
30	1

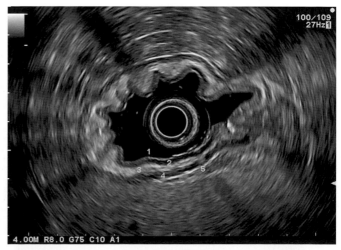

Figure 1 Normal gastric wall with five layers. Electronic radial scope. (1) interface between the gastric lumen and the epithelium, (2) mucosa including muscularis mucosae, (3) submucosa, (4) muscularis propria, (5) serosa and interface with the perigastric fat.

- Video-EUS (Fig. 2) for the study of the esophagus, stomach, duodenum, pancreaticobiliary region, anal canal, rectum and colon, with the option of simultaneously visualizing the ultrasound image and the endoscopic image. There are two types of radial video-EUS:

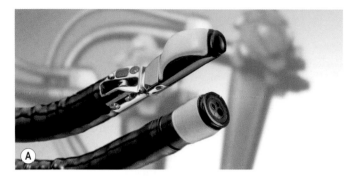

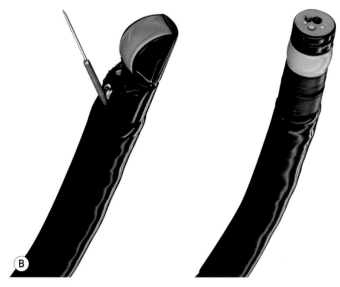

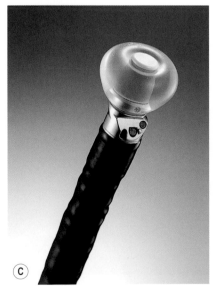

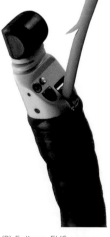

Box 1 Blind probe (Olympus GIF-MH908)

For the esophagus, use a transnasal or pediatric gastroscope, which can pass through the stenosis without previous dilation. Aspirate the air present in the gastric lumen, position a 0.035 inch guidewire in the stomach, withdraw the endoscope, slide the blind probe onto the guidewire and insert, under the stenosis, moderately inflating the balloon to facilitate its passage. Then advance the probe into the stomach (celiac region). The examination is performed by withdrawing the probe under ultrasound control as far as the cervical esophagus.

- Rotating mechanical: this is the oldest type (developed in the early 1980s). It is used increasingly rarely and Doppler studies are not possible.
- Electronic in B-mode. The three companies that manufacture echoendoscopes supply this type of apparatus. The endoscopic view is either end-viewing (Pentax, Fig. 2A, or Fujinon, Fig. 2B), or oblique-forward (Olympus, Fig. 2C). The instruments produce several frequencies (5–12 MHz) and thus allow Doppler studies and power Doppler sonography. The latest instruments, which are connected to very sophisticated ultrasound consoles, allow contrast harmonic ultrasound after intravenous injection of ultrasound contrast agents.
- Rigid probes are designed for examination of the anal canal and its sphincters and the lower and mid-rectum. Both rotating mechanical or electronic transducers are available.
- Miniprobes (Fig. 3) can be introduced into the operating channel of conventional endoscopes, and are particularly suited to the use of very high frequencies (20 and 30 MHz). They were developed in the mid-1990s, and are used before curative endoscopic treatment of superficial flat cancers of the digestive tract (0–IIa, b, c) and high-grade dysplasia; these very high frequency miniprobes allow accurate patient selection for curative endoscopic treatment of superficial cancers whether for endoscopic mucosectomy, submucosal dissection, photodynamic therapy or radiofrequency ablation.
- Mid-way between the miniprobe and the echoendoscope, is the 'blind' probe (Fig. 4; Box 1), a

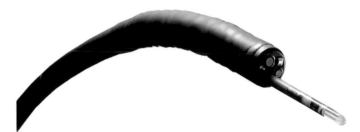

Figure 2 (A) Pentax EUS scopes, radial and linear. (B) Fujinon EUS scopes, radial and linear. (C) Olympus EUS scopes, radial and linear.

Figure 3 Olympus high frequency (mechanical radial) miniprobe (30 MHz) used through a standard gastroscope.

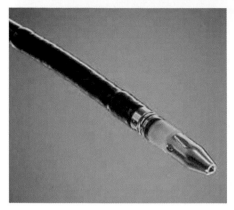

Figure 4 Olympus blind probe MH 908 (mechanical radial 7.5 MHz).

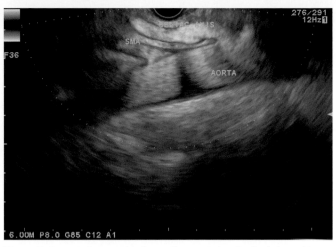

Figure 5 Aorta. 3–5 cm under the cardia seen in longitudinal view with celiac and superior mesenteric artery (SMA) take-off. Olympus linear scope coupled with Aloka α10 console.

flexible instrument with a small diameter (7.8 mm) and lacking endoscopic optics, with a miniature transducer at its end; it uses the rotating mechanical radial technique, emitting at 7.5 MHz, and is tapered at its end (3 mm). The blind probe can be passed over a guidewire previously positioned under endoscopic control. It is intended for the examination of stenotic esophageal or rectal lesions.

2.2.2. Curved linear array (Fig. 2)

The ultrasound image obtained in electronic B mode is a sagittal image (Figs 5, 6) provided by an electronic transducer. The plane of the image is parallel to the axis of the endoscope.

The main advantage of this technique is the ability to carry out intra- or transmural EUS-guided FNA (Fig. 7) as the path of the needle to the target can be followed in real time on the ultrasound image.

As a result of this option, therapeutic EUS uses echoendoscopes with a large operating channel.

The drawback of this type of equipment is the nature of the sagittal images as these are inappropriate for studying the circumference of the GI tract and thus assessing locoregional involvement prior to treatment or surveying cancers of the GI tract.

Two types of instrument use this technique: video-echoendoscopes and rigid probes.

- Video-echoendoscopes can be used to study the esophagus, stomach, duodenum, pancreaticobiliary region, anal canal, rectum, and colon. They are less suited to examining the esophagus, common bile duct, anal canal and rectum than instruments using the radial technique, because of the nature of the images obtained. They are also more difficult to use for the stomach and duodenum. On the other hand, they allow very satisfactory examination of the pancreas and the peripancreatic region, particularly its vascular aspect, and the posterior mediastinum.

- Rigid probes are designed for examination of the anal canal and rectum. Although the image obtained is not very practical for studying the anal sphincters and the pre-treatment assessment of rectal and anal cancers, it nevertheless allows an accurate measurement of the distance between the lower margin of a rectal cancer, the pelvic floor and the internal anal sphincter, thus providing valuable information on whether intersphincteric resection is indicated for low rectal cancers. Rigid probes are also very well suited to dynamic studies in patients with pelvic floor disorders since they allow the simultaneous examination of the lower part of the anterior rectal wall, the anal sphincters, the urethra and bladder, and the rectovaginal septum. Hitachi consoles can provide a useful three-dimensional evaluation of the mesorectal region.

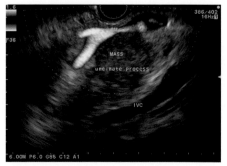

Figure 6 Pancreatic cancer located within uncinate process, invading the posterior side of the SMV. IVC, inferior vena cava. Electronic linear scope.

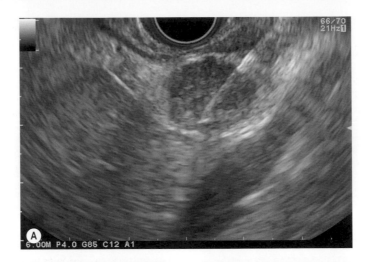

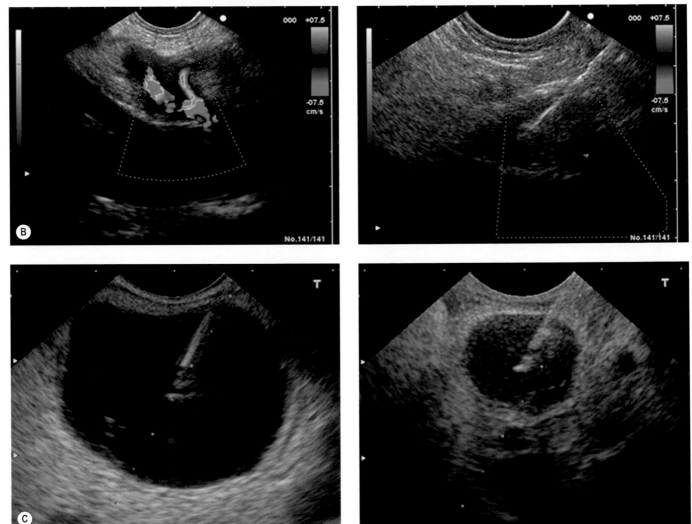

Figure 7 (A) EUS-guided FNA of a malignant (15 mm in diameter) lymph node located along the liver under the cardia. (B) Pancreatic adenocarcinoma located within the body with involvement of the celiac axis (left) with EUS-guided FNA (right) using a Pentax linear scope coupled with a Hitachi console. (C) EUS-guided FNA of a pancreatic cystic lesion (left) and a malignant lymph node (right), using a Fujinon scope coupled with a Toshiba console.

2.3. Sedation analgesia and general anesthesia

EUS, even if performed without FNA sampling, usually requires intravenous sedation or light general anesthesia because the procedures can be prolonged and require the patient to remain completely still. The use of a benzodiazepine (Midazolam) may be sufficient for examination of the esophagus, stomach and mediastinum. Combining this with an opiate or Propofol, to produce short-term general anesthesia may be necessary for pancreaticobiliary examination or for any EUS-FNA, depending on local custom. This means that EUS needs to be performed at centers with appropriate outpatient facilities.

In contrast, endorectal or endoanal ultrasound without FNA may be performed without sedation (except for painful cancer of the anal canal, or perianal abscess or fistula).

2.4. How to position the patient, doctor, and console

2.4.1. Patient position

- For gastroesophageal or duodenal examination, the left lateral decubitus position is usual. The patient's head and chest may be raised if water is instilled into the stomach or duodenum.
- For pancreaticobiliary examination, left lateral decubitus, tilted forwards by 30°–45°, is the best position (Fig. 8A). The left shoulder should therefore be moved back and the right leg brought to the front. If the patient is very thin, it is often useful to have him/her lie almost prone, to examine the common bile duct and pancreatic head.
- For anorectal examination, supine is the simplest position. Instilled water pools at the most dependent point and therefore indicates the posterior wall of the lower and mid-rectum at the bottom of the screen, and the anterior wall at the top of the screen, the right wall to the right of the screen and the left wall to the left of the screen.

2.4.2. Examiner's position

- If there is a second monitor in addition to the console screen and this is positioned behind the patient's back, the examiner is usually facing the patient, at an angle of 45° facing the patient's feet when he has to use an open handle position, or at an angle of 45° facing the patient's head when he has to use a closed handle position. This is the most ergonomic position for the examiner, regardless of the position of the console which can be positioned either close to the patient's head or by the patient's legs.
- If there is no second TV monitor, the examiner's position will depend on the position of the console (see below).

2.4.3. Position of the echoendoscope handle

Definitions concerning the position of the echoendoscope handle:

- The neutral position (Figs 8B, 9) is where the front of the handle is facing the patient.
- The open position (Figs 8C, 9) is where the front of the handle is facing the patient's feet. It is reached by turning anti-clockwise through 90° from the neutral position.
- The closed position (Figs 8D, 9) is the opposite of the open position. It is reached by turning clockwise through 90° from the neutral position.
- The extreme closed position (Figs 8E, 9) is reached by continuing to turn the handle clockwise through a further 90° by shoulder rotation, bringing the handle opposite the neutral position.

- The neutral and open positions account for at least 75% of the positions used for pancreaticobiliary and rectal examination.
- The closed position is used to examine the pancreatic tail and is one of the three positions used to examine the uncinate process of the pancreas.
- The extreme closed position is used for pancreatic tail biopsy and is one of the three positions used to biopsy the uncinate process of the pancreas.
- When the ultrasound console is at the patient's head (Fig. 10), the closed position of the handle (facing the console) is used for examination of the posterior mediastinum: the spine and the aorta (posterior) being at the bottom of the screen and the left atrium (anterior) at the top of the screen; the right side of the screen then corresponds to the left of the posterior mediastinum and the left side of the screen to the right of the posterior mediastinum.
- When the console is at the patient's feet, the open position (Fig. 11) of the handle (which is facing the console) is used (Fig. 8F) for examination of the posterior mediastinum: the spine and aorta (the back) are at the top of the screen and the left atrium (the front) is at the bottom of the screen; the right side of the screen then corresponds to the right side of the posterior mediastinum and the left side of the screen to the left of the posterior mediastinum.

2.4.4. Console position

- The console position is unimportant if there is a second monitor positioned behind the patient's back. If not, you can choose between the top and bottom of the patient.
- The majority of endosonographers place the console (and therefore the screen) at the patient's head (Fig. 10), i.e. to the right of the examiner when he/she is facing the patient. As such, the most natural position of the handle is facing the screen, which corresponds to the closed position described. For the handle to face the patient, i.e. in the neutral position, it must be turned anti-clockwise through 90° from the most natural position and this is not problematic. On the other hand, it is difficult to continue to turn the handle anti-clockwise through a further 90° to reach what is described as the open position because the screen is then 180° opposite this position.
  - It is because the neutral position and the open position account for three-quarters of the positions that are useful for pancreaticobiliary and rectal examination that this console position has not been considered.
- It is advisable to place the console alongside the patient's legs (Fig. 11). The open position of the handle (Fig. 8C,F) is therefore the natural position, because the examiner is then positioned at an angle of 45° in relation to the screen. The neutral position (Fig. 8B) is easy because the examiner is then facing the patient. The closed position (Fig. 8D) is easy because the left hand, which is holding the endoscope handle, is up against the examiner's right clavicle and you are facing

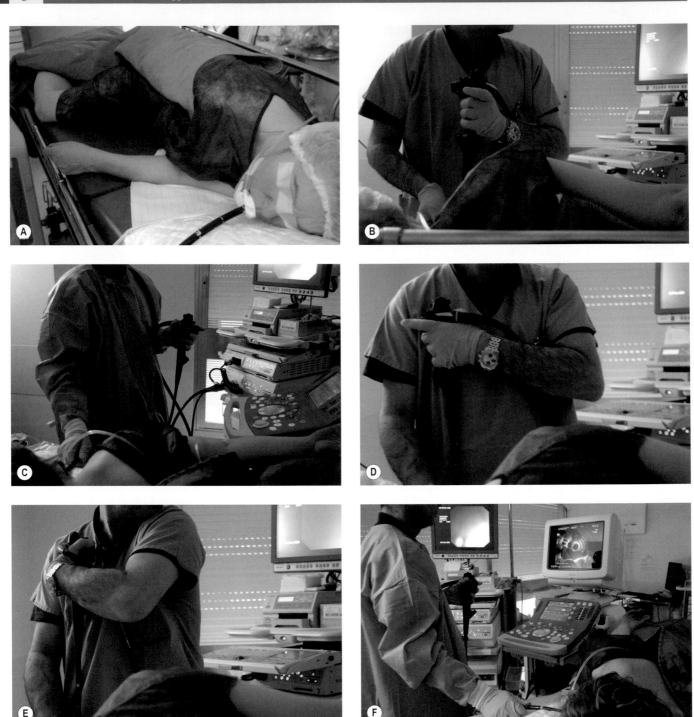

Figure 8 (A) Position of the patient for pancreaticobiliary examination. (B) The neutral position of the echoendoscope handle: the front of the handle is facing the patient. (C) The open position of the echoendoscope handle. (D) The closed position of the echoendoscope handle. (E) The extreme closed position of the echoendoscope handle. (F) The open position facing the console located at the patient's feet is used for the examination of the posterior mediastinum.

the patient. Only one handle position is uncomfortable for the examiner when the console is placed at the patient's feet: this is the extreme closed position (Fig. 8E), i.e. with the handle opposite the patient. It is then difficult to see the screen positioned along the patient's legs, while maintaining this extreme closed position for any length of time. This handle position is useful only for biopsying certain tumors of the uncinate process and pancreatic tail. In these two situations, it is

advisable to change the position of the console and place it at the patient's head.

- In summary:
  - It is best to have a second monitor positioned behind the patient's back
  - Otherwise, it is best to position the console beside the patient's legs, since this facilitates pancreaticobiliary and rectal examination (Fig. 12) in which the extreme closed position is rarely used

Position of the echoedoscope handle for EUS

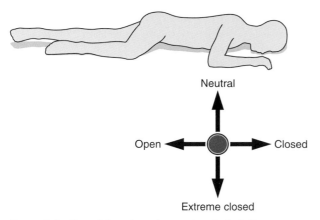

Neutral

Open ← ● → Closed

Extreme closed

Figure 9 Position of the echoendoscope handle for EUS.

Console adjacent to the patient's head

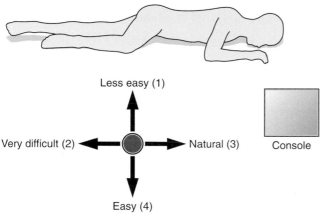

Less easy (1)

Very difficult (2) ← ● → Natural (3)   Console

Easy (4)

Figure 10 Console adjacent to the patient's head. The closed position (3) is the most natural. The extreme closed position (4) is easy to obtain. The neutral position (1) is easy to obtain. The open position (2) is very difficult to sustain for any length of time. Passing from the neutral to the open position has to be very precise. This position is used when biopsying the tail or neck of pancreas.

and since this does not complicate esophageal or mediastinal examination; on the contrary, the right side of the screen corresponds well to the right part of the patient's mediastinum and the left side of the screen to the left part of the patient's mediastinum.

3. General EUS examination technique

3.1. General technique

EUS examination uses two different methods that are sometimes combined to obtain a satisfactory acoustic window between the transducer and the gut wall, as well as the surrounding region. The first is the balloon method, and the second is the instillation of water through the operating channel of the echoendoscope.

- The balloon technique is often essential for the examination of the esophagus, the adjacent mediastinum, the duodenum and the adjacent

Console adjacent to the patient's legs

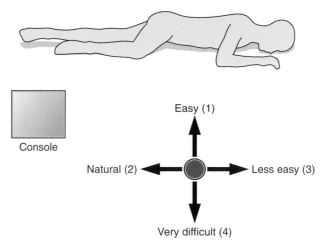

Console

Easy (1)

Natural (2) ← ● → Less easy (3)

Very difficult (4)

Figure 11 Console adjacent to the patient's legs. The open position (2) is the natural position. The neutral position (1) is very easy to obtain. The closed position (3) is easy to obtain. The extreme closed position (4) is very difficult to sustain for any length of time. Passing from the closed (3) to the extreme closed position (4) has to be very precise. This position of the console is used for 90% of EUS procedures.

Examination of the rectum and anus

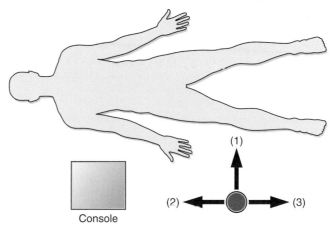

Console

(1)

(2) ← ● → (3)

Figure 12 Examination of the rectum and anus. Patient in supine position. Console next to the patient's abdomen, alongside their right arm. The positions of the handle that are used are the neutral (1) and the open positions (2). (3) closed position of the handle, is used to pass the scope through the junction sigmoid rectum.

pancreaticobiliary region, but also for the anal canal, rectum and sigmoid colon as well as of the surrounding pelvic area. The balloon method is also used alone for the stomach after aspiration of the air present, for examination of the antrum, where this technique is sufficient, but also for examination of the pancreatic neck, body and tail, the left liver lobe or the spleen.
- The instillation of water into the gut lumen is a technique used mainly in the stomach for the examination of the gastric wall, body and fundus, and for the characterization of wall lesions (thickened gastric folds, cancer, lymphoma or submucosal tumor). It is also useful for the examination of minor lesions of the duodenum or the ampulla of Vater region.

- The use of deaerated water (i.e. boiled and cooled beforehand) is preferred for the examination of small superficial lesions in the stomach, because the acoustic window is far better. Water instillation is required for examination of rectal lesions, since this allows the endoscope to reach and pass the rectosigmoid junction (where the examination should begin) without the need for air instillation, i.e. without the need to view the wall endoscopically during progression, being guided simply by the stream of water instilled into the rectum, so as not to impair the ultrasound examination. The use of deaerated water is particularly useful for villous tumors or superficial cancers.

3.2. Examination technique using miniprobes

The miniprobes are introduced into the endoscope operating channel and slid in endoscopic view over the lesion to be studied:

- For the stomach, 100–150 cc of deaerated water should be instilled. Examination is easy, the images are very clear and interpretation is usually easy, except for the angularis incisura which should be examined after positioning the patient prone.
- For the esophagus, an ultrasound interface needs to be created between the miniprobe and the esophageal wall. This can be done with either a purpose-designed disposable balloon (Olympus) which requires the use of an endoscope with a large operating channel, or a condom fixed to the end of the endoscope; the condom can then be filled with water using a catheter previously attached along the endoscope. The best technique is to flood the esophagus with deaerated water, which requires tracheal intubation of the patient beforehand. Paralysis of esophageal peristalsis is often necessary, using intravenous atropine or glucagon.
- Examination of the bile and pancreatic ducts has also benefited from the introduction of miniprobes. Miniprobes are available mounted on a guidewire, and these can be introduced into the desired duct without previous sphincterotomy. This type of technique can be used only in an interventional endoscopy room equipped with fluoroscopy and with the ability to produce X-ray images.
- The blind probe used in cases of stenotic esophageal or rectosigmoid cancers requires prior introduction of a guidewire through the stenosis, under endoscopic control. The air introduced during endoscopy must be carefully aspirated, because the blind probe has no suction channel. The probe is then advanced over the guidewire into the stenosis and positioned beyond it. Examination takes place as the probe is progressively withdrawn.

Box 2 Indications for EUS-FNA

- Pancreatic masses.
- N1 or M1 lymph nodes (LN) in patients with primary esophagogastric cancer.
- Evaluation of pancreatic cystic lesions.
- Mediastinal LN (N2 or N3) in patients with known or suspected lung cancer.
- Mediastinal masses of unknown etiology.
- Retroperitoneal LN or masses.
- Perirectal LN or masses.
- Lesions in the left lobe of liver.
- Left adrenal masses.
- Subepithelial masses.
- Thickened gastric or intestinal wall with negative mucosal biopsies.

4. EUS-guided FNA

4.1. Indications and contraindications

There is a broad range of indications for EUS-FNA and these are outlined in Box 2.

These indications will continue to evolve, especially with advances in oncology, e.g. restaging after neoadjuvant therapy or to provide tissue for molecular genetic analysis to guide treatment and/or prognosis.

4.1.1. Contraindications

These are few and are listed in Box 3.

4.1.2. Needles

The needles are disposable and designed for single use.

- 22 G Needle. A 22-gauge needle is used for pancreatic and lymph node fine-needle biopsy (if the lymph nodes are small) and for pancreatic cystic tumors.
- 19 G Needle. A 19-gauge needle is recommended when biopsying a submucosal tumor of the digestive tract, or a large mediastinal lymph node. A 19-gauge needle can be used to obtain a true core biopsy, which is useful if a stromal tumor or lymphoma is suspected since this helps histological interpretation. The 19-gauge needle is difficult to use because it is fairly stiff and usually cannot be used for transduodenal biopsy. The stylet must be routinely withdrawn by 5 mm to pass through the wall.
- 25 G Needle. 25-gauge needles have recently become available, and are mainly indicated for sampling tumors of the uncinate process of the pancreas which

Box 3 Contraindications to EUS-FNA

- Severe coagulopathy or thrombocytopenia.
- Inability to visualize lesion clearly.
- Large interposed vessels.
- Risk of tumor seeding, e.g. resectable pancreatic body or tail lesion.

are sometimes difficult to reach in the short position and require a long position with extreme angulation in the second part of the duodenum. They can also be used for hypervascular tumors and particularly for biopsying renal cancer metastases or endocrine tumors. These needles provide better, less hemorrhagic cytological smears and they are therefore preferred when working without a specialist cytopathologist. On the other hand, the sample obtained for a cell block preparation is poor. The 25 G needle is not widely used in Europe, where it is unusual to have a cytologist present in the examination room and where cytologists are usually cytopathologists who prefer to work on high-quality cell blocks.

- Tru-Cut 19 G Needle. A 19-gauge Tru-Cut needle is available (Cook Medical), which provides a true core biopsy. It is indicated for submucosal tumors, lymph nodes when lymphoma is suspected, and in the pancreas when autoimmune pancreatitis is suspected. It cannot normally be used in the duodenum owing to its rigidity. The path of the lesion to be biopsied must be at least 20 mm long for it to be biopsied safely. Unfortunately, this device has not been as effective as it could be, it is costly and for this reason it has not replaced the 19 G needle in many centers.

4.2. General aspects

EUS-FNA requires adequate sedation or general anesthesia and patient monitoring for at least 4–6 h afterwards. Many factors influence the success of EUS-FNA (Box 5).

The lesions can be located using either radial or linear EUS. The linear scope is then used to perform EUS-FNA. A balloon is not useful in this setting.

Upwards deflection of the scope tip keeps the transducer tip pressed against the wall and creates a shallow exit angle for the needle. The needle is advanced from its sheath and applied against the gut wall at an exit angle pre-determined by the endoscope being used. The path of the needle towards the target must take account of this predetermined angle making pre-positioning of the echoendoscope in relation to the target essential. Once pre-positioned against the wall, it may be necessary (depending on the needle type) to retract the small central stylet by 5 mm (if there is a blunt end) in order to be able to pass through the wall, especially with 19-gauge needles.

The latest generation Olympus and Pentax echoendoscopes have an elevator and are therefore easier to handle than older echoendoscopes, because the angle of passage through the digestive wall to the target can be adjusted. This is particularly useful for lesions that are difficult to access, notably those of the uncinate process, for lesions remote from the digestive wall (more than 15 mm away), or for very small lesions (≤1 cm in diameter). The Fujinon echoendoscope has a virtual target line (Fig. 7C) that shows the operator the path the needle will take. The exit angle of the needle is very shallow and is comparable, without an elevator, to that provided by Olympus and Pentax instruments when used with their elevators.

4.3. Antibiotic prophylaxis

The value of intravenous antibiotic prophylaxis is debatable for solid lesions unless indicated for prevention of infective endocarditis. Antibiotic prophylaxis is essential for biopsy of a cystic lesion, whether of the pancreas or digestive wall. It is also required if the patient is using gastric antisecretory drugs (PPI) since this type of product encourages gastroduodenal microbial overgrowth. Antibiotic prophylaxis is also required for transrectal FNA. The antibiotic therapy must be continued orally for 3 to 5 days.

 Warning!

Before undertaking EUS-FNA, check by power Doppler imaging that there is no vessel in the intended path of the needle. Before removing the needle from the sheath, check endoscopically that the sheath around the needle is visible, but only barely visible.

4.4. Pancreatic cancer biopsy

A 22 G needle is advanced under ultrasound control into the tumor. Once in position, the stylet, if it has been partially retracted, is pushed back into the needle so that any fragment of the digestive wall present at the tip of the needle will not obstruct it; the stylet is then removed completely and a 10–20 cc syringe, preferably with a continuous negative pressure instrument, is fitted to the needle. Once continuous negative pressure has been obtained, the needle should be moved slowly to and fro several (about 20) times in the lesion without hurrying, without removing the needle from the lesion, and trying, if possible, to change the angle of penetration of the lesion; this is helped by having an elevator, if the target is small and close to the lesion or if the lesion is soft, which is rare in cancer of the pancreas; if, as is more common in pancreatic cancer, the lesion is large, far from the probe or hard, angulation of the endoscope should be adjusted (from up to down angulation) to change the path of the needle in the lesion.

The needle must always be monitored in real time on the screen, during these movements, to avoid vascular or organ injury. To be sure that the needle is correctly centered in the lesion during aspiration, make small clockwise and anticlockwise movements of the handle. Avoid penetrating any vascular and particularly arterial structures which may be present between the digestive wall and the target. Power Doppler imaging should be used for this purpose. On the other hand, unexpected passage through intramural or adjacent collateral venous circulation does not usually cause any significant complications if the vein is <3 mm in diameter. As little healthy pancreatic tissue should be traversed as possible, in order to limit the risk of acute pancreatitis. It is also advisable to avoid penetrating the common bile duct and main pancreatic duct, particularly if the latter is dilated upstream of a tumor, since the risk of acute pancreatitis is then increased. Do not puncture the gallbladder or the common bile duct above the pancreas owing to the risk of biliary leakage. Once the biopsy has been completed, release the negative pressure otherwise tumor cells may be deposited in the needle tract as it is withdrawn. Once negative pressure has been released, the needle is withdrawn into its protective sheath and the EUS-FNA needle is removed from the operating channel of the echoendoscope, which is left in position over the lesion. The biopsy sample is then checked. It is ideal to have a cytologist present in the biopsy room since he/she can immediately assess the quality of the sample. If there is no cytologist available, several biopsy passes (two to three on average) should be made in the tumor. The sample should preferably be placed in a tube containing formaldehyde or formalin so that histology can be performed on a cell block preparation. For this purpose, the stylet is advanced through the needle, gradually expelling the sample. Once a sufficient sample has been obtained for histological study, the remainder is divided, giving preference to smears (two to three slides should be prepared), and the rest is placed in CytoLyt medium for liquid-based cytology. This is particularly useful if the sample is poor or liquid, as in cystic tumors of the pancreas. Liquid-based cytology involves the automated concentration of the cells and produces a slide that is easy to process with a thin, even layer of cells. Liquid-based cytology can also be used for immunohistochemistry, unlike slide smears. Once the three types of sample have been obtained, the stylet should be withdrawn and the needle purged, using a 10 cc syringe filled with air, onto slides, yielding a further 1–3. The inside of the needle should be purged with 30 cc of physiological saline between biopsies. If the same patient with pancreatic cancer has several targets, the procedure should start with a biopsy of a hepatic metastasis, then a lymph node biopsy and finally the tumor itself. For lymph node biopsies, start with the lymph node least likely to be involved by tumor and end with the most suspicious.

The biopsy procedure must be stopped if blood is aspirated into the syringe.

If the pancreatic cancer is very hard and the sample is very poor (just some serous fluid) and there is no cytologist available in the examination room, a 50 cc or 60 cc suction syringe should be used. For cancer of the pancreatic body or tail, the needle can also be changed for a 19 G needle combined with a 50 cc or 60 cc suction syringe.

4.5. Biopsy of a cystic lesion

For a cystic lesion biopsy, puncture only once to avoid introducing infection. A cystic lesion should be punctured boldly and cleanly by quick, firm pressure so as not to tear the wall (this can happen if you push in the needle slowly while the patient's respiratory movement causes the lesion to move). After withdrawing the stylet, attach a 10 or 20 cc suction syringe, according to the volume to be aspirated. If no fluid is visible after a few seconds, check that the needle is positioned correctly. If it is, wait because this means that the fluid is viscous (IPMN or mucinous cystadenoma).

Where possible, i.e. if the cystic lesion is not too large, it should be drained completely, in particular if it is a cystic lesion of the pancreas. Cystic lesions of the mediastinum, esophagus or rectum should not be punctured since several cases of abscess formation and in particular mediastinitis have been reported in the literature. The same applies to infected necrosis following acute pancreatitis.

4.6. Lymph node biopsy

For lymph node biopsy, adjust the needle and sampling technique according to the suspected nature of the lymph node and its size.

- For a large lymph node with suspected lymphoma or sarcoidosis in the mediastinum or around the stomach, use a 19 G needle, moving it back and forth a number of times (about 20) without suction, then end with suction with a 10 cc syringe for just a few movements. Give preference to cell block preparation and place part of the sample in an appropriate fluid for the study of lymphocyte populations by flow cytometry.

- For a lymph node that is a suspected metastasis from a gastrointestinal or pancreatobiliary (non-endocrine) cancer, use a 22 G needle adopting the same procedure for the first pass as described for the 19 G needle. If the sample from the first pass is poor, use a 20 cc suction syringe for the second pass and begin to aspirate after just a few back and forth movements without suction and carry out about 30 back and forth movements with suction. Preference should be given to liquid-based cytology if the sample is poor and to cell block preparation if the sample is hemorrhagic. If the sample is rich (presence of whitish material), smears and cell block preparation should be preferred.
- If a lymph node metastasis from an endocrine tumor is suspected, use a 22 G or 25 G needle (depending on whether you are working with a cytopathologist or a cytologist), carry out numerous back and forth movements without suction, then aspirate with a 2 cc or 5 cc syringe during a few back and forth movements. If the sample is very hemorrhagic and a 22-gauge needle has been used, use a 25-gauge needle for the second pass with even less or no suction at all. If the sample is poor, use a 10 cc suction syringe and aspirate more vigorously (10–20 back and forth movements).

4.7. Difficult biopsies

Some lesions are difficult to biopsy, for example some benign or malignant pancreatic tumors, either because they are hard (or very fibrotic) or because they are very small (usually endocrine tumors), because they are far from the gut wall, or because they are in areas where the needle has little penetration force.

4.7.1. Biopsy of the uncinate process of the pancreas

In this case, the endoscope is sometimes looped in the long position in the second part of the duodenum so that the biopsy path avoids the dilated common bile duct or the dilated pancreatic duct, or because it is the only way to approach the target with the echoendoscope. Looping the echoendoscope in the second part of the duodenum prevents the needle leaving its protective sheath and reduces the exit angle of the needle, so that the combination of these two factors limits penetration force into the lesion. This technical problem is best solved by using echoendoscopes with a large operating channel (therapeutic echoendoscope), using new latest-generation Teflon-coated needles with lower friction, or by using 25 G needles.

Clinical Tip

During FNA sampling of hard lesions or where the tip of the echoendoscope is acutely angulated, the needle may become bent, making it difficult to visualize during further passes. Always check the needle and reshape it so that it is straight between passes.

4.7.2. Biopsy of the pancreatic neck

Patients with a long stomach usually require more than 50 cm of the echoendoscope to be introduced so that it is positioned in the stomach over the lesion. The biopsy path towards the target is then at a tangent to the gut wall (distal lesser curve), which reduces penetration force and causes, when the needle is advanced, the gastric wall and the lesion to move, without the needle penetrating the lesion. The echoendoscope, which is lying along the posterior side of the lower vertical lesser curve, tends to withdraw to the greater curve as the needle attempts to puncture the wall. An elegant way of resolving this problem is to accelerate the puncture of the needle through the wall into the lesion, using a sudden, firm thrust, having previously measured the distance between the wall and the lesion, so as to limit the penetration of the needle by means of the adjustable lock on the handle. This avoids accidentally passing through the target. An alternative effective way of biopsying neck tumors is to position the echoendoscope in the duodenal bulb and hyper-inflate the balloon then withdraw the echoendoscope to 50 cm from the incisors, leaving the tip in position in the bulb. The neck and the lesion then appear under the transducer, and the needle exits immediately upstream of the pylorus into the distal antrum. Full penetration of the needle can then be obtained either by pushing the needle progressively towards the tumor or using a sudden, hard thrust.

4.8. Renal cancer metastases and endocrine tumor

The biopsy technique for a pancreatic mass suspected of being an endocrine tumor or a renal cancer metastasis must be different as regards the suction force exerted. Make several back and forth movements without suction, then lightly aspirate using a 2 cc syringe for 1–2 s. Cells from this type of cancer, which are very fragile, thus remain analyzable. This also lowers the risk of post-biopsy hematoma (see Fig. 138) associated with these hypervascular tumors.

4.9. Complications of EUS-FNA

- EUS without FNA can be performed on patients receiving anticoagulant treatment in the therapeutic range. It does not require specific antibiotic prophylaxis. Provided the duodenal anatomy is normal and compliant, diagnostic EUS has no specific complications compared with conventional upper GI endoscopy.
- The main complications of EUS-FNA are superinfections of pancreatic cystic lesions, pseudocysts and other cystic lesions (bronchogenic or foregut duplication cysts). Bleeding and, in particular, hematomas in the gut wall or in biopsied cystic lesions have also been described, but without major consequences. A few cases of pancreatitis have been described, mainly after biopsy of a benign pancreatic lesion (cystic tumor, IPMN of the uncinate process or endocrine tumor), where it was necessary to pass through healthy pancreatic tissue, whereas the risk of pancreatitis is very low in pancreatic cancer biopsy. Complications of EUS-FNA occur in 2–6% of cases. These complications are very rarely severe, for example

complicated acute pancreatitis. Mortality is estimated at 0.2% and is observed almost exclusively in EUS-FNA of benign pancreatic lesions.

To summarize, EUS-FNA is an invasive technique with low morbidity but it is nevertheless associated with a small number of severe complications.

The indication for performing EUS-FNA should thus be considered carefully and based on an assessment of the risk-benefit ratio – the patient should be fully informed of this.

 Warning!

BEWARE! Do not perform FNA of mediastinal cystic lesions: abscess or mediastinitis can occur.

5. How to examine tumors of the esophagus and mediastinum

5.1 General points

After upper endoscopy (EGD) to identify the location of the tumor (distance from the incisors, length, circumferential involvement, degree of stenosis and ulceration), EUS begins in the stomach, 45–50 cm from the incisors, over the posterior side of the lesser curve, at the junction between the upper and middle thirds of the lesser curve. The echoendoscope must be pressed (by up angulation) against the lesser curve, between the liver (segment II) and the junction between the pancreatic neck and body. The air present in the stomach must have been completely aspirated beforehand, especially if EGD has been carried out previously.

The celiac region and the subcardial and left gastric artery lymph node areas are examined by progressively withdrawing the echoendoscope, keeping the transducer pressed against the wall by up angulation of the scope tip.

The anterior subcardial lymph node areas between the anterior surface of the upper part of the stomach and the apex of the left lobe of the liver should also be examined. The splenic hilum should also be examined; this can be a drainage region, in the event of subcardial involvement by esophageal cancer, following the splenic artery and vein to the spleen. If a suspicious lymph node is discovered in the celiac region, the examination should be continued as far as the second part of the duodenum, to examine the retroduodenopancreatic and lumbar aortic lymph node areas and the hepatic pedicle, which may be affected.

By withdrawing the instrument into the posterior mediastinum, the esophagus and peri-esophageal region can be visualized:

- Over the lower third, i.e. below the left atrium, between 40 and 35 cm from the incisors
- Over the left atrium, between 35 and 30 cm from the incisors
- Over the subcarinal region, the carina and the arch of the aorta, between 30 and 23 cm from the incisors
- In the supra-aortic and upper thoracic region between 23 and 20 cm from the incisors
- In the cervical region (Fig. 13A,B) between 20 and 16 cm from the incisors.

Generally speaking, the lymph node drainage areas of esophageal cancers are often ipsilateral (right or left) to the predominant spread of the cancer on one or other of the lateral walls.

Five major regions should be examined very closely for metastatic adenopathy. They are, from the top down:

- The cervical region, below the thyroid lobes, in the right and left tracheo-esophageal angle
- In the upper thorax, latero-esophageal region and tracheo-esophageal angle (Fig. 13C) between 18 and 22 cm from the incisors above the aortic arch
- In the aortopulmonary window (Fig. 13D), below the inside edge (right) of the aortic arch between the left side of the esophagus, the anterior part of the origin of the descending aorta, the left pulmonary artery, the termination of the trachea and the origin of the left main bronchus
- In the subcarinal region (Fig. 13E), behind the right pulmonary artery, which crosses the anterior side of the esophagus, and behind the upper part of the left atrium
- Over the lower third and the junction between the middle third and the lower third of the esophagus, and the peri-esophageal region, particularly the posterior part.

Tumor stenoses are impassable in only a few cases if a gastroscope has passed through beforehand. If a stenosis is impassable, a blind probe, capable of passing through almost 95% of malignant stenoses, should preferably be used. If a blind probe is unavailable, cautious dilation can be considered. Dilation up to a diameter of 13 mm is usually sufficient to allow the latest generation echoendoscopes to pass through. This type of dilatation is usually safe. The use of a 7.5 or 12 MHz miniprobe is a less satisfactory alternative to a blind probe.

5.2. Special features of radial examination

While studying an esophageal tumor using a radial echoendoscope fitted with a balloon, the balloon should be inflated moderately so that the endoscope can be advanced and retracted without creating an oblique image. The endoscope should be kept angulated so that the transducer remains perpendicular to the lesion examined. This means making sure that the muscle layer is visible through 360° around the lesion examined. For a small lesion, the inflated balloon should be positioned between the lesion and the transducer, with the aid of sufficient angulation so that it is not pressed against the lesion.

Box 7 Examination of the esophagus with a radial instrument

- Left lateral decubitus.
- Use a moderately inflated balloon (15–20 mm in diameter).
- Begin the examination in the stomach over the celiac region.
- Bring the scope up to the cricoid cartilage (landmark for the start of the esophagus).

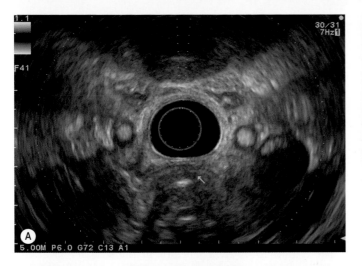

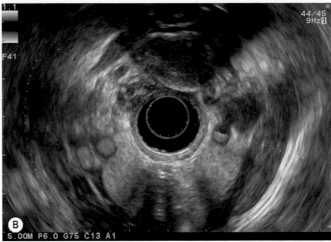

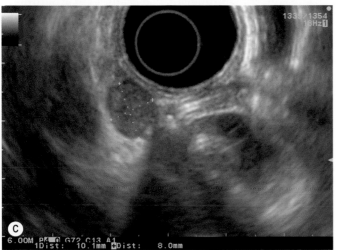

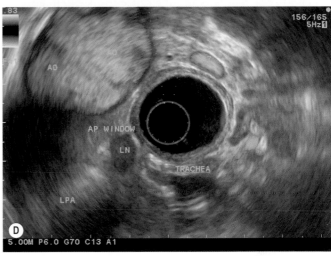

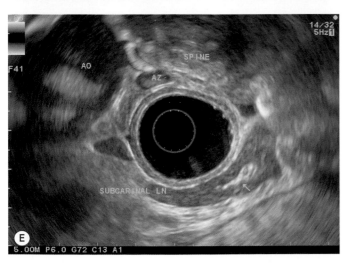

Figure 13 (A) Radial examination of the esophagus in the cervical region with visualization of the cricoid cartilage (white arrow), with the console positioned beside the patient's feet using the open position of the echoendoscope handle. (B) Radial examination of the esophagus in the cervical region with visualization of the thyroid lobes and the common carotid arteries on both sides of the trachea. (C) Small metastatic lymph node (M1a) in the upper thorax in the left tracheo-esophageal angle in a patient with an esophageal cancer at 35 cm arising in Barrett's esophagus. (D) Small metastatic lymph node in the aorto-pulmonary window in a patient with squamous lung cancer. (E) Subcarinal lymph node. Note the triangular shape and the central area (white arrow) highly suggestive of benign appearance.

5.3. Special features of linear examination

5.3.1. General points

Examination of an esophageal cancer or a submucosal tumor of the esophagus is not optimal with a linear instrument because the entire lesion does not appear on the same image when it is advanced or withdrawn, and the endoscope handle has to be rotated in addition to the forwards and backwards movement. This is tedious if the tumor is of a considerable length and is near-circumferential, which is almost always the case if the patient is dysphagic. On the other hand, linear examination has the advantage of being able to differentiate better between a celiac or left gastric location of a suspected malignant lymph node located in front of the abdominal aorta, and clearly allows it to be biopsied. It is therefore preferable to perform this after a radial examination if lymph node biopsy is indicated.

The transducer must be pressed against the wall for lymph node examination and separated from the wall by the inflated balloon for examination of the lesion, particularly if it is small. Serosal involvement of the cancer or the originating layer of a submucosal tumor should be interpreted only if the image plane is perpendicular to the lesion, in the craniocaudal direction, i.e. if the muscle layer is clearly visible, longitudinally, above, over and below the lesion, of consistent thickness, and in the axis of the lesion. This technique requires far more training than radial EUS.

5.3.2. Examination of the celiac region

The celiac region is examined by inserting from the cardia, where the aorta should be located longitudinally, then descending 3–6 cm along the vertical lesser curve, along the aorta with small clockwise and anti-clockwise movements of the endoscope handle, since the celiac trunk often takes off laterally from the anterior face of the aorta. After locating the origin of the celiac trunk, follow it to the origin of the left gastric artery (see Fig. 52) which can be seen climbing vertically along the stomach then as far as the bifurcation of the hepatic artery and the splenic artery (see Fig. 52). The upper margin of the pancreatic body appears 1 cm below this bifurcation (see Fig. 53). The celiac lymph nodes are

sometimes located in this bifurcation, sometimes along the lateral sides of the celiac trunk, which is examined by turning the endoscope handle clockwise and anti-clockwise in front of its origin. The left gastric lymph nodes are closer to the stomach along the left gastric artery, which is examined by following it upwards while withdrawing the echoendoscope from its origin at the celiac trunk.

5.3.3. Examination of the posterior mediastinum with linear instruments

The lymph node areas of the posterior mediastinum and the celiac and mesenteric region should be examined in patients with cancer of the esophagus and cardia, when assessing bronchogenic cancer or in patients with benign or malignant mediastinal masses.

The examination always begins in the stomach over the celiac region. The left adrenal gland, readily located by turning the endoscope handle clockwise from the celiac trunk, should then be examined. The left lobe of the liver is easy to locate by turning the handle anti-clockwise from the celiac trunk.

The endoscope is then brought up to the cardia (40 cm from the incisors), following the aorta longitudinally. At this point the suprahepatic venous confluence at the inferior vena cava (Fig. 14A) and the dome of the liver, which is

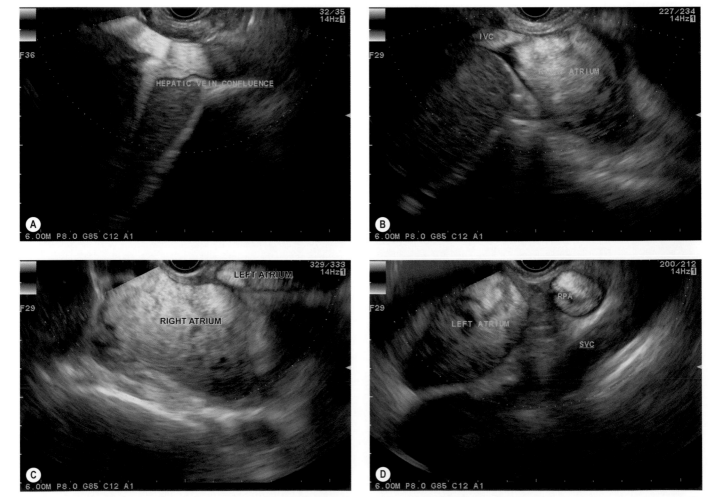

Figure 14 (A) Suprahepatic venous confluence seen with a linear scope. (B) Right atrium seen with a linear scope. (C) Right atrium and left atrium seen with linear scope. (D) Subcarinal region with the left atrium, the right pulmonary artery (RPA) and the superior vena cava (SVC) seen with linear scope.

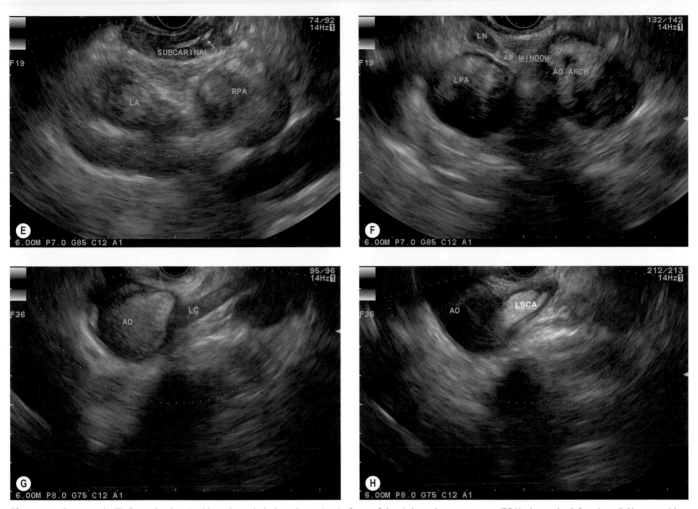

Figure 14 Continued. (E) Central subcarinal lymph node below the carina in front of the right pulmonary artery (RPA) above the left atrium (LA) seen with linear scope. (F) Aorto-pulmonary window (AP window) between the aortic arch (AO arch) and the left pulmonary artery (LPA) seen with a linear scope. (G) Left common carotid artery (LC) branching from the aortic arch (AO) seen with a linear scope. (H) Left subclavian artery (LSCA) branching from the aortic arch (AO) seen with a linear scope.

located around it, can be observed by turning the handle clockwise and anti-clockwise, then climbing along the inferior vena cava as far as the right atrium (Fig. 14B). When the right atrium disappears on withdrawal of the endoscope (35 cm from the incisors), the left atrium (Fig. 14C) can be examined by making small clockwise or anti-clockwise turns of the handle, and the endoscope is brought up along the central part of the left atrium (the largest part) as far as its upper margin (28–30 cm from the incisors). On withdrawal, the subcarinal region then appears and the screen shows, below the transducer, from top to bottom, the air present in the trachea and carina, the subcarinal region, the right pulmonary artery in cross-section (Fig. 14D) and the upper part of the left atrium. Turning the handle clockwise and anti-clockwise then allows all the subcarinal lymph nodes (Fig. 14E) to be examined (the right group, which is close to the large azygos vein, the central group between the esophagus and the right pulmonary artery, and the left group near the descending aorta).

With maximum up angulation, withdrawing the endoscope 1–2 cm and turning the handle anti-clockwise, the aortopulmonary window (region IVL) will become visible between the aortic arch, round in section, at the top of the screen, and the left pulmonary artery, round in section, at the bottom of the screen (Fig. 14F).

Continuing withdrawal of the endoscope reveals the supraaortic (left paratracheal and para-esophageal) region with the left common carotid artery (Fig. 14G) and the left subclavian artery (Fig. 14H), then the origin of the left vertebral artery and the left retroclavicular lymph node region, finally, above the left thyroid lobe.

If the handle is turned clockwise from the aortic arch, the trachea, then the supra-azygos region (above the arch of the azygos vein), and if the endoscope is retracted keeping the same image plane, the brachiocephalic trunk will appear followed by its bifurcation into the right subclavian and right carotid artery, the origin of the right vertebral artery, then the right thyroid lobe.

6. How to examine the stomach

6.1. Introduction

It is advisable to almost always start with a radial instrument. It is far easier and more comprehensive. The linear instrument can be used first only if the examiner has to biopsy a large submucosal tumor suspected of being a GIST. By contrast with conventional teaching, it is advisable to instil water into the stomach only very rarely, because it is usually ineffective and may cause pulmonary aspiration.

6.2. Examination of the stomach with a radial instrument

For malignant or suspected malignant tumor disease, the examination begins in the duodenum, as for pancreaticobiliary examination, looking for retropancreatic and interaortocaval metastatic adenopathy, particularly at the base of the posterior segment of the hepatic pedicle. Returning into the bulb allows examination of the preportal (pyloric) hepatic chain. Moving into the stomach allows examination of the left gastric, celiac and cardiac lymph node regions. Each part of the stomach should be examined systematically, the antrum, body and fundus, to be sure you have examined the lymph node areas adjacent to these regions. The liver is the key landmark anteriorly, the pancreas is the key landmark posteriorly, the spleen for the greater curve, and the lesser curve can be readily located at the junction between the posterior and anterior walls (Fig. 15).

The key to success when performing EUS of the gastric wall is to try to obtain a study of the layers of the wall so that they are perpendicular to the ultrasonic beam (Fig. 1). EUS is not possible across the whole circumference of the stomach simultaneously. In other words, once the anomaly to be examined has been located roughly on one wall of the stomach, focus on this anomaly so that the layers of the wall over and below the anomaly, but also at its edges, are clearly individualized. It is only by proceeding in this manner that you can be sure that the EUS abnormalities are real and not due to an 'oblique image' which may be misinterpreted (overlapping of several structures creating false images that suggest serosal involvement of a tumor or wrongly attributing the anomaly to a layer other than the one in which it is actually located). Examination of the fundus is sometimes difficult when the lesion in question is small. It is sometimes easier to perform the examination without instillation of

water, after aspirating all the air present. It is sometimes necessary to work with the echoendoscope in retroflexion to visualize the anomaly if it is small. Examination of the body of the stomach is easy, and examination of the antrum is equally easy for the horizontal portion. On the other hand, examination of the incisura is more problematic. The best solution is to inflate the balloon immediately upstream of the pylorus, maintaining maximum up angulation, to check that the gallbladder is facing the anterior side, which means that the lesser curve is then at the bottom of the screen and the greater curve at the top. Once this has been confirmed, withdrawal of the echoendoscope, with the balloon inflated and up angulation, usually means that it can remain perpendicular to the lesser curve, whether in the horizontal portion, the incisura itself or the vertical portion immediately above the incisura. Examination of an immediate prepyloric lesion is difficult because it is often impossible to avoid oblique images of the pylorus itself which will give the impression that there is a submucosal tumor in the muscle layer. This is a frequent cause of false positive results for stromal tumors. This type of error obviously occurs only with small tumors, since large tumors are usually clearly visible, regardless of the image plane used.

6.3. Examination of the stomach with a linear instrument

It is advisable to use a linear instrument only to biopsy a submucosal tumor whose exact location has already been determined by UGIE or by a radial examination performed immediately beforehand.

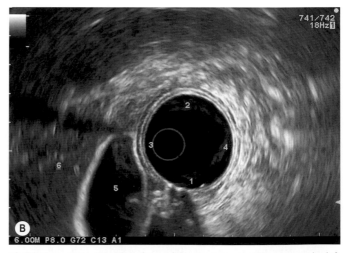

Figure 15 (A) Radial examination of the lesser curve (1), between the posterior side (2), the anterior side (3), in front of the greater curve (4) between the left lobe of the liver (6) and the body of the pancreas (5). (B) Radial examination of the gastric antrum. The scope being pushed immediately upstream the pylorus maintaining maximum up angulation. The lesser curve (1) is between the anterior side of the antrum which is facing the gallbladder (5) and the liver (6). (4) posterior side and the antrum. (2) greater curve of the antrum.

7. How to examine the pancreaticobiliary region

7.1. Essential anatomic knowledge for correctly performing a pancreaticobiliary examination

Familiarity with the celiac and mesenteric anatomy is required:

- The celiac trunk takes off from the anterior side of the aorta, 3–4 cm below the cardia. The celiac trunk sometimes takes off to the front perpendicular to the aorta, but it usually runs at an oblique angle to the right and front and sometimes, very rarely, it runs first diagonally to the left before bending to the right. Its first branch is the left gastric artery towards the top; this is not clearly visible in its initial portion in a radial image, although it is very clearly visible on linear imaging. It then splits into the splenic artery and the hepatic artery.
- The hepatic artery heads right, usually horizontally, and then becomes the gastroduodenal artery and the hepatic artery proper. The gastroduodenal artery is the key landmark for the anterior part of the pancreatic head. A tumor located to the right of the origin of the gastroduodenal artery can be resected only by Whipple's pancreaticoduodenectomy, whereas a tumor located to the left of the origin of the gastroduodenal artery can be resected by middle pancreatectomy or by left pancreatectomy. The gastroduodenal artery is visible behind the duodenal bulb. It is therefore examined best through the duodenal bulb. This artery leads into the anterior and superior pancreatico-duodenal artery, which in turn becomes an arterial branch that descends along the second part of the duodenum to the region of the ampulla of Vater. This arterial branch is therefore usually parallel to the path of the common bile duct and Doppler imaging can distinguish the artery path from the bile duct, if the latter is narrow.
- The splenic artery, at its origin, may head slightly right before turning left. Its path is almost always downwards initially, before turning left and following a more upwards route to the left. The splenic artery extends along the upper edge of the body-tail of the pancreas, it has a snake-like sinuous path and is visible in radial images in only small portions.
- The splenic vein usually runs over the posterior segment of the pancreatic body and tail. It extends horizontally and a long segment of the vein can be examined in a radial imaging. There is usually some pancreatic parenchyma visible, between the stomach and the splenic vein, but the central segment of the pancreatic body and tail is usually below the level of the splenic vein, so that the pancreatic duct which is in the central segment of the pancreatic gland appears horizontally in a transverse radial image, when the splenic vein is no longer visible.
- The right hepatic artery, which branches off from the hepatic artery proper, generally crosses the common bile duct below the hilum. It may indent the common hepatic duct, causing an appearance of pseudostenosis on MRCP. This artery, which is often infiltrated in the presence of cholangiocarcinoma of the common hepatic duct, normally takes off from the hepatic artery proper in the middle part of the hepatic pedicle. It may take off early and intersect the portal trunk prematurely, then run along its right edge, parallel to the common bile duct before intersecting it at the top right and entering the hilum of the liver.
- In 15% of cases the right hepatic artery takes off from the superior mesenteric artery. It then extends initially into the area known as the retroportal region, when it is visible between the right edge of the portal vein and the common bile duct. The retroportal region is a very important region for assessing the spread of cancers of the pancreatic head, which cause jaundice. This region is located between the posterior side of the portal vein in front, the superior mesenteric artery to the left and the anterior side of the inferior vena cava to the rear.

  After crossing the retroportal region, the right hepatic artery, which is a branch of the superior mesenteric artery, intersects the posterior right edge of the portal vein and then extends along the right edge of the portal vein, along the common bile duct (between the portal vein and the common bile duct), before intersecting the common hepatic duct at the top right, and then entering the hilum of the liver.

  To summarize, when you see an arterial structure at the right edge of the portal vein, between this and the bile duct, on a radial EUS image that passes through the common bile duct examined longitudinally at the common hepatic duct and the cystic duct-common bile duct junction and through the portal vein (likewise in a linear image), this is the right hepatic artery. If you see the right hepatic artery here, i.e. distinctly under the hilum of the liver, this means that the artery takes off either prematurely from the hepatic artery proper (which is rare), or from the superior mesenteric artery (which is usually the case).
- The ampulla of Vater is the extreme right posterior segment of the pancreatic head. The uncinate process is located below and behind the ampulla of Vater, and the posterior segment of the pancreatic head is located above it. If you can see the common bile duct running towards the ampulla of Vater, you are over the posterior segment of the pancreatic head; if the common bile duct disappears into the duodenal wall, you are in the region where the uncinate process begins. This is therefore the lowest and most posterior segment of the pancreatic head.
- The common bile duct follows a retropancreatic path, i.e. it is very posterior to the pancreatic head, even its most posterior segment. It terminates in an intrapancreatic path measuring no more than 15 mm in height in front of the duodenal wall. This means that, if necessary, an experienced surgeon can detach the anterior side of the common bile duct from the channel in which it runs in the posterior part of the pancreatic head, with a view to sectioning the bile duct at the point where it enters the pancreatic head. This type of surgery is sometimes performed during liver transplants for primary sclerosing cholangitis to

minimize the length of the residual biliary stump and to reduce the subsequent risk of bile duct cancer. It is also performed in order to resect the common bile duct in patients with choledochal cysts.

- The cystic duct terminates at the right wall of the hepatic duct to form the common bile duct in 85–90% of cases. In 10% of cases, there is a low insertion of the cystic duct and common bile duct, i.e. located in the retropancreatic segment of the common bile duct.

Clinical Tip

In 10–15% of cases, the cystic duct intersects the common bile duct, terminating at its left edge. This is why the cystic duct does not terminate in the place where you might expect (at the right edge of the common bile duct) in one in 10 cases, in a radial image. It is therefore important to be aware of this possibility and to try to create ultrasound images which show the intersection of the cystic duct with the bile duct.

- The gallbladder has three segments: the fundus, the body, and the left segment which is the infundibulum. The infundibulum is hook-shaped. It is the most frequent site of small stones that have gone undetected during percutaneous ultrasound. The gallbladder fundus is sometimes best examined through the antrum by pushing the echoendoscope with the balloon inflated towards the pylorus. Gallstones are generally located in the fundus of the gallbladder, and are therefore sometimes visible only when the echoendoscope is placed in the antrum, pushing towards the pylorus. The gallbladder may be bilobed, i.e. with a partial septum in the middle segment of the body which separates the gallbladder fundus from the infundibulum. This encourages formation of stones in the gallbladder.
- The main pancreatic duct, which is known as Wirsung's duct in the absence of pancreas divisum, runs along the central segment of the pancreatic gland, i.e. in the middle of the pancreas along the tail, body and neck. In the pancreatic head, however, the main pancreatic duct extends first along the anterior segment of the head, then along the middle of its right segment, and finally along its posterior segment, towards the ampulla of Vater, which is the most posterior segment of the pancreatic head. The main pancreatic duct thus lies in the path of pancreatic cancers that can cause jaundice, as 70% are located in the posterior segment of the pancreatic head. This is why cancer of the pancreatic head causing jaundice is almost always accompanied by dilation of both the bile duct and the pancreatic duct. Paradoxically, this dilation of both ducts sometimes does not occur in cases of tumor of the ampulla of Vater since this may be located purely in the biliary segment of the ampulla, leaving the termination of the main pancreatic duct unaffected. The main pancreatic duct can be visualized through the duodenal bulb using EUS, starting at the pancreatic neck and advancing to the right part of the pancreatic head. From this point on, the duct can sometimes be seen, in

10–15% of cases, terminating horizontally in the upper segment of the pancreatic head, while the common bile duct is still visible in the hepatic pedicle, and the gallbladder is still visible. If you see the pancreatic duct terminating in or running very close to the duodenal wall while the bile duct is still visible in its suprapancreatic course and has not yet begun its retropancreatic path, this is known as a dominant dorsal main pancreatic duct, which in most cases indicates the presence of pancreas divisum. Pancreas divisum may of course be incomplete, i.e. there may be a small passage between this dominant dorsal duct and the main pancreatic duct, which is in the ventral pancreas, but this passage is often extremely narrow and may not be detected by EUS or MRCP. On the other hand, if the main pancreatic duct is followed into the pancreatic head then appears parallel to the bile duct, running towards the ampulla of Vater, this means that the main pancreatic duct that you saw in the upper segment of the pancreatic head, coming from the neck, and that can be followed towards the ampulla of Vater, is the main pancreatic duct (also known as 'Wirsung's duct'), and that the ventral and dorsal segments of the pancreatic gland have fused, which in turn indicates that there is no pancreas divisum. A simple way to determine this using EUS is to find the main pancreatic duct in the upper part of the pancreatic head, which is usually bright and echogenic, corresponding to the dorsal pancreas, and then observe the pancreatic duct entering the hypoechoic segment of the pancreatic head, corresponding to the ventral segment from the embryological standpoint. If the pancreatic duct extends from the echogenic segment of the pancreas to the hypoechoic segment of the pancreas, it can be concluded that there is no pancreas divisum.

- The pancreatic tail is usually located above the pancreatic body. The pancreas extends diagonally from right to left and bottom to top. In 10–15% of cases, however, the pancreatic tail is lower than the pancreatic body, in which case it is at a distance from the stomach and is not clearly visible with a radial echoendoscope. In this specific case, you cannot be sure whether the whole of the distal end of the pancreatic tail has been examined. This is clearly visible on CT scans. In the vast majority of cases, the pancreatic tail is easily seen close to the posterior side and the greater curve of the stomach, but the pancreatic tail is sometimes remote from the posterior side and the greater curve of the stomach, and it is easy to understand why it is difficult to examine it completely with a radial echoendoscope. In this case, switch to a linear echoendoscope, which allows visualization, in 100% of cases, of the entire pancreatic tail, even in patients in whom it is remote from the stomach.
- Liver segments I, II and III are visible via the stomach using a radial instrument. The liver segment that is visible around the gallbladder through the duodenum is a part of segment IV. When the right kidney becomes visible on advancing the echoendoscope into the duodenum, the liver segments in contact with the right kidney are segment V and segment VI. Segment VII,

Box 9 Pancreaticobiliary and duodenal examination with a radial instrument

- Left lateral decubitus, tilted towards the examination table at an angle of 30–40°.
- Use a moderately inflated balloon.
- Begin the examination in the stomach 45–50 cm from the incisors, to examine the body and tail region.
- After advancing through the pylorus under endoscopic control, proceed from the bulb to the second part of the duodenum by pushing the echoendoscope gently under ultrasound control, turning the handle clockwise if the superior duodenal angle is open, then push the echoendoscope in the long position towards the ampulla of Vater, adding up angulation. Use the ERCP withdrawal maneuver under endoscopic control, from the apex of the bulb if the superior duodenal angle is closed (thin patient), and allow the head of the echoendoscope to fall into the second duodenum, then push the tip over the ampulla of Vater, in the long position, and start the examination at this point.

segment VIII and the anterior part of segment IV can never be viewed with a radial instrument.

7.2. Radial EUS pancreaticobiliary examination

The vascular structures are the anatomical landmarks for the examination of the pancreaticobiliary region (Fig. 16).

7.2.1. Examination of the pancreatic head and the common bile duct

There are three ways of examining the head of the pancreas and the common bile duct:

- Start in the duodenal bulb, with the handle in the neutral position, and advance the echoendoscope under ultrasound control, turning the handle clockwise (which brings it to the closed position). Proceed from the duodenal bulb to the superior duodenal angle and then add up angulation to bring the echoendoscope in front of the ampulla of Vater. The gallbladder can then

be visualized above the bulb, then the common bile duct, the portal vein and the mesenteric-portal vein confluence, followed by the superior mesenteric vein, the posterior segment of the pancreatic head, the main pancreatic duct parallel to the common bile duct and finally the ampulla of Vater, between 9 and 8 o'clock on the duodenal circumference.

- Start over the aorta and inferior vena cava viewed in transverse section, in the 'long' position (Fig. 17), i.e. with the tip of the echoendoscope pushed immediately below the ampulla of Vater region, with up angulation, and the handle in the neutral position (Fig. 18A). The spine (Fig. 18B) is to the rear (top of the screen), and the right kidney may be visible to the right of the inferior vena cava (right of the screen). The liver is sometimes to the front (bottom of the screen) if it overlaps extensively. The gallbladder, which is distended in obstructive jaundice, can also be visualized to the front (bottom of the screen) in this plane. A pancreatic segment is sometimes visible in this image, at the bottom left of the screen. This is the lower anterior segment of the pancreatic head and uncinate process. In this transverse section (Fig. 18B), the top of the screen corresponds to the back, the bottom corresponds to the front, and the right and left correspond to the right periduodenal and left periduodenal regions, respectively. The mesenteric vessels are often visible (arteries and veins) in a transverse image, to the left of the duodenum.

By withdrawal of the instrument (Fig. 19), with maximum up angulation, and turning the handle anti-clockwise, which advances the tip into the inferior duodenal angle bringing it upright (Fig. 20), you can see in succession at the top of the screen or the top and right: the aorta (Fig. 21), in a longitudinal image, then the superior mesenteric artery, also in a longitudinal image (to the left on the screen), and the left renal vein in a transverse image between the aorta to the rear and the superior mesenteric artery over and to the front. By withdrawing the echoendoscope a little more, turning anti-clockwise, with up angulation, this image is

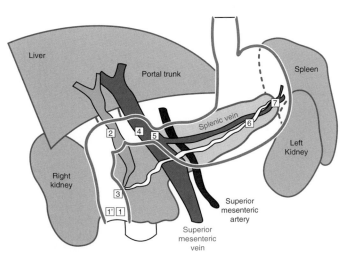

Figure 16 General view: The numbers in the graphic refer to the various positions of the head of the radial endoscope for an examination of the pancreaticobiliary region.

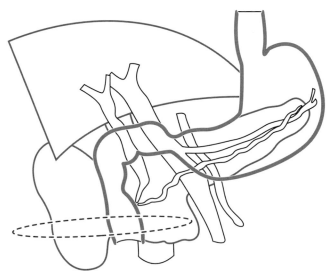

Figure 17 Transducer being advanced to D2 with the bending section of the endoscope all the way up.

replaced by a image through the inferior vena cava (Fig. 22), which, like the aorta, occupies the top right of the screen, above the duodenum, the superior mesenteric artery being replaced by the superior mesenteric vein and the mesenteric-portal vein confluence. The segment of the pancreatic head adjacent to the duodenum, between the duodenum, inferior vena cava and superior mesenteric vein, corresponds to the uncinate process of the pancreas then to the posterior segment of the pancreatic head when the echoendoscope is retracted above the ampulla of Vater region. This region is located by the termination of the bile and pancreatic ducts but also by the junction between the two echogenically different regions of the pancreatic head (Fig. 23), present in 75% of patients. These are the hypoechoic right posterior juxta-duodenal area corresponding to the ventral pancreas, and the more echogenic left anterior juxta-mesenteric region corresponding to the dorsal pancreas.

The secret of pancreaticobiliary examination is, while continuing to withdraw the endoscope, to obtain

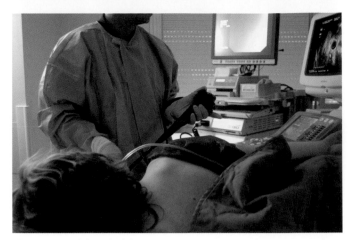

Figure 19 Withdrawal of the scope, maximum up angulation, turning the handle anti-clockwise.

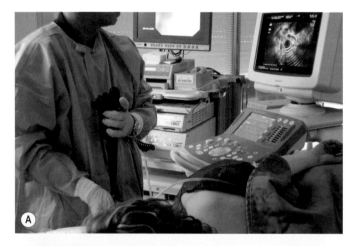

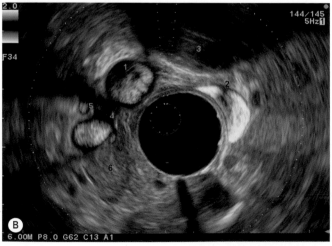

Figure 18 (A) The echoendoscope is pushed into the long position in D2 (90 cm from the incisors), the tip of the scope is positioned at the level of the ampulla of Vater, with the echoendoscope handle in neutral position, with up angulation. (B) EUS scope in D2 in front of the ampulla of Vater, neutral position, up angulation of the handle. (1) aorta, (2) inferior vena cava, (3) spine, (4) superior mesenteric vein, (5) superior mesenteric artery, (6) uncinate process.

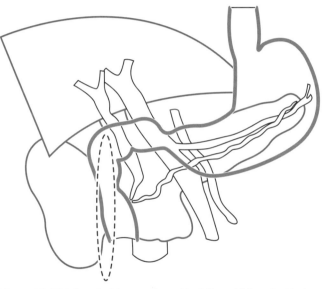

Figure 20 Withdrawal of the transducer (tip deflected fully up) with the handle rotated anti-clockwise in order to image the inferior neck of pancreas vertically.

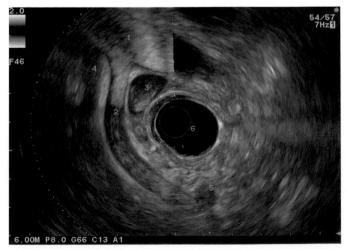

Figure 21 Because of the withdrawal of the scope, the tip is now at the 'inferior genu' (6), allowing imaging the SMA in long section (2) branching of the aorta (1), the left renal vein (3). The celiac axis take-off is visible (4).

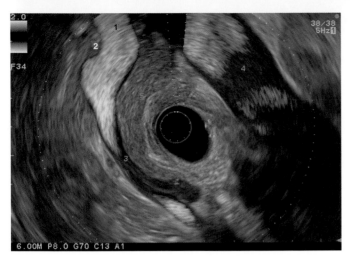

Figure 22 (1) portal vein (PV), (2) hepatic artery (HA), (3) SMV, (4) IVC, (5) uncinate process.

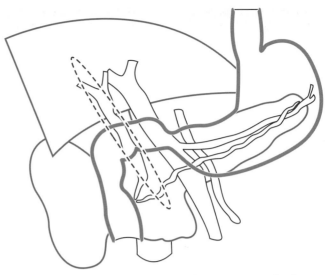

Figure 24 Transducer at the inferior neck (the image is verticalized).

a long view of the mesenteric-portal vein confluence and the common bile duct (Figs 24, 25), which is the non-vascular ductal structure located closest to the duodenal wall. If you obtain an image lengthwise through the common bile duct and the mesenteric-portal vein confluence, what appears on the left of the screen is in fact at the front left, what is on the right of the screen is at the back left, what is at the top corresponds to the hepatic hilum and the liver, and what is at the bottom corresponds to the ampulla of Vater region. The segment of the pancreas between the duodenum and the superior mesenteric vein and the mesenteric-portal vein confluence is the posterior segment of the head.

The ampulla of Vater region can be examined in several ways: the simplest is to push the endoscope gently, following the common bile duct, once it has been brought into vertical view during the initial withdrawal of the instrument (Fig. 26). When trying to follow the common bile duct, turn the echoendoscope handle gently clockwise from the open position to the

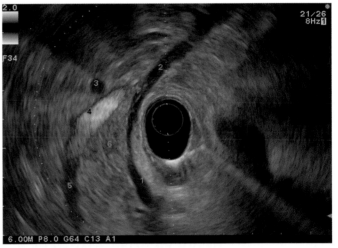

Figure 25 (1) CBD, (2) common hepatic duct (CHD), (3) HA, (4) portal vein confluence, (5) SMV, (6) posterior segment of the head.

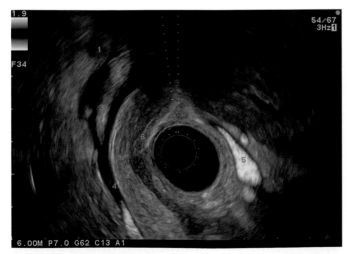

Figure 23 (1) HA, (2) PV, (3) portal vein confluence, (4) SMV, (5) IVC, (6) ventral segment of the head, (7) dorsal segment of the head.

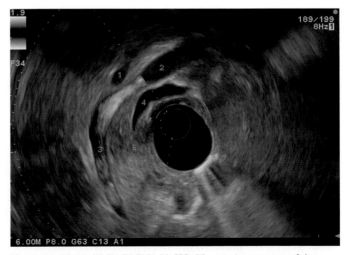

Figure 26 (1) HA, (2) PV, (3) SMV, (4) CBD, (5) posterior segment of the head.

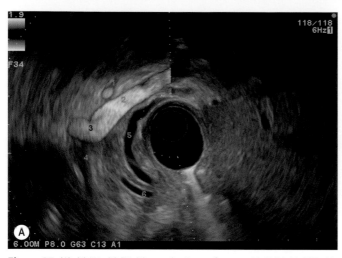

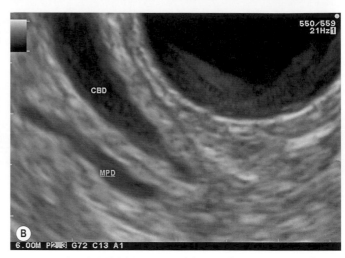

Figure 27 (A), (1) HA, (2) PV, (3) portal vein confluence, (4) SMV, (5) CBD, (6) main pancreatic duct (MPD). (B) Pancreatico-biliary confluence. CBD, common bile duct; MPD, main pancreatic duct.

neutral position while pushing the instrument. Once you can see the bile duct close to the duodenal wall (Figs 27, 28) slight up angulation should be added which causes the bile duct to disappear and the terminal main pancreatic duct to appear (Fig. 29). The ampulla of Vater is then visible between 8 and 9 o'clock in contact with the balloon (Figs 28, 30, 31). An important point to note is that the ampulla is not satisfactorily visible until the bile duct disappears into the duodenal wall.

There is another way of visualizing the ampulla of Vater, but it is fairly difficult because the echoendoscope tends to withdraw rather too quickly during the maneuver. It involves starting from the long position with the handle in the neutral position and withdrawing the echoendoscope with up angulation, turning the handle anti-clockwise, or angulation to the left, which amounts to the same. After visualizing the superior mesenteric vessels in longitudinal section, at the point when the mesenteric vein appears on the

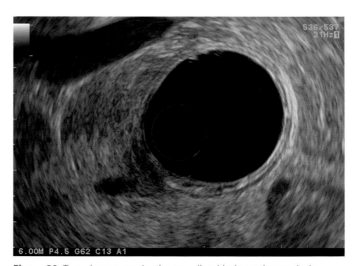

Figure 29 Transducer opposite the ampulla with the endoscope's tip deflected upward.

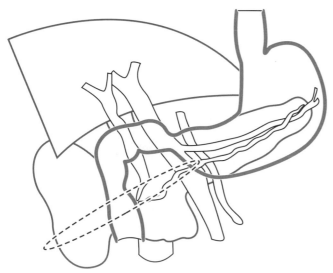

Figure 28 Transducer adjacent to the ampulla of Vater (tip deflected up).

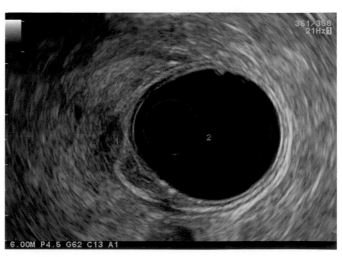

Figure 30 (1) Ampulla of Vater, (2) D2.

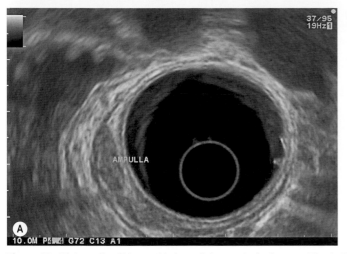

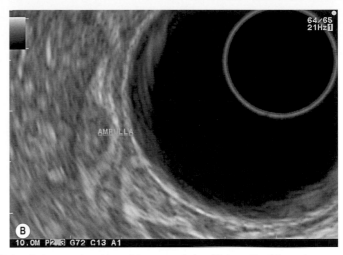

Figure 31 (A) Ampulla of Vater, with the radial scope in the long position in D2, handle in neutral position with up angulation. (B) Ampulla of Vater, the scope and handle position are the same: oval, hypoechogenic small nodule visualized in the submucosa of the internal (left) side of D2.

screen (Fig. 22), the termination of the main pancreatic duct is usually visible in contact with the duodenal wall (Fig. 29), which means that the ampulla of Vater is exactly over the transducer. Stop withdrawing and advance again slightly so that you can see the last cm of the pancreatic duct along with its penetration point in the duodenal wall, which is then an indication of the presence of the ampulla of Vater between 8 and 9 o'clock on the duodenal circumference (Figs 30, 31).

- The third way of examining the pancreatic head and the common bile duct is by *specific* withdrawal. Unlike the withdrawal described previously (*classic* withdrawal), specific withdrawal starts from the long position, with maximum up angulation of the echoendoscope and above all maximum angulation to the right, turning the echoendoscope handle clockwise towards the closed position, i.e. by pressing the endoscope against the top right part (Fig. 32A) of the

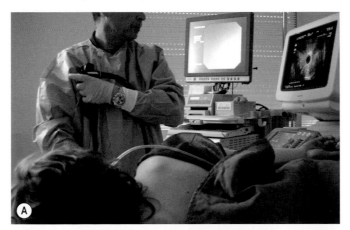

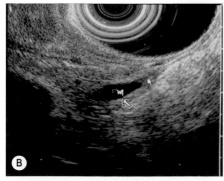

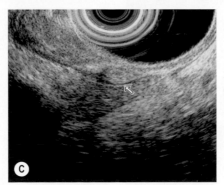

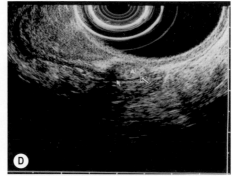

Figure 32 (A) Withdrawal of the scope, starting in long position in D2 in front of the ampulla, EUS scope handle in closed position, up angulation. (B) Junction of the ventral hypoechogenic segment of the head and the dorsal hyperechogenic segment of the head and the duodenal wall. The area of the ampulla is identified by the visualization of the end of the MPD at 6 o'clock. (C) The ampulla within the submucosa of the duodenal wall is visualized by slightly pushing the scope when the image 32B is seen. (D) Cross-section of the ampulla of Vater with visualization of the muscularis propria (white arrow), seen on the entire circumference of the duodenum (which means that the ultrasonic beam is perpendicular to the ampulla. This section allows you to accurately stage a small ampullary tumor (T1 vs T2 tumor).

examiner's chest, withdrawing the echoendoscope in this way will place it in the short position. This is the same maneuver that is carried out with a duodenoscope to place it in the short position, but in this case the maneuver is started from a long position. You will see the aorta first of all, followed by the inferior vena cava at the bottom left of the screen, then the junction between the two echogenically different regions of the pancreatic head (ventral and dorsal) between 5 and 6 o'clock and the main pancreatic duct (Fig. 32B) at about 6 o'clock, which means that the ampulla of Vater is visible at this point, if you stop withdrawal and push the echoendoscope again slightly. The ampulla of Vater appears as a small swelling (Fig. 32C) in the duodenal wall, surrounded on all sides by a little submucosa and separated from the pancreatic head by a hypoechoic border corresponding to the muscle layer of the ampulla of Vater (Fig. 32D). This is the best way of examining tumors of the ampulla of Vater and determining whether the submucosa has been infiltrated. This is also the best way of examining the uncinate process of the pancreas and the last 2 cm of the common bile duct and the main pancreatic duct.

- Examination of the gallbladder. The gallbladder can be examined after entering the bulb by inflating the balloon and pushing the transducer towards the superior duodenal angle, handle in the neutral position. The gallbladder is then visible above the balloon (Fig. 33); it disappears as you press on the apex of the bulb and the neck is the last part of the gallbladder visible. If you continue pushing, the bile duct and portal vein then become visible in the left half of the screen (Fig. 34).

  If the superior duodenal angle is compliant (rarely the case in slim patients under 40, or in very thin patients of any age), the bile duct can be followed (Fig. 35) to the ampulla of Vater, advancing the endoscope by turning the handle clockwise, with neutral angulation then adding up angulation.
- Large diverticula in the medial duodenal wall hinder the examination of the pancreatic head, the ampulla of

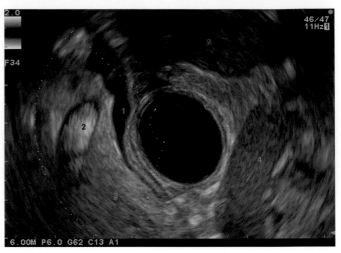

Figure 34 (1) CBD, (2) portal vein confluence, (3) posterior segment of the head, (4) right kidney, (5) segment IV of the liver.

Vater region and the terminal common bile duct. Instillation of water into the second part of the duodenum usually allows the diverticulum to be filled temporarily and its presence confirmed. If there is no fluid in the diverticulum, it appears as hyperechoic harmonic air gap between the transducer and the pancreatic head, over the region where the pancreatic duct and the common bile duct terminate.

- Pneumobilia also hinders the examination of the common bile duct. If it is related to previous endoscopic sphincterotomy, it is usually possible to visualize the bile duct termination by instilling water into the second part of the duodenum, over the ampulla of Vater region. This procedure is brief but usually allows a distinction to be made between residual stones and air in the lower common bile duct. Air remains pressed against the duodenal side of the common bile duct, whereas stones tend to sink against the opposite or pancreatic side of the common bile duct. The common bile duct is usually invisible in the hepatic pedicle in patients with choledochoduodenal anastomosis, despite the instillation of water through the anastomosis.

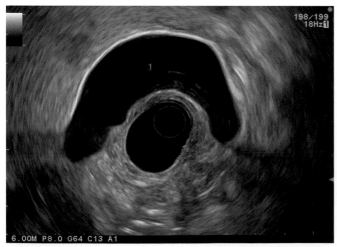

Figure 33 The gallbladder (1) seen through the duodenal bulb. The gallbladder is kept at the top of the screen after intubating the pylorus, while pushing the scope slowly.

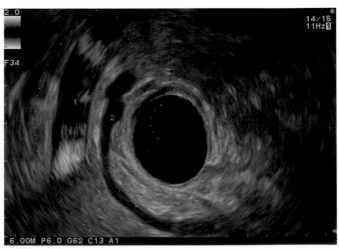

Figure 35 (1) Portal vein, (2) CBD, (3) posterior segment of the head.

- Examination of the common hepatic duct. The upper part of the common bile duct, i.e. the common hepatic duct and the biliary confluence, can be examined if the diameter of the duct is 5 mm or more. There are two complementary ways, which means that they are rarely both effective in the same patient and depend on his/ her specific anatomy.
  - The simplest way is to start from a neutral handle position, in the duodenal bulb, and advance the echoendoscope, keeping the gallbladder or liver above the balloon and observing the appearance of the common bile duct. At this point, rather than turning the handle clockwise to advance to the second part of the duodenum, turn the handle anti-clockwise to the open position and push the instrument against the superior duodenal angle. You can then see the bile duct running toward the liver: this is the common hepatic duct (Fig. 36) and the superior biliary confluence, often intersected at this point by the right hepatic artery.
  - If this method is ineffective, you can push the echoendoscope to the long position in the second part of the duodenum and carry out specific withdrawal (Fig. 32). Once the ampulla of Vater has been visualized at 6 o'clock, release right angulation and partially release up angulation, and continue withdrawal of the echoendoscope, with the handle in the closed position.

The common bile duct appears horizontal under the duodenum (Figs 37A, 37B). The cystic duct joins the common bile duct from below if you continue withdrawal very gently by adjusting the path of the common hepatic duct, keeping it horizontal by means of up angulation under the duodenum, aiming at the liver which is on the left of the screen. The vessel in this image, which is parallel to the common bile duct visible below it, is the inferior vena cava.

This also allows examination of the gallbladder (Fig. 38), which is to the left of the screen between the liver and the duodenum, turning the handle anti-clockwise

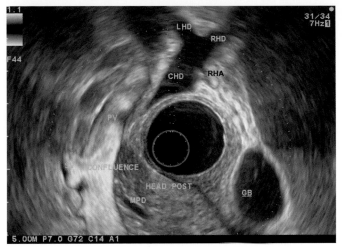

Figure 36 CHD, common hepatic duct; LHD, left hepatic duct; RHD, right hepatic duct; RHA, right hepatic artery; GB, gallbladder; MPD, main pancreatic duct.

from the neutral position and adding up angulation. The gallbladder fundus is at the top of the screen in this image, and the neck level with the balloon with its characteristic hook shape. The cystic duct can be followed from the gallbladder neck to the hepatic duct.

- Examination of the anterior side of the pancreatic head and neck. The following image, continuing to withdraw the instrument, reveals the portal vein in a transverse plane in the place of the common bile duct, under the balloon, with the hepatic artery in a transverse image extending in front and above it, almost in contact with the bulb wall (Fig. 39).

This view, which visualizes the portal vein below the transducer (Fig. 39), shows the anterior and superior segment of the pancreatic head between the bulb wall and the anterior side of the splenoportal vein confluence. At this point there is usually a bifurcation between the hepatic artery and the gastroduodenal artery, which can be followed to the rear of the bulb

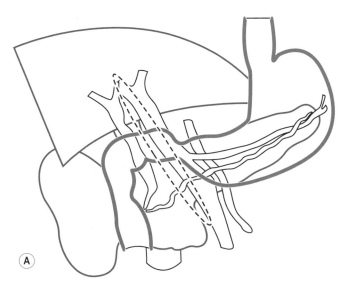

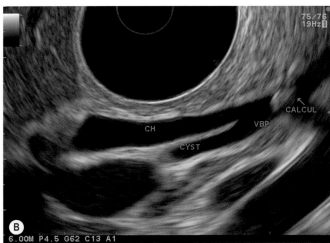

Figure 37 (A) Transducer in the duodenal bulb with the endoscope's bending section up, while the endoscope is being withdrawn. (B) CH: common bile duct, cyst: cystic duct, VBP: CBD, calcul: CBD stone.

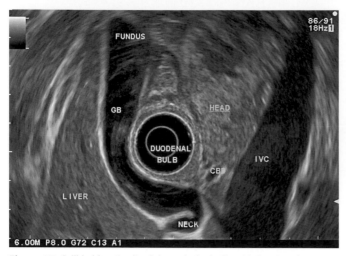

Figure 38 Gallbladder visualized through the bulb, withdrawing the scope turning the handle anti-clockwise with up angulation.

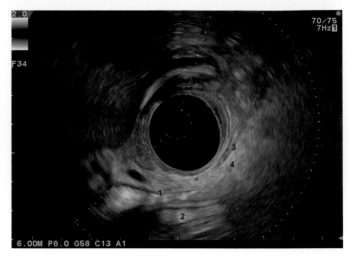

Figure 41 (1) Portal vein, (2) IVC, (3) gastroduodenal artery, (4) anterior segment of the head.

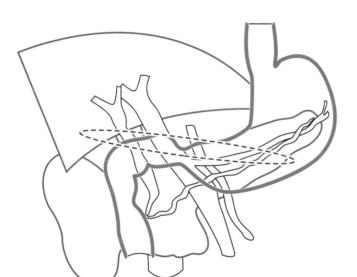

Figure 40 Transducer in the duodenal bulb under traction with the balloon inflated and the bending section up.

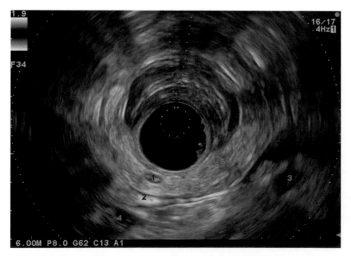

Figure 39 (1) Hepatic artery, (2) portal vein, (3) SMA, (4) IVC, (5) anterior segment of the head.

wall (i.e. below the bulb wall on the screen) by making back and forth movements advancing then withdrawing the endoscope, with up angulation, handle in the closed position (Figs 40, 41).

7.2.2. Examination of the pancreatic neck and body

If you continue progressive withdrawal of the echoendoscope, with the balloon very inflated, into the bulb, inverting the pylorus, you will see the pancreatic neck between the pylorus and the anterior side of the splenoportal confluence, below and to the right of the balloon. The landmark which indicates that you are opposite the neck is the superior mesenteric artery which is then visualized below the mesenteric-portal vein confluence (Figs 42, 43), in a transverse image. The main pancreatic duct in the neck is visible between the duodenal wall and the portal confluence.

Entering the stomach, continuing to retract the instrument, with the handle in the neutral position and up angulation, usually positions the instrument in the middle of the gastric body (between 45 and 50 cm from the incisors), over the pancreatic body (Figs 44, 45), with the handle in the neutral position. If you angulate to the right and slightly down, the echoendoscope is pressed against the posterior side of the stomach, which usually allows the left portion of the pancreatic body and tail to be examined, along with the splenic vein (Fig. 46). If you angulate up, this usually places the echoendoscope along the vertical part of the lesser curve, and this allows the right part of the pancreatic body to be examined at its junction with the neck (Fig. 47).

Changing from one of these positions to the other is usually done by slightly withdrawing the echoendoscope 1–2 cm to examine the left side of the pancreatic body and tail (Figs 48, 49A,B) and slightly advancing the endoscope 2 cm to visualize the right segment of the pancreatic body and neck (Fig. 49C). Apply slight up or neutral angulation when descending to the neck, and neutral or slight down and right angulation when withdrawing the echoendoscope to examine the pancreatic tail.

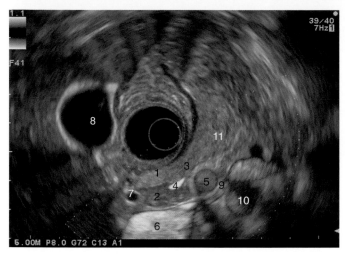

Figure 42 (1) Dorsal segment of the anterior part of the head, (2) ventral segment of the head, (3) neck of the pancreas, (4) portal vein confluence, (5) SMA, (6) IVC, (7) CBD, (8) gallbladder, (9) left renal vein, (10) aorta, (11) body of the pancreas.

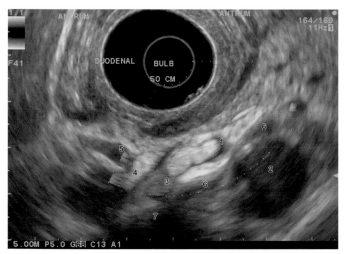

Figure 43 (1) SMA, (2) aorta, (3) right hepatic artery, (4) portal vein confluence, (5) hepatic artery, (6) left renal vein, (7) IVC.

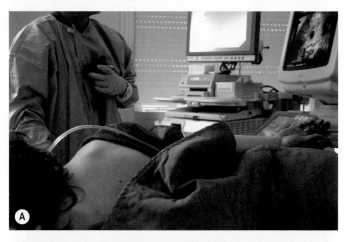

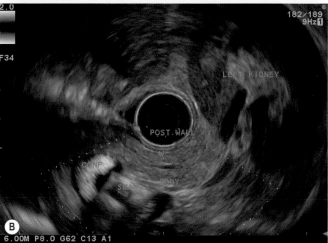

Figure 45 (A) Neutral position for the examination of the body and the tail of the pancreas. (B) Conf, portal vein confluence; SMA, superior mesenteric artery; W, Wirsung duct.

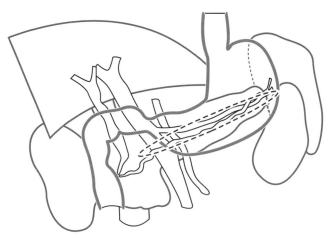

Figure 44 Transducer between 45 and 55 cm from the incisors and pressed against the posterior side of the stomach.

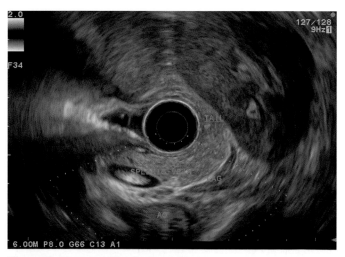

Figure 46 AO, aorta; LAG, left adrenal gland.

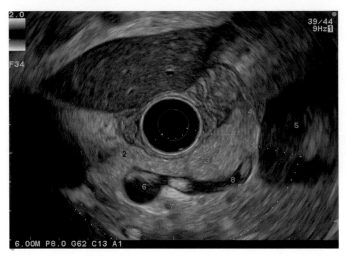

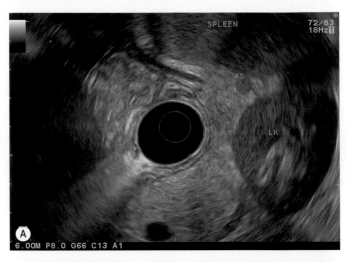

Figure 47 (1) Left lobe of the liver, (2) neck of the pancreas, (3) body of the pancreas, (4) tail of the pancreas, (5) left kidney, (6) portal vein confluence, (7) SMA, (8) splenic vein.

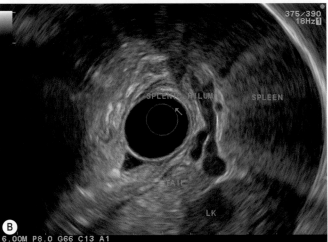

An important point is that it is as easy to examine the whole of the neck, body and tail, including the angle of the main pancreatic duct (Fig. 49C), through the stomach in women (shorter stomach) as it is difficult to visualize the neck and the junction between the neck and the head through the stomach in men. The junction between the neck and the head can thus be visualized (50 cm from the incisors) under the transducer through the bulb (Fig. 42), with the balloon very inflated pulling on the pylorus, with maximum up angulation, and with the handle in the closed position.

The celiac region can be examined immediately above the neck by withdrawing the instrument 1 cm, with maximum up angulation, and the handle in the neutral position (Fig 50A,B). An alternative method of examining the celiac region is to follow the aorta from the cardia, descending along the lesser gastric curve (Fig. 50C).

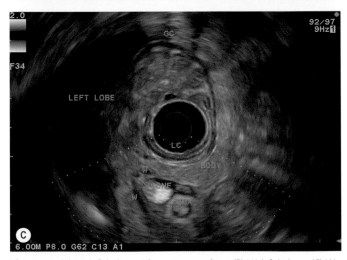

Figure 49 (A) LK, left kidney; AS, accessory spleen. (B) LK, left kidney. (C) W, Wirsung duct; LC, lesser curve; GC, greater curvature; SMA, superior mesenteric artery; conf, portal vein confluence.

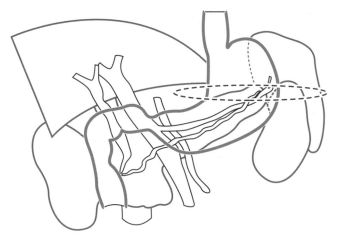

Figure 48 Transducer 45 cm from the incisors, pressed against the greater curvature.

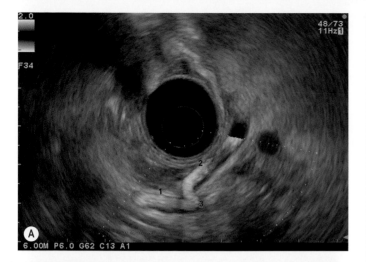

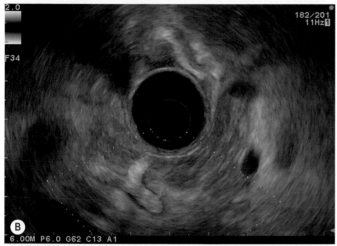

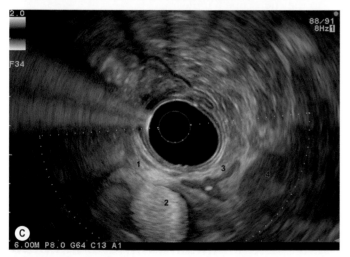

Figure 50 (A), (1) hepatic artery, (2) splenic artery, (3) celiac axis. (B), (1) hepatic artery, (2) splenic artery, (3) celiac axis. (C), (1) celiac axis, (2) aorta, (3) left adrenal gland, (4) left kidney.

7.3. Linear EUS pancreaticobiliary examination

7.3.1. Positioning the console, the patient, and the examiner

For a diagnostic examination of the pancreaticobiliary region, the console, the patient, and the examiner should be in the same position as for the radial instrument. If, however, you know that the examination will be followed by EUS-guided FNA, the console position will differ according to the location of the biopsy target. If the target is in the uncinate process or the juxta-ampullary segment of the head or pancreatic tail, the console should be positioned alongside the patient's head, with the examiner perpendicular to the patient's head facing the console, and with the endoscope handle also facing the console (handle in the closed position) or sometimes pressed against the upper right part of the examiner's chest (extreme closed position).

If the target is in the anterior segment of the head, in the posterior segment of the hepatic pedicle (retrobiliary or pre-caval lymph node), at the junction between the neck and head or in the pancreatic body, the console should be positioned parallel to the patient's lower limbs with the examiner facing the patient, and the endoscope handle facing the patient or sometimes in the open position, i.e. facing the console.

In contrast, with an examination performed with a radial instrument, which frequently uses clockwise and anti-clockwise rotation of the handle and where the hand holding the endoscope shaft just advances or retracts the instrument, examination with a linear instrument obviously uses clockwise or anti-clockwise rotation of the handle but this may sometimes be insufficient and the hand holding the shaft also has to be used to apply torque in a clockwise or anti-clockwise direction while advancing or withdrawing the instrument.

7.3.2. Examination of the neck and body-tail segment of the pancreas

This examination is carried out through the stomach. Examining the pancreatic and retroperitoneal anatomy is less routine with a linear instrument than with a radial instrument. It is even more crucial with this technique to follow the main vascular and duct landmarks in order to locate the various segments of the pancreatic gland. It is possible to study almost the entire pancreas through the stomach with the linear instrument, not just the neck, body and tail. Only the ampullary and periampullary region, the juxta-duodenal

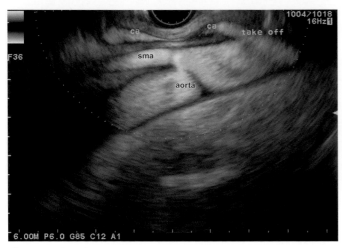

Figure 51 Ca, celiac axis; sma, superior mesenteric artery.

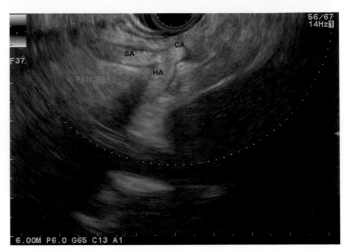

Figure 53 CA, celiac axis; SA, splenic artery; HA, hepatic artery.

segment of the head and uncinate process cannot be examined by the transgastric route.

There are two approaches to pancreaticobiliary examination through the stomach:

- Follow the aorta from the cardia region to the celiac trunk. Locate the aorta at the cardia, then position it in a longitudinal plane and advance the endoscope following the aorta lengthwise. While following it, locate the origin of the celiac trunk (Fig. 5) and immediately below it the origin of the superior mesenteric artery (Fig. 51). The celiac trunk can be followed longitudinally downwards, allowing visualization of the bifurcation into the splenic and hepatic arteries after observing the takeoff of the left gastric artery (Fig. 52) which climbs to the right of the screen. The pancreatic body appears below the bifurcation of the splenic artery and the hepatic artery (Fig. 53). If the endoscope handle is turned clockwise, the pancreatic gland can be followed towards the tail. If the handle is turned anti-clockwise, the right segment of the pancreatic body is visualized; descending a little, the pancreatic neck and the junction between the neck and the anterior segment of the pancreatic head

become visible (Fig. 54). The pancreatic duct can be followed at the genu and it can then be seen descending to the bottom of the screen to the right, then to the posterior segment of the pancreatic head. The origin of the duct of Santorini can sometimes be seen, descending to the left of the screen, extending towards the duodenum, located by air present in the duodenal lumen. By turning the endoscope handle clockwise, withdrawing the instrument slightly upwards, the pancreas can be followed to the left segment of the pancreatic body (Fig. 55A), then the pancreatic tail (Fig. 55B), thus arriving at the splenic hilum (Fig. 55C). It is often necessary to add clockwise torque to the endoscope shaft to increase the clockwise rotation, which is often insufficient when applied only to the endoscope handle.

- Alternatively, begin the examination by following the left lobe of the liver with the endoscope handle in the open position (anti-clockwise); the left lobe of the liver appears in the bottom half of the screen and you will see the left portal branch in the left lobe. You can then advance the endoscope and follow this left portal branch to the hilum of the liver where it receives the

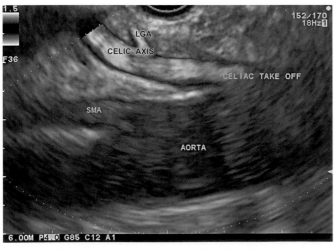

Figure 52 SMA, superior mesenteric artery; LGA, left gastric artery.

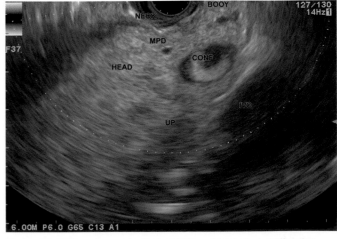

Figure 54 MPD, main pancreatic duct; UP, uncinate process; IVC, inferior vena cava; conf, portal vein confluence.

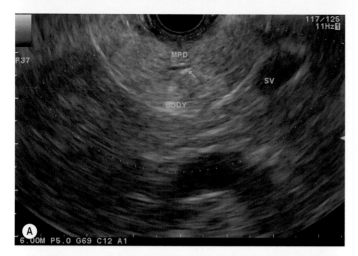

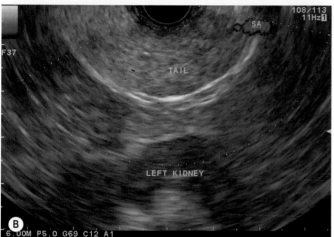

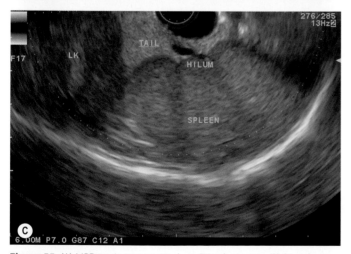

Figure 55 (A) MPD, main pancreatic duct; SV, splenic vein. (B) SA, splenic artery. (C) LK, left kidney.

right portal branch to form the portal vein. By advancing the endoscope and following the portal vein, the superior mesenteric vein appears (Fig. 56) by turning the endoscope handle clockwise (moving it from the open position to the neutral position). Once you have found the superior mesenteric vein, which has a horizontal path on the screen, the uncinate process and the posterior segment of the pancreatic

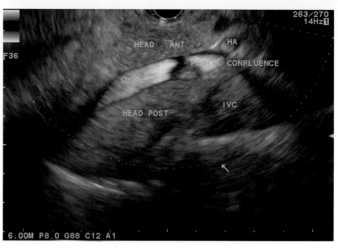

Figure 56 HA, hepatic artery; IVC: inferior vena cava.

head can be visualized below the superior mesenteric vein. By withdrawing the echoendoscope and turning the handle anti-clockwise, you can return to the portal vein then to the hepatic hilum, whereas if you retract the endoscope, while turning clockwise, you can follow the splenic vein (Fig. 57) to the splenic hilum. The superior mesenteric artery is easy to find from the aorta located at the cardia. Once the origin of the superior mesenteric artery has been observed, you can follow its longitudinal path by advancing the endoscope and maintaining suitable angulation, until you arrive over the uncinate process. It is then easy to find the superior mesenteric vein (Fig. 58), which runs parallel to the superior mesenteric artery, by applying anti-clockwise rotation. The hepatic artery can also be followed from the bifurcation of the celiac trunk, usually by advancing the endoscope with anti-clockwise rotation, whereas the splenic artery can usually be followed by straightening the endoscope into the up position and applying clockwise rotation.

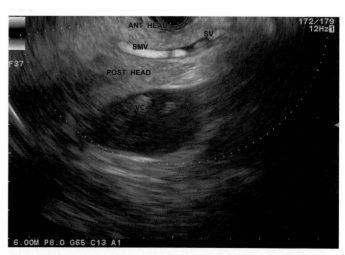

Figure 57 SMV, superior mesenteric vein; SV, splenic vein; IVC, inferior vena cava.

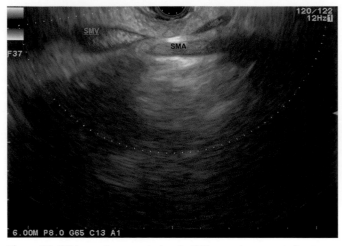

Figure 58 SMV, superior mesenteric vein; SMA, superior mesenteric artery.

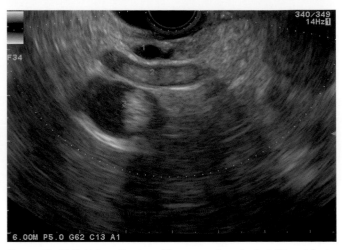

Figure 60 (1) Right hepatic artery, (2) common hepatic duct, (3) portal vein.

7.3.3. Transduodenal examination of the pancreaticobiliary region

The gallbladder (Fig. 59) is easy to observe through the duodenal bulb by turning the endoscope handle anti-clockwise. Once it has been visualized, the common bile duct can be located by advancing the endoscope slightly into the duodenal bulb and applying clockwise rotation. The common bile duct then appears between the duodenum and the right hepatic artery and the mesenteric-portal vein confluence (Fig. 60). If you continue to advance the endoscope, maintaining clockwise rotation, you will follow the common bile duct to the rear of the pancreatic head (Fig. 61) then see it enter the pancreatic head (Figs 62, 63) and terminate at the ampulla of Vater in the duodenum (Fig. 64). The appearance of the main pancreatic duct (Fig. 62) will have been observed in parallel, and can be followed in the same movement (Fig. 63) to its termination at the ampulla (Fig. 64). The reverse maneuver from the ampullary region, i.e. withdrawing the endoscope gently with anti-clockwise rotation, is sufficient to follow the bile duct as far as the hilum (Fig. 65). An alternative method of examining the common bile duct is to put the endoscope in the long position over the ampulla of Vater, then retract it progressively, maintaining maximum up

angulation, pressed against the ampullary region and turning the handle clockwise. In this way the uncinate process can be seen located within the angle between the inferior vena cava and the superior mesenteric vein, below and behind the end of the main pancreatic duct and CBD (Fig. 66A). When the

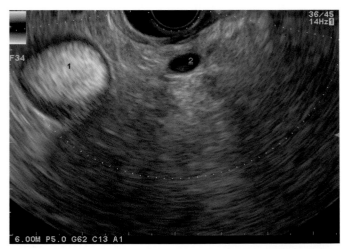

Figure 61 (1) Inferior vena cava, (2) CBD.

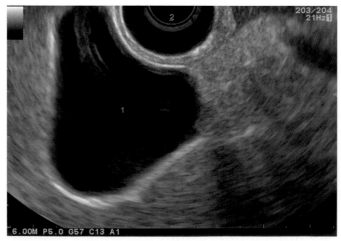

Figure 59 (1) Gallbladder, (2) duodenal bulb.

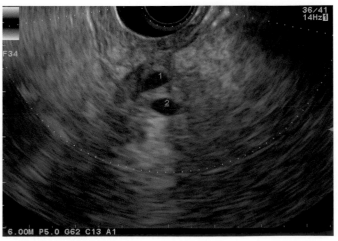

Figure 62 (1) CBD, (2) MPD.

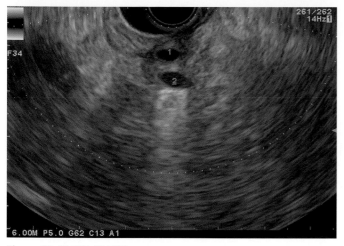

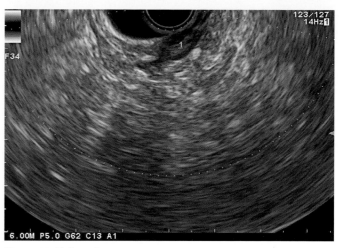

Figure 63 (1) CBD, (2) MPD.

Figure 64 (1) Ampulla.

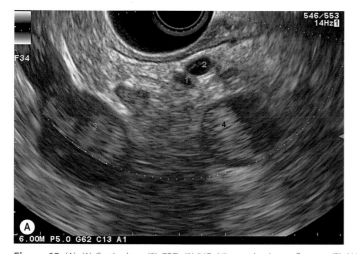

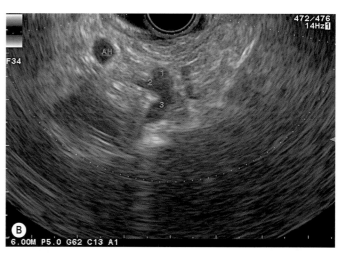

Figure 65 (A), (1) Cystic duct, (2) CBD, (3) IVC, (4) portal vein confluence. (B) AH, right hepatic artery; (1) common hepatic duct, (2) right hepatic duct, (3) left hepatic duct.

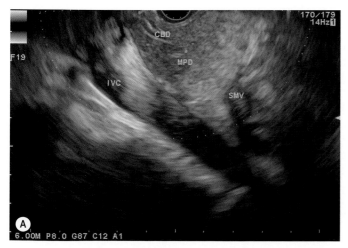

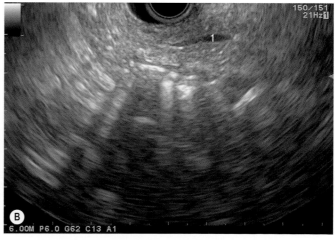

Figure 66 (A), IVC, inferior vena cava; CBD, common bile duct; MPD, main pancreatic duct; SMV, superior mesenteric vein. (B), (1) MPD.

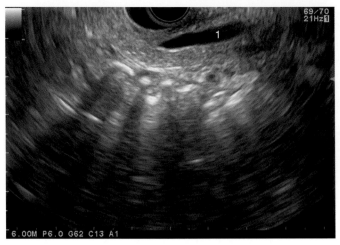

Figure 67 (1) CBD.

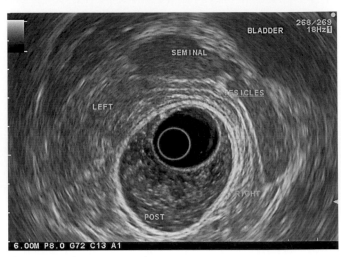

Figure 69 Mid-rectum in a male.

endoscope has reached the short position, you will see the termination of the pancreatic duct appear first (Fig. 66B), then the termination of the common bile duct, which can be followed for 2 or 3 cm (Fig. 67), i.e. along its intrapancreatic path.

8. How to examine the anorectal region

8.1. Anatomy

The patient is examined either supine or in left lateral decubitus. It is advisable to position the US console near the patient's head so the examiner is therefore standing alongside the patient's right thigh (Fig. 12).

The urogenital organs are the preferred landmarks for examination of the anorectal region for the lower and middle rectum, if the endoscope handle is held in the open position facing the console screen. The prostate (Fig. 68) and the seminal vesicles (Fig. 69) on the one hand, and the vagina (Fig. 70), cervix uteri and uterus on the other, are usually positioned at the top right of the screen, while the sacrum and coccyx are at the bottom left.

The seminal vesicles are usually located between 7 and 9 cm from the anal verge and constitute the limit between the lower and middle rectum. The line of reflection of the rectovesical pouch is located immediately above the seminal vesicles. It can thus be determined whether a cancer of the anterior wall of the rectum in a man is subperitoneal or above the rectovesical pouch.

In a woman, the rectovaginal septum separates the vagina from the anterior wall of the lower rectum; it continues upwards between the posterior vaginal fornix, which is behind the cervix uteri, and the lower part of the middle rectum, then upwards between the uterus (Fig. 71), also called the neck of the uterus, and the upper part of the middle rectum. The recto-uterine pouch, which is located to the rear of the uterus, begins above the rectovaginal septum.

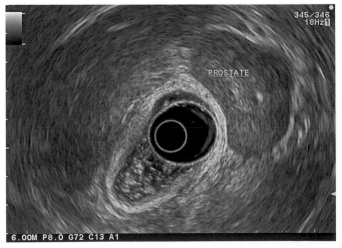

Figure 68 Lower rectum in a male.

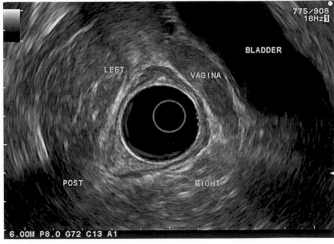

Figure 70 Lower rectum in a female.

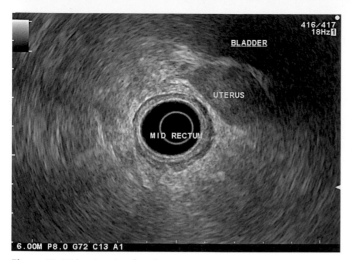

Figure 71 Mid-rectum in a female.

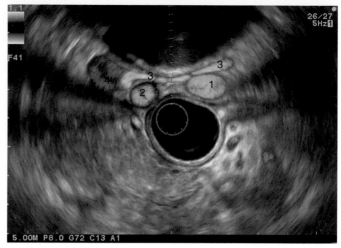

Figure 72 Cross-section of the promontory. (1) Left iliac artery, (2) right iliac artery, (3) left iliac vein, (4) right iliac vein.

Box 11 Examination of the rectum

- Performed in the supine or left lateral decubitus position.
- Introduce 100 cc of water into the rectum to flatten the angle between the middle and upper rectum.
- Try to reach the distal sigmoid colon, following the curves of the rectum, without insufflating air, to start the examination over the sacral promontory.

8.2. Anorectal examination

Examination of the lymph nodes in cancer of the rectum or anal canal should begin at the rectosigmoid junction, which should be reached while avoiding viewing the rectum endoscopically. To achieve this, about 100 cc of water should be instilled into the rectum to flatten the upper part of the rectum and advance the echoendoscope, moving progressively from the open position to the closed position, following the rectal curve revealed. Examination of the lymph

nodes therefore begins over the sacral promontory where the spine is visualized at the front along with the vascular structures (Fig. 72), which bifurcate and continue along the withdrawal path of the instrument to the lower rectum, advancing and withdrawing again whenever a round hypoechoic structure appears so as to clearly differentiate a lymph node from a vascular structure: the latter can be followed for a short distance and has a Doppler signal.

The instrument is therefore retracted progressively with anti-clockwise rotation moving from the closed to the open handle position on the way down from the upper rectum to the middle and lower rectum. The mesorectum and its external margin (the fascia recti) is clearly visible in patients when it is sufficiently fatty (Fig. 73).

The internal sphincter consists of a clearly visible, circular, hypoechoic band at least 2–3 mm thick (Fig. 74), in the anal canal. The striated external sphincter is less visible; over the anorectal junction and the lower part of the rectum, there is a longitudinal strip which surrounds the anorectal junction from the rear and extends anteriorly along both sides of the anorectal junction (Fig. 74). This is the puborectalis portion

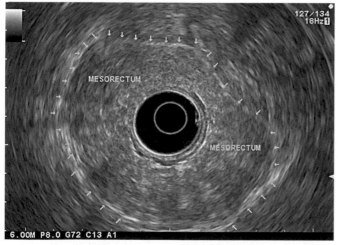

Figure 73 Mesorectum all around the upper part of the mid-rectum: white arrows: fascia recti (outer margin of the mesorectum).

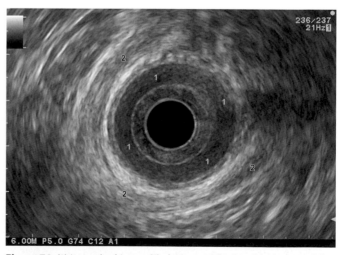

Figure 74 (1) Internal sphincter, (2) elevator ani (horizontal segment of the pubo-rectalis muscle).

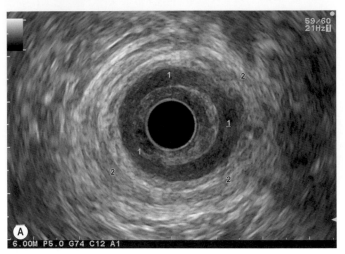 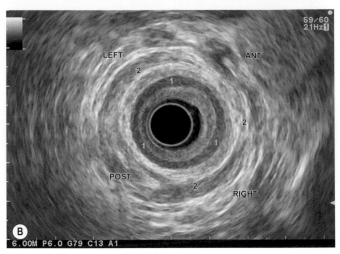

Figure 75 (A), (1) Internal sphincter, (2) circumferential segment of the external sphincter. (B) Anatomy of the male anal sphincter. (1) Internal sphincter, (2) circular striated sphincter.

of the levator ani and forms a circular sling around the internal sphincter (Fig. 75A). The sphincter anatomy is easy to locate in men (Fig. 75B) and more difficult in women, since the anterior side of the circular striated sphincter is usually fairly short.

9. Ultrasound terminology

9.1. Structure of the digestive wall and basis for interpretation in digestive oncology

At a frequency of 5, 7.5 or 12 MHz, endosonography shows that the wall of the esophagus, stomach, duodenum, rectum and colon consists of five layers (alternately hyper- and hypoechoic) (Fig. 1). Seven layers can sometimes be visualized, particularly in the rectum but also sometimes in the stomach and proximal esophagus in normal individuals (Fig. 76), or in the lower esophagus, particularly in those with a primary motor disorder such as achalasia. The significance of these layers has been determined by *in vivo* but mainly in *ex-vivo* studies and is now clearly established.

9.1.1. Wall with five layers (Fig. 76A)

*   The first echogenic layer is the interface between the GI tract lumen and the epithelium, to which the balloon is added when it is applied against the wall.
*   The second layer, which is hypoechoic, is the mucosa and perhaps part of the submucosa. The muscularis mucosae is included in this second layer and cannot therefore be identified separately.
*   The third layer, which is hyperechoic, forms the middle layer and corresponds to the submucosa, or at least to the majority of the submucosa, but also to the interface which separates the submucosa from the muscle layer.
*   The fourth layer, which is hypoechoic, is the muscularis propria.
*   The fifth layer, which is echogenic, is the interface between the muscularis propria and the peridigestive fat and is therefore equivalent to serosa or adventitia, depending on the organ.

9.1.2. Wall with seven layers (Fig. 76B)

The first three layers are the same as those visualized in a five-layer wall. The fourth layer is divided into three layers by a thin hyperechoic band which corresponds to the interface between the inner circular muscle layer and the outer longitudinal muscle layer, and both these layers are hypoechoic. The echogenic seventh layer is equivalent to the fifth layer of a five-layer wall, and thus corresponds to the interface between the muscularis propria and the peridigestive fat.

9.1.3. Wall with nine layers

By using (Fig. 77) very high frequency miniprobes (20 and especially 30 MHz) and the zoom on electronic radial 10 MHz instrument (Fig. 78), nine concentric layers can be visualized in the gut wall in the esophagus, but also the stomach.

*   The first layer is an echogenic layer, corresponding to the interface between the digestive lumen and the epithelium.
*   The second layer is hypoechoic and corresponds to the epithelium.
*   The third layer is echogenic and corresponds to the interface between the epithelium and the lamina propria, as well as the lamina propria itself.
*   The fourth layer, which is hypoechoic, corresponds to the muscularis mucosae.
*   The fifth layer, which is echogenic, corresponds to the submucosa.
*   The sixth layer, which is hypoechoic, corresponds to the inner circular muscle layer.
*   The seventh layer, which is echogenic, corresponds to the interface between the two layers of the muscularis propria.
*   The eighth layer, which is hypoechoic, corresponds to the outer longitudinal muscle layer.
*   The ninth layer, which is echogenic, corresponds to the interface between the muscularis propria and the peridigestive fat, and is equivalent to serosa or adventitia.

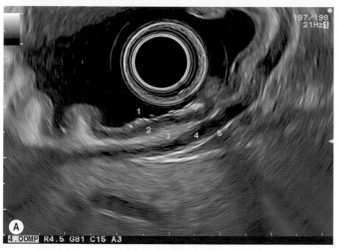

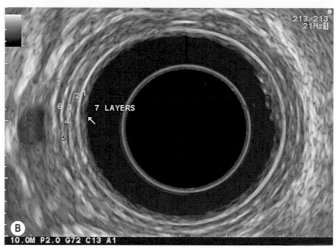

Figure 76 (A) Stomach wall with 5 layers. (1) interface between the gastric lumen and the epithelium, (2) mucosa including muscularis mucosae, (3)submucosa, (4) muscularis propria, (5) serosa. (B) Esophageal wall: seven layers are visualized with 10 MHz, electronic radial scope. (1) Balloon and epithelium, (2) mucosa including muscularis mucosae, (3) submucosa, (4) internal (circular) layer of the muscularis propria, (5) interface, (6) external (longitudinal) layer of the muscularis propria, (7) adventitia.

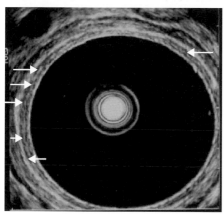

Figure 77 Esophageal wall: nine layers are visualized with the 30 MHz Olympus mechanical radial high frequency miniprobe covered with the Olympus balloon. Muscularis mucosae is visible (arrows) within the mucosa.

9.2. Tumor terminology

The endosonographic classification of GI tract cancers is based on the TNM classification. The cancer usually appears as a hypoechoic mass. The involvement of the wall will be determined based on the persistence or disruption of the echogenic layers, i.e. the echogenic middle third layer which corresponds (in a wall with five or seven layers) to the submucosa, and the echogenic outer-fifth layer, which corresponds, or is equivalent, in a five-layer wall, to serosa or adventitia (this also applies to the echogenic peripheral seventh layer of a seven-layer wall).

9.3. T1 tumor

A tumor that leaves all or part of the echogenic middle third layer intact (in a five- or seven-layer wall) is a T1 tumor (Fig. 79), i.e. a superficial tumor. With the frequencies currently in use (5–12 MHz), it is impossible to distinguish within the T1 category between a tumor located in the mucosa (T1m), which has a generally very low risk of lymph node involvement regardless of the organ affected, and a T1 tumor which has already invaded the submucosa (T1sm). These have a

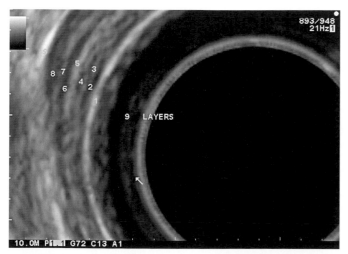

Figure 78 Esophageal wall: nine layers are visualized with a 10 MHz electronic radial scope using the zoom. (1) Interface between the digestive lumen and the epithelium. (2) Epithelium. (3) Interface between the epithelium and the lamina propria, as well as the lamina propria. (4) Muscularis mucosae. (5) Submucosa. (6) Inner circular muscle. (7) Interface between the two layers of the muscularis propria. (8) Outer longitudinal muscle layer. (9) Serosa or adventitia.

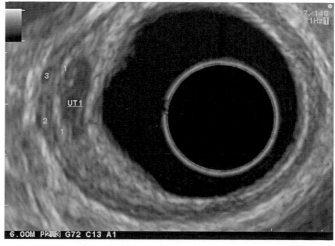

Figure 79 Nodular UT1 squamous esophageal cancer. (1) Submucosa, (2) interface, (3) external (longitudinal) layer of the muscularis propria.

Table 2   Risk of lymph node involvement according to submucosal involvement

	Squamous esophageal cancer	Esophageal adenocarcinoma	Gastric cancer	Colon cancer	Rectal cancer
Risk of lymph node involvement for T1sm tumors (%)	19–45	3–15	5–15	3–10	5–15

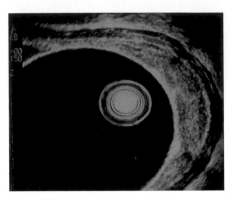

Figure 80   Nodular (O-Is) uT1 m3 squamous esophageal cancer.

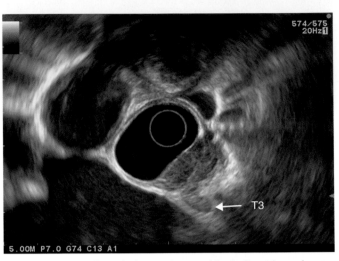

Figure 83   UT3 esophageal adenocarcinoma arising in Barrett's esophagus.

distinctly poorer prognosis as there is a significant risk of lymph node involvement, which varies depending on the tumor site (Table 2), degree of differentiation and the presence of lymphovascular invasion.

By using very high frequency miniprobes (20–30 MHz), it is possible to stage these lesions more accurately and select those that may benefit from endoscopic resection or ablation.

From an endosonographic perspective, with regard to the esophagus and stomach, tumors eligible for curative endoscopic treatment are conventionally those that have not infiltrated the muscularis mucosae (hypoechoic fourth layer), if it has been correctly located in the nine layers visualized using a very high frequency miniprobe (preferably 30 MHz) (Figs 77, 80).

9.4. T2 tumor

In a wall with five or seven layers, a cancer accompanied by the disappearance of the echogenic middle third layer but leaving the echogenic peripheral fifth layer (or the echogenic peripheral seventh layer in a wall with seven layers) intact theoretically corresponds to a T2 cancer (a cancer that has invaded the muscularis propria) (Figs 81, 82). In 10% of cases, a cancer accompanied by the disappearance of the echogenic middle third layer (submucosa) is overstaged as T2 when it is really a T1 cancer because the submucosa can be entirely invaded by the tumor, without the muscle layer being involved (sm3).

9.5. T3 and T4 tumor

In a wall with five or seven layers, the disappearance of the fifth or the seventh layer corresponds to a T3 tumor (Fig. 83). In such cases T2 tumors are overstaged as T3 in 5–10% of cases. A tumor is staged T4 when the cancer is invading a neighboring organ.

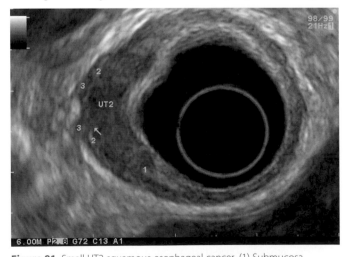

Figure 81   Small UT2 squamous esophageal cancer. (1) Submucosa, (2) Interface between the circular and the longitudinal part of the muscularis propria, (3) External (longitudinal) layer of the muscularis propria.

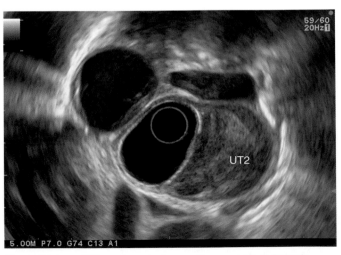

Figure 82   Large UT2 esophageal adenocarcinoma arising in Barrett's esophagus.

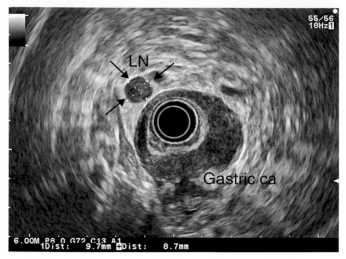

Figure 84 Typical small (9 mm) metastatic lymph node (LN), spherical, hypoechogenic, well demarcated, with smaller diameter >5 mm.

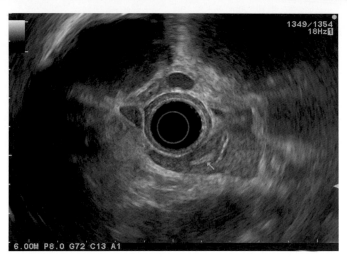

Figure 86 Large (25 mm) benign subcarinal lymph node. Triangular shape and hyperechogenic center (arrow).

9.6. Regional lymph nodes

9.6.1. Lymph node appearances

Metastatic lymph nodes usually appear as round, hypoechoic, finely heterogeneous, spherical structures, i.e. round in all planes and with a well-defined border (Fig. 84). They are sometimes more echogenic (Fig. 85), but this is observed only if the tumor itself is relatively echogenic, since the echostructure of the metastatic lymph node is comparable with that of the primary tumor. They are sometimes very hypoechoic and even anechoic, but in this case their echostructure is also comparable with that of the primary tumor. The presence of readily identifiable lymph nodes in areas that are usually unaffected is an important indicator of malignancy in these lymph nodes, particularly if the lymph node area in question drains directly from the primary tumor (usually on the same side, particularly in the mediastinum). Silicosis (as regards the posterior mediastinum) and some lymph node diseases such as sarcoidosis, histoplasmosis, lymph node tuberculosis or malignant non-Hodgkin's lymphomas may be accompanied by lymph node

anomalies affecting numerous subdiaphragmatic or posterior mediastinal areas, thus mimicking massive lymph node involvement where associated with esophageal, stomach or lung cancer. It is very rare for a digestive tract or lung cancer to coexist with a lymph node disease causing massive enlargement of the peridigestive lymph nodes, but the possibility should not be disregarded.

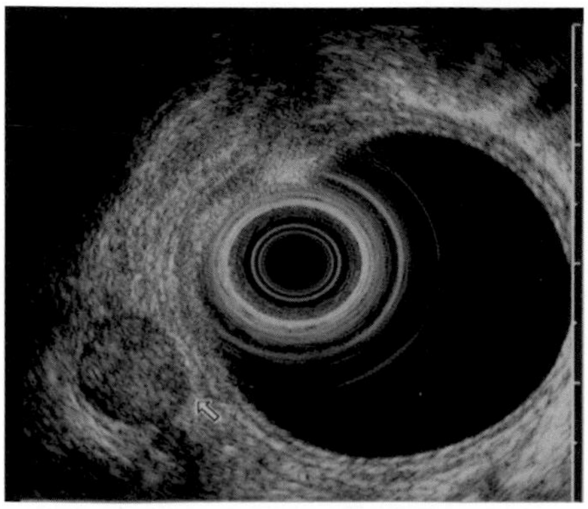

9.6.2. Lymph node size

Lymph node size is a criterion of malignant or benign disease. Having a maximum diameter greater than or equal to 1 cm for an oval or round, spherical lymph node (i.e. as large in height as in transverse section) is a very good criterion of malignancy. Having a minimum diameter ≥5 mm for an oval or round, spherical lymph node is also a very good criterion of malignancy.

Very small non-metastatic lymph nodes (reactive or physiological) may be either very hypoechoic, homogeneous, with a distinct border, but are flat (not spherical). They are usually relatively hyperechoic, oval, but not spherical (flat) or triangular, and they are more echogenic than the primary tumor. The presence of calcification, particularly in the subcarinal region and hepatic pedicle, is a sign of benign disease, when the calcifications remain central and are not disorganized. The presence of a linear hyperechoic band (known as a lymph node sinus) in the middle of the lymph node (Fig. 13E) or apparently aiming towards the center of the lymph node (Fig. 86) from its periphery is also a sign of benign disease when a lymph node is enlarged. The interpretation of this phenomenon is that the cause of the enlargement has not had the effect of disrupting the lymph node architecture as an invasive tumor would do. This obviously does not exclude the presence of micrometastasis.

9.7. EUS-FNA

The advent of fine-needle biopsy and EUS-FNA (Fig. 87) has totally altered the debate concerning the specificity of

Figure 85 Small (7 mm) metastatic hyperechogenic lymph node.

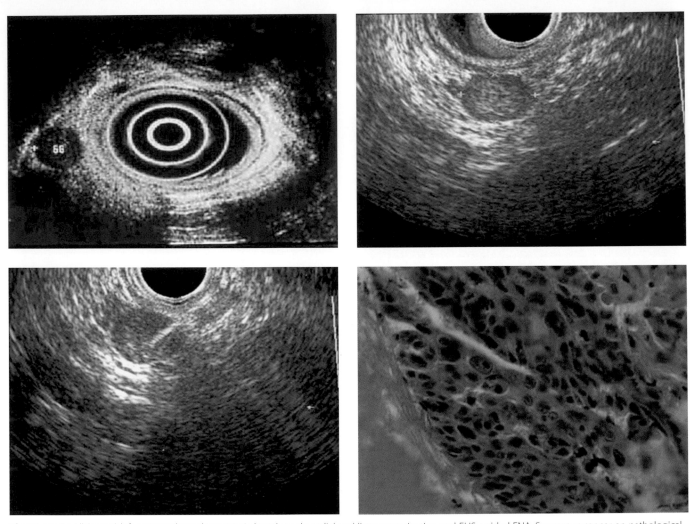

Figure 87 Small (7 mm) left paraesophageal metastatic lymph node, radial and linear examination and EUS-guided FNA. Squamous cancer on pathological examination obtained with 22 G needle.

endosonographic appearances of lymph nodes for a diagnosis of malignancy, regardless of whether they are periesophageal posterior mediastinal or perigastric and in particular celiac or perirectal lymph nodes. The diagnostic accuracy of EUS-FNA of accessible lymph nodes is 90%, which is clearly higher than that obtained by analysis of the EUS morphological features, which varies from 60% to 75% depending on the cancer examined. This improvement in the diagnostic accuracy is related to an improvement in specificity, which is close to 100%. The positive predictive value of malignancy is therefore close to 100%. On the other hand, the sensitivity of EUS-FNA depends on the diameter of the lymph node examined. It is approximately 70% for lymph nodes measuring less than 10 mm in short axis, whereas it is more than 90% for lymph nodes measuring ≥10 mm. This lack of sensitivity explains the negative predictive value for malignancy (ability of the method to strictly exclude a malignant diagnosis) which is approximately 75% (50% when the short axis diameter is <10 mm, 80% when it is ≥10 mm). In other words, when EUS-FNA of a lymph node measuring <10 mm does not yield any evidence of malignancy, there is a 50% chance that this is true, whereas when it yields evidence of malignancy, this is almost always the case. In some locations, the sensitivity and specificity of the EUS image of a spherical hypoechoic lymph node measuring >1 cm and with a distinct border, are greater for a diagnosis of malignancy than the result of EUS-guided FNA; this applies mainly to lymph nodes in the celiac region when they are associated with esophageal cancer.

10. Endosonography in gastrointestinal oncology

10.1. Introduction

Gastrointestinal endosonography has two roles in the diagnosis of cancer of the digestive tract: linitis plastica (where the endosonographic appearance is characteristic) and in assessing the etiology of rectal or esophageal strictures where pathology has been non-diagnostic. In these cases identification of an intraparietal mass by endosonography confirms that these strictures are malignant in origin.

With these exceptions, EUS is not used to diagnose digestive cancers, as the diagnosis of malignancy relies exclusively on histological analysis of biopsies obtained at conventional endoscopy.

10.2. Assessment of GI cancers prior to neoadjuvant therapy or surgery

An imaging technique such as endosonography is useful for assessing locoregional involvement of accessible gastrointestinal cancers prior to treatment only in patients for whom a therapeutic option exists and in whom an accurate assessment of locoregional involvement will influence management.

In contrast, EUS is not useful for assessing pre treatment locoregional involvement of these cancers when it will not alter management (e.g. in colon cancer where surgery is indicated immediately, regardless of locoregional involvement – Dukes A–C), where there is only one curative option or when, for one reason or another (advanced age, co-morbidity, obvious metastatic involvement, etc.) palliative treatment or supportive therapy is more appropriate.

Endosonography is not equally useful for all tumors and its role can be separated into two parts:

10.2.1. Decision-making

For guiding the choice of therapy, for example when the detection of aortic involvement in a patient with cancer of the middle third of the esophagus contraindicates primary resection, when the detection of submucosal involvement as far as the middle third of the esophagus of a cardiac cancer will require subtotal esophagectomy, when preoperative radiotherapy is indicated if involvement of the perirectal fat is found in a patient with rectal cancer inaccessible to digital examination, or when localized transanal resection or endoscopic mucosal resection is indicated with involvement limited to the mucosa or at most the submucosa without suspicious lymph nodes in a small rectal cancer.

10.2.2. Monitoring

The pre-therapeutic examination serves as a reference and will allow an assessment of the therapeutic efficacy of non-surgical treatment (i.e. in gastric lymphoma, anal cancer or linitis plastica, for example) or neoadjuvant treatment (i.e. radiotherapy or chemotherapy in esophageal cancer, prior to surgery).

Box 12   Esophageal cancer

How is a full assessment of the locoregional involvement of esophageal cancer carried out with endosonography?

- Start with high definition UGI endoscopy for an accurate assessment of the location in relation to the incisors, the length of the tumor, whether it is stenotic, and the Paris classification for early cancer (see Chapter 3 for details). Lugol's staining should be performed for squamous cell cancer, or staining with acetic acid and indigo carmine for adenocarcinoma arising in Barrett's esophagus. If the stenosis is impassable with a videoendoscope, use a nasogastroscope.
- Use radial EUS to assess the T and N stage, including the celiac region, and if this is affected, continue into the duodenum to look for lumbar aortic, retroduodenopancreatic and hepatic lymph node involvement.
- If lymph node involvement is suspected, use a linear echoendoscope to perform EUS FNA of all suspicious lymph nodes if involvement is exclusively regional (N1), beginning with the most remote lymph nodes (M1a), if present.
- If the radial echoendoscope will not pass through the stenosis, use an Olympus MH 908 blind probe, a 7.5 MHz miniprobe or a linear echoendoscope that is used for EUS FNA.
- If none of these options are possible, dilate the stenosis to 13 mm, if a videoendoscope 10 mm in diameter has passed through it.
- If the stenosis was impassable with a 10 mm videoendoscope, do not dilate and conclude that the EUS examination cannot be completed.

10.3. Esophageal cancer

It has been acknowledged for more than 10 years, that endosonography is superior to all the imaging techniques available for assessment of locoregional (parietal and lymph node) involvement in esophageal cancers, when the instrument can pass through the tumor. The endosonographic TNM stage correlates better with the prognosis in particular with 5-year survival than the stage determined by CT, and correlates very well with the pTNM stage.

10.3.1. Performance

Overall, the diagnostic accuracy of endosonography for parietal involvement is 85% (Figs 79, 81–83, 88), whereas

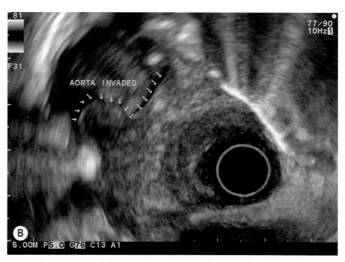

Figure 88 (A) Large squamous esophageal cancer with invasion of the anterior side of the descending aorta (ao). (B) Large squamous esophageal cancer with a large nodule invading (arrows) the descending aorta.

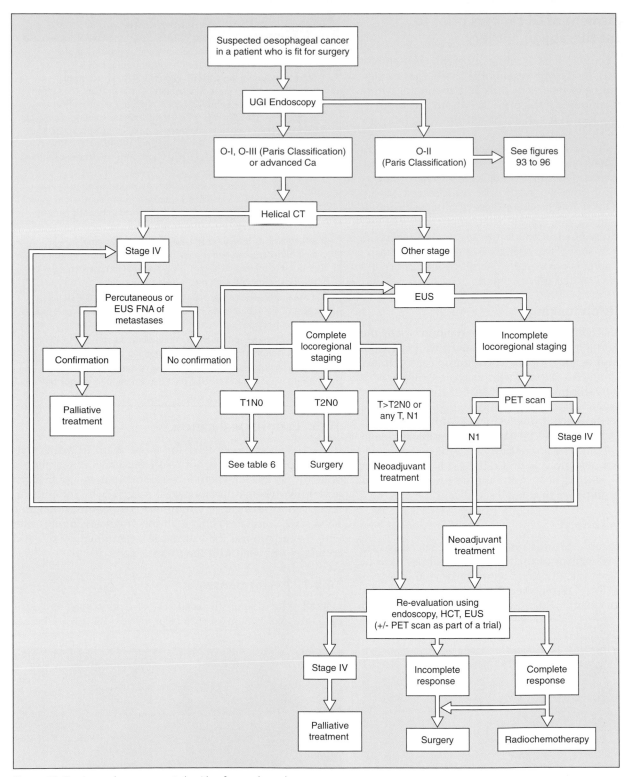

Figure 89 Staging and management algorithm for esophageal cancer.

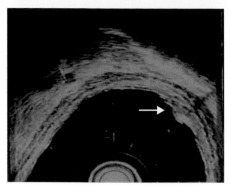

Figure 90 Early flat slightly elevated (0–IIa), squamous esophageal cancer, uT1m2 visualized with 30 MHz Olympus high frequency miniprobe.

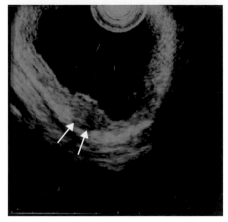

Figure 92 Early uT1sm1 squamous esophageal cancer visualized with the Olympus 30 MHz miniprobe.

the diagnostic accuracy for lymph node involvement is 80%. The diagnostic accuracy is comparable from one T stage to another, although it is not quite as good for stage T2.

The role of endosonography in relation to CT of the chest and abdomen is now well established. CT scanning is used to assess for any hepatic and pulmonary metastases, while endosonography is used for assessment of locoregional involvement if there is no evidence of distant metastases. The role of positron emission tomography (PET scan) is not yet clear, however, owing to its cost and accessibility and to the results of studies of its advantages compared with helical CT and EUS, it makes sense to limit its use to prospective trials or cases in which it is impossible to carry out a full assessment by EUS (Fig. 89).

10.3.2. Squamous HGD and early esophageal squamous cell cancers

Curative endoscopic treatment of early squamous cell cancer of the esophagus applies to tumors with a very low risk of

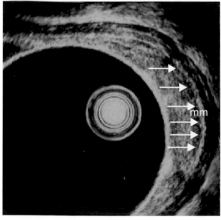

Figure 91 Early uT1m3 squamous esophageal cancer visualized with the Olympus 30 MHz miniprobe. mm: muscularis mucosae.

lymph node involvement, which have not spread to the muscularis mucosae.

Owing to the advent of very high frequency miniprobes, the muscularis mucosae can now be visualized in a high percentage of significant cases. If this technique is applied to a squamous cell cancer with an endoscopic appearance of a flat tumor, it yields a diagnostic accuracy of 85% for detecting infiltration confined to the mucosa, accessible to curative endoscopic mucosal resection (0–3% of metastatic lymph node involvement in this type of cancer). Diagnostic errors are almost always overestimates (demonstration of involvement of the submucosa when the muscularis mucosae has not been infiltrated), related to peritumoral inflammation. Standard EUS should be performed routinely to confirm that the tumor is T1 (the submucosa has not been infiltrated) and N0 (with no apparently metastatic lymph nodes in the peridigestive region). If the patient is operable, he or she may be referred to a practitioner with experience of very high frequency miniprobes once the tumor has been classified as usT1N0 using a standard echoendoscope, so that only usT1mN0 patients are offered endoscopic mucosal resection (EMR) or endoscopic mucosal dissection (ESD) (Figs 90–92), since these techniques are not without significant complications. The use of very high frequency miniprobes is clearly essential before the use of photodynamic therapy and radiofrequency ablation for the treatment of high-grade dysplasia and intramucosal carcinoma with visible lesions, since these destructive techniques do not yield histological confirmation (as after EMR or ESD) of the effectiveness of the treatment. Figures 93 and 94 show the indications of EUS for early squamous cell cancers.

10.3.3. Early Barrett's cancer

The role of EUS is summarized in Figures 95 and 96.

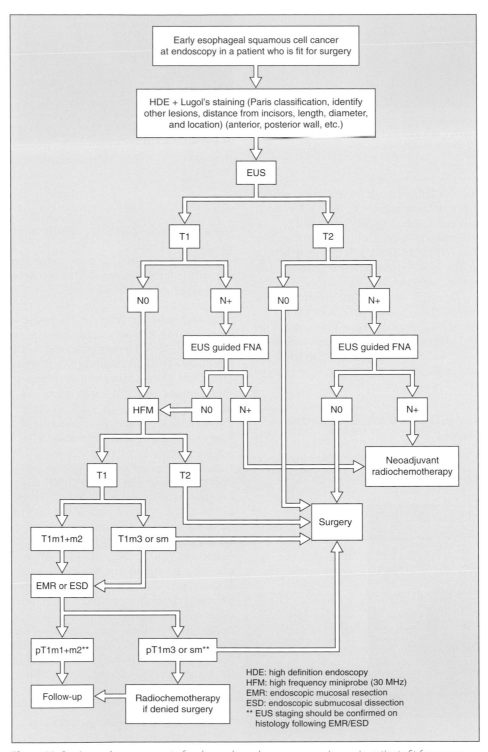

Figure 93 Staging and management of early esophageal squamous carcinoma in patients fit for surgery.

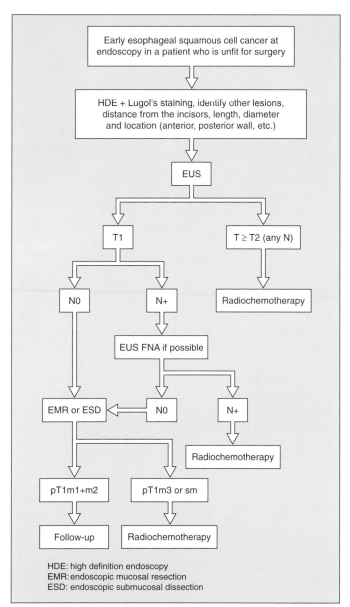

Figure 94 Staging and management of early esophageal squamous carcinoma in patients not fit for surgery.

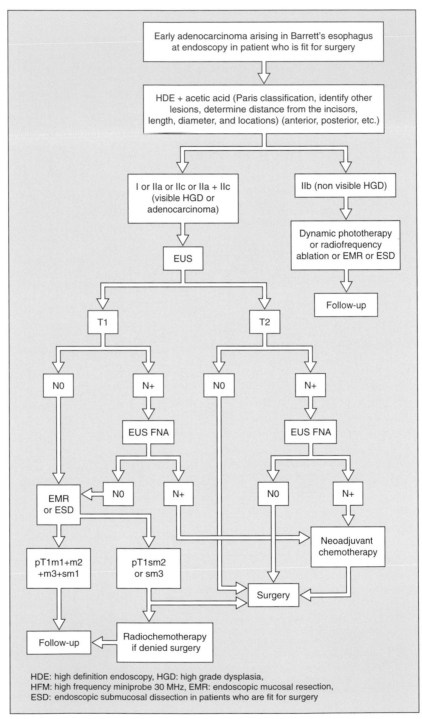

Figure 95   Staging and management of early esophageal adenocarcinoma in patients fit for surgery.

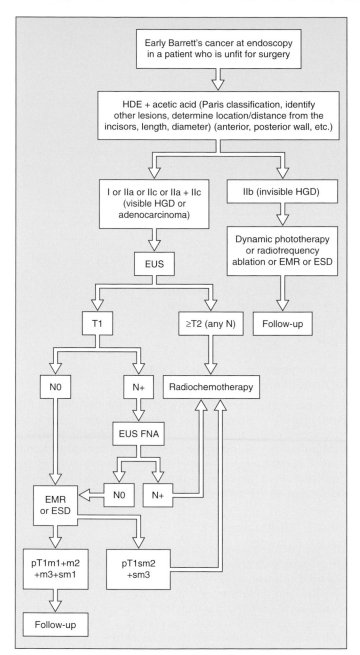

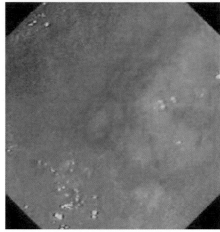

Figure 97 Early flat slightly elevated (Paris classification O–IIa) gastric adenocarcinoma.

Since the advent of preoperative neoadjuvant therapy, the use of EUS after CT is far commoner (Figs 101, 102) in order to select patients who may be immediately operable (usT2N0M0) and those who should receive neoadjuvant treatment (Fig. 93) (us T >T2 or any T N+).

Overall, the diagnostic accuracy of endosonography is 80% for parietal T involvement and 70% for lymph node involvement. Errors involve overstaging T1 tumors as T2 and T2 tumors as T3. This occurs in gastric cancers owing to the frequency of ulcerating cancers which are responsible for particularly extensive peritumoral fibrous and inflammation, leading to over-estimation of the depth of the tumor involvement.

10.4.1. Junctional/cardia cancers

Junctional cancer has two features which complicate management compared to other stomach cancers:

- If there is significant esophageal involvement (Sievert type I), esophagectomy with mediastinal dissection is performed with a thoracotomy by either the left or right route depending on the length of esophageal involvement, which is combined with a gastrectomy
- Peri-esophageal posterior mediastinal metastatic lymph node involvement is observed in 20% of cases, particularly in the subcarinal region, which then

Figure 96 Staging and management of early esophageal adenocarcinoma in patients not fit for surgery.

10.4. Gastric cancer

Until recently, preoperative endosonographic assessment of locoregional involvement of gastric cancer was not routinely considered, as it was for esophageal cancer, because unlike esophageal cancer, gastric cancer was considered above all a surgical cancer and as such an EUS assessment was indicated only if the information obtained was likely to alter the therapeutic strategy, i.e.:

- To guide the surgical resection (for cardiac cancer)
- To avoid excessive resection for a small tumor in a patient at high surgical risk (Figs 97, 98)
- To exclude inappropriate curative surgery for a large tumor in a patient with impaired general health and suspected extensive locoregional involvement (Figs 99, 100).

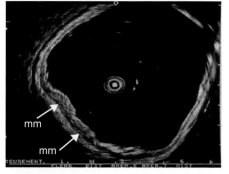

Figure 98 Same patient as Figure 79. Early uT1m2 gastric cancer visualized with the 30 MHz Olympus high frequency miniprobe. mm: muscularis mucosae.

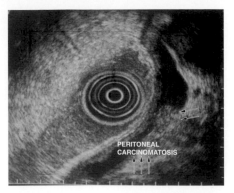

Figure 99 Gastric cancer with peritoneal carcinomatosis located within the lesser sac.

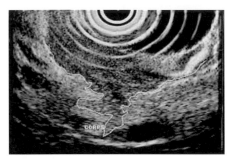

Figure 100 Advanced gastric cancer with invasion of the pancreatic body.

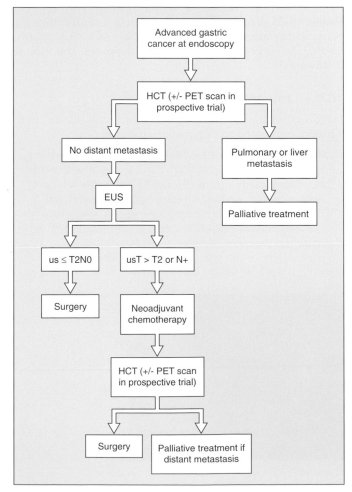

Figure 101 Stage-directed management of advanced gastric cancer.

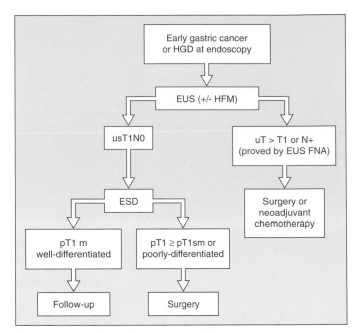

Figure 102 Stage-directed management of early gastric cancer.

requires esophagectomy and mediastinal node dissection by right thoracotomy.

Neither endoscopy with biopsy, CT nor barium studies have proved satisfactory for determining the esophageal involvement of cardiac cancers and visualizing posterior mediastinal lymph node involvement. On the other hand, endosonography has proved effective in resolving these two problems. It is therefore essential in the pre-therapeutic assessment of this type of cancer.

10.4.2. Linitis plastica

Linitis plastica is often difficult to diagnose (>50% of cases are missed) with endoscopy and biopsies. The entirely characteristic endosonographic appearance of this disease makes EUS the best diagnostic technique (Figs 103, 104). Besides its role in the differential diagnosis of benign hypertrophic gastritis (Figs 105, 106) and linitis plastica, gastric endosonography is capable of detecting minimal ascites which indicates

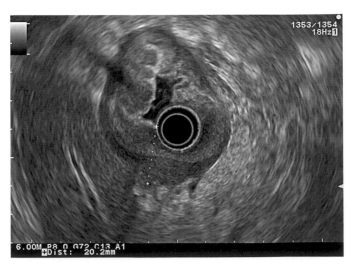

Figure 103 Linitis plastica uT3.

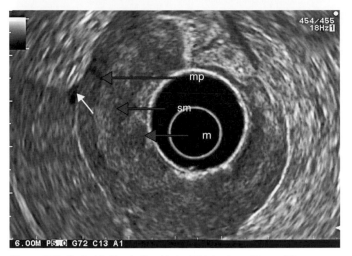

Figure 104 Typical linitis plastica. Marked thickening of the wall layers. m, Mucosa; sm, submucosa; mp, muscularis propria. Small amount of ascitis highly suggestive of peritoneal carcinomatosis (white arrow).

peritoneal carcinosis, undetected by other imaging techniques (Fig. 104). It is also useful for demonstrating infiltration of adjacent organs, in particular the corporeo-caudal region of the pancreas (usually between 45 and 50 cm from the incisors facing the posterior side), or the transverse mesocolon (under the pancreatic body facing the horizontal greater antral curve). The same applies for detecting submucosal involvement upwards to the esophagus or downwards to the duodenal bulb. The results of EUS FNA for the diagnosis of linitis plastica are poor (sensitivity <30%).

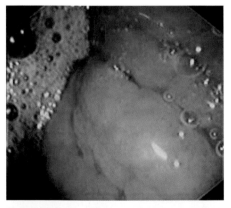

Figure 105 Giant folds gastritis. Ménétrier's disease.

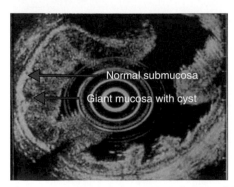

Figure 106 Ménétrier's disease. Typical aspect of this benign disease with giant gastric folds: huge thickening of the mucosa with normal submucosa.

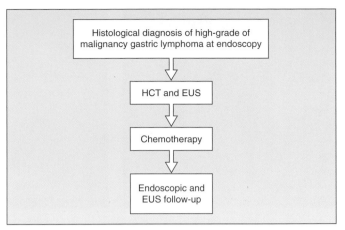

Figure 107 Management of high-grade gastric lymphoma.

10.4.3. Gastric lymphomas (Figs 107, 108)

There are several EUS features (Figs 109–111) of gastric lymphomas: flat, large folds, nodular or polypoid, or infiltrated pseudolinitis. None of these features are specific for the diagnosis, despite what was initially described. The diagnosis of lymphoma is a histological diagnosis obtained easily from biopsies performed during endoscopy. The main benefit of endosonography is thus in assessing locoregional involvement. Endosonography is very effective for

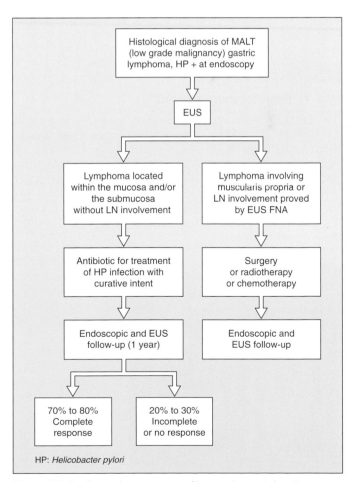

Figure 108 Staging and management of low-grade gastric lymphoma (MALToma).

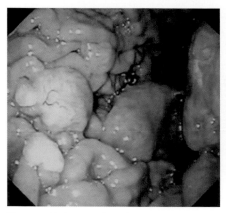
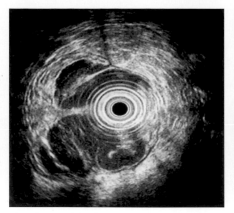
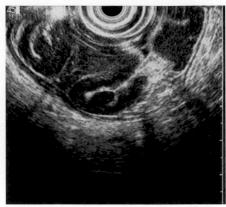

Figure 109 Low-grade malignancy arising in a MALT lymphoma of the fundus. Endoscopic view of giant gastric folds. Hypoechogenic thickening well confined to the mucosa.

this purpose with a diagnostic accuracy in the order of 90% for T staging and 80% for N staging. In low-malignancy MALT lymphoma, endosonography is the most reliable predictor of a response to *Helicobacter pylori* eradication. In addition to the efficacy of antibiotic treatment on *H. pylori* eradication, two pre-therapeutic endosonographic criteria are highly predictive of a good response, and these are infiltration confined to the mucosa or the superficial part of the submucosa (tumor thickness <5 mm) and the absence of lymph node involvement detectable by EUS. If both these criteria are met, the response rate (complete remission) 18 months after successful *H. pylori* eradication is 70–80%.

10.5. Rectal cancer

10.5.1. Parietal involvement

The diagnostic accuracy of endosonography for the parietal involvement of rectal cancers according to the TNM classification varies from 75–95%. It is in the order of 95% for T1 tumors (Figs 112, 113), 75% for T2 tumors (Fig. 114), 90% for T3 tumors (Fig. 115) and 95% for T4 tumors. The distinction between a T1 tumor and greater involvement (T2 to T4) is 95%. The distinction between a tumor located in the wall (T1, T2) and a tumor that has reached the fat or an adjacent organ (T3, T4) is 90%.

10.5.2. Lymph node involvement

Lymph node involvement is correctly predicted in 70% of cases (Fig. 116). Round (splenical) shape, hypoechogenic, well demarcated, >5 mm in smaller diameter are criteria suggesting malignancy.

10.5.3. In summary

Endosonography is significantly superior to clinical examination and CT for assessing parietal and lymph node involvement. Comparisons have also shown that endosonography is superior to MRI for assessing the spread of localized tumors to the wall, equivalent for assessing the spread of advanced tumors (T3)), and equally sensitive for assessing lymph node involvement. Furthermore, EUS FNA can be carried out if necessary (which improves the specificity of the method). MRI seems to be more accurate than EUS in case of T4 cancer of the upper rectum. The management of early rectal cancer is summarized in Figure 117. Actually, since the last 2 years, the management of advanced rectal cancer has changed because of the better efficacy of the neo-adjuvant chemoradiation therapy in comparison with radiotherapy

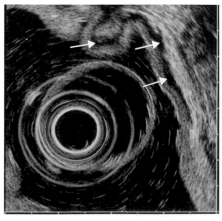

Figure 110 Low-grade malignancy arising in a MALT lymphoma. Hypoechogenic thickening of the inner part of the submucosa.

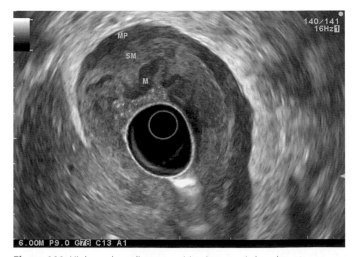

Figure 111 High-grade malignancy arising in a gastric lymphoma. Considerable thickening of the different wall layers which are still visible. M, mucosa; SM, submucosa; MP, muscularis propria.

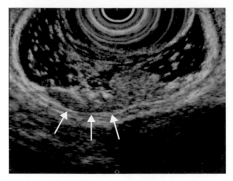

Figure 112 uT1 Rectal cancer confined to the mucosa. Submucosa is intact (white arrows).

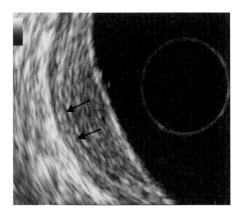

Figure 113 T1 rectal cancer confined to the mucosa. Muscularis mucosae is well visualized (black arrows), but not invaded.

alone. The indications of neoadjuvant chemo-radiation therapy have dramatically increased. Any rectal cancer which is staged by EUS or MRI as T >T2 receives neoadjuvant chemoradiation therapy whatever the circumferential margin is more or less than 1 mm. Moreover, any lymph node visualized by EUS or MRI leads to chemoradiation therapy. Thus, the specific indications of MRI (i.e. to determine the circumferential margins of the rectal cancer staged as T3 using EUS) have now disappeared.

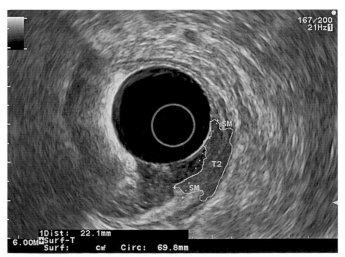

Figure 114 T2 rectal cancer.

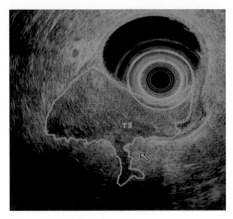

Figure 115 T3 Rectal cancer.

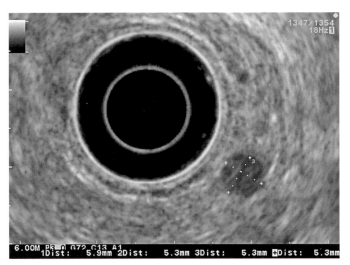

Figure 116 Small malignant perirectal lymph node.

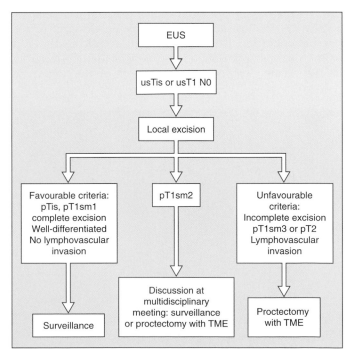

Figure 117 Role of local treatment for early rectal cancer: recommendations for clinical practice.

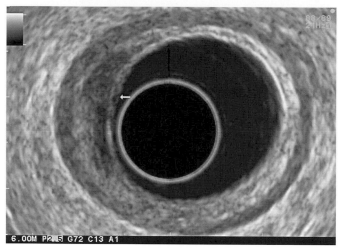

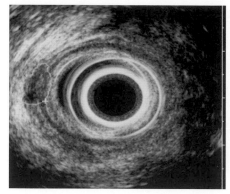

Figure 120 Small nodular recurrence located within the internal sphincter 1 year following completion of treatment for anal canal cancer.

Figure 118 Small uT1 squamous anal cancer confined to the mucosa and the submucosa.

Given the very significant difference in the cost of these two methods, rectal endosonography remains the method of choice for the pre-therapeutic assessment of both early tumors and advanced cancers and MRI is mandatory to stage very fixed cancer of the lower and mid rectum with suspicion of T4 lesions at EUS and advanced stenotic cancer of the upper rectum.

10.6. Anal cancer

The depth of the involvement of the anal canal and the rectal wall and the presence of metastatic lymph nodes around the rectum are major prognostic factors as regards the response to radiotherapy or radiochemotherapy. Anorectal endosonography should be considered essential for the treatment of patients with squamous cell cancer of the anal canal (Figs 118, 119); it has, in fact, been shown that endosonographic staging (T1 no invasion of the rectal muscle layer or the internal sphincter, T2 invasion of the rectal muscle layer or the internal sphincter, T3 invasion of the peri-rectal fat or the striated sphincter, T4 invasion of the vagina or

rectovaginal septum, invasion of the prostate) is a significantly better predictor of response to treatment than the use of the clinical TNM classification. EUS is particularly useful for cT1 or cT2 tumors in the clinical UICC classification as 20–30% of these tumors are classified uT3 by endosonography. Furthermore, the sensitivity of endosonography for detecting N1 invaded lymph nodes (perirectal) is significantly superior to clinical examination (UICC classification). Finally, EUS FNA can easily be performed if necessary (in contrast with CT, MRI and PET scans).

10.7. Post-therapeutic monitoring of digestive cancers

Post-therapeutic monitoring has been shown to be clearly advantageous in rectal cancer after surgery and probably advantageous for cancers which have not been treated surgically (anal canal or lymphoma). Its value is debatable after neoadjuvant treatment of esophageal cancers. Generally speaking, the post-therapeutic monitoring of digestive cancers treated medically is far more difficult than pre-therapeutic assessment or the post-therapeutic monitoring of cancers after surgery, since residual parietal and peridigestive anomalies detected by EUS are common and they are particularly difficult to interpret (scar or recurrence) (Fig. 120). This underlines the importance of sending these patients to referral centers with experience in this form of monitoring.

11. Pancreatic disease

11.1. Introduction

The two main reasons why transabdominal ultrasound is less effective in assessing the pancreas and bile ducts than it is in the liver and gallbladder can be overcome by using an echoendoscope in the stomach and duodenum. The distance separating the transducer from the target structure is reduced to a few millimeters, and the result is not subject to disturbance by peridigestive fat and intradigestive air, regardless of the morphology of the patient examined. The use of high frequencies (6–10 MHz) yields images with unequalled spatial resolution, despite major progress made since the mid-1990s and above all the mid-2000s in external image imaging, whether by CT or high-definition MRI, including

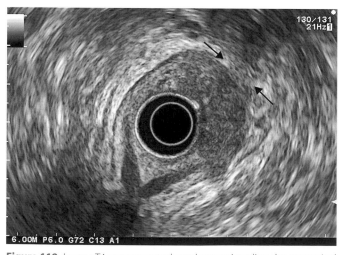

Figure 119 Large uT4 squamous anal canal cancer invading the anovaginal septum (black arrows).

MRCP. For example, the detection threshold for EUS for common bile duct or gallbladder stones is 0.5 mm, whereas it is 2–3 mm for solid intrapancreatic tumors (as has been demonstrated in patients with multiple endocrine neoplasia type I).

In pancreatic disease, particularly tumors (solid or cystic), there is now no doubt that conventional diagnostic EUS is strongly rivalled by CT and MRCP. However, the advent of EUS FNA toward the end of the 1990s and the development of therapeutic EUS during the 2000s have once again made EUS a key tool in the diagnostic and therapeutic management of pancreatic diseases.

11.2. Diagnosis and assessment of locorectional involvement in pancreatic cancer

11.2.1. How does EUS perform in the diagnosis of pancreatic cancers?

EUS can be used to examine the whole of the pancreatic gland from the uncinate process to the tail in almost all patients, regardless of their morphology. The head cannot be completely examined in patients with impassable duodenal stenosis, or gastrectomy with Billroth II anastomosis. A history of endoscopic sphincterotomy or the presence of a metal stent may hinder the examination of the pancreatic head. Generally speaking, EUS should be performed if possible, whether for diagnostic or histological purposes, before inserting a stent in the common bile duct, if the examination is to be as effective as the best results published in the literature. Examination of the caudal pancreas is unsatisfactory or incomplete in 10% of cases, in my experience, when the radial technique is used because the distance between the greater curve of the stomach and the pancreatic tail is too great. It is then necessary to change to an electronic linear echoendoscope.

The sensitivity of EUS in the diagnosis of pancreatic cancers exceeds 95%, even for small cancers (Fig. 121) with a diameter of 2 cm or less (these cancers are rare but unfortunately represent the vast majority of cancers curable by surgical resection). These small cancers are not detectable by MDCT

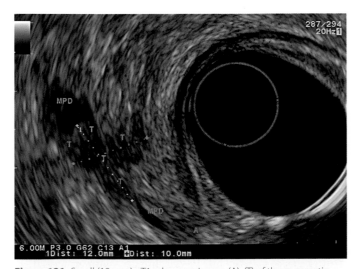

Figure 121 Small (12 mm) uT1 adenocarcinoma (A), (T) of the pancreatic head with slight dilatation (4 mm) of the main pancreatic duct (MPD) revealed by an episode of acute pancreatitis. This small cancer was not demonstrated by MDCT or MRI and was suggested but not visualized by MRCP.

Box 13 Contrast-enhanced EUS

- Requires specific contrast enhancement harmonic (CEH-EUS) software.
- Uses different US contrast agents (UCA).
- In Europe, the most widely used UCA is Sonovue (sulphur hexafluoride).

In CEH-EUS

- Ductal adenocarcinomas of the pancreas are very hypovascular compared to the parenchyma, in the various injection phases (Fig. 122).
- Endocrine tumors of the pancreas are hyper- (Fig. 123) or isovascular (Fig. 124) with a hypervascular rim in relation to the adjacent parenchyma, in the arterial phase (8–20 seconds after the injection).
- Focal pancreatitis is slightly less vascularized or as vascularized as the adjacent parenchyma (Figs 125, 126), during the arterial and the venous phase. It is more vascularized than adenocarcinoma and less vascularized than endocrine tumor.
- Adenoma (mural nodule in the case of IPMN or a tumor of the ampulla of Vater) is isovascular in relation to the adjacent parenchyma.

---

in 30% of cases because they remain isodense after the injection of contrast medium.

EUS remains superior in terms of diagnostic performance to the best imaging techniques including MDCT and MRI. Its sensitivity, close to 100% for the diagnosis of small cancers, and a resulting negative predictive value of more than 95% mean that EUS remains the reference examination for the detection of a focal lesion of the pancreas when it has not been conclusively identified by modern imaging. Furthermore, a normal EUS examination of the pancreas almost certainly rules out a diagnosis of pancreatic cancer, which is impossible with MDCT and MRI.

Nevertheless, subject to the results of current studies on the use of contrast media (Box 13) and elastography (Box 14), two new methods of tissue characterization whose results are promising, none of the EUS characteristics of pancreatic masses has a sufficient positive or negative predictive value for satisfactorily discriminating between a malignant tumor and an area of pancreatitis. It has, moreover, been shown that in the case of chronic advanced pancreatitis

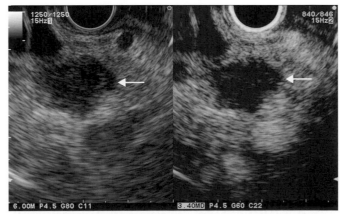

Figure 122 Contrast-enhanced EUS of a small (17 mm) adenocarcinoma (right image) of the head of the pancreas. Typical aspect of a hypovascular, nodular lesion in the various injection phases.

Elastography is a means of measuring tissue stiffness. Malignant tissue is harder than benign tissue and elastography may be able to differentiate between both. The technology is based on the detection of small structure deformations within the B-mode image caused by compression, so that the strain is smaller in hard tissue than in soft tissue. The degree of deformation is used as an indicator of the stiffness of the tissue. Different elasticity values (on a scale of 1–255) are shown as different colors. The system is set up to use a hue color map (red-green-blue), in which hard tissue areas are shown in dark blue, medium-hard tissue areas in cyan, intermediate hardness tissue areas in green, medium-soft tissue areas in yellow, and soft tissue areas in red.

EUS-elastography has been used for the diagnosis of pancreatic cancer and malignant lymphadenopathy with variable sensitivity, specificity, and accuracy in different studies. More recently, specially designed software has been available for computerized analysis of EUS-elastography images and videos. This has allowed quantification of tissue hardness by calculating hue histograms of each individual elastographic image, rather than qualitative analysis of the EUS images.

Elastography may allow differentiation of focal chronic pancreatitis (CP) from pancreatic cancer or, when the latter occurs on a background of CP, it may allow accurate targeting of the best area for FNA biopsy. Results of further studies are awaited.

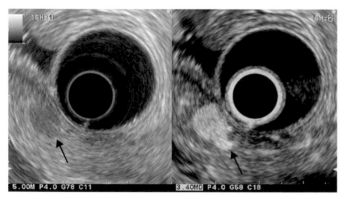

Figure 123 Contrast-enhanced EUS of a small (8 mm) insulinoma of the body of the pancreas. Typical aspect of a hypervascular (right image) nodular lesion in the arterial phase.

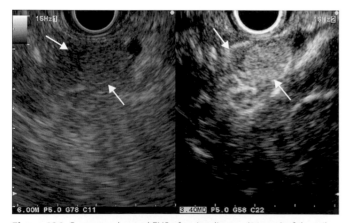

Figure 124 Contrast-enhanced EUS of an insulinoma (14 mm) of the tail of the pancreas. Isovascular (right image) compared to the adjacent parenchyma in the arterial phase, well circumscribed by the hypervascular ring (white arrows). This insulinoma was isoechogenic to the adjacent parenchyma using EUS (left image), and was not visible on MDCT or MRI.

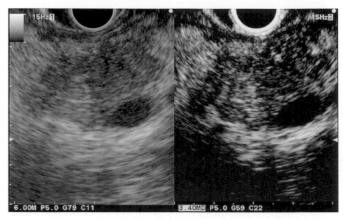

Figure 125 Contrast-enhanced EUS of a pseudotumor in a patient with auto-immune pancreatitis of the tail of the pancreas. First second after injection: the focal mass (right image) is hypoechogenic compared to the normal parenchyma.

or after a recent episode of severe acute pancreatitis, EUS may miss a pancreatic cancer.

EUS-FNA has, according to the latest studies, a sensitivity of between 85 and 95% and a specificity in the order of 100% for the diagnosis of malignant pancreatic tumors. Nevertheless, the negative predictive value never exceeds 80%, which means that a negative biopsy does not rule out a diagnosis of cancer. If malignancy is strongly suspected, based on biochemical or morphological clinical criteria, do not hesitate to carry out a second EUS-FNA of a focal pancreatic image, so as not to miss the opportunity for surgical resection which remains the only method likely to cure a patient with pancreatic cancer.

In summary, EUS, combined if necessary with FNA, is essential for the diagnosis of pancreatic cancer when imaging methods (MDCT and MRI) do not provide any certainty (see Fig. 132).

11.2.2. How does EUS perform in the assessment of locoregional involvement in pancreatic cancers?

Definition

- Pancreatic cancer is considered unresectable if there are metastases to organs (liver, peritoneum or lung) or to

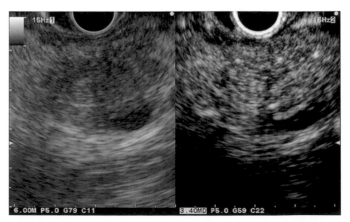

Figure 126 Same patient as Figure 125. The pseudotumor (right image) is isovascular to the adjacent parenchyma 6 seconds after injection.

the left supraclavicular lymph nodes or if the tumor is locally advanced.

- Pancreatic cancer is considered locally advanced if unresectable vascular involvement is present. This is defined as:
  - Involvement of the superior mesenteric vein, the mesenteric-portal vein confluence and the portal vein, if a thrombosis with or without a cavernoma is present (see below)
  - Involvement of the hepatic artery, superior mesenteric artery or celiac trunk
  - This is also the case if there are lymph node metastases remote from the tumor (in the lumbar aortic, superior mesenteric, pyloric, celiac or posterior mediastinal location).

At diagnosis, almost 50% of pancreatic cancers have hepatic or peritoneal metastases, 30% are locally advanced, and 15% to 20% are resectable. Surgical resection is currently the only treatment that can cure a small percentage of patients: approximately 20% of patients with pancreatic cancers, who have undergone curative surgery (R0 resection), are still alive 5 years later, which means that there are 5% survivors at 5 years after a diagnosis of pancreatic cancer. The incidence, i.e. the number of new cases annually of this cancer, is equal to its prevalence, i.e. the total number of surviving patients affected, which means that almost all patients die within a year of diagnosis. The few patients who survive are those who had no lymph node involvement in the resection tissue (N0 patients). It has recently been demonstrated that moderate involvement, affecting the portal vein, the superior mesenteric vein or the mesenteric-portal vein confluence, could undergo curative R0 surgical resection (at the cost of a vascular procedure, and thus greater morbidity) without worsening the prognosis, in other words obtaining approximately 20% survivors at 5 years as if there had been no vascular involvement, however this percentage was obtained only if there was no lymph node involvement in the resection tissue (N0). It has also been shown that even in the absence of recovery, R0 surgical resection is the most effective palliative method in terms of survival and quality of life. It has finally been demonstrated that owing to progress in chemotherapy and endoscopic drainage, the palliative non-surgical management of patients with locally advanced cancer improved the duration and quality of their survival, and that 10% of these patients became eligible for curative surgical resection.

Several studies and teams have, in recent years, proposed laparoscopy as the final stage in diagnosing the resectability of pancreatic head cancers, before curative pancreaticoduodenectomy. The success rate of laparoscopy in these studies after performing a preoperative imaging assessment to diagnose resectability ranged from 20% to 75%, depending on the quality of the preoperative assessment. A recent study has shown that when the assessment of resectability of a cephalic adenocarcinoma included thin section pancreatic MDCT and high-quality EUS, the benefit of routine laparoscopy barely exceeded 10%, confirming that this benefit was inversely proportional to the quality of the preoperative assessment.

Between 1990 and 1997, EUS was regarded as the reference examination for assessing the lymph node and vascular involvement of pancreatic cancers, superior to both CT and angiography. Thin section MDCT centered on the pancreas

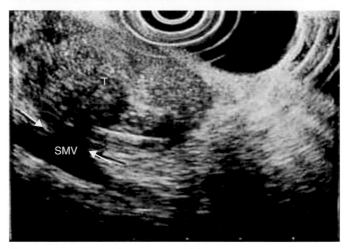

Figure 127 3 cm uT3 adenocarcinoma of the uncinate process, slightly invading the posterior side of the superior mesenteric vein (SMV).

currently has a diagnostic sensitivity of 80% for venous invasion and 90% for arterial invasion. The specificity of this examination for the diagnosis of vascular non-resectability is close to 100% (excluding malignant IPMN). Combined with the fact that the diagnosis of hepatic metastases is correct in almost 90% of cases, this means that thin section MDCT is sufficient to optimally determine the management of almost 70% of patients with pancreatic cancer. The sensitivity of thin section MDCT for the diagnosis of moderate disease of the superior mesenteric vein, the mesenteric-portal vein confluence or the portal vein is, nevertheless, unsatisfactory, while its sensitivity for the diagnosis of lymph node involvement remains poor and has not improved. Small subcapsular metastases, which are one of the features of pancreatic cancers, remain difficult to detect and peritoneal carcinosis remains undetectable in the majority of cases. These limitations of thin section MDCT are residual indications of EUS for the assessment of locoregional involvement. The method should therefore be used only in patients who have been filtered by thin section MDCT.

In summary

- The sensitivity of EUS for the diagnosis of moderate involvement of the mesenteric-portal vein confluence in patients with pancreatic cancer with a diameter ≤3 cm is close to 100% (Figs 127, 128)

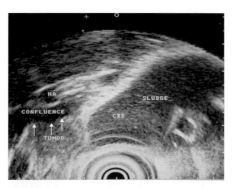

Figure 128 14 mm, uT3, adenocarcinoma of the upper and posterior part of the head of the pancreas, slightly invading the posterior and right side of the portal vein confluence (white arrows). HA, hepatic artery; CBD, common bile duct.

- The sensitivity of EUS for the diagnosis of remote metastatic lymph nodes (N2) is close to 80% (Fig. 129), and it allows EUS FNA which provides histological confirmation of metastasis
- EUS is capable of detecting and confirming by biopsy small subcapsular metastases of segment II and segment I that are invisible or cannot be biopsied during MDCT (Fig. 130)
- EUS is the most sensitive method of detecting slight ascites suggesting peritoneal carcinosis, allowing a cytological study by FNA (Fig. 131).

After carrying out a thin section pancreatic MDCT, EUS currently remains essential for the optimal management of a large proportion of patients with pancreatic cancer:

- Patients in whom the diagnosis has not been confirmed by MDCT or MRI (Fig. 132)
- Patients without hepatic metastases, considered eligible for resection after MDCT (Fig. 133)

- Patients in whom a histological diagnosis is essential and who have no hepatic metastases accessible to percutaneous biopsy (Figs 134, 135).

11.2.3. Indications and results of EUS-FNA of solid pancreatic masses

EUS is the only method of biopsying all parts of the pancreatic gland, including the uncinate process and the tail. Any pancreatic mass with a minimum diameter ≥5 mm can be biopsied. Owing to improvements in echoendoscopes and techniques for cytology and histology (use of immunohistochemistry, P53, Ki67, K ras, etc.), their sensitivity for the diagnosis of malignant pancreatic tumors exceeds 90% and their specificity is close to 100%, whether for adenocarcinoma or a tumor with a less common histology and a better prognosis, such as pancreatic metastases, neuroendocrine cancers or lymphomas.

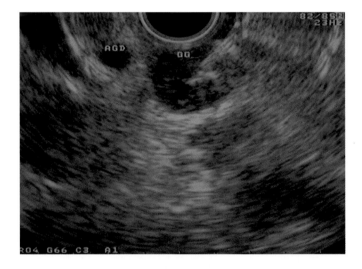

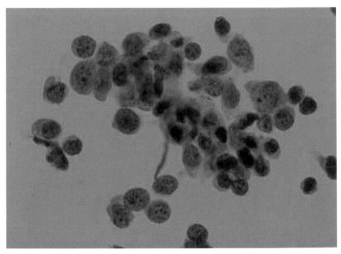

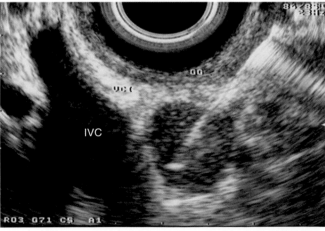

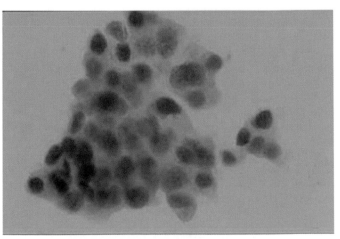

Figure 129 EUS-guided FNA (22 G needle) of a small (1 cm) malignant lymph node (upper left image), close to the hepatic artery (this is an N2 node if the primary is in the pancreatic head). Cytology (upper right image) was positive for adenocarcinoma. EUS-guided FNA (22 G needle) of a small (12 mm) lumbar aortic malignant lymph node (lower left image) in front of the inferior vena cava (IVC). Cytology (lower right image) was positive for adenocarcinoma.

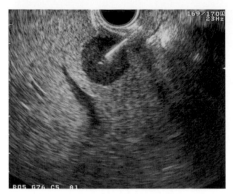

Figure 130 EUS-guided FNA (22 G needle) of a small (12 mm) subcapsular liver metastasis in segment II.

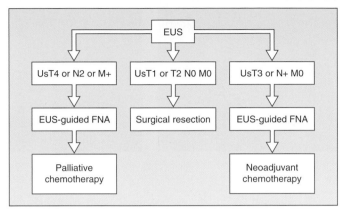

Figure 133 Resectable cancer at MDCT.

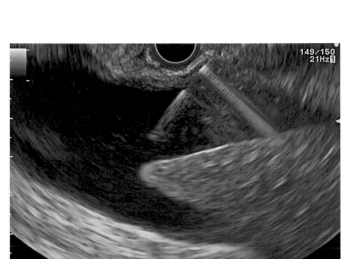

Figure 131 EUS-guided FNA (22 G needle) of ascitis in a patient with pancreatic body cancer. Positive liquid phase cytology for adenocarcinoma.

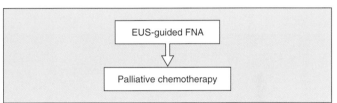

Figure 134 Unresectable cancer at MDCT without liver metastasis.

The rate of complications is low, comprising mainly acute pancreatitis which occurs almost exclusively when benign tumors are biopsied through healthy pancreatic tissue. The risk of peritoneal or parietal spread along the biopsy path is lower than with the percutaneous route, owing to the proximity between the echoendoscope and the tumor (which rarely exceeds a few mm). Furthermore, for a transduodenal biopsy of a potentially resectable tumor (diagnosis of a small cephalic pancreas tumor carried out exclusively by EUS), there is no risk of spread because the biopsy path is removed during pancreaticoduodenectomy. A study has shown that the risk of peritoneal carcinomatosis caused by EUS-FNA was very significantly lower than after CT-guided percutaneous FNA. One explanation for this difference, apart from the

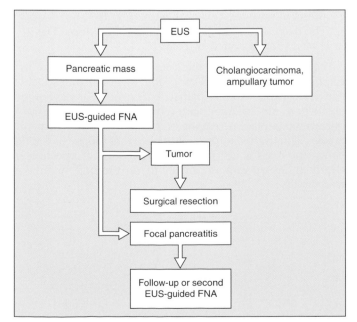

Figure 132 No pancreatic mass at MDCT.

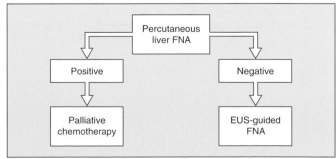

Figure 135 Pancreatic cancer with liver metastasis at MDCT.

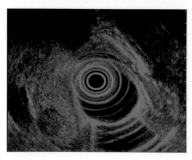
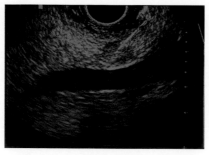
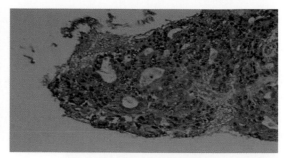

Figure 136 Radial EUS and EUS-guided FNA (22 G needle) of a small (11 mm) uT1 pancreatic cancer of the uncinate process only visualized by EUS in a patient with hereditary pancreatic cancer. The histology was positive for adenocarcinoma.

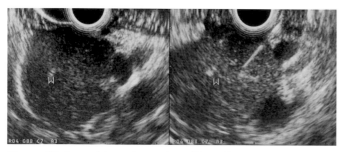

Figure 137 A pseudotumor in a patient with autoimmune pancreatitis (AIP) who presented with jaundice. The main pancreatic duct with a hyperechogenic wall (W) is well seen within the mass. EUS-guided FNA with 22 G needle. Cell block histology revealed an inflammatory process with numerous IgG 4 plasmocytes, compatible with type I AIP.

length of the biopsy path, is the use of a different needle diameter in each of the two methods: a 22-gauge or 25-gauge needle is sufficient to diagnose malignant disease in more than 90% of cases using an echoendoscope, whereas a 19-gauge needle is necessary to obtain 90% sensitivity by the percutaneous route (the percutaneous use of a 22-gauge needle rarely achieves a sensitivity of >70%).

The validated indications of EUS-FNA are:

- The cytohistological diagnosis of pancreatic masses invisible to MDCT or MRI, detected only by EUS (Fig. 136)
- A differential diagnosis between pancreatic adenocarcinoma and a pancreatitis nodule, in particular in patients with chronic calcifying pancreatitis or a clinical and biochemical picture compatible with pseudotumoral pancreatitis (autoimmune pancreatitis) (Fig. 137)
- A differential diagnosis between pancreatic adenocarcinoma and a pancreatic metastasis of a synchronous or metachronous cancer (in order of frequency: kidney, breast, lung, colon, etc.) (Fig. 138)
- The cytohistological diagnosis of unresectable non-metastatic locally advanced cancers (Figs 134, 139–143) or cancers with hepatic metastases not accessible percutaneously (Fig. 135). A biopsy is essential in these cases before palliative treatment is started, because pancreatic adenocarcinomas account for only 85–90% of pancreatic cancers, with 5–10% being neuroendocrine cancer, 5% a metastasis, and 1–2% lymphoma
- The cytohistological diagnosis of the adenocarcinomatous nature of a resectable tumor before its inclusion in a preoperative chemotherapy protocol for neoadjuvant therapy (Fig. 133)
- The diagnosis of an asymptomatic solid tumor (Figs 144–148) discovered by chance.

The commonest of all these indications is of course the cytohistological diagnosis of locally advanced unresectable pancreatic cancers before palliative treatment. In view of the excellent results obtained with very low morbidity, EUS-FNA promises to replace percutaneous biopsy for solid pancreatic masses. Finally, it is important to note that biopsy of a solid pancreatic mass is not indicated when surgical resection is clearly indicated (no doubt about its tumoral nature or resectability).

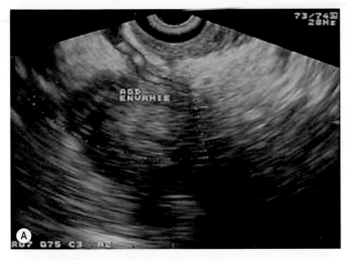

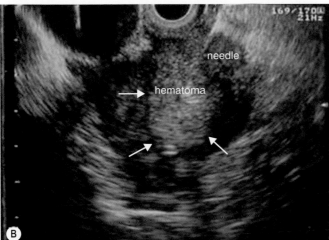

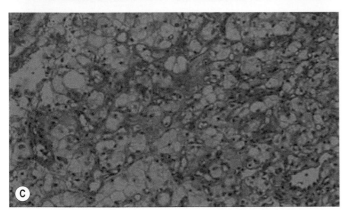

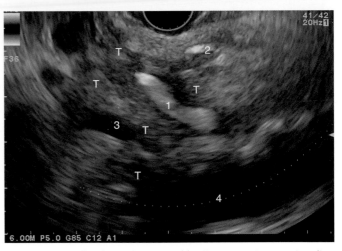

Figure 139 Locally advanced, unresectable uT4 pancreatic cancer invading the celiac axis (1), left gastric artery (2), superior mesenteric artery (3) and aorta (4).

Figure 138 3 cm pancreatic head mass, invading the gastroduodenal artery (A). EUS-guided FNA (22 G needle) of the mass (B) which was complicated by a hematoma (white arrows) due to the hypervascular nature of the mass. Histology was positive for renal cell cancer metastases on cell block (C).

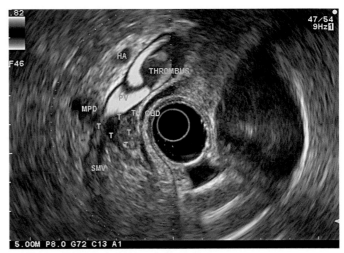

Figure 140 Small (20 mm), locally advanced, unresectable uT4 pancreatic head cancer invading the portal vein confluence with partial thrombosis of the portal vein.

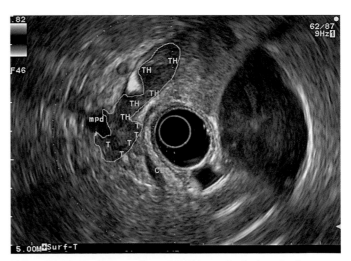

Figure 141 Same patient as Figure 140. TH, portal vein thrombosis, T, tumor, MPD, main pancreatic duct.

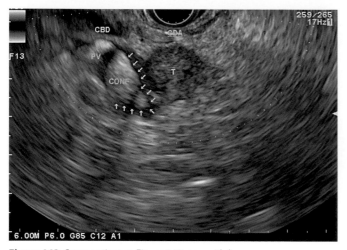

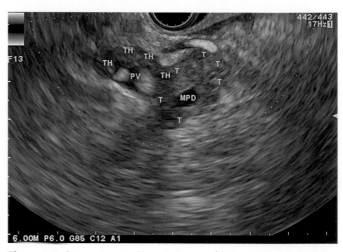

Figure 142 Same patient as Figure 140 seen with linear scope.

Figure 143 Same patient as Figure 140 seen with linear scope. Note the tumor (T) involving the main pancreatic duct (MPD) and portal vein (PV) with portal vein thrombosis (TH).

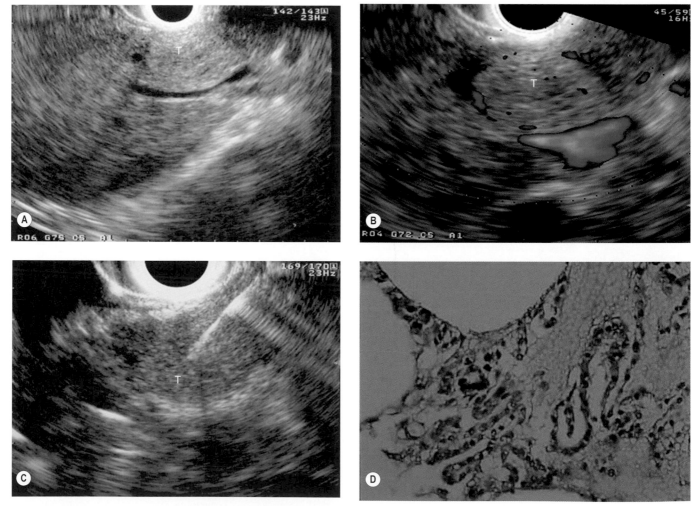

Figure 144 Pseudosolid serous cystadenoma (T) of the pancreatic neck. (A) Radial examination. (B) Note that the tumor is encorbelled by vessels. (C) EUS-guided FNA with 22 G needle. (D) Histological aspect of serous cystadenoma.

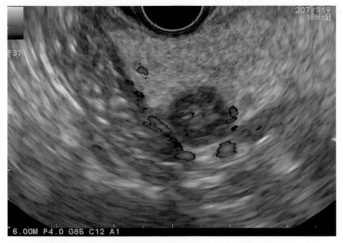

Figure 145 Small (9 mm) solid incidentaloma of the pancreatic head.

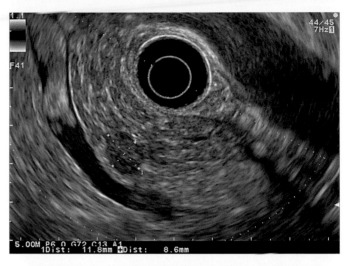

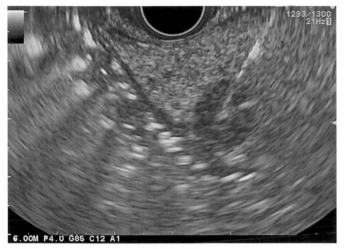

Figure 146 Same patient as Figure 145, with EUS-guided FNA (22 G needle).

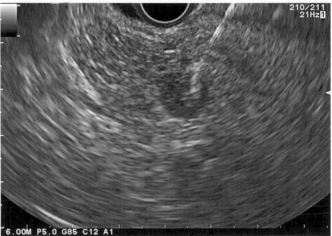

Figure 148 Small incidentaloma (11 mm) of the uncinate process in a young male. EUS-guided FNA (22 G needle) demonstrated a solid pseudo-papillary tumor.

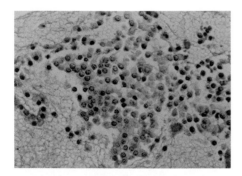

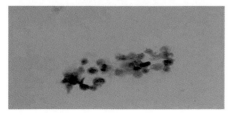

Figure 147 Same patient as in Figures 145 and 146. The cell block demonstrated positive immunohistochemical staining with chromogranin A (upper image) consistent with a neuroendocrine tumor. Immunohistochemical quantification of the proliferation marker KI 67 evaluated at 20% on liquid phase cytology suggesting a small malignant endocrine cancer (lower image), which was confirmed on histology of the resected specimen.

11.3. Pancreatic neuroendocrine tumors

Ever since the 1980s, EUS has been the reference examination for determining the preoperative location of secretory endocrine tumors potentially of pancreatic or duodenal origin, and in particular the two commonest forms, insulinoma and gastrinoma. When the method is performed by an experienced EUS operator, the diagnostic accuracy of the method for locating pancreatic gastrinomas or insulinomas exceeds 90%, whereas in combination with somatostatin receptor scintigraphy, its sensitivity is 90% for duodenal gastrinomas (Figs 149–157).

The detection threshold of a pancreatic endocrine tumor by EUS is approximately 2 mm. EUS is capable of locating almost 80% of pancreatic endocrine tumors in patients with multiple endocrine neoplasia type I. An endocrine tumor is typically round or oval with a distinct boundary, hypoechoic, very homogeneous, surrounded by a very thin hypoechoic ring (Fig. 149). It yields peripheral signal enhancement, indicating hypervascularization. In Doppler energy imaging, it is laced with small vessels that penetrate it (Figs 150, 151); it is a very pretty tumor. It is sometimes isoechoic (Fig. 152) with the parenchyma, and difficult to locate. Its echostructure is more homogeneous than the adjacent parenchyma

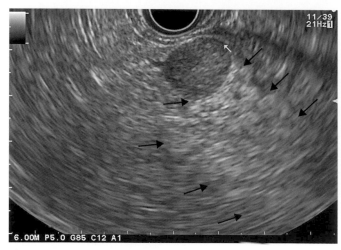

Figure 149 Typical aspect of a pancreatic endocrine tumor located within the tail of the pancreas. Thin hypoechogenic ring (white arrow) with peripheral signal enhancement (black arrows).

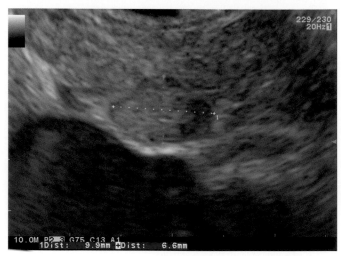

Figure 152 Isoechogenic pancreatic insulinoma seen only with EUS. The tumor is visualized because of the more homogeneous echostructure compared to the adjacent parenchyma, thin hypoechoic ring and peripheral signal enhancement.

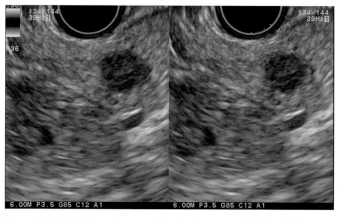

Figure 150 Small (6 mm) pancreatic endocrine tumor. On the right image vessels can be seen surrounding the tumor.

and it can then be located by peripheral signal enhancement (Fig. 153) or by peripheral vascularization (Figs 154, 155). It is sometimes heterogeneous, with partial attenuation of the ultrasound beam indicating areas of fibrosis. There are sometimes small calcifications. Sometimes it is cystic. If it is large, multiple rather central small cystic areas are fairly common. If it is small and cystic, the antral cystic area accounts for the majority of the tumor volume, the tumor being confined to the wall of the cyst which is fleshy, homogeneous (Figs 157, 158), and covered with small vessels on Doppler energy imaging.

EUS FNA is very effective, with a sensitivity close to 100% using immunohistochemistry. It is the standard examination

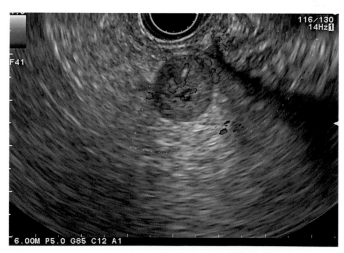

Figure 151 Pancreatic endocrine tumor with peripheral signal enhancement with vessels which surround and penetrate the tumor.

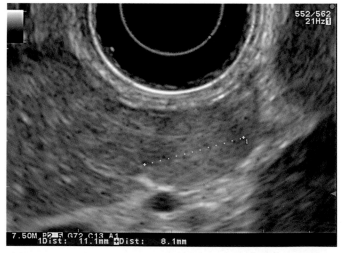

Figure 153 Isoechogenic insulinoma of the tail of the pancreas only seen with EUS. The tumor is visualized because of the more homogeneous echostructure compared to the adjacent parenchyma and the peripheral signal enhancement.

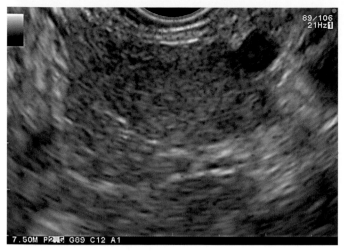

Figure 154 Same tumor as Figure 124.

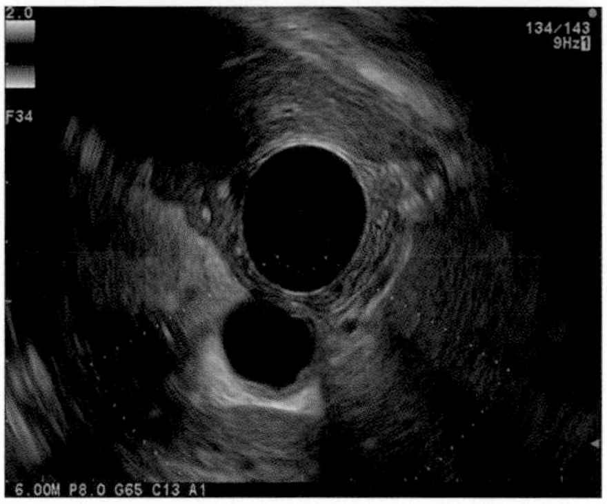

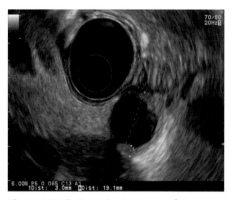

Figure 157 Cystic endocrine tumor of the pancreas.

for confirming a diagnosis of non-functional endocrine tumor when it has been discovered by chance and in the absence of somatostatin receptor scintigraphy. The histoprognosis based on EUS-FNA correlates well with that obtained by resection. The opportunity for immunohistochemical quantification of the proliferation marker Ki67 and the mitotic index is very helpful when decision-making is difficult. The role of EUS and EUS FNA in the management of pancreatic endocrine tumors is summarized in Figures 159–161.

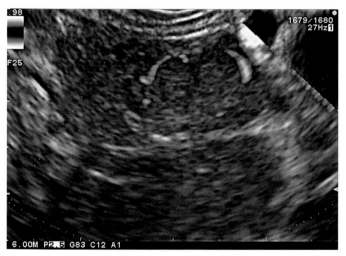

Figure 155 Same tumor as Figure 124 with the vessels surrounding it.

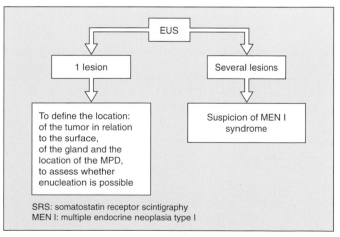

Figure 158 Cystic endocrine tumor of the pancreas.

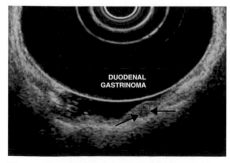

Figure 156 Small (2.5 mm) duodenal gastrinoma in a patient with Zollinger–Ellison syndrome.

Figure 159 Clinical and biological features of functional NET without localization of the tumor by MDCT, MRI, and SRS.

337

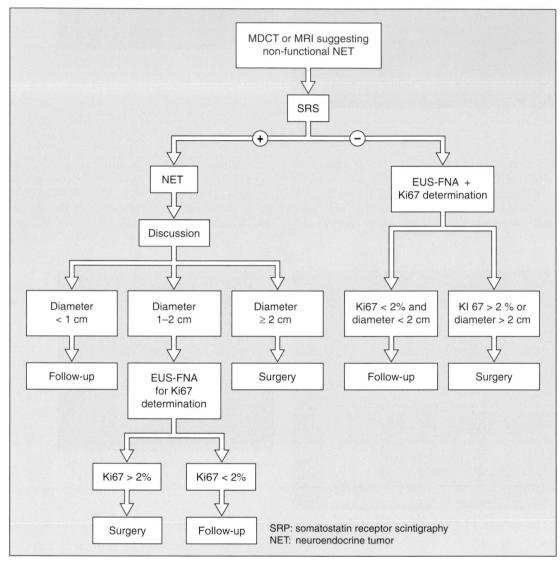

Figure 160 Staging and management of non-functional pancreatic neuroendocrine tumors (NET).

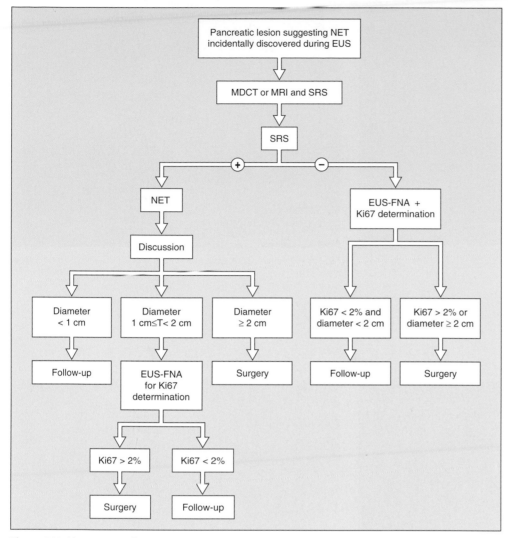

Figure 161 Management of pancreatic neuroendocrine tumors discovered coincidentally at EUS.

11.4. Cystic pancreatic tumors

EUS is very useful for examining cystic lesions of the pancreas when their nature has not been clarified by a combination of percutaneous ultrasound and spiral CT or MRI with MRCP. It facilitates the diagnosis of serous cystadenomas (Fig. 162) if it reveals microcysts in an apparently solid tumor (Fig. 163) or in a predominantly macrocystic tumor (these are macrocystic serous cystadenomas (Fig. 164), the frequency of which is probably greatly underestimated). EUS facilitates the diagnosis of mucinous cystadenoma if it detects parietal thickening and thick septa (Fig. 165), or eggshell calcifications (Figs 166, 167A), the presence of a solid component or a mural nodule (Fig. 167B,C) developed from the wall or septal thickening, or if the cyst contents are thick (Fig. 168) or have a fluid-fluid level (Figs 166, 167). It confirms the diagnosis of cystadenocarcinoma if it detects invasion of the adjacent parenchyma from a tumoral solid component or a tumoral thickening of the cyst wall (Fig. 169). It is very effective in the diagnosis of intraductal papillary-mucinous neoplasia of the pancreas, whether it is the form located in the main duct where diagnosis is fairly

easy (Figs 170–173) or the form located in the secondary ducts when it shows several fluid images (Fig. 174A–D), distributed through all or part of the pancreatic gland, adjacent to the pancreatic duct, duct-shaped (much longer than it is wide), with or without clearly visible communication with the pancreatic duct with or without dependent droplets of mucus (Fig. 174E). The diagnosis is confirmed when mucus is identified emerging from the major or accessory papilla (Figs 175, 176).

When diagnostic uncertainty persists as regards the mucinous or non-mucinous nature of a cystic tumor, or when diagnostic doubt persists between a mucinous cystadenoma and a pseudocyst, it is then useful to carry out FNA of the cystic fluid, with a very low risk of spread along the path, to allow a biochemical analysis (Table 3) (amylase and lipase) and a study of tumor markers (CEA is the most discriminating, while CA 19–9 and CA 72–4 are less effective).

Cytology is helpful in 40–50% of cases, and more effective if liquid phase cytology is used, particularly if there is a nodule to biopsy (sensitivity >80%). The combination of the EUS appearance and the information yielded by biochemical

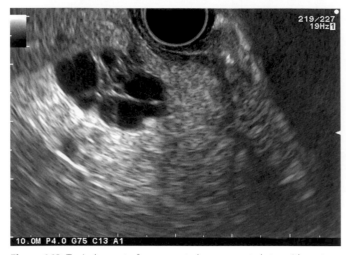

Figure 162 Typical aspect of serous cystadenoma: central star with septa originating from it and microcysts within it.

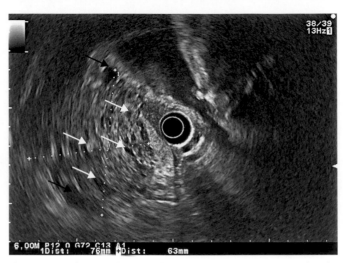

Figure 163 Other typical aspect of serous cystadenoma: large (8 cm) ovale mass of the head of the pancreas. Hyperechoic mass with numerous microcysts (white arrows) and peripheral minicysts (black arrows).

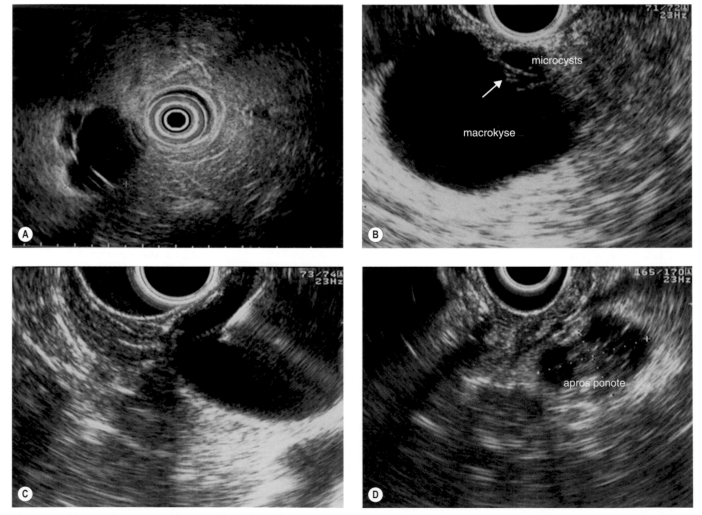

Figure 164 Macrocystic serous cystadenoma. (A) peripheral thin septa; (B) some microcysts within a peripheral star; (C) EUS-guided FNA for CEA level; (D) after EUS-FNA and aspiration, the typical appearance of a serous cystadenoma can be seen with a central star and microcysts within it.

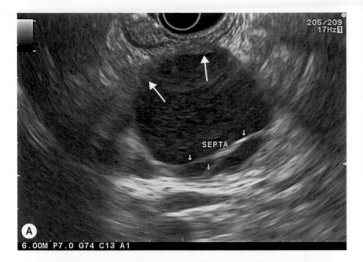

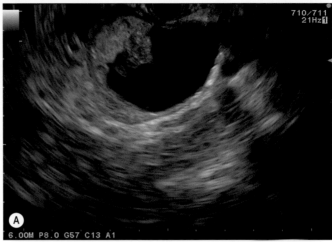

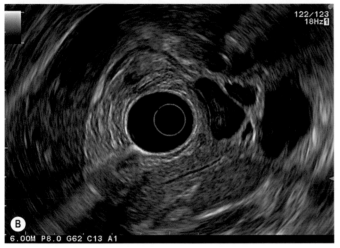

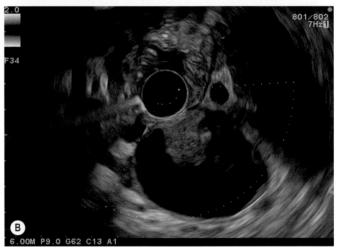

Figure 165 (A) Typical aspect of a mucinous cystadenoma: round cystic lesion with thick wall and septa. (B) Typical aspect of a mucinous cystadenoma of the tail of the pancreas with thick septa.

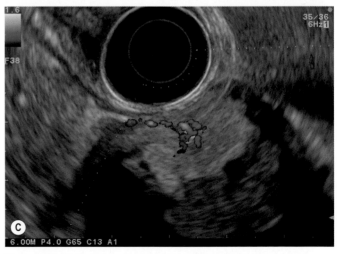

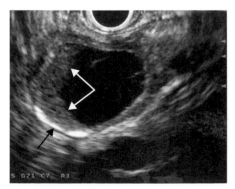

Figure 166 Typical small (2.5 cm) mucinous cystadenoma with eggshell calcifications (black arrow) and thick dependent content (white arrows).

Figure 167 (A) Typical mucinous cystadenoma with thick dependent content, and eggshell calcifications. (B) Typical mucinous cystadenoma with solid component (mural nodule) and droplet of mucus. (C) Same patient, with vessels in the stalk of the polypoid mural nodule.

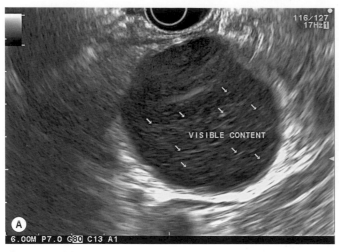

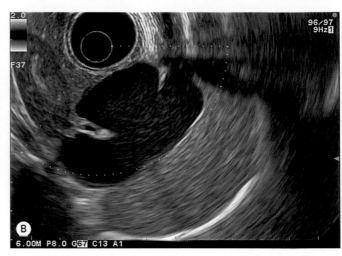

Figure 168 (A) Mucinous cystadenoma with thick visible content. (B) Mucinous cystadenoma with thick septa and visible thick content.

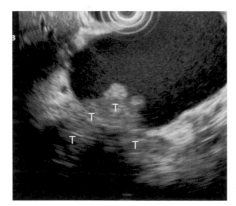

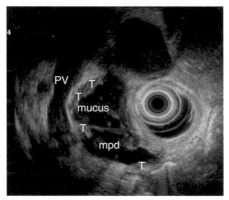

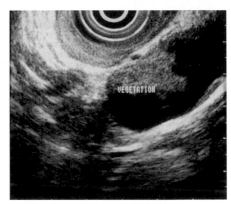

Figure 169 Mucinous cystadenoma with solid component with invasion of the adjacent pancreatic parenchyma (T).

Figure 170 Main duct type IPMN of the head of the pancreas with tumour involving (T) the wall (<3 mm) of the main pancreatic duct (mpd) and mucus within the lumen.

Figure 171 Main duct type IPMN with the presence of a mural nodule, with height >5 mm, indicating at least borderline tumor and more often severe dysplasia.

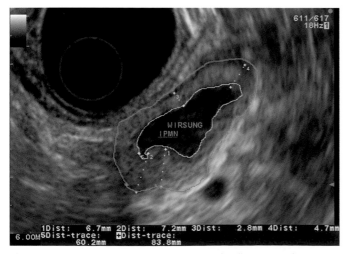

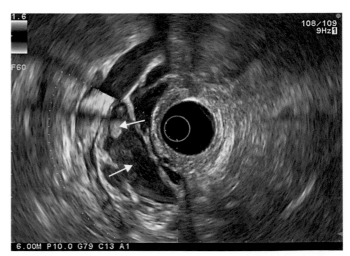

Figure 172 Main duct type IPMN with thickened wall >3 mm indicating at least borderline tumor and more often severe dysplasia.

Figure 173 Mixed type IPMN of the head of the pancreas with thick mucus within the lumen (thin white arrow) and mural nodule (thick white arrow).

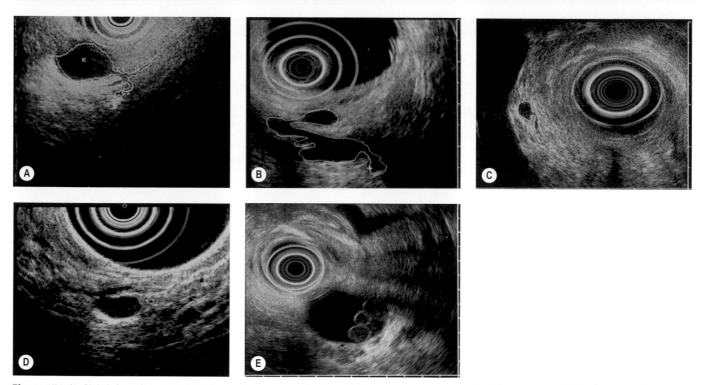

Figure 174 (A–D) Side branch type IPMN with or without communication with the main pancreatic duct. (E) Side branch type IPMN with several dependent droplets of mucus (white arrow).

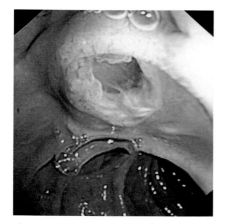

Figure 175 Endoscopic view of the patulous papilla with mucus.

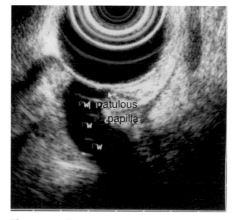

Figure 176 Same patient: EUS image of the patulous papilla and the dilated main pancreatic duct (w).

Table 3 Reassessment of the value of biochemical and tumor markers in cyst fluid in the diagnosis of 130 cystic lesions of the pancreas

Marker	Cut-off value	Diagnosis	Sensitivity		Specificity		PPV		NPV	
			n	(%)	n	(%)	n	(%)	n	(%)
Amylase	>5000 U/L	PC	93	94	82	74	86	85	91	88
Ca 19.9	>50 000 U/mL	MC/MCAC	72	75	84	90	63	67	88	90
CEA	>400 ng/mL	MC/MCAC	57	50	99	100	96	100	85	85
CEA	<5 ng/mL	SC	92	100	87	86	61	54	98	100
Ca 72.4	>40 U/mL	MC/MCAC	73	63	99	98	96	95	84	85
Mucins M1	>1200 U/mL	MC/MCAC	41	30	93	100	71	100	79	79

PC, pseudocyst; MC, mucinous cystadenoma; MCAC, mucinous cystadenocarcinoma; SC, serous cystadenoma. PPV, positive predictive value; NPV, negative predictive value.
Serous cystadenomas, n=24; mucinous cystadenomas and cystadenocarcinomas, n=36; pseudocysts, n=70.
Data obtained in Beaujon Hospital in 1998.
(From Hammel P. Gastrointest Endosc Clin N Am 212:791, 2002.)

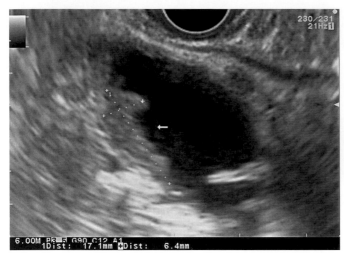

Figure 177 Mural nodule (height >5 mm) in a side branch IPMN.

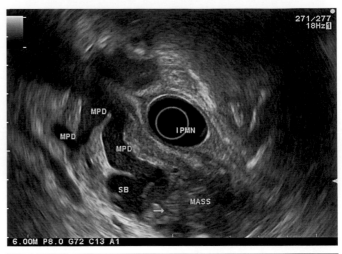

study, cytology and tumor markers can predict the nature of the cystic lesion in 90% of cases. In the specific case of intraductal papillary-mucinous neoplasia of the pancreas, besides its diagnostic contribution which is now rivalled very effectively by MRI with MRCP, EUS is essential for the management of these patients since it has been demonstrated that it is by combining all these imaging techniques that a real picture can be obtained of the longitudinal spread of the disease to guide resection, and of the degree of malignancy. The degree of malignancy is correlated with the extent of parietal thickening in the main duct (Figs 170, 172) or in the secondary ducts and with the presence of a mural nodule (Figs 171, 173, 177), two components that are detected better by EUS than by MDCT and MRI. An MPD diameter >10 mm, parietal thickening >3 mm and a mural nodule height >5 mm are highly predictive of severe dysplasia (Figs 172, 173, 177). In the branch duct type, a diameter <3 cm and the absence of parietal thickening and a mural nodule are highly predictive of low-grade dysplasia. Obviously, the presence of a mass is highly suggestive of invasive carcinoma (Fig. 178).

Given the frequency of totally asymptomatic IPMN located in the secondary ducts, distributed throughout the gland, found in particular in the female population over the age of 60, and discovered by chance (due to progress in non-invasive imaging), and given the low risk of degeneration of this type of IPMN (<10% at 5 years), if there are no predictive signs of malignancy, close monitoring is now the recommended method of treatment. This is based on annual MRI with MRCP, with EUS at intervals of not more than 3 years, since this is the only examination capable of the early detection of changes in the aspect of the secondary ducts in terms of parietal thickening or small mural nodules. Such changes then constitute a convincing argument for prophylactic surgical resection. A significant change in the diameter of a branch duct during the follow-up is also an indication for surgery in a patient who is fit for surgery.

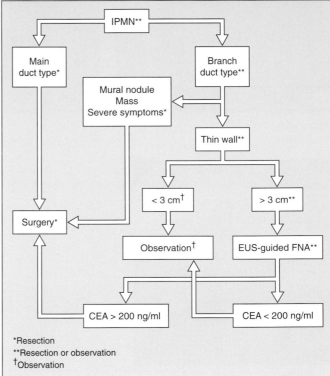

Figure 178 (A) Mixed type IPMN. Presence of a mass highly suggestive of invasive carcinoma. (B) Management of intraductal papillary mucinous neoplasia (IPMN).

11.5. Chronic pancreatitis (alcoholic or hereditary)

Although ultrasound and CT scanning has long been used routinely to diagnose chronic calcifying pancreatitis, ERCP remained until recently the gold standard for the diagnosis of early chronic pancreatitis (non-calcifying), using a classification of main duct and secondary duct anomalies (Cambridge classification). Several studies in the 1990s showed that EUS, by virtue of its resolving power on pancreatic parenchyma and the pancreatic ducts, correlated well with pancreatographic anomalies to diagnose the absence of chronic pancreatitis and to diagnose moderate to severe

---

Box 15   EUS criteria for the diagnosis of chronic pancreatitis

Parenchymal criteria

- Hyperechoic foci
- Hyperechoic strands
- Hypoechoic lobules
- Cyst.

Ductal criteria

- Dilated main pancreatic duct
- Irregular main pancreatic duct
- Dilated side branches
- Hyperechoic pancreatic duct wall
- Calculi.

Diagnosis of chronic pancreatitis

- 0–1 criteria have >90% chance of having an ERCP with no evidence of chronic pancreatitis
- ≥6 criteria have >80% chance of having an ERCP compatible with chronic pancreatitis
- The threshold for diagnosing chronic pancreatitis based on EUS features varies with most clinicians using ≥5 criteria for older individuals and ≥4 criteria for younger person.

Box 16   Rosemont classification for chronic pancreatitis

Major criteria

- Hyperechoic foci with shadowing (A).
- Main pancreatic duct calculi (A).
- Lobularity with honeycombing (B).

Minor criteria

- Cysts.
- Dilated ducts ≥3.5 mm.
- Irregular pancreatic duct contour.
- Dilated side branches ≥1 mm.
- Hyperechoic duct wall.
- Strands.
- Non-shadowing hyperechoic foci.
- Lobularity with non-contiguous lobules.

Diagnosis of chronic pancreatitis using Rosemont criteria

Consistent with chronic pancreatitis

- 1 major A feature + ≥3 minor features.
- 1 major A feature + major B feature.
- 2 major A features.

Suggestive of chronic pancreatitis

- 1 major A feature + <3 minor features.
- 1 major B features + ≥3 minor features.
- ≥5 minor features.

Indeterminate for CP

- 3–4 minor features, no major feature.
- Major B features alone or with <3 minor features.

Normal

- ≤2 minor features, no major feature.

Terminology	Definition
Hyperechoic foci with shadowing	Echogenic structures ≥2 mm in length and width that shadow.
Lobularity	Well circumscribed, ≥5 mm structures with enhancing rim and relatively echo-poor center.
With honeycombing	Contiguous ≥3 lobules.
Without honeycombing	Non-contiguous lobules.
Hyperechoic foci without shadowing	Echogenic structures foci ≥2 mm in both length and width with no shadowing.
Cysts	Anechoic, rounded/elliptical structures with or without septations.
Stranding	Hyperechoic lines of ≥3 mm in at least two different directions with respect to the imaged plane.
MPD calculi	Echogenic structure(s) within MPD with acoustic shadowing.
Irregular MPD contour	Uneven or irregular outline and ecstatic course.
Dilated side branches	Three or more tubular anechoic structures each measuring ≥1 mm in width, budding from the MPD.
MPD dilation	≥3.5 mm body or ≥1.5 mm tail.
Hyperechoic MPD margin	Echogenic, distinct structure greater than 50% of entire MPD in the body and tail.

From: Catalano MF, Sahai A, Levy M, et al EUS-based criteria for the diagnosis of chronic pancreatitis: the Rosemont classification. Gastrointest Endosc 69(7): 1251–1261, 2009.

---

chronic pancreatitis (Fig. 179). On the other hand, correlation was poor for the diagnosis of minor chronic pancreatitis and uncertainty concerning the specificity of minor EUS anomalies (fewer than five criteria) was normal for almost 10 years.

EUS (Box 15) is, in fact, more sensitive than ERCP since almost 70% of chronic alcoholic patients with symptoms of pancreatic disease and who had minor EUS anomalies and normal retrograde pancreatography, eventually had a definite pancreatographic diagnosis of chronic pancreatitis (after 3–5 years). The EUS criteria for a diagnosis of chronic pancreatitis are summarized in Box 15. An alternative method of defining chronic pancreatitis is to use the Rosemont criteria. These criteria were developed by an international consensus panel which was convened in Rosemont, Illinois (Box 16).

Although EUS is not advantageous for the diagnosis of chronic pancreatitis where there is already calcification, it is useful in the management of several of the complications associated with chronic pancreatitis.

In patients with duodenal stenosis, EUS is the standard examination for diagnosing cystic dystrophy of the duodenal wall developed on aberrant pancreas (Fig. 180), which is the leading cause of symptomatic duodenal stenosis in alcoholic chronic pancreatitis. This complication, which often goes unrecognized because it is incorrectly interpreted in cross sectional imaging, is observed in 5–10% of cases of alcoholic chronic pancreatitis and is more frequent with a clinical picture of severe pancreatitis in terms of pain, weight loss and vomiting. EUS is also useful if retrograde pancreatography shows a filling limit in a duct downstream of an area of segmental acute pancreatitis, when it can detect a stone that is not yet calcified, invisible to MDCT, at the junction between the normal pancreatic duct and the diseased area (Fig. 181).

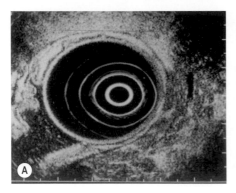

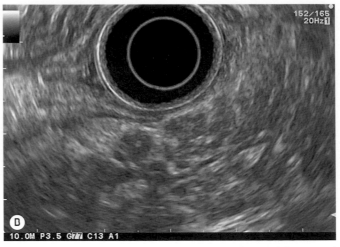

Figure 179 (A) EUS image of the tail of the pancreas suggestive of early alcoholic chronic pancreatitis: lobularity with honeycombing (major criteria B), strands, non-shadowing hyperechoic foci, hyperechoic pancreatic duct wall (three minor features), using Rosemont classification. (B) EUS image of the body of the pancreas consistent with early alcoholic chronic pancreatitis: shadowing hyperechoic foci (major criteria A) lobularity with honeycombing (major criteria B), strands and hyperechoic duct wall, using Rosemont classification.

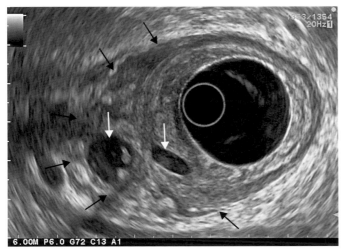

Figure 180 Cystic dystrophy of the duodenal wall developed on an aberrant pancreas in the descending duodenum. Thickening of the duodenal wall (black arrows) and small cyst within the submucosa and the muscularis propria (white arrows).

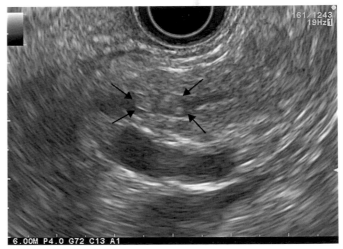

Figure 181 Non-calcified intraductal pancreatic stone (black arrows), non-visible on MDCT and MRCP and misdiagnosed as a tumoral stenosis on ERCP.

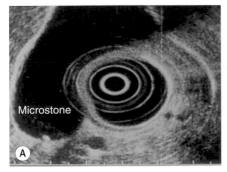

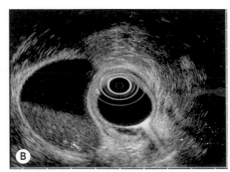

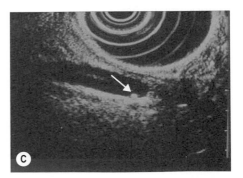

Figure 182 Microlithiasis. (A) Microstone (1 mm in size) within the gallbladder; (B) microstone (white arrow) within biliary sludge; (C) microstone (white arrow) within the CBD.

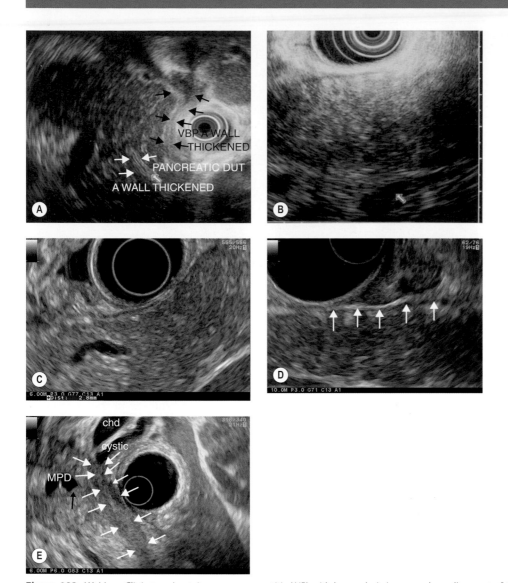

Figure 183 (A) Mayo Clinic type I autoimmune pancreatitis (AIP) with hypoechoic 'sausage shaped', aspect of the gland, ductitis (white arrow), i.e. main pancreatic duct (MPD) narrowing with hyperechoic thickening of the MPD wall, and autoimmune cholangitis (black arrows), i.e. diffuse thickening of the CBD wall. (B) Mayo Clinic type I AIP with heterogeneous hypoechoic 'pepper and salt' 'sausage shaped' aspect of gland. (C) Mayo Clinic type II AIP with hypoechoic 'sausage shaped' aspect of the gland and ductitis, i.e. hypoechoic thickening of the MPD wall. (D) Hypoechoic peripheral rim (white arrows) around the pancreatic body in AIP. (E) Mayo Clinic type I AIP in a young (15 years old) female with stenosis of the MPD (black arrows) and autoimmune cholangitis of the distal CBD (white arrows).

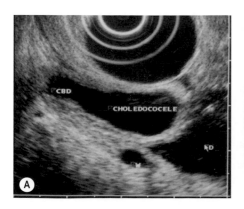

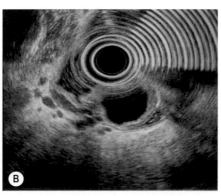

Figure 184 (A) Choledochocele. D, duodenal lumen filled of water; CBD, common bile duct. (B) Other aspect of a choledochocele.

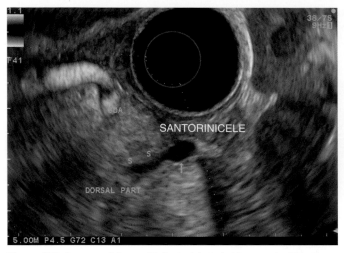

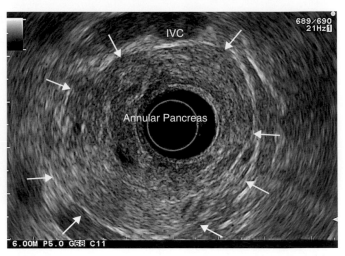

Figure 185 Pancreas divisum with Santorinicele (white arrow) within the minor papilla and the distal part of the Santorini duct (S) within the dorsal part (bright echostructure) of the head of the pancreas. GDA, gastroduodenal artery.

Figure 187 Annular pancreas (white arrows) imaged in the first part of the descending duodenum. IVC, inferior vena cava.

11.6. Acute pancreatitis

Although it is probably very sensitive, EUS has never been validated in the diagnosis of acute pancreatitis which relies on a combination of clinical signs, laboratory tests and characteristic CT features. EUS has also never been validated for assessing the severity of acute pancreatitis, although its ability to detect minimal peripancreatic areas of inflammation is excellent. It has, however, now been clearly demonstrated that EUS is very useful when it has not been possible to determine the origin of acute pancreatitis from questioning the patient, the usual morphological examinations such as ultrasound and MDCT, and specialized laboratory tests.

11.6.1. Acute biliary pancreatitis

EUS has clearly been established as the most accurate technique for identifying an unrecognized biliary cause, which accounts for almost half of all acute cases of pancreatitis of indeterminate origin at the initial assessment. Its sensitivity for the diagnosis of gallbladder microlithiasis in the absence

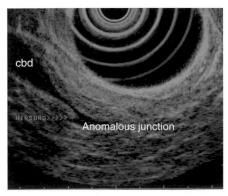

Figure 186 Anomalous junction of the biliary duct (cbd) and pancreatic duct (Wirsung).

of stones detectable on ultrasound exceeds 90% (Fig. 182) and it is significantly superior to the microscopic study of bile collected by duodenal intubation after cholecystokinin stimulation. EUS is also, as we shall see in the chapter on biliary disease, the standard method for the diagnosis of stones in the common bile duct which are known to be present in one-quarter of all cases after acute biliary pancreatitis (Fig. 182C). EUS is therefore particularly useful before laparoscopic cholecystectomy after mild or moderate acute biliary pancreatitis to ensure the common bile duct is unobstructed. To detect gallbladder microlithiasis, EUS should be performed if possible within 48 h of acute pancreatitis so that fasting will not distort the interpretation of any sludge visualized in the gallbadder. If the examination is performed some time after the episode of acute pancreatitis, it is better to wait for about 2 weeks after resuming eating so that interpretation of the images of the gallbladder are really informative.

11.6.2. Chronic pancreatitis

EUS is, as we have seen, extremely sensitive for the diagnosis of early non-calcifying chronic pancreatitis which is the second highest cause of acute pancreatitis of indeterminate origin (Fig. 179). Since the consequences of edematous acute pancreatitis for the parenchyma are different from the aspect of chronic pancreatitis, there is no reason to delay EUS in a patient with unexplained acute pancreatitis. In severe acute pancreatitis with parenchymatous necrosis, the lesions may persist for several months or even years, and it is usually impossible to make a diagnosis of the etiology of pancreatitis.

11.6.3. Acute pancreatitis of tumoral origin

EUS is the most sensitive technique for diagnosing a small tumor causing an episode of obstructive acute pancreatitis (Fig. 121), and it is also the standard examination for the diagnosis of IPMN, now a very classic etiology which should be investigated routinely in patients with unexplained acute pancreatitis, particularly if there has been recurrent acute pancreatitis.

11.7. Autoimmune pancreatitis

Finally, EUS strongly suggests a diagnosis of autoimmune pancreatitis when it shows a diffuse, very great increase in the volume ('sausage shaped')of the pancreatic gland, which usually has a hypoechoic (Fig. 183A) or heterogeneous hypoechoic 'salt and pepper' (Fig. 183B) echostructure, along with a pancreatic duct that is invisible or visible only in places; this aspect is known as ductitis, with hypoechoic (Fig. 183C) or hyperechoic (Fig. 183A) thickening of the wall in the areas where it is invisible or at the junction between an area where it is visible and one where it is invisible, and this is probably specific to this disease. Hypoechoic peripheral rim (Fig. 183D) when observed is also specific. Significant hypoechoic thickening of the bile duct wall (Fig. 183A), particularly in its distal section, is further evidence of an autoimmune origin, given the frequency of an association between autoimmune pancreatitis and autoimmune cholangitis in Mayo Clinic type I AIP. EUS FNA can yield additional support for the autoimmune nature of the disease. EUS FNA is essential if the autoimmune pancreatitis is localized to the pancreatic head, causing a picture of pseudotumoral pancreatitis with obstructive jaundice and a large cephalic mass (Fig. 137). Generally speaking, Mayo Clinic type II AIP is not well classified using HISORt classification, because of the lack of increased level of IgG 4 in the serum, absence of IgG4 plasmocytes in the biopsy specimen of the pancreas and of the papilla and difficulty to obtain typical histology of AIP using 19 G Tru-Cut EUS-guided biopsy. Typical EUS features of AIP including ductitis could be an additional criterion helpful for the diagnosis of Mayo Clinic type II AIP.

11.8. Embryological anomalies

Finally, EUS is very effective for the diagnosis of congenital pancreaticobiliary anomalies, whether for choledochocele (Fig. 184), pancreas divisum (Fig. 185), as EUS is equivalent to MRI with MRCP, or rarer anomalies such as an anomalous junction of the pancreatobiliary duct (Fig. 186) or an annular pancreas (Fig. 187).

In conclusion, EUS is essential to assess the etiology of acute pancreatitis of indeterminate origin. It can be carried out early to determine whether the etiology is biliary, tumoral or inflammatory. It is useful in severe acute pancreatitis only at a very early stage, to detect stones in the gallbladder and common bile duct.

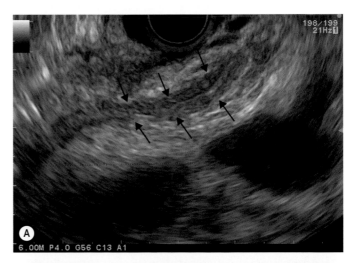

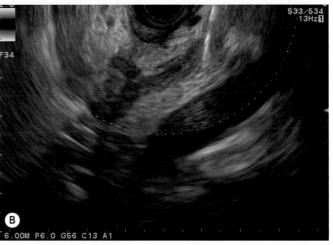

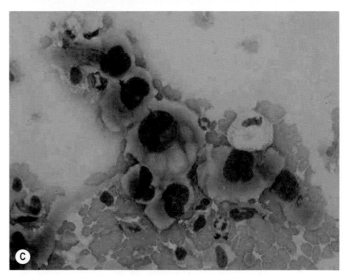

Figure 189 (A) Cholangiocarcinoma (black arrows) of the distal CBD. (B) EUS-guided FNA through the upper part of the descending duodenum of a cholangiocarcinoma of the distal CBD looking as PSC. (C) Cytology of a cholangiocarcinoma.

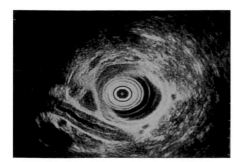

Figure 188 Primary sclerosing cholangitis.

12. Biliary EUS

12.1. Performance

The performance of biliary EUS is now clearly established. The resolving power is <1 mm and the common bile duct can be examined lengthwise in its entirety, including from the hepatic duct to the ampulla of Vater; the gallbladder can be visualized in its entirety, including at its neck and the origin of the cystic duct, and this can be followed as far as the cystic duct–common bile duct junction.

12.2. Limitations

The limitations of biliary EUS have also been clearly established:

- EUS is poor at identifying obstructing lesions in the hilum
- Very poor visualization of the distal segment of the common bile duct if the pancreas is very calcified, or in patients with severe necrotic acute pancreatitis
- It is impossible to carry out a correct biliary examination in patients with gastrectomy with Billroth type II gastroenterostomy
- It is impossible to examine the hepatic duct correctly in patients with pneumobilia caused by choledochoduodenal anastomosis or sphincterotomy and it is impossible to examine the ampulla of Vater correctly in patients who have undergone sphincterotomy
- It is difficult to make a differential diagnosis between primary sclerosing cholangitis (Fig. 188) and infiltrating non-polypoid cholangiocarcinoma if it is limited to the wall of the bile duct (Fig. 189) because these two diseases appear as a regular thickening of the common bile duct wall in EUS
- It is difficult to make a differential diagnosis between gallbladder cancer and lithiasic pyocholecystitis after a course of antibiotics.

12.3. Results

12.3.1. Common bile duct stones (Tables 4–6; Fig. 190)

EUS is the standard technique, superior to ERCP, perioperative opacification and MRCP, for the diagnosis of common bile duct stones with a diagnostic accuracy of 95% and a negative predictive value, i.e. the ability to rule out a diagnosis of common bile duct stones, of >95% (Figs 191, 192).

Table 4 EUS in CBD stones

Radial EUS				
Prospective blind/cholangiography studies				$n = 10$
Retrospective blind/cholangiography studies				$n = 1$
Patients at risk of CBDS				$n = 1470$
Patients with CBDS on gold standard exam				$n = 656$ (45%)
Se (%)	Sp (%)	Ac (%)	PPV (%)	NPV (%)
95	97	97	97	96

Linear EUS				
Prospective blind/cholangiography studies				$n = 1$
Patients at risk of CBDS				$n = 134$
Patients with CBDS on gold standard exam				$n = 91$ (68%)
Se (%)	Sp (%)	Ac (%)	PPV (%)	NPV (%)
93	93	94	98	87

Table 5 EUS vs ERC

	Overall		<4 mm stones	
	EUS	ERC	EUS	ERC
Sensitivity (%)	91[a]	75	90[a]	23
Specificity (%)	100	100	100	100
Accuracy (%)	92[a]	87	98[a]	89
PPV (%)	99	98	95.7[a]	59.1
NPV (%)	93[a]	82	98.8	95.3

[a]$p < 0.05$.
Randomized blind study – RCT with 120 patients undergoing EUS (first) and ERC (second) vs ERC only.
(From Karakan T, Cindoruk M, Alagozlu H, et al. EUS versus endoscopic retrograde cholangiography for patients with intermediate probability of bile duct stones: a prospective randomized trial, Gastrointest Endosc 2009; 69:244–252.)

Table 6 Outcomes. Prospective randomized controlled trial comparing EUS prior to ERC vs ERC alone for suspected CBD stones or significant biliary pathology

	Karakan 2009 (GIE)		Lee 2008 (GIE)		Polkowski 2007 (Endoscopy)	
	EUS/ERC	ERC	EUS/ERC	ERC	EUS/ERC	ERC
n	60	60	32	33	50	48
Endoscopic procedures per patient	1.4	1.6	1.3	1.1	1.4	1.3
Complications (%)	1.6	10	6	12.5	8	40

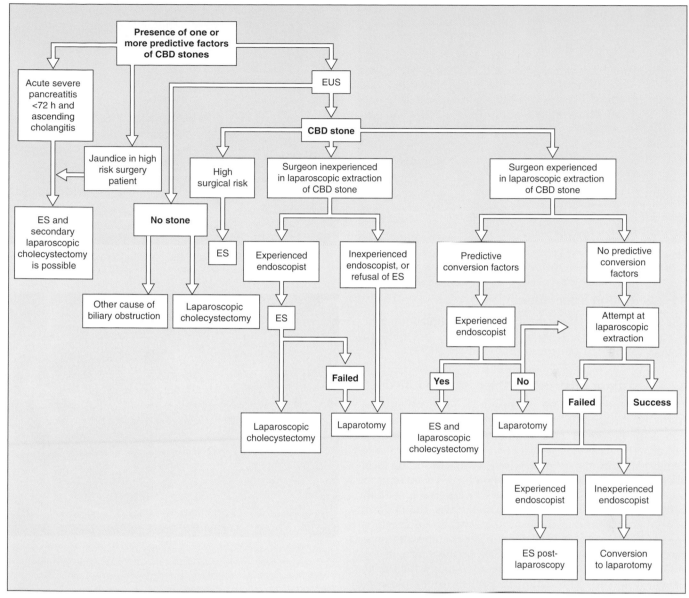

Figure 190 Algorithm on the usefulness of EUS when there is suspicion of CBD stone prior to laparoscopic cholecystectomy. ES: endoscopic sphincterotomy.

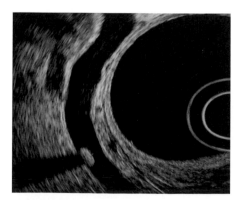

Figure 191 Small CBD stone (3 mm) within a non-dilated (5 mm) distal CBD.

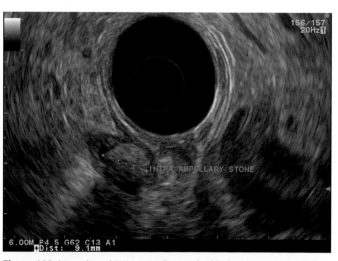

Figure 192 Large (1 cm) intra-ampullary embedded stone responsible for a pseudoneoplastic jaundice.

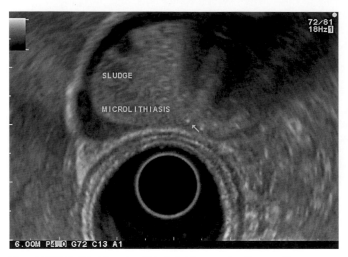

Figure 193 Gallbladder microlithiasis (white arrow), with acoustic shadowing within biliary sludge.

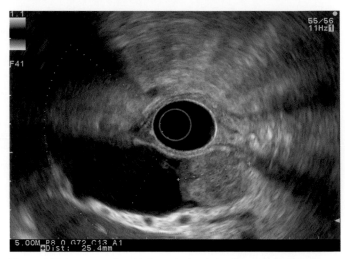

Figure 195 Intra-ampullary high-grade dysplasia villous adenoma.

12.3.2. Gallbladder stones

The sensitivity of EUS for the diagnosis of gallbladder stones is close to 100%. It is 90% for gallbladder microlithiasis undetected by percutaneous ultrasound (Fig. 193).

12.3.3. Tumor obstructing the common bile duct

The sensitivity of EUS for the diagnosis of cholangiocarcinoma of the subhilar bile duct (Fig. 194), cancer of the pancreatic head and intra-ampullary tumor of the ampulla of Vater (Figs 195–197) is close to 100% when local anatomical conditions are met. Given its diagnostic performance, EUS is the standard examination for assessment of the locoregional involvement of these cancers. For potentially operable patients without hepatic metastases, the performance of EUS in the diagnosis and assessment of locoregional involvement makes it ideal for the pre-therapeutic assessment of patients who have jaundice possibly related to a subhilar tumor, to determine more accurately which might benefit from surgical resection and which from endoscopic drainage. EUS should, generally speaking, be performed before any endoscopic drainage procedure since drainage may affect the result of the method.

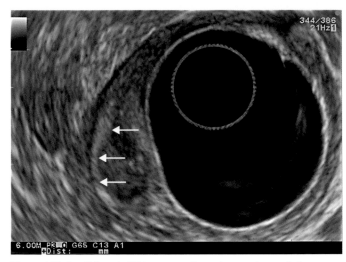

Figure 196 Small (1 cm) uT1 intra-ampullary adenocarcinoma. Submucosa is still visible (white arrows) around the tumor. It is impossible to know if submucosa is invaded (30% of lymph node involvement) or not (0% of lymph node involvement).

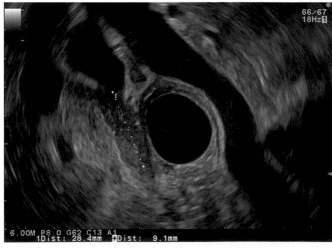

Figure 194 uT2 cholangiocarcinoma of the distal CBD.

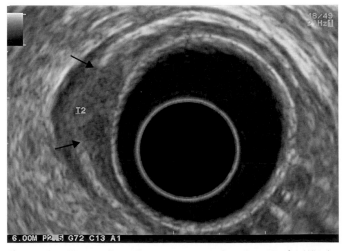

Figure 197 uT2 ampullary adenocarcinoma confirmed as pT2 after Wipple resection. Submucosa is interrupted (black arrows) and muscularis propria is invaded.

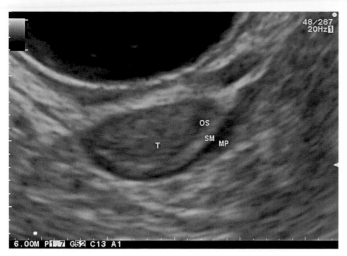

Figure 198 Intra-ampullary mucosal adenocarcinoma classified as uT1m by EUS. Oddi sphincter (OS) is not passed. Thus, submucosa (SM) is not invaded. The image of the ampulla is obtained using the specific withdrawal of the EUS scope. MP, muscularis propria.

In patients with tumor of the ampulla of Vater, EUS is essential for selecting patients with a usT1N0 tumor (Figs 196, 198), since they may possibly benefit from curative ampullectomy. Where possible, the use of a very high frequency miniprobe (20 MHz) mounted on a guidewire should be considered to improve the T staging and to rule out ampullectomy for patients in whom submucosal involvement has been detected, since the risk of lymph node involvement is then close to 30%.

12.3.4. Indications of biliary EUS

The indications of biliary EUS depend on the performance and limitations of the technique in biliary disease but also on the clinical context and results of hepatobiliary ultrasound, MDCT and, if necessary, MRCP.

- If endoscopic treatment is considered immediately.
  - If the diagnosis is strongly suspected, whether of a benign disease such as common bile duct stones (presence of progressive cholangitis or severe acute pancreatitis with signs of progressive biliary obstruction) or a malignant disease (apparently neoplastic obstruction on ultrasound or a CT scan) in an inoperable patient, it is clear that EUS has only a limited role compared with therapeutic ERCP. EUS is, in fact, carried out increasingly, despite all of this, immediately prior to ERCP, in the interventional endoscopy room, because even if it is not essential to the management of patients of this type, it assists ERCP and endoscopic treatment by determining exactly the nature and location of the obstruction and, in particular, the site of the biliary obstruction in relation to the ampulla of Vater. Furthermore, all the prospective studies concerning stone-like obstructions in the common bile duct have shown that in 10–15% of cases, the disease was not, in fact, due to stones and was easily accessible to EUS diagnosis, thus allowing correction of a diagnostic error which may have been prejudicial to the patient. EUS FNA is, moreover, very often

indicated in an inoperable patient with a tumor mass on MDCT, regardless of the reason, and we have previously seen, its performance is significantly better if it is carried out before insertion of a biliary stent.
- Before laparoscopic cholecystectomy (Fig. 190)
  - EUS is indicated in a patient with symptomatic gallbladder stones whenever there are factors predicting common bile duct stones, and biliary drainage is not urgent (no progressive cholangitis). Economic studies devoted to this condition and prospective randomized trials have shown that EUS performed in the interventional radiology room before ERCP, is the most cost-effective examination strategy (Table 6).

If obstruction by a tumor is suspected or already confirmed by ultrasound and MDCT, and if the patient is operable, with a view to resection, we have seen in the chapter on pancreatic diseases that it should go further in terms of the assessment of locoregional involvement, in particular of the vessels or lymph nodes.

- If a tumor-related obstruction is suspected or has been confirmed by ultrasound and MDCT in a patient who appears to be borderline from a surgical point of view, and if there is a difficult therapeutic choice between palliation by insertion of a biliary stent or surgical resection, further support for either one of these solutions should be obtained without causing morbidity. The tumor size, its precise location and its locoregional involvement, as well as its histological nature which can be obtained by EUS FNA, are often factors that will determine this choice. EUS is then the imaging technique that best meets the requirements of efficacy and low morbidity needed in this situation.
- Where there is diagnostic doubt about a possible obstruction, for example unexplained anomalies in hepatic tests, in particular cholestasis, associated in some cases with biliary duct dilation, the diagnosis of the obstruction (which is usually small in this case) should be confirmed or ruled out. EUS is in this case too the key examination, owing to its unrivalled spatial resolution.
- In patients who have undergone a cholecystomy, or in whom ultrasound does not show gallbladder stones, who have apparently biliary pain, EUS is again the ideal examination, owing to its resolving power of less than a mm, for confirming or ruling out a diagnosis of residual stones or unrecognized gallbladder microlithiasis. Given a clinical and biochemical picture suggesting migration, in the absence of stones, it is an elegant way of diagnosing sphincter of Oddi dysfunction without the risk of causing morbidity.

13. Assessment of submucosal tumors of the digestive tract

13.1. Introduction

EUS is very effective (>95%) for distinguishing between a true submucosal tumor in the digestive tract wall and extrinsic compression by a normal or pathological peridigestive structure and for locating large subcardiac intraparietal varices which may mimic a submucosal tumor. It is therefore indicated whenever a subepithelial swelling is visualized during endoscopy to determine its origin (Fig. 199). Some submucosal tumors have a characteristic appearance on EUS, for example lipoma (Fig. 200), aberrant pancreas (Fig. 201), duplication (Fig. 202), bronchogenic cyst of the lower esophagus (Fig. 203) and cystic dilatation of the submucosal glands of the esophagus (Fig. 204).

The positive diagnosis of stromal tumors, which are the most frequent mesenchymatous submucosal tumors in the stomach and the duodenum, is easy because they are a round or oval hypoechoic tumor, usually originating in the hypoechoic 4th layer (Fig. 205) which corresponds to the muscularis propria, or the echogenic 3rd layer which corresponds to the submucosa. They are well vascularized on Doppler study (Fig. 206) and contrast harmonic enhancement (Fig. 207). Their echostructure is largely homogeneous. Several criteria have been established to distinguish between stromal tumors that are entirely benign (Fig. 205), and stromal tumors that are malignant or potentially malignant.

- The presence of intratumoral cystic cavities (Fig. 208), or a tumor with outer borders that are irregular or spread out (Fig. 209)
- Size <3 cm, a homogeneous echostructure and regular borders are criteria highly predictive of a completely benign lesion (Figs 205–207).

EUS FNA with a 19-gauge needle (Fig. 210) is indicated to distinguish between leiomyoma and stromal tumor if surgery is not conclusively indicated (tumor <4 cm, no ulceration of the mucosa, patient over 60 years old), or if the tumor is awkwardly positioned (posterior side of the fundus or the subcardiac region). It is important to remember that in the esophagus (Fig. 211) and cardia (Figs 212, 213), >90% of hypoechoic tumors originating in the muscle layer are leiomyomas, since GISTs are very rare and 100% of hypoechoic tumors of the muscularis mucosae are leiomyomas (Fig. 210).

In the stomach, unlike in the esophagus, GISTs represent 85% of hypoechoic tumors originating in the muscularis propria, while leiomyomas and schwannomas represent only 15% of these lesions.

In the rectum, they are usually GISTs, and usually aggressive, and resection is a requirement in this location.

The classification, location in the digestive tract and principal endosonographic characteristics of submucosal tumors are summarized in Tables 7–9.

- Mostly leiomyomas (98%)
- Mostly GISTs (80%), leiomyomas (15%), schwannomas (5%)
- GISTs or leiomyomas.

The algorithm for the management of asymptomatic gastric submucosal tumors is shown in Figure 214.

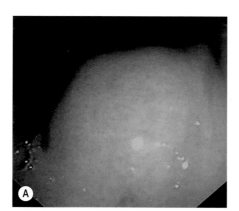
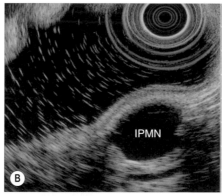
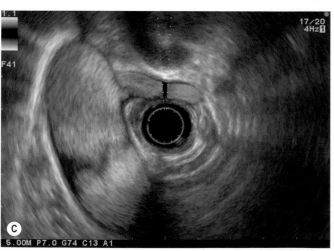

Figure 199 (A,B) Pseudo-tumorous submucosal bulge of the stomach due to an IPMN side branch type of the body of the pancreas. (C) Pseudo-tumorous submucosal bulge of the esophagus due to retroesophageal right subclavian artery.

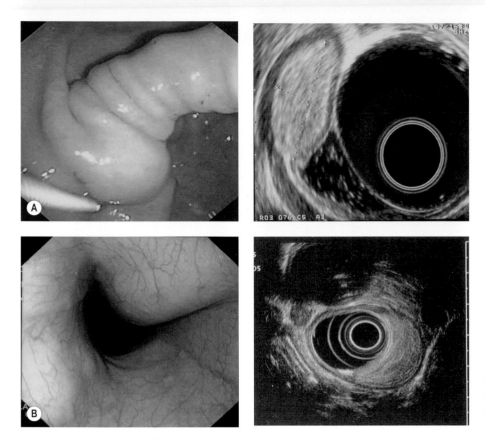

Figure 200 (A) Gastric lipoma located in the antrum. Pillow sign on the left, hyperechoic well-demarcated mass within the submucosa on the right. (B) Esophageal lipoma.

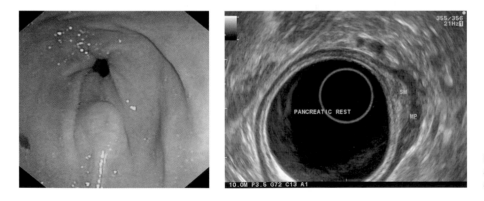

Figure 201 Pancreatic rest located in the antrum, developed within the submucosa (SM) and the muscularis propria (MP).

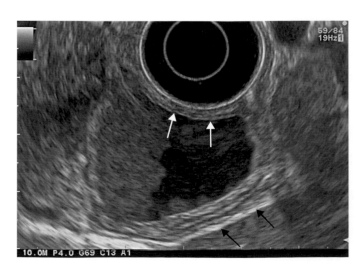

Figure 202 Duodenal duplication: five layers on the duodenal side (white arrows) and nine layers on the pancreatic side (black arrows). Dependant sludge is visible within the duplication.

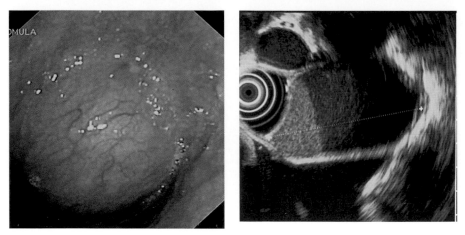

Figure 203 Bronchogenic cyst of the right side (always the right side) of the inferior part of the esophagus.

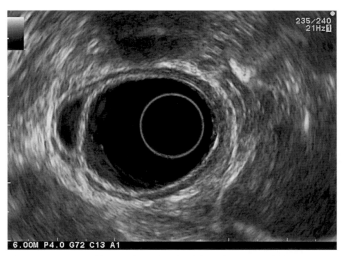

Figure 204 Cystic dilation of the glands of the submucosa of the lower esophagus.

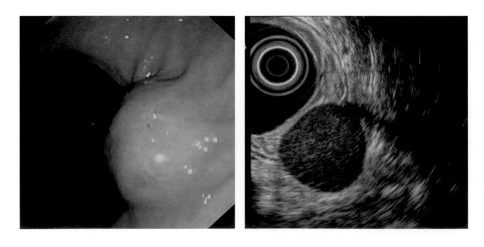

Figure 205 Small benign GIST located in the posterior part of the antral angle of the lesser curve. Hypoechoic, homogeneous, well demarcated, <3 cm in diameter round mass originating from the muscularis propria.

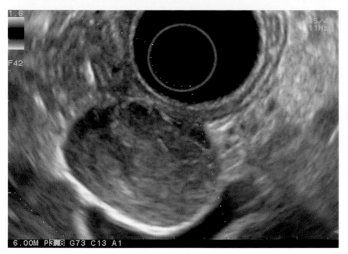

Figure 206 Small benign GIST developed outside the gastric wall, attached to the muscularis propria. See the vessels originating from the gastric wall, entering the tumor.

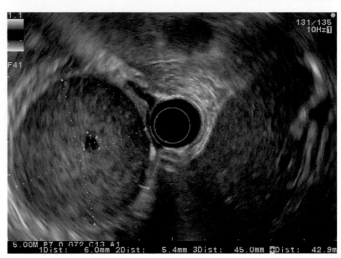

Figure 208 4.5 cm gastric GIST with central cystic image suggesting that the tumor is not benign.

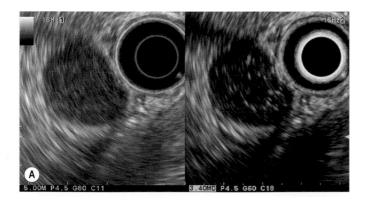

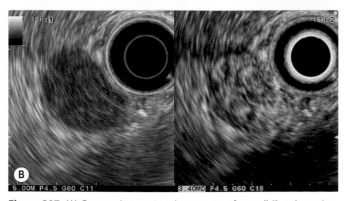

Figure 207 (A) Contrast harmonic enhancement of a small (3 cm) gastric GIST. 16 s after intravenous of 2.4 ml of Sonovue, the microvascularization starts to be visible with the tumor (on the right). (B) Same patient as A, image obtained 29 s after intravenous injection of Sonovue. See the hypervascularization of the tumor (right image).

Table 7 Classification of submucosal lesions

Neoplastic lesion	Non-neoplastic lesion	
GIST		
Leiomyoma	Cyst:	Duplication cyst
Leiomyosarcoma		Bronchogenic cyst Submucosal cyst
Schwannoma	Giant varix	
Granular cell tumor	Lymphangioma	
Carcinoid	Pancreatic rest	
Lipoma	Brunner's gland hamartoma	
Glomus tumor	Inflammatory fibroid polyp	
Metastatic deposit	Rectal endometriosis	

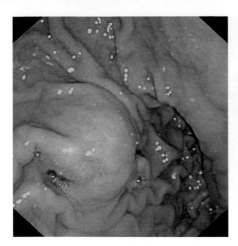
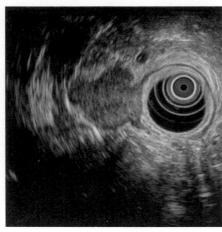

Figure 209 3.5 cm gastric GIST with irregular outer margin suggesting that the tumor is not benign.

Table 8 Main EUS features of submucosal tumors or lesions

SMT	EUS layer (organ)	EUS features
Benign lesions		
Leiomyoma	2nd or 4th (esophagus, cardia)	Hypoechoic, round or oval, well demarcated
Schwannoma	3rd or 4th (stomach)	Hypoechoic, round or oval, well demarcated
Lipoma	3rd (stomach, rectum)	Hyperechoic, smooth margins
Cysts, duplication cyst	Variable (mostly 3rd) (esophagus, stomach, duodenum)	Anechoic, compressible, round or oval (3 or 5 layer wall suggests duplication)
Bronchogenic cyst	4th (lower part of the esophagus)	Large, round, anechoic or hypoechoic, compressible mass, with beam enhancement, no Doppler signal
Lymphangioma	3rd (duodenum)	Anechoic
Pancreatic rest	2nd, 3rd or 4th (antrum, bulb)	Hypoechoic or mixed echogenicity, Ductal structure possible
Varices	2nd or 3rd (fundus)	Anechoic, serpiginous or linear with venous Doppler signal
Granular cell tumor	2nd or 3rd (lower esophagus)	Oval, small (thickness <1 cm) hypoechoic
Brunner's gland hyperplasia	2nd and 3rd (bulb)	Hyperechoic, smooth margins, possible hypoechoic dilated gland duct
Inflammatory fibroid polyp	2nd (antrum, bulb)	Polypoid, hypoechoic, covered by a thin mucosa
Potentially malignant lesions		
GIST	4th (stomach)	Hypoechoic, round, <3 cm, homogeneous with smooth margins: likely benign
		>3 cm, heterogeneous with cystic spaces and irregular extraluminal border: likely borderline or malignant
Lymphoma	2nd, 3rd or 4th (stomach)	Hypoechoic
Carcinoid	2nd or 3rd (fundus, rectum)	Hypoechoic
Sarcoma	4th (esophagus, stomach)	Hypoechoic, round, often heterogeneous with irregular extraluminal border or invasion of neighboring organs

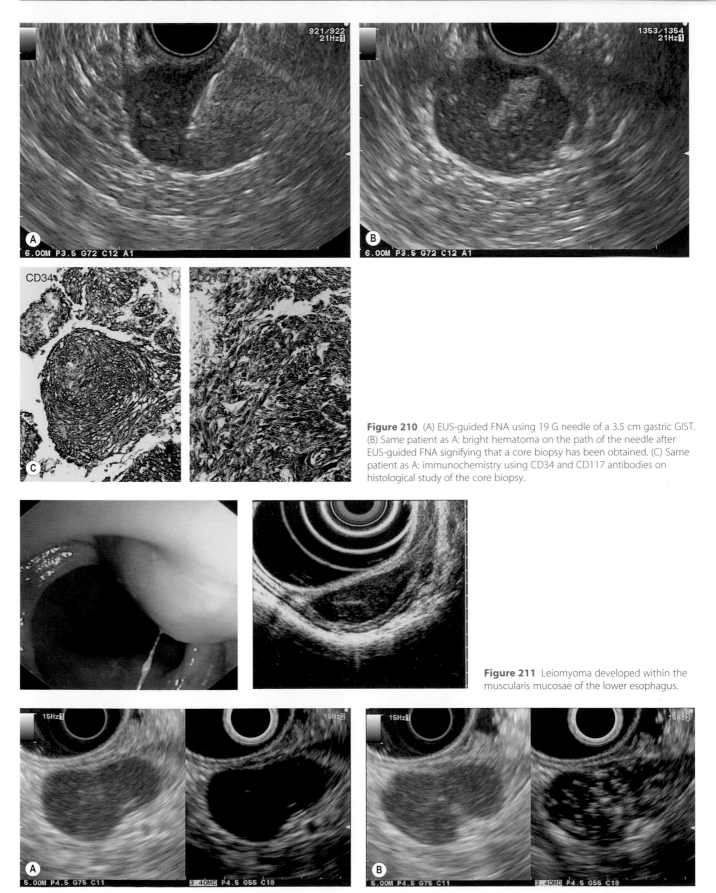

Figure 210 (A) EUS-guided FNA using 19 G needle of a 3.5 cm gastric GIST. (B) Same patient as A: bright hematoma on the path of the needle after EUS-guided FNA signifying that a core biopsy has been obtained. (C) Same patient as A: immunochemistry using CD34 and CD117 antibodies on histological study of the core biopsy.

Figure 211 Leiomyoma developed within the muscularis mucosae of the lower esophagus.

Figure 212 (A) Contrast harmonic enhancement of a leiomyoma developed in the cardia. 1 second after IV injection of 2.4 mL of Sonovue, the tumor is very hypoechoic. (B) Same patient as A: image obtained 15 s after IV injection. The microvascularization is less important and more heterogeneous than in GIST (see Fig. 207).

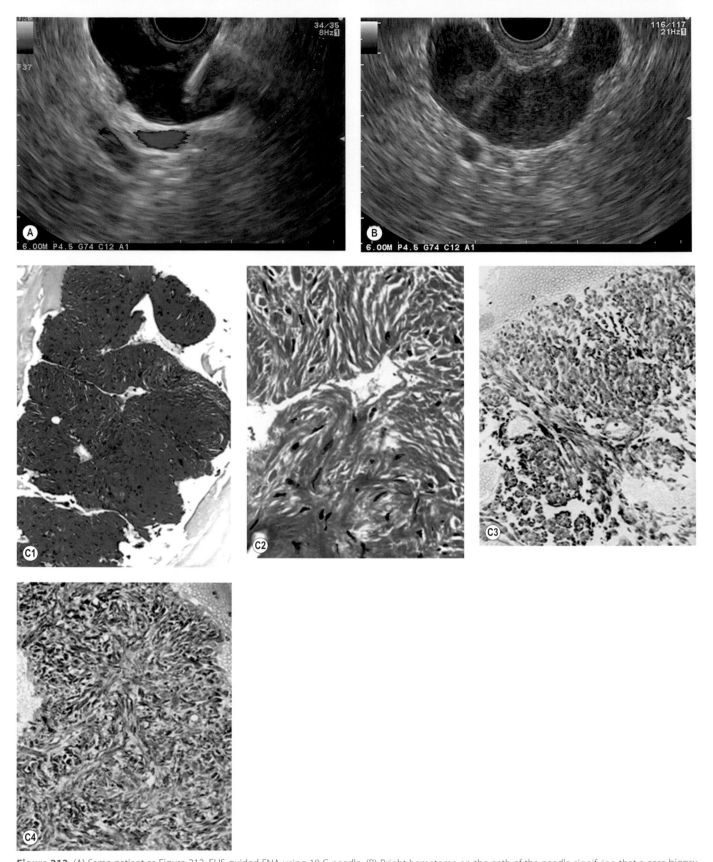

Figure 213 (A) Same patient as Figure 212. EUS-guided FNA using 19 G needle. (B) Bright hematoma on the path of the needle signifying that a core biopsy has been obtained. (C), (1,2) and top right: core biopsy with 19 G needle showing spin cells, with low nuclear density; (3) immunohistochemistry using H cadesmone antibodies demonstrating leiomyoma; (4) immunohistochemistry using desmin antibodies demonstrating leiomyoma.

Table 9 Frequency (%) of various submucosal lesions in relation to the location in the GI tract (histologically confirmed lesions only)

	Esophagus	Stomach	Duodenum	Rectum
GISTs or tumors formerly known as smooth muscle neoplasms	77[a]	54[b]	17[b]	14[c]
Pancreatic rest	0	16	2	0
Carcinoid	0	3	17	43
Lipoma	1	5	14	14
Cysts	1	9	19	0
Granular cell tumor	13	1	0	0
Lymphangioma or hemangioma	5	1	2	13
Brunner's gland hyperplasia	0	0	19	0
Other lesions	2	11	10	16

a, mostly lesiomyomas (98%)
b, mostly GIST (80%), leiomyomas (15%), schwannomas (5%)
c, GIST or leiomyoma

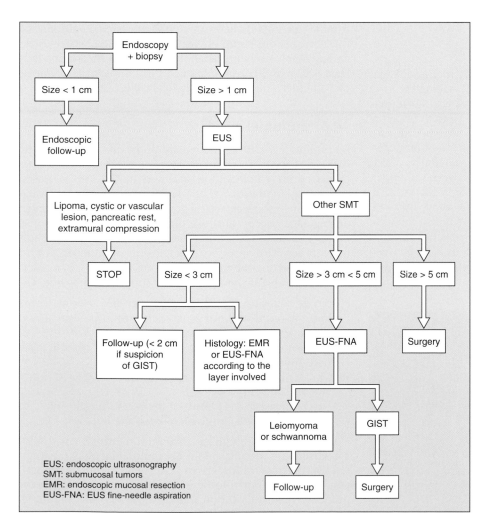

EUS: endoscopic ultrasonography
SMT: submucosal tumors
EMR: endoscopic mucosal resection
EUS-FNA: EUS fine-needle aspiration

Figure 214 Evaluation of asymptomatic gastric submucosal tumors.

14. Assessment of other GI disorders

14.1. Assessment of incontinence

The management of anal incontinence has been improved over the last 10 years by the use of anal endosonography which has become the standard examination for detecting sphincter defects, whether of the internal or external sphincter. Anal endosonography is therefore routinely indicated as the first-line examination for the diagnostic assessment of anal incontinence. It is also indicated to assess the quality of sphincter repair.

14.2. Anorectal inflammatory diseases

Endosonography, preferably performed with a sagittal electronic transducer, is very informative for the management of complex Crohn's fistulas and abscesses. Identifying the exact location of the primary orifice, which is sometimes clinically undetectable in the case of an anal fistula, is a very good indication for endosonography with a radial instrument. Insufflation of air into the anal canal during the examination facilitates the procedure.

14.3. Esophageal motor disorders

The endosonographic aspect of idiopathic megaesophagus is fairly characteristic in many cases (70%), taking the form of a very distinct thickening of the internal circular muscle layer (Fig. 215), which is clearly separated from the external longitudinal muscle layer by the interface which then appears to be very visible. This thickening, usually 2–3 mm, predominantly affects the lower-third of the esophagus and is found to a lesser degree at the junction between the upper- and middle-thirds, i.e. at the upper edge of the aortic arch. The esophageal wall is then entirely normal above this area. This thickening of the internal muscle layer is also found in diffuse esophageal spasm. Endosonography is the standard examination in doubtful cases for distinguishing between idiopathic megaesophagus and pseudomegaesophagus sec-

ondary to the presence of periesophageal infiltration, whether of gastric, pancreatic or metastatic origin (uterus or prostate).

14.4. Portal hypertension

Endosonography is more accurate than endoscopy for the diagnosis of gastric varices and congestive gastropathy of portal hypertension. This does not apply to the study of esophageal varices which are compressed by the balloon and may be invisible if they are low grade. Endosonography has been proposed to predict the risk of recurrent bleeding after the endoscopic treatment of esophageal varices. The risk of recurrence is believed to be higher in patients with extensive peri-esophageal collateral venous circulation after endoscopic treatment. Extensive collateral venous circulation in the periesophageal posterior mediastinum is believed to be an independent predictive factor of hemorrhagic recurrence.

14.5. Large (giant) fold gastritis

EUS is recommended in patients with endoscopic or radiological hypertrophic gastritis to distinguish malignant hypertrophic gastritis, where there is consistent submucosal thickening, from benign hypertrophic gastritis, where thickening is exclusively mucosal. If the mucosal thickening is at least 5 mm and it contains microcystic images, a diagnosis of Ménétrier's disease is highly likely (Fig. 106).

14.6. Endometriosis

Endometriosis is a recent but major indication for diagnostic EUS, given the increasing prevalence of this disease. Endometriosis of the rectal wall is observed in 10–25% of cases, depending on the study. The lesions (affecting the rectovaginal septum or the rectovesical pouch) are usually inaccessible during laparoscopy and are difficult to diagnose because none of the external imaging techniques, even MRI, are sufficiently sensitive or specific. Diagnosing endometriosis with certainty and quantifying its severity are essential when determining therapeutic and particularly surgical management.

- Single adhesion (adherences between the endometriosis and the rectal wall but no invasion into the muscle layer)
- Slight invasion of a small part of the rectal muscle layer (<10 mm in diameter)
- Moderate invasion of the rectal muscle layer (>10 mm and <15 mm in diameter)
- Severe invasion (>15 mm) of the rectal muscle layer
- Invasion of the submucosa or even the mucosa.

The surgical treatment of rectal endometriosis consists of a laparoscopic approach alone or combined with a transvaginal approach for minor lesions (<10 mm, submucosa intact), combined with laparotomy with excision of the nodule for moderate disease (>10 mm and <15 mm, submucosa intact), and laparotomy with rectal resection for severe disease or when the submucosa is involved.

The sensitivity of EUS is close to 100% for detecting lesions of the rectal wall (Figs 216, 217), its specificity is also excellent and, above all, the method can predict whether the endometrial lesions can be resected completely

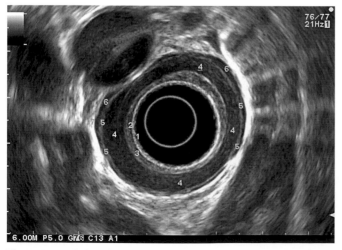

Figure 215 Achalasia. See the thickening of internal layer (4) of the muscularis propria. (5) interface between the internal, circular (4) and the external longitudinal (6) layer of the muscularis propria.

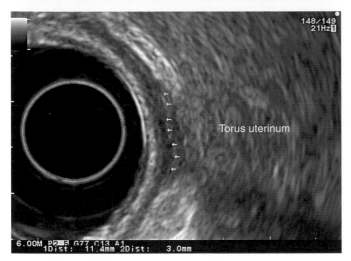

Figure 216 Endometriosis of the upper part of the rectovaginal septum behind the torus uterinum. The muscularis propria of the rectal wall is not invaded (white arrows). This kind of rectal involvement can be treated by laparoscopic approach without rectal resection.

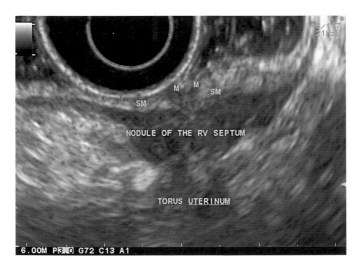

Figure 217 Endometriosis of the upper part of the rectovaginal septum, behind the torus uterinum invading the muscularis propria, the submucosa (SM) and the deeper part of the mucosa (M) of the rectal wall. This kind of rectal involvement justifies anterior rectal resection.

laparoscopically. The examination should therefore be recommended routinely before surgical treatment of the disease, in combination with other methods, notably MRI, which is effective for ovarian and anterior locations.

15. Celiac plexus neurolysis (EUS-CPN)

15.1. Introduction

The celiac plexus is composed of two groups of ganglia, usually located anterior and lateral to the aorta at the level of the celiac trunk (Fig. 218). This is usually around the level of the L1 vertebra but may vary from T12 to L2. The right ganglia are, on average, a few millimeters cephalad compared with those on the left and they can be identified as 1–5 oblong echopoor structures about 0.5–1.0 cm distal to the origin of the celiac artery.

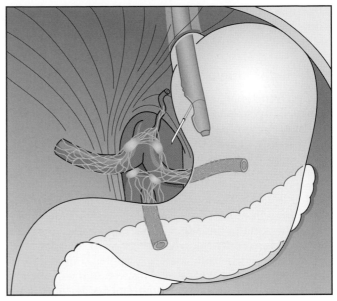

Figure 218 Schematic illustration of EUS-guided celiac plexus neurolysis procedure. The ganglia are approached at EUS from an anterior aspect, via the lesser curve of the stomach.

Box 17 Drugs used for celiac plexus neurolysis/block
CPN
• 20 mL 99% alcohol.
• 10 mL 0.25–0.5% bupivacaine.
CPB
• 20 mL 0.25% bupivacaine.
• 80 mg triamcinolone (4 mL).

Box 18 CPN/CPB: contraindications and difficult situations
• Inability to visualize anatomical landmarks/ensure correct needle tip placement:
◦ Previous surgery
◦ Large tumor mass
◦ Eccentric origin of celiac artery
◦ Ectatic aorta.
• Loss of soft tissue space between gastric wall and aorta in cachectic patients.
• Coagulopathy or severe thrombocytopenia.

Celiac plexus *neurolysis* (CPN) refers to permanent ablation of the celiac plexus and is usually performed with phenol or alcohol for malignant disease. Celiac plexus *block* (CPB) refers to temporary inhibition of pain using corticosteroid and long-acting local anesthetic (Box 17), usually for chronic pancreatitis.

CPN/CPB rarely relieve pain completely but may reduce opioid dosage and side-effects. The procedure should be regarded as part of an overall management strategy and discussed carefully with patients and other team members; other factors potentially contributing to pain in cancer patients (e.g. constipation, depression) should also be considered and treated. There are few contraindications to CPN/CPB (Box 18).

Injection of alcohol is painful despite sedation so a long-acting local anesthetic is also used, most commonly 10–20 mL of 0.25% bupivacaine.

15.2. Technique of CPN/CPB

The procedure is performed under conscious sedation with the patient in the left lateral position. Some advocate broad-spectrum antibiotics (e.g. ciprofloxacin 200 mg IV during the procedure and 250–500 mg twice daily orally for the next 3 days) if steroids are being injected into patients with chronic pancreatitis because of case reports of peripancreatic abscess.

Using a CLA echoendoscope, the region of the celiac plexus is visualized from the lesser curve of the gastric body by following the aorta to the origin of the main celiac artery and traced, using counter-clockwise rotation, to its bifurcation into splenic and hepatic arteries. Doppler control can be useful in some cases. With careful inspection it will often be possible, using slight rotational movements, to identify the celiac ganglia as several elongated hypoechoic structures.

A 22 G or 19 G EUS-FNA needle is usually used but in some countries a dedicated 20 G 'spray' needle with multiple sideholes is available and allows solutions to spread over a greater area. The caliber of larger needles also means less force is required to inject the relatively large volumes required. The stylet is withdrawn, the needle flushed with saline to remove air and then the gastric wall is punctured as for an FNA procedure (Fig. 219). The tip is placed slightly anterior and cephalad to the origin of the celiac artery or directly into the ganglia if these can be identified as discrete structures. Aspiration is first performed to exclude vascular puncture. Bupivacaine is injected first, followed by alcohol (or triamcinolone for CPB) and an echogenic 'blush' can usually be seen during injection. For injection, one of two strategies can be used in cases where the ganglia cannot be clearly seen. Injection of the entire solution into the area cephalad of the celiac trunk can be performed or else the echoendoscope is rotated to one side of the celiac artery and half of the solution is injected. The other half is then injected

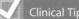
on the opposite side of the celiac artery origin: there is little evidence to support one method over another.

Resistance to injection of solutions is significant when using a 22-gauge needle. If no resistance is encountered, the possibility of vascular puncture should be considered. Using a 19-gauge needle, little if any resistance is encountered and injection is quicker to perform. It is important to realize that while injecting alcohol for CPN, needle visibility is obscured because of the hyperechoic appearance of the solution resulting in a 'snow storm' effect. Accurate needle tip placement prior to injection is, therefore, crucial.

Patients should be observed for 2–4 h after the procedure for fever or pain and with careful blood pressure monitoring. Postural hypotension is usually temporary and responds to intravenous fluids. Pain may worsen temporarily requiring higher analgesics doses and transient diarrhoea, reflecting sympathetic blockade, usually settles spontaneously or with antidiarrheal agents. Patients should be warned about the importance of reporting any lower limb weakness or numbness although neurological damage has not been reported following EUS-CPN/CPB. It may be helpful to document pain scores before and after the procedure to decide whether or not it has been successful.

15.3. Superior hypogastric plexus block

This technique involves injecting absolute alcohol opposite the sacral promontory below the aortic bifurcation (Fig. 220). The indication for this technique is chronic

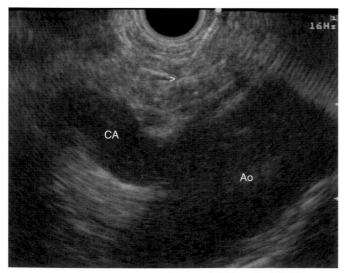

Figure 219 EUS-CPN. The needle tip (arrowhead) is positioned just cephalad and anterior to the origin of the celiac axis (CA) as it arises from the aorta (Ao).

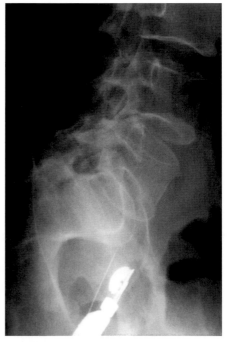

Figure 220 Hypogastric block: endoscopic ultrasound probe and alcohol needle in place in front of the promontory.

Acute pancreatic fluid collection (PFC)

- Occur early after acute pancreatitis.
- Thin or no wall, no solid component and almost always sterile.
- Resorb spontaneously and rarely require treatment.

Pseudocysts

- Occur ≥4 weeks after acute pancreatitis or in the course of chronic pancreatitis.
- Well-defined wall and high amylase content due to communication with pancreatic duct.
- No necrosis and duct disruption may spontaneously seal off with resolution.
- In chronic pancreatitis duct disruption rarely seals off and drainage should be considered in the presence of symptoms, or size ≥6 cm.

Walled-off pancreatic necrosis (WOPN)

- May be sterile or infected and occur after acute necrotizing pancreatitis.
- Presence of gas on CT, fever or clinical evidence of sepsis mandate treatment as does presence of severe symptoms.
- Differentiation from a simpler pseudocyst is essential in treatment planning and both MRI and EUS may be required.

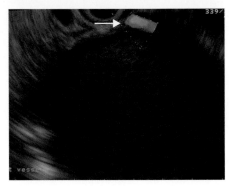

Figure 221 Pancreatic pseudocyst. The cyst contents are homogeneous and hypoechoic with no evidence of solid matter or necrosis. Doppler flow identifies an interposed vessel at the site of intended puncture (arrow).

Box 20   Indications for drainage of pancreatic pseudocysts

- Pain.
- Obstruction – biliary or gastric outlet.
- Sepsis.
- Tail lesion with segmental portal hypertension (risk of spontaneous splenic rupture).

morphine-dependent pelvic pain in the presence of recurrent rectal cancer, and more rarely infiltration secondary to urogenital malignancy. Locating the aortic bifurcation after positioning the echoendoscope in the sigmoid is simple and use of fluoroscopy allows for an anterior injection into the plexus without risk of vascular puncture or the use of contrast media, thus reducing the risk of infection. The mean duration of efficacy is 10 weeks and considering the prevalence of this type of pain syndrome this procedure may eventually be performed more often than CPN.

16. Drainage of pancreatic fluid collections (PFC)

16.1. Classification and terminology

Before considering endoscopic drainage of pancreatic fluid collections it is essential to have a clear understanding of the different types of fluid collection and these are classified as (see Box 19 for more details):

- Acute peripancreatic fluid collections
- Pseudocysts
- Walled-off pancreatic necrosis.

There are two types of pancreatic pseudocysts:

- Retention pseudocysts, which complicate chronic calcific pancreatitis
- Pseudocysts secondary to acute pancreatitis, which may be primary (e.g. biliary) or acute-on-chronic pancreatitis.

Endoscopic drainage can be either transpapillary or transmural and is subject to very specific indications (Box 20), which are the same regardless of the approach used.

16.1.1. Pseudocysts occurring in chronic pancreatitis

For these transpapillary drainage at ERCP should be attempted first. Transmural drainage is indicated if transpapillary drainage fails (e.g. ductal stones).

16.1.2. Pseudocysts secondary to acute pancreatitis

Only mature pseudocysts are amenable to drainage (the presence of a defined wall or capsule should be apparent on CT). The contents must be fluid and contain little or no necrotic debris (Figs 221, 222). CT is an inadequate method for assessment of the nature of cyst contents and transabdominal ultrasound or MRI should be used instead. EUS with FNA using a 19-gauge needle is probably best for this and can be used prior to definitive drainage. Transpapillary drainage is best avoided as communication between the pancreatic duct and cyst is common and there is a risk of infecting the cyst contents.

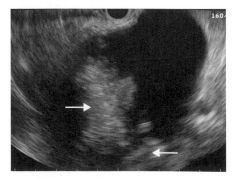

Figure 222 This pseudocyst contains a large amount of solid debris and necrotic material (arrows).

Transmural drainage of PFC is minimally invasive, reasonably safe and has traditionally been performed at endoscopy using a therapeutic gastroscope or duodenoscope and fluoroscopic assistance ('conventional transmural drainage', CTD) with variable success. For CTD, a visible endoscopic bulge in the stomach or duodenum is necessary and this occurs in only 50% of patients. Perforation rates of 2–5% and major bleeding in 10% are potentially serious complications. Bleeding usually occurs because of puncture of interposed vessels between the gut wall and cyst cavity, often related to the presence of varices resulting from splenic vein thrombosis and segmental portal hypertension.

✓ Clinical Tip

Contraindications to EUS pseudocyst drainage
- Absence of mature walled cyst.
- Cyst >1 cm away from the gastric or duodenal wall.
- Pseudoaneurysm.

In recent years numerous studies have demonstrated the potential advantages of EUS (Table 10). EUS is used either to assess the pseudocyst prior to CTD, in which case the nature, location and size of the cysts are carefully documented, alternative diagnoses are excluded (e.g. cystic neoplasm), the presence of solid debris within the cyst is excluded and the optimum site for drainage is marked by tattooing, or for mucosal biopsy. Cyst fluid contents can be aspirated by EUS-FNA for microbial culture as well as measurement of fluid amylase, lipase and CEA concentrations. The echoendoscope is then replaced by a therapeutic gastroscope or duodenoscope and CTD performed. If the cyst is relatively small, a 0.035 inch guidewire is coiled within the cyst after it has been punctured with a 19 G EUS-FNA needle. Care must be taken as there is a risk of guidewire dislodgement during endoscope exchange or if the patient is repositioned during the procedure.

16.2. One-step EUS-guided pseudocyst drainage

This approach has been increasingly adopted in most centers in recent years and offers a number of advantages compared to CTD (Table 10).

A therapeutic echoendoscope with a large (3.7–3.8 mm) operating channel is essential. This scope allows placement of 8.5–10 French stents and a nasocystic drain if the cyst contains thick debris and in cases of abscess (Figs 223–225). Other equipment required for one-step EUS guided PFC drainage is detailed in Box 21.

16.3. Technique

The separate steps in the procedure are outlined in Figure 226. After EUS–guided puncture of the cyst cavity with a 19 G needle and aspiration of fluid contents for analysis, a 0.035 inch guidewire is coiled within the cyst, confirmed fluoroscopically. To facilitate stent deployment it is essential to dilate up the puncture tract and a number of different methods to achieve this have been described. Some rely on the use of electrocautery with pure cutting current. This is

Table 10 Comparison of conventional and EUS-guided drainage of pancreatic pseudocysts

Advantages	Disadvantages
Conventional drainage (CTD)	
Better optical view. Large instrument channel – suctioning large fluid volumes; deployment of 10 F stents. Potential for pancreatogram or debridement if required.	Only possible if endoscopic bulge seen. Requires two procedures or scope exchange for EUS. No EUS imaging at time of puncture. Risk of guidewire displacement. Longer procedure time.
One-step EUS-guided drainage	
Allows confirmation that it is a pseudocyst and not a cystic tumor. Precise measurement of distance between gut wall and cyst lumen (must be <1 cm). Endoscopic bulge not required. Selection of optimum site for transmural puncture. Possible for difficult/unusual puncture sites, e.g. cardia. Identification of pseudoaneurysms. Accurate detection of necrosis/solid debris. Detection of interposed vessels or gastric varices. Direct visualization of cyst puncture. No scope exchange.	Oblique-forward viewing optics. Tangential accessory path through gastric wall. Smaller instrument channel (3.8 mm) hinders passage of 10 F stents; cannot pass 10 F stent if guidewire alongside in channel.

performed using either a wire-guided needle knife or a 10 F cystotome and is relatively straightforward but perhaps increases the risk of perforation. As such some experts prefer to dilate the tract with an ECRP cannula or a Soehendra dilator and then biliary dilation balloons to facilitate stent deployment, avoiding the need for electrocautery. There is no good evidence that one technique is superior to the other and the choice should depend on operator experience.

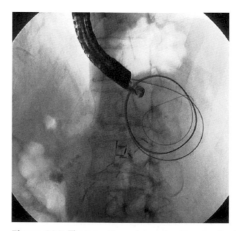

Figure 223 Therapeutic endoscopic ultrasound using a probe with a wide operating channel and a guidewire looped in the pseudocyst. A guide catheter that is looped on the guidewire is also used.

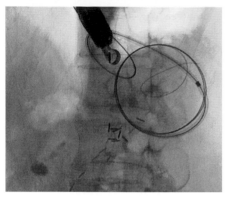

Figure 225 Endoscopic ultrasound probe in place; placement of a 10 French dual-pigtail stent.

16.3.1. Drainage of abscesses or walled-off pancreatic necrosis (WOPN)

To ensure adequate drainage of thick, purulent material, multiple stents, a nasocystic catheter for intensive irrigation or even endoscopic transmural necrosectomy (ETN) may be necessary. To allow these complex procedures to be performed, multiple guidewires need to be inserted into the cyst. A number of slightly different techniques have been described, including the use of a prototype 3-layered kit consisting of a 22 G FNA needle inside a 5 F Teflon catheter,

Box 21	Equipment required for EUS-guided PFC drainage

- CLA echoendoscope with instrument channel ≥3.7 mm.
- 19 G EUS-FNA needle.
- 0.035 inch guidewires.
- Tract dilation devices:
  - 4–5 F ERCP cannula
  - 10 F Soehendra dilation catheter
  - Over-the-wire needle knife catheter
  - 10 F cystotome.
- Biliary balloon dilator (6–8 mm) or 12 mm CRE balloon.
- 7 F or 10 F double pigtail stents.
- Nasocystic catheter if suspicion of infection/necrosis.

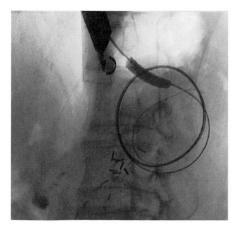

Figure 224 Endoscopic ultrasound probe in place, balloon dilatation for 6 mm of the path.

 Clinical Tips

Steps prior to pseudocyst drainage

- Ensure diagnosis has established this is a pseudocyst and not a pancreatic cystic tumor.
- Wait for pseudocyst to mature or resolve (4–6 weeks or longer).
- Define any communication with pancreatic duct (MRCP).
- Use transpapillary approach first except for pseudocysts occurring in acute pancreatitis.
- Identify any intracystic pseudoaneurysm (CT and/or EUS).
- Look for segmental portal hypertension associated with gastric varices.
- Exclude any collateral vessels between gut wall and cyst.
- Verify pseudocyst is closely applied to gastric or duodenal wall (<1 cm).
- Check for necrosis /solid debris in pseudocyst (EUS or MRI).
- Check for blood in the pseudocyst by FNA prior to drainage.

which is in turn inside a 8.5 F Teflon outer catheter. Alternatively a 10 F cystotome device can be used. With this a wire-guided inner needle knife with electrocautery is used under EUS guidance to puncture the cyst. The needle knife is withdrawn leaving the wire in place and the inner 5.5 F catheter advanced into the cyst over the wire. The outer 10 F catheter is then advanced over this with electrocautery and a second guidewire placed through the 10 F catheter after the inner 5.5 F catheter is removed.

Sequential dilation is performed with ERCP cannulae, Soehendra dilators or biliary balloons as described above. Finally, a new prototype forward viewing therapeutic echoendoscope has been developed with a larger working channel and may become more available for this type of procedure in the near future.

The nasocystic catheter is continuously irrigated with 1–1.5 L of saline every 24 h for 2–3 days and also flushed with 100–200 mL of saline by syringe lavage four times daily. When there is organized necrosis, ETN may be performed by experts with great care. This requires a mature collection with a thick wall which is no more than 1 cm away from the gastric wall. One week after the initial EUS drainage procedure, the procedure is repeated with balloon dilatation of the tract up to 15–20 mm. Thereafter, a therapeutic gastroscope may be used to enter the cavity and solid material can be gently grasped and removed using a Dormia basket, Roth net or endoscopic snare. Great care is required to prevent arterial bleeding from the friable wall. Free perforation is also a risk and air embolism has been reported as a result of insufflation of excess air. Carbon dioxide is therefore recommended as it is much more rapidly absorbed. ETN usually requires multiple sessions, repeated every 1–4 days to clear all necrotic tissue and full back-up facilities must be available – intensive care, surgery, and radiology.

EUS-guided drainage of PFC is time consuming, challenging and not without risk. It should only be undertaken by endoscopists experienced in both EUS and ERCP techniques. The full range of EUS, ERCP and radiology facilities need to be available as do expert anesthesia, intensive care and pancreaticobiliary surgery. Before embarking on these procedures the indication, appropriateness and choice of technique all need to be carefully considered and discussed

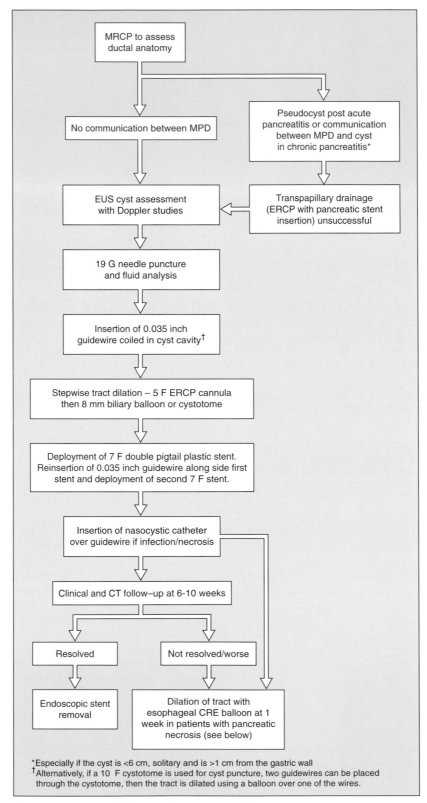

Figure 226 EUS-guided drainage of pancreatic pseudocysts.

in a multidisciplinary setting so that the goals of treatment are carefully understood by all concerned. Endoscopic transmural necrosectomy remains an investigational technique and should probably only be undertaken by a limited number of endoscopists working in tertiary referral centers.

17. EUS fine-needle injection and fiducial placement

17.1. EUS fine-needle injection

EUS fine-needle injection (EUS-FNI) is used to mark tumors for resection. This is particularly useful for neuroendocrine tumors or those that will be resected laparoscopically. EUS-FNI is performed in the same manner as EUS-FNA. A 22 G needle is inserted proximal to the lesion under direct visualization. 2–4 mL of sterile purified carbon particles (GI spot) or indocyanine green in injected under direct visualization. India ink has also been used; however, it has been associated with sterile abscesses and it is not recommended. Injection is continued as the EUS-FNA needle is withdrawn leaving an inked tract but care must be taken to avoid intraperitoneal injection. Peri-procedural intravenous ciprofloxacin is usually given and continued orally for 3 days.

17.2. EUS-guided fiducial placement

Stereotactic radiotherapy is being increasingly used to treat pancreatic adenocarcinoma. The ability to accurately target a lesion is a key component of this treatment. EUS-FNI can be used to place three to five gold fiducials (Fig. 227) which can be seen with X-ray.

The stylet is removed from a 19 G EUS-FNA needle. The 5 mm long fiducial embedded in a small piece of sterile wax

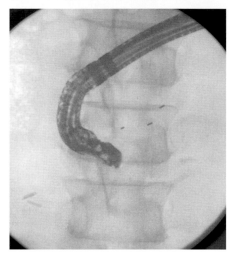

Figure 227 Three gold fiducials have been placed by EUS in a mass in the head of pancreas.

is backloaded into the tip of the needle; 3 mm fiducials can also be used; however, they are more difficult for the radiation oncologists to visualize. The stylet is then reinserted so that it is just proximal to the fiducial. The needle is then inserted into the tumor. Once the needle is in an adequate position, the stylet is advanced, releasing the fiducial from the needle and into the tumor. The needle is then withdrawn and the process repeated. A minimum of three fiducials should be placed at the edges of the tumor. A clip should be placed on mucosa closest to the area to be irradiated, allowing the radiation oncologist to avoid irradiating this area.

Further Reading

ASGE. Guideline: Complications of EUS, *Gastrointest Endosc* 61(1):8–12, 2005.

ASGE. Guideline: The role of endoscopy in the diagnosis and the management of cystic lesions and inflammatory fluid collections of the pancreas, *Gastrointest Endosc* 61(3):363–370, 2005.

ASGE Technology Committee: Technology evaluation status report. Echoendoscopes, *Gastrointest Endosc* 66(3):435–440, 2007.

ASGE Technology Committee: Technology evaluation status report. EUS accessories, *Gastrointest Endosc* 66(6):1076–1081, 2007.

Jhala D, Jhala N: a cytology primer for endosonographers. In Hawes RH, Fockens P, editors : *Endosonography*, ed 2, London, 2010, Elsevier, pp 234–251.

Collins D, Penman I, Mishra G, Draganov P: EUS-guided celiac block and neurolysis, *Endoscopy* 38(9):935–939, 2006.

Dancygier H, Lightdale CH, editors: *Endosonography in gastroenterology*, New York, 1999, Thieme.

Diagnostic and interventional endoscopic ultrasound. 6th International symposium on endoscopic ultrasonography, *Gastrointest Endosc* 69(2):Supplement, 2009.

Hawes RH, Fockens P, editors: *Endosonography*, ed 2, London, 2010, Elsevier.

Karakan T, Cindoruk M, Alagozlu H, et al: EUS versus endoscopic retrograde cholangiography for patients with

intermediate probability of bile duct stones: a prospective randomized trial, *Gastrointest Endosc* 69(2):244–252, 2009.

Sahai AV, Banerjee, P: How to perform EUS-guided FNA. In: Hawes RH, Fockens P, editors: *Endosonography*, ed 2, London, 2010, Elsevier, pp 265–272.

Seewald S, Ang, TL, Teng KYK, et al: Endoscopic ultrasound-guided drainage of abdominal abscesses and infected necrosis, *Endoscopy* 41:166–174, 2009.

Sobin L, Gospodarowicz M, Wittekind C, editors: *International Union against Cancer (UICC) TNM Classification of cancer*, ed 7, London, 2009, Wiley-Blackwell.

Endoscopic retrograde cholangiopancreatography

Jean Marc Canard, Anne Marie Lennon, Jean-Christophe Létard, Jacques Etienne, Patrick Okolo

10.1 Introduction

Introduction

Although almost all endoscopic retrograde cholangiopancreatography (ERCP) is undertaken with a view to a therapeutic intervention, an understanding of the basic concepts is essential before progressing to therapeutic ERCP. This chapter is divided into two sections. The first section introduces the basic techniques required to selectively cannulate the common bile duct or pancreatic duct, as well as the equipment required for ERCP; how to ensure that you obtain the optimum images from the procedure; and what pitfalls to watch out for in image interpretation. The second part of the chapter discusses therapeutic procedures and the complications associated with ERCP.

Photodynamic therapy was written by Jacques Etienne.

©2011 Elsevier Ltd.
DOI: 10.1016/B978-0-7020-3128-1.00010-9

Key Points

- The commonest cause of litigation in ERCP is that the procedure was not indicated.
- Diagnostic ERCP should be avoided, and has been replaced by EUS and MRI.
- If EUS is indicated, it should be performed before ERCP, as a sphincterotomy or stent placement limits the ability to adequately visualize the ampullary region.

Introduction

It is essential that an endoscopic retrograde cholangiopancreatography (ERCP) is undertaken for an appropriate indication. The commonest cause of litigation in ERCP is that the procedure was not indicated. Consensus and association guidelines are available and can be found in the further reading section. ERCP is primarily a therapeutic procedure. Non-invasive imaging (EUS or MRI) should be performed if an intervention is unlikely to be required. If EUS is indicated, it should be performed before ERCP when possible, as a sphincterotomy or stent insertion greatly limits the ability to assess the papilla and distal common bile duct.

1. Indications

1.2. Biliary

- *Choledocholithiasis*: Routine ERCP is not indicated for assessment of common bile duct stones in patients undergoing laparoscopic cholecystectomy, where there is a low probability of having choledocholithiasis. ERCP is indicated in patients with a high suspicion of choledocholithiasis (jaundice, dilated common bile duct, cholangitis, or acute pancreatitis secondary to choledocholithiasis).
- *Malignancy*: ERCP is useful in assessing ampullary lesions. It can be used to acquire tissue in patients with biliary or pancreatic malignancy, although it is not always diagnostic. ERCP can be used to palliate malignant biliary obstruction.
- *Biliary strictures*: ERCP is effective in treating benign bile duct strictures.
- *Bile duct leak*: ERCP should be the first procedure used to treat bile duct leak.
- *Sphincter of Oddi dysfunction (SOD)*: ERCP with sphincterotomy is indicated in type I. Patients with type II SOD should undergo manometry and may benefit from sphincterotomy if elevated pressure (>40 mmHg) is found.

1.3. Pancreatic

- *Acute pancreatitis*: ERCP has no role in acute pancreatitis, with the exception of acute pancreatitis associated with choledocholithiasis. ERCP is indicated in patients with acute recurrent pancreatitis to assess and treat the cause.
- *Chronic pancreatitis*: ERCP is useful for treating symptomatic strictures, pancreatic duct stones, and for draining pseudocysts.
- ERCP is useful for the management of pancreatic duct leak or duct disruption.

Further Reading

Adler DG, Baron TH, Davila RE, et al: ASGE guidelines: the role of ERCP in diseases of the biliary tract and the pancreas, *Gastrointest Endosc* 62:1, 2005.

Cohen D, Bacon BR, Berlin JA, et al: National Institutes of Health state-of-the-science conference statement: ERCP for diagnosis and therapy, *Gastrointest Endosc* 56:803, 2002.

10.3 Drugs used in ERCP

Key Points

- Glucagon decreases peristalsis and can be used to decrease duodenal motility.
- Secretin stimulates secretion of pancreatic juice and can be used to facilitate identification of the ampulla of Vater and the accessory papilla.

Introduction

In addition to the usual medications used for sedation (see Ch. 2.3), glucagon and secretin are sometimes use to aid identification of the major or minor papillae or assist cannulation.

1. Glucagon

Glucagon causes transient relaxation of the smooth muscles of the GI tract, thus decreasing motility. Glucagon has an onset of action of 1 min, with a duration of effect of 20–30 min. It should be avoided in patients undergoing sphincter of Oddi manometry.

Dose

- The initial dose is 0.25–0.5 mg IV.

Side-effects

- Nausea, vomiting
- Hypertension, hypotension, tachycardia
- Hypersensitivity or allergic reaction.

Use with caution

- Adrenal insufficiency
- Chronic hypoglycemia
- Elderly
- Chronic obstructive airways disease (COAD).

Contraindications

- Phaeochromocytoma
- Insulinoma
- Known hypersensitivity to glucagon.

Use in pregnant women

- FDA Category B (see Ch. 2.3)

Interactions

- Patients on beta-blockers may have an exaggerated increase in heart rate and blood pressure.

Reversal agent

- None.

2. Secretin

Secretin causes stimulation of pancreatic secretions and can be used to facilitate identification of the ampulla of Vater and the accessory papilla. Secretin has a rapid onset of action, with levels returning to baseline within 90 min.

Dose

- The initial dose is 0.2 μg/kg over 1 min IV (Reconstitute using 8 mL of sodium chloride. Each reconstituted mL contains 2 μg of secretin.)

Side-effects

- Nausea, vomiting
- Flushing
- Abdominal pain.

Contraindications

- Known hypersensitivity to secretin
- Acute pancreatitis.

Use in pregnant women

- FDA Category C (see Ch. 2.3).

Interactions

- Anticholinergic drugs may decrease the response to secretin.

Reversal agent

- None.

10.4 Equipment

Key Points

- All equipment should be available in duplicate.
- A therapeutic duodenoscope is used for the majority of procedures.
- A forward viewing endoscope may be required in patients with altered anatomy.
- Short wire systems have been developed which allow for rapid exchange, control of the wire by the endoscopist and avoid the need for an experienced assistant.
- All baskets should be compatible with a lithotripter.
- High quality radiological equipment is essential.

1. Endoscopes

1.1. Video duodenoscope

- Almost all ERCPs are performed with a 'therapeutic' duodenoscope which has a 4.2 mm operating channel. This duodenoscope can be used for both diagnostic and therapeutic procedures. This size instrument channel allows insertion of all accessories and as well as performing cholangioscopy.
- A 'diagnostic' duodenoscope is thinner and has a smaller instrument channel. The instrument channel will only allow the passage of an 8½ Fr stent. As their diameter is slimmer, they are useful where there is altered anatomy (i.e. Billroth I), a stricture, or if an ERCP is being performed in a child or young adult.

1.2. Forward viewing endoscope

- For patients with Billroth II, start with a standard duodenoscope; however, ensure that a forward viewing endoscope is available. Options include using an enteroscope by itself, or augmented enteroscopy with a single balloon, double balloon or Spirus overtube (see Ch. 5.2). A pediatric colonoscope can also be used.

2. ERCP equipment

2.1. Catheters

The choice of whether to start with a catheter or a sphincterotome is based on endoscopist preference, and also on whether a sphincterotomy is likely to be made. In cases where this is unlikely, or where a sphincterotomy has already been performed, a catheter is often used to cannulate. There are several types of catheters available. A standard catheter has a graduated, precurved tip with a single channel, which can be used for either contrast or a wire. A triple lumen catheter has two channels which allow contrast to be injected while keeping a wire in place. A taper-tip catheter has a shorter, 5 mm tip. The taper-tip catheter is sometimes useful for cannulating a stenosed or minor papilla. There is a slightly increased risk of submucosal injection with this type of catheter.

2.2. Sphincterotomes

The sphincterotome consists of a metal wire covered by an insulating sheath, with the distal 20–30 mm of wire exposed, and a short radio-opaque, tapered tip (5 mm). Cannulation is usually attempted with a sphincterotome if a sphincterotomy is likely. The angle of the tip of the sphincterotome can be altered, by asking the assistant to 'tense' the sphincterotome, which is also useful if cannulation is difficult.

Several different types of sphincterotomes are available. A double-lumen sphincterotome allows either injection of contrast or a guidewire (Fig. 1A). A triple lumen sphincterotome (Fig. 1B) allows injection of contrast without removing the guidewire. A tapered tip (5 mm tip) (Fig. 1D) is sometimes used if the papilla is stenotic or to cannulate the minor papilla. In patients in whom the orientation of the biliary and pancreatic ducts are reversed (i.e. Billroth II), a special sphincterotome is available which is orientated in the opposite direction to the regular sphincterotome (Fig. 1E). Where sphincterotomy fails, a needle-knife sphincterotome with a retractable wire or blade with guidewire option (Fig. 1C) can be used. Sphincterotomes with long cutting wires (Fig. 1G) are no longer used due to an increased risk of bleeding and perforation. The sphincterotome with a long tip nose (Fig. 1F) was used prior to guidewire cannulation, but is rarely used now.

2.3. Balloon catheters

Balloon catheters are used to remove either small or medium-sized stones or sludge. They can also be used to obtain a cholangiogram where there is a very dilated duct or following a sphincterotomy. Balloon catheters come either in a single size or with three different attachments which alter the size of the balloon. They are also available as wire guided if required.

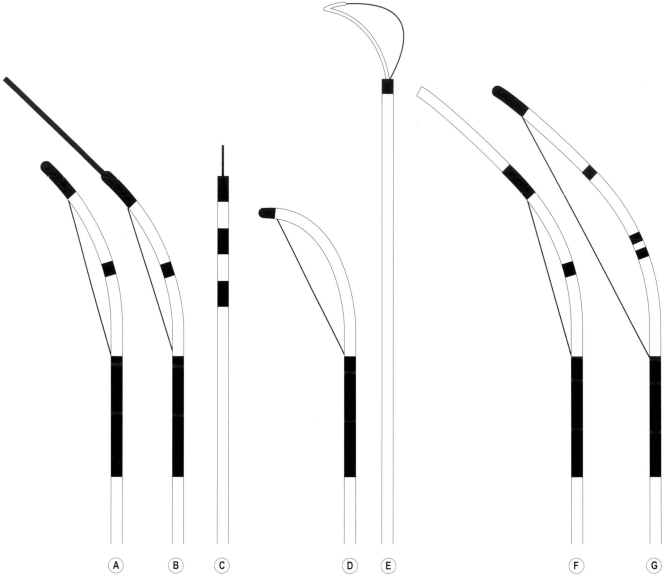

Figure 1 Different types of sphincterotomes. (A) A double-lumen sphincterotome allows either injection of contrast or a guidewire. (B) A triple lumen sphincterotome allows injection of contrast without removing the guidewire. (C) A needle-knife sphincterotome with a retractable wire or blade. (D) A tapered tip (5 mm tip) is sometimes used if the papilla is stenotic or to cannulate the minor papilla. (E) In patients in whom the orientation of the biliary and pancreatic ducts are reversed (i.e. Billroth II), a special sphincterotome is available which is orientated in the opposite direction to the regular sphincterotome. (F) Sphincterotome with a long tip nose was used prior to guide wire cannulation, but is rarely used now. (G) Sphincterotomes with long cutting wires are no longer used due to an increased risk of perforation bleeding and perforation.

2.4. Brushes

Wire guided brushes are available and are used to obtain tissue from suspicious strictures.

2.5. Forceps

Regular biopsy forceps should be available. These can be used to biopsy the ampulla where an ampullary cancer is suspected or where autoimmune pancreatitis is a possibility. They can also be used to biopsy bile duct strictures after a biliary sphincterotomy. Pediatric biopsy forceps (6 Fr) are sometimes used. These are easier to insert into the bile duct than regular biopsy forceps; however, they provide smaller samples. There may be a slightly decreased risk of complications compared with paediatric biopsy forceps than with regular biopsy forceps.

Jumbo forceps should also be available. These are used to remove stents. Stents are easier to grasp with the jumbo forceps than a snare; however, the stent cannot be removed through the operating channel, necessitating removal and reinsertion of the duodenoscope.

2.6. Snare

A snare is used to remove stents. It takes a little more practice to use than the jumbo forceps; however, the stent can usually be removed through the instrument channel of a therapeutic duodenoscope avoiding removal and reinsertion of the duodenoscope.

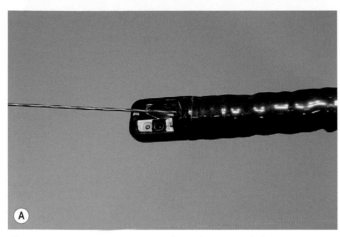

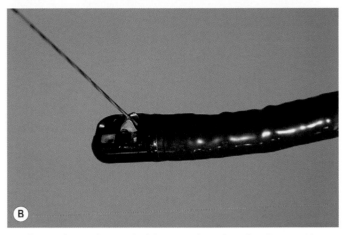

Figure 2 V-Scope. (A,B) Demonstrate how the V-shaped elevator captures the wire, allowing for rapid removal of devices without formal exchange with an assistant. (From Shah R et al. Short-wire ERCP systems. Technology status evaluation report. Gastrointestinal Endoscopy 2007;66:650-655.)

✓ Clinical Tip

How to remove a stent with a snare

Take time to position the scope. Insert the snare and open it just above or below the distal end of the stent. If you are going to remove it though the instrument channel, place the snare as close to the distal end of the stent as possible, close the snare and withdraw it through the instrument channel. If the stent has partially migrated out of the bile duct, grasp the side flap with the snare and gently push the stent back into the bile duct. Once this is done, the distal end of the stent can be snared and the stent removed.

✓ Clinical Tip

How do you exchange over a wire?

The endoscopist sets the pace of the exchange and watches the monitor to ensure that the wire does not move. The assistant should watch the hands of the endoscopist and move at the same speed. Most wires are made in two colors so that it is easy to see if the wire is moving. The distal end of the wire are often made of a different color (i.e. yellow and black with a pure black distal end) so that if a wire has moved significantly it will be obvious before it comes out of the duct. If it does move, stop, check the position of the wire with fluoroscopy, and once the wire is in a secure position, restart the exchange.

2.7. Wires

Wires are an essential part of the ERCP armamentarium. A wire consists of a nitinol or stainless steel core with a smooth coating. The type of coating determines the performance characteristics of the wire. A hydrophilic wire consists of a nitinol core with a polyurethane coating covering the entire length of the wire. Hydrophilic wires are often used for difficult cannulations (i.e. stricture at the hilum). They are excellent at navigating tight, difficult strictures but their hydrophilic coating means that they are more difficult to handle for the assistant. Hybrid wires combine regular wire with a hydrophilic section. The aim of these wires is to give the ease of use of the non-hydrophilic wire, with the ability to traverse a tight stricture of the hydrophilic wires. PTFE or Teflon coated wires were used in the past, but are rarely used nowadays, as they must be removed prior to performing a sphincterotomy due to the risk of conducting current.

Wires come with a variety of tips. A straight tip is usually used; however, an angled tip is useful if a tight stricture is encountered. They also come in different widths: 0.035 inch is the most commonly used, though a 0.025 inch or 0.018 inch may be required to pass a tight stricture.

2.7.1. Short wire system

The classic system is a 'long' wire which is manipulated by an assistant. This is exchanged by the assistant advancing the wire at the same rate as the physician withdraws the instrument (see clinical tip box). With the long wire system, an experienced assistant is essential to the success of the procedure. Short wire systems have been developed which allow rapid exchange over the wire and give control of the wire to the endoscopist. The potential advantages of the short wire system include:

- Rapid exchange
- No need for an experienced assistant
- Control of the wire by the endoscopist.

They are three components to the short wire system:

- Short wires (185–270 cm vs 400–460 cm)
- Locking device for the wire
- Devices designed to be exchanged over the short wire platform.

There are currently three short wire systems. The V system (Olympus, Toyko, Japan), contains the 'V' locking device. This is an elevator with a V-shaped groove on the elevator, which acts as an internal wire lock (Fig. 2), securing the wire and allowing devices to be removed over the wire without exchanging with an assistant.

Both the Fusion System (Cook Endoscopy; Winston Salem, NC) and the RX Biliary System (Boston Scientific, Natick, MA) consist of short wire systems with external wire locking systems. They both have specially designed biopsy caps,

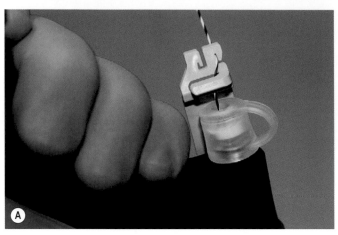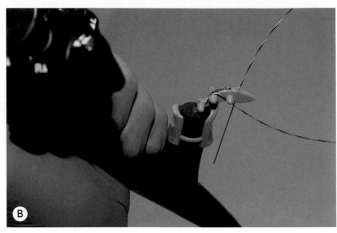

Figure 3 RX System and Fusion System. (A) The RX System has an anti-leak biopsy cap and wire locking device. (B) The Fusion System has a specially designed biopsy cap and a locking device which can hold up to two wires. (From Shah R et al. Short-wire ERCP systems. Technology status evaluation report. Gastrointestinal Endoscopy 2007;66:650-655.)

which prevent leaking of air or bile. The Fusion System incorporates a wire lock with port cap (Fig. 3B), while the RX Biliary System has a separate anti-leak biopsy cap, and a wire lock which is attached to the handle of the endoscope and allows fixation of two wires (Fig. 3A). A large variety of compatible devices are available (see Shah et al 2007, for information on available devices) including sphincterotomes and stents.

2.8. Other equipment

A selection of other equipment should be available. This includes:
- A selection of Dormia baskets in various shapes and sizes should be available; the small and medium sizes are the most used. Rigid baskets which do not deform, are preferred to flexible ones (baskets made of nitinol do not deform). All baskets should be compatible with a lithotripter
- Nasobiliary and nasopancreatic drains
- Small and large snares if an ampullectomy is being performed
- Clips
- Epinephrine (adrenaline) and injection needle
- Mechanical lithotripter
- Electrohydraulic lithotripter
- Electrocautery unit.

3. Radiology suite and equipment

Ideally the ERCP room should be an integral part of the endoscopy suite, thus avoiding the need to move equipment and personnel. The ERCP room should be an adequate size to allow for the amount of equipment and personnel required, and should be provided with equipment to allow propofol or general anesthesia if necessary. It is essential that high quality radiological equipment is used. The ideal equipment is a digital remote-control table operated by a radiographer.

3.1. General radiology equipment

- Articulated arm supplying fluids and electrical current over the video console (with several power points, two suction inlets, one oxygen point, one nitrous oxide point)
- An X-ray generator with continuous and pulsed exposure capability (most now have high frequency generators which provide excellent exposure reproducibility and automatic brightness control)
- Bifocal X-ray tube
- Collimation and filtration
- High definition image intensifier
- Digital image recording and display using a minimum of two display screens
- The patient table should minimize X-ray attenuation while providing sufficient strength to support large patients. The configuration most commonly used in GI is a mobile C-arm with an under table X-ray tube
- Standard radiation protection aprons, eye shielding and standard radiation protection systems, including lead barriers between the patient and operator
- Foot pedal to acquire images.

Further Reading

Kethu SR, Adler DG, Conway JD, et al:
ERCP cannulation and sphincterotomy devices, *Gastrointest Endosc* 71:435–445, 2010.

Shah RJ, Somogyi L, Petersen BT, et al:
Short-wire ERCP systems. Technology status evaluation report, *Gastrointest Endosc* 4:650–657, 2007.

10.5 Checklist before starting an ERCP

Key Points

- Always ensure that you have reviewed the patient notes and imaging.
- Check the duodenoscope and equipment before starting.

1. Patient checklist

- Patient preparation (see Chapters 2.1, 2.2 and 2.3)
- Admission notes
- Previous imaging
- Liver function tests (AST, ALT, GGT, alkaline phosphatase, and bilirubine)
- Pancreatic tests (amylase and lipase)
- Anaesthetic review
- Informed consent
- INR, platelets
  - Usually only required in patients with evidence of a bleeding disorder, liver disease, malnutrition, prolonged therapy with antibiotics associated with clotting factor deficiencies, prolonged biliary obstruction or in patients who are receiving anticoagulation therapy
- Venous access in right arm
- Antifoam solution is sometimes given prior to the procedure.

2. Endoscopist checklist

- Check that the endoscope is aspirating, blowing air and water correctly, and that white balancing has been performed
- Make sure that endoscopy recording equipment is available and working.

3. Patient positioning

- The patient is placed in the left lateral decubitus position with their left arm at their back
- Patients should preferably be placed in a supine position, if access to the minor papilla is required or in cases of hilar stenosis, to allow optimal visualization of the biliary tree.

10.6 Basic ERCP technique

Key Points

- Patience is key to successful cannulation.
- The major papilla usually has a 'neck tie' appearance.
- The minor papilla is usually 2 cm proximal and anterior to the major papilla and is usually most easily identified and cannulated with the patient supine.
- ERCP in patients with altered anatomy is associated with lower success rates and higher complication rates. It is essential to know what type of surgery has been performed. Augmented enteroscopy, with single/double balloon or spiral enteroscopy, is sometimes required.

Box 1 Short versus long scope position

- In a short scope position, the duodenoscope is straight with no gastric loop, and is normally between 50 and 70 cm from the incisors.
- In the long scope, a gastric loop is left in the stomach with 70+ cm of the duodenoscope inserted.

1. Inserting the duodenoscope and positioning over the papilla

How to intubate and position the duodenoscope in front of the papilla is illustrated in Figure 1. Gently insert the duodenoscope to the upper esophageal sphincter. The esophagus is intubated blindly with gentle forward pressure and slight clockwise rotation. If there is resistance STOP, and change to a forward viewing gastroscope to exclude anything which may cause difficulties with intubation (i.e. Zenker's diverticulum/stricture). Due to the side-viewing nature of the duodenoscope, a full view of the esophagus is not possible. Once the duodenoscope passes the gastroesophageal junction, make a half turn clockwise and follow the lesser curve to the pylorus. As the duodenoscope is side viewing, the duodenum is entered by placing the pylorus in the 'setting sun' position, so that the upper half of the pylorus is visible at the 6 o'clock position. Check that the shaft of the scope is at the 12 o'clock position when intubating the pylorus as this ensures optimum positioning in front of the papilla. The duodenoscope is then inserted into the second part of the duodenum. Two maneuvers are performed in succession: first turn the big wheel anticlockwise and the small wheel clockwise, thus deflecting the tip of the scope up and right, then withdraw the endoscope to 50–70 cm from the incisors to reduce the gastric loop.

1.1. Problems with intubation

- Unable to intubate the esophagus:
  - STOP. DO NOT PUSH. Withdraw the duodenoscope and insert a forward-viewing scope to exclude a

pharyngeal pouch or stricture. A guidewire can be left in the stomach to guide insertion with the duodenoscope if required.
- The duodenoscope coils in the fundus:
  - Ensure the patient is fully in the left lateral decubitus position. If necessary, place a bolster under the patient. Withdraw to the cardia then deflect slightly to the right after advancing through the cardia once again. Follow the vertical folds along the lesser curvature to the pylorus.
  - Avoid over-inflating the stomach.
- The duodenoscope advances as far as the superior flexure of the duodenum facing upwards:
  - Rotate the scope to the right through 90°, by turning from facing the patient to facing the monitor video and be perpendicular to the patient (Fig. 7) patient. This will present the second part of the duodenum.

2. Locating the papilla

The major papilla should now be in the field of vision. The major papilla consists of a frenulum, a hood, infundibulum, and orifice (Fig. 2). It is often a different color from the rest of the duodenum. The papilla should be inspected for evidence of stone passage (gaping or inflamed orifice), edema or papillary adenoma. The major papilla is then classified depending on its appearance (Fig. 3). This is important when assessing how far a sphincterotomy may be extended and to do a diathermic puncture of biliary infundibulum.

2.1. Problems identifying the major papilla

The papilla is normally found on the medial wall of the duodenum, but can be located anywhere from the duodenal

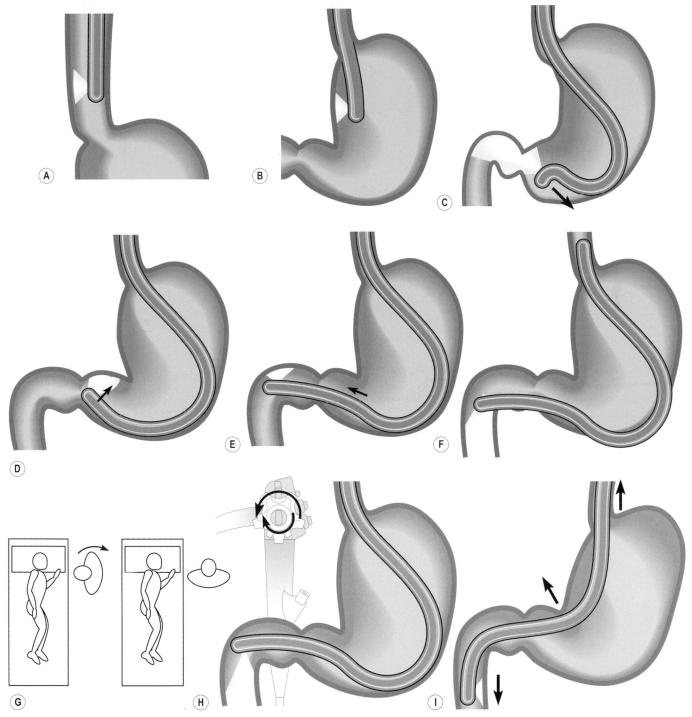

Figure 1 Inserting the duodenoscope and positioning over the papilla. (A) Duodenoscope advancing blind into the esophagus. (B) Advancing along the lesser curvature. (C) The endoscope rests on the greater curvature and faces the pylorus. (D) Deflection upwards, before advancing through the pylorus. (E) The apparatus advances to the superior flexure. (F) The endoscopist turns to his right through 90°. (G) The endoscopist has turned to his right through 90°. (H) Deflection upwards and to the right by turning the small wheel clockwise and the big wheel anti-clockwise. (I) Withdrawal of the endoscope to approximately 70 cm which removes the gastric loop.

bulb to the mid-descending duodenum. If the papilla is not visible after performing the maneuvers described above, the following should be tried:

- Wait a little before changing position
- Improve visualization with antifoam solution (i.e. simethicone)
- Give glucagon to decrease duodenal motility

- Search for the papilla by gently lifting the mucosal folds with a catheter and look for the frenulum, infundibulum, or hood
- There is usually only one longitudinal fold in the second part of the duodenum – the major papilla is usually located at the end of this fold. This is often described as having a 'neck tie' appearance (Fig. 4)

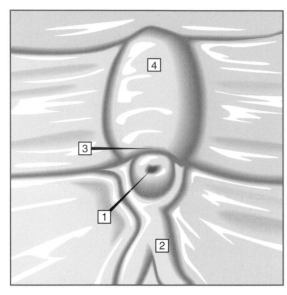

Figure 2 Normal papilla. (1) Papillary orifice. (2) Frenulum. (3) Hood. (4) Infundibulum.

- Occasionally, the papilla is located in the third part of the duodenum. This can be reached using the long scope position (>70 cm)
- The infundibulum can be divided into four types (Type 0–3; Fig. 3). This system is useful if a pre-cut sphincterotomy is required. A Type 0 infundibulum is not suitable for pre-cut, while Types 2 or 3 have the ideal configuration for pre-cut sphincterotomy.

In cases where there is difficulty identifying the major papilla, look for the 'neck tie' appearance with a longitudinal fold (Fig. 4) in the second part of the duodenum.

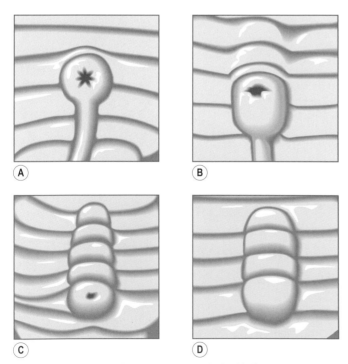

Figure 3 Classification of the various types of infundibulum. Type 0: no infundibulum. Type 1: the infundibulum extends to the limit of visibility. Type 2: a prominent infundibulum. Type 3: a large infundibulum which covers the papilla.

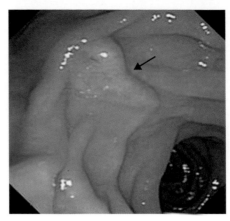

Figure 4 Neck tie appearance of the major papilla (arrow).

2.2. Locating the minor papilla

The minor papilla is smaller (Fig. 5), and is usually located 2 cm proximal and anterior to the major papilla in the second part of the duodenum. It can be difficult to locate. In these cases consider the following:

- Use a long scope position: this is usually the optimum position to see the minor papilla
- Place the patient in the supine position
- Give secretin. Some authors recommend spraying the second portion of the duodenum prior to giving secretin.

3. Cannulating the major papilla

Flush the catheter or sphincterotome with dye prior to commencing the procedure to prevent any injection of air. Prior to attempting cannulation, optimize conditions and ensure there is an adequate view of the papilla by ensuring:

- Duodenal hypotonia: give glucagon if necessary
- No bubbles or mucus: use antifoam solution (simethicone)
- Take time to optimally position the duodenoscope and ensure that the orifice is at the center of the image
- Wait a little for the orifice to open.

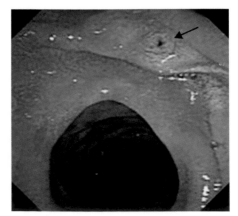

Figure 5 Minor papilla (arrow).

3.1. Cannulating the bile duct and pancreatic duct

To selectively cannulate the bile duct, the side-viewing duo-denoscope should be placed below the major papilla. Place the catheter slightly below the papilla and direct the catheter vertically towards 11–12 o'clock (Fig. 6) in the right upper quadrant. Cannulation of the pancreatic duct requires the duodenoscope to be placed *en-face*, and slightly to the left of the papilla. The catheter should be placed on the right side of the papilla between 1 and 3 o'clock, with the catheter moving from left to right. If the os is difficult to catheterize, the catheter can initially be introduced a few millimeters, then directed towards the biliary or pancreatic orifice. The catheter is then introduced as far as possible into the chosen duct.

In obese patients, those with malignant pancreatic disease, particularly where there is a lesion in the genu of the pancreas, it can be difficult to properly centre the major papilla. In these cases, a long scope position may be required, and the endoscopist may need to position themselves in the opposite of the classic position (i.e. at 90° to the patient's face).

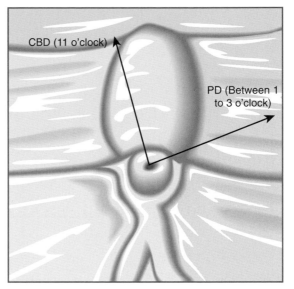

Figure 6 Orientation of the pancreatic and bile duct. Using the face of a clock for orientation, the pancreatic duct is found between 1 and 3 o'clock position, while the bile duct is found at 11 o'clock.

- ■ Use fluoroscopy to check the position of the endoscope and the direction of the catheter. To cannulate the bile duct, check that the tip of the endoscope is slightly under the papillary orifice, with the catheter pointing towards 11 o'clock (Fig. 7). For the pancreatic duct, the tip of the endoscope should be placed in the same area as the papillary orifice, with the catheter directed towards 1–3 o'clock (Fig. 7).
- The pancreatic and biliary orifices are separate:
  - ■ If the pancreatic duct is repeatedly cannulated, look above the cannulated orifice for the biliary orifice.
- The catheter is in the correct direction for the bile duct, but deep cannulation cannot be achieved:
  - ■ This is because the catheter is up against the anterior wall of the ampulla or the common bile duct. Withdraw the endoscope slightly: when the papilla has disappeared from the visual field, push the catheter forward into the bile duct.
- Use a hydrophilic guidewire to cannulate the desired duct (Fig. 8).

4. Failure to cannulate the desired duct

- Check that the catheter is in the correct orientation to cannulate the desired duct:

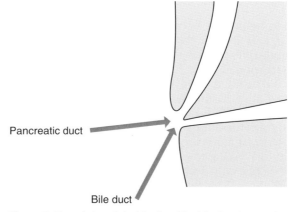

Figure 7 Cannulation of the bile duct. The bile duct is cannulated going from inferior to superior while directing the catheter towards 11 o'clock. The pancreatic duct is cannulated in an *en face* position, directing the catheter from left to right and towards 1 o'clock.

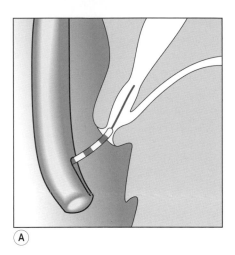
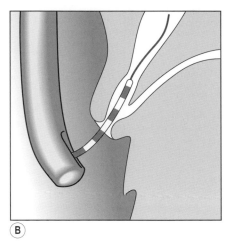

Figure 8 Selective cannulation with a wire. A wire can be used to selectively cannulate either the bile duct. (A) Note the position of the duodenoscope below the papilla or the pancreatic duct. (B) Once the correct duct has been cannulated with the guidewire, the sphincterotome is then inserted over it.

- Change the catheter to a sphincterotome:
  - The sphincterotome can be tensed, which allows for maximum elevation to assist biliary cannulation.
- The papilla is stenotic:
  - A tapered catheter or sphincterotome is sometimes useful.
- If the pancreatic duct is repeatedly entered, a wire can be left in the pancreatic duct. This prevents further pancreatic duct cannulation. It also identifies the direction of the pancreatic duct. Once this is known, the direction of the bile duct can be determined. Alternatively, a pancreatic duct stent can be inserted, with subsequent cannulation of the common bile duct.
- Cholecystokinin can sometimes be used. This causes the gallbladder to empty with subsequent opening of the papillary orifice.

Needle knife pre-cut sphincterotomy should not be used to access the biliary or pancreatic duct, except in an emergency. If the above maneuvers fail, the procedure should be discontinued and a repeat attempt made 24–48 h later. This allows the edema to settle, and the second procedure is often successful.

5. Cannulating the papilla beside a diverticulum

Diverticulae frequently occur in the second part of the duodenum, especially in elderly individuals. In these cases, look for the papilla at the edges or inside the diverticulum (Fig. 9). Occasionally it is hidden by the duodenal folds, which should be lifted using a catheter. If the papilla cannot be identified, identify the frenulum and hence the papilla. Cannulating a papilla located at the edge, inside or in the middle of a diverticulum is usually possible. The difficulty arises when the papilla is located inside the diverticulum and with the os also facing towards the inside of the diverticulum. In these cases, the following can be tried:

- Evert the papilla by pressing with a catheter on the edge of the diverticulum without insufflating it too much.
- Saline has been used raise the papilla from the diverticulum (Fig. 10A,B); however, this can be associated with pancreatitis.

- Gently tease the papilla outside the diverticulum with a biopsy forceps (Fig. 10C).
- It is sometimes possible to place the tip of the endoscope into the diverticulum to center it.
- Percutaneous transhepatic wire can be inserted through the ampulla (see section 8.11).

6. Cannulating a stricture

Traversing a difficult stricture requires patience, skill and optimum X-ray control. When a difficult stricture is encountered the following should be tried:

- Consider using a fully hydrophilic wire for difficult strictures (Fig. 11). Also an angled tip is sometimes

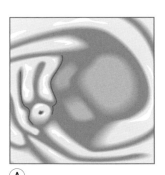
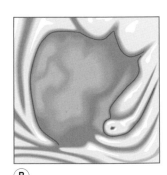
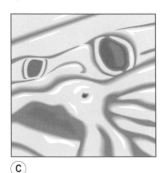
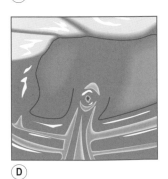

Figure 9 Location of papilla in the presence of a diverticulum. The papilla is located at the left (A) or right (B) edge of a large diverticulum. This is the most common presentation. (C) Papilla between two small diverticula. (D) Papilla in the centre of large diverticulum.

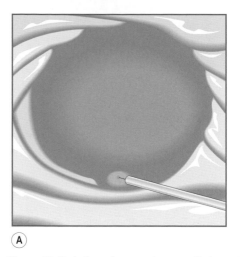
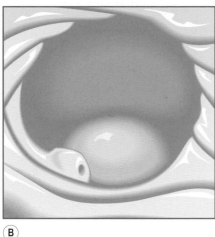
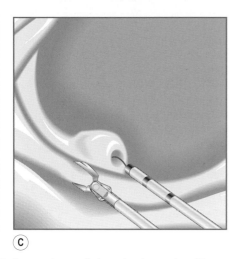

Figure 10 Techniques for accessing a papilla located within a diverticulum. Saline can be injected (A) which raises the papilla from the diverticulum (B). However, this is associated with an increased risk of pancreatitis. Biopsy forceps can also be used to tease the papilla out of the diverticulum (C).

useful. Repeat forward and back movements while simultaneously twirling the wire. Occasionally, a 0.025 or 0.018 inch guidewire is needed. An ultratapered sphincterotome or cure-tipped 5–6 Fr cannula may also be useful. Once the stricture has been traversed, the sphincterotome is advanced across the stricture and the guidewire should be exchanged for a regular guidewire as this facilitates dilation or stent placement.

- The left hepatic duct is usually more difficult to cannulate. Bounce the guidewire off the lateral wall to cannulate the left hepatic duct. A swingtip or Haber Ramp catheter is occasionally useful in difficult cannulation.
- Cannulate the right hepatic duct by placing the sphincterotome at the level of the bifurcation and direct towards the right hepatic duct.
- Distortion of the second part of the duodenum by tumour can hinder the correct centering of the papilla. If cannulation of the papilla is difficult, determine if this is a technical problem or a low

stenosis. Review pre-ERCP imaging (ideally MRC or EUS) to determine whether there is a low stenosis near the papillary orifice. In this case, use a sphincterotome mounted on a guidewire to find the orifice of the stenosis. Pre-cut sphincterotomy or diathermy loop excision of the infundibulum may be necessary.

- Make a loop with the guidewire (Fig. 12). Once the loop moves in the desired direction, advance the sphincterotome over the guidewire to the apex of the loop. Then withdraw the guidewire until the wire is straight. Reinsert the guidewire, forming a loop if necessary. This is repeated until the stricture is traversed.
- Advance stepwise if the stenosis has several angulations. The guidewire is advanced to the end of the first angulation (Fig. 13A). The sphincterotome is advanced over the guidewire to this point (Fig. 13B). The guidewire is advanced to the end of the second angulation, followed by the sphincterotome (Fig. 13C). This is repeated until the stricture is crossed (Fig. 13D).

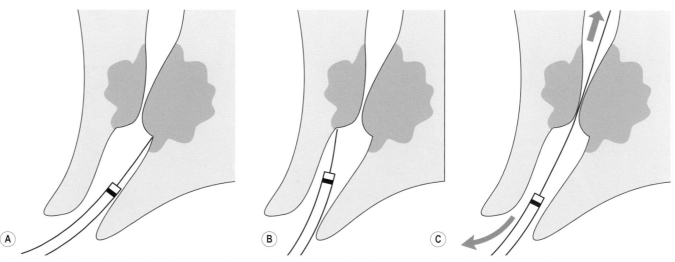

Figure 11 Inserting a guidewire through a stricture. Strictures should be crossed initially using a guidewire. If the guidewire is hitting the side walls (A,B), withdraw the sphincterotome slightly (C). This maneuver allows optimal alignment of the guidewire with the stricture.

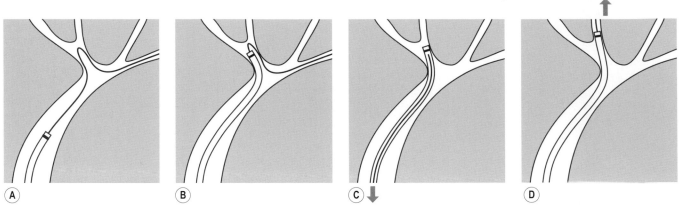

Figure 12 How to manipulate the wire into the correct hepatic duct. (A) Produce a loop with the guidewire. (B) Insert the catheter to the end of the loop. (C) Undo the loop formed by the guidewire. (D) Insert the guidewire through the catheter lying in the correct direction. Withdraw the guide catheter to change the direction of the guidewire if the guidewire fails to pass through the stenosis.

- Changing the patient position can help. For complex hilar strictures, placing the patient in the dorsal decubitus position is often useful.
- Placing an inflated retrieval balloon below the stricture can stretch the bile duct and alter the angle aiding guidewire cannulation.

7. Cannulating the minor papilla

The accessory or minor papilla is usually located 2 cm proximal and anterior to the major papilla in the second part of the duodenum. The os is often very small (2 mm), with the duct of Santorini running from the 5 o'clock to the 11 o'clock position. The easiest position to cannulate the minor papilla is in the 'long' scope position, with the patient supine. Patience is essential. Wait for the orifice to open before attempting cannulation. Cannulation is usually performed initially with wire, following with the sphincterotome once the duct has been cannulated. This is usually possible with a regular sphincterotome, however a tapered sphincterotome can be required if the os is very small or stenosed. Care should be taken to avoid submucosal injection. If the minor papilla is difficult to locate or cannulate, placing the patient

in the supine position is often useful helpful. Secretin can be used to aid identification and to encourage the os to open.

8. ERCP in patients with altered anatomy

8.1. Post-surgical anastomoses

Performing ERCPs in patients who have undergone gastroenteric anastomoses is becoming increasingly common as more patients undergo gastric bypass surgery for obesity. It is important to know what type of surgery has been performed before commencing the ERCP, as this will determine the type of endoscope used, as well as the difficulty of the procedure. Some of these procedures, such as post-duodenopancreatectomy (Whipple's) are technically demanding, and are often best referred to a tertiary referral centres.

8.2. Which endoscope to use?

A duodenoscope is usually used where possible, as the presence of the elevator facilitates cannulation. In addition, the side viewing assists location of the ampulla (Fig. 14A).

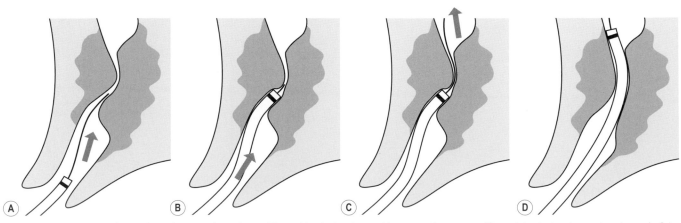

Figure 13 Inserting a guidewire through a complex stricture. The guidewire is advanced in a stepwise manner. The guidewire is advanced to the end of the first angulation (A). The sphincterotome is advanced over the guidewire to this point (B). The guidewire is advanced to the end of the second angulation, followed by the sphincterotome (C). This is repeated until the stricture is crossed (D).

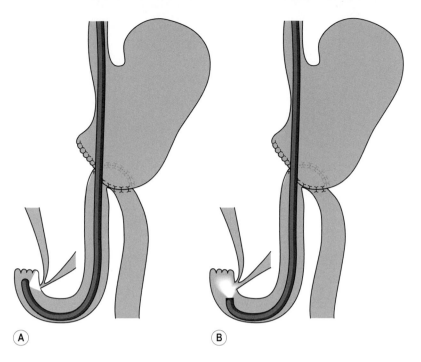

(A)   (B)

Figure 14 View of the ampulla in a patient with altered anatomy with a duodenoscope or forward viewing scope. In patients with altered anatomy, the ampulla can be reached with a duodenoscope or a forward viewing endoscope. The duodenoscope is side viewing and allows good visualization of the ampulla (A). The ampulla can be slightly more difficult to visualize with a forward viewing endoscope (B).

However, it is sometimes not possible to reach the papillary area due to the length of the afferent loop. In these cases, a forward viewing scope should be used. Reaching the ampulla is often successful with a forward viewing scope; however, the ampulla can be more difficult to visualize (Fig. 14B), and the lack of an elevator can make cannulation or exchanging over a guidewire difficult. The choice of forward viewing scope depends on what is available in the unit and the experience of the endoscopist. Options include a pediatric colonoscope, a single or double balloon enteroscope, or an enteroscope with Spirus overtube. Where a forward-viewing endoscope is used, but cannulation has failed, it is possible to leave a wire and then backload this wire onto a duodenoscope.

8.3. Pyloroplasty and Billroth I surgery

The major papilla can be reached with a duodenoscope, and the common bile duct or pancreatic duct is cannulated as normal.

8.4. Gastroenteric anastomosis with a preserved pylorus

In cases of gastroenteric anastomosis, a duodenoscope can be used if the pylorus is patent. However, the pylorus often becomes stenosed. In these cases, the afferent loop should be used to access the papilla.

8.5. Choledochoduodenal anastomosis

For patients with a choledochoduodenal anastomosis (Fig. 15A), a forward-viewing endoscope is sometimes required. The anastomosis is usually located on the anterior side of the bulb. If the anastomosis is patent, the endoscope can be introduced into the bile duct. If it is an end-to-side

choledochoduodenal anastomosis (Fig. 15B), i.e. if the segment underlying the anastomosis is closed, access to the papilla should be gained using a duodenoscope.

> ☑ **Clinical Tip**
>
> **Sump syndrome**
>
> 'Sump syndrome' is a rare complication of a side-to-side choledochoduodenostomy (Fig. 15A). The common bile duct between the anastomosis and the ampulla of Vater acts as a reservoir in which debris and stones collect. This can result in abdominal pain, cholangitis, biliary obstruction or pancreatitis. ERCP findings include dilated bile or pancreatic duct, and signs of chronic pancreatitis.

8.6. Pancreaticoduodenectomy (Whipple's)

The classic pancreaticoduodenectomy described by Whipple consists of removal of the pancreatic head, duodenum, first 15 cm of the jejunum, common bile duct, and gallbladder, as well as a partial gastrectomy (Fig. 16). There is a side-to-side gastrojejunostomy, often with a long afferent loop and a variety of placements for the pancreatico- and hepatico-jejunostomies. In a pylorus preserving pancreaticoduodenectomy, the gastric antrum, pylorus, and proximal 3–6 cm of the duodenum are preserved, with an end-to-side pylorojejunostomy. The pancreaticojejunostomy is usually located at the apex of the loop, with the hepatic-jejunotomy about half way down the afferent loop. In these patients, pancreatic and biliary anastomoses can rarely be reached with a duodenoscope and a forward viewing endoscope should be used.

8.7. Gastrojejunal anastomosis (Billroth II)

A Billroth II was often performed in patients with peptic ulcer disease or gastric antral carcinoma and consists of a

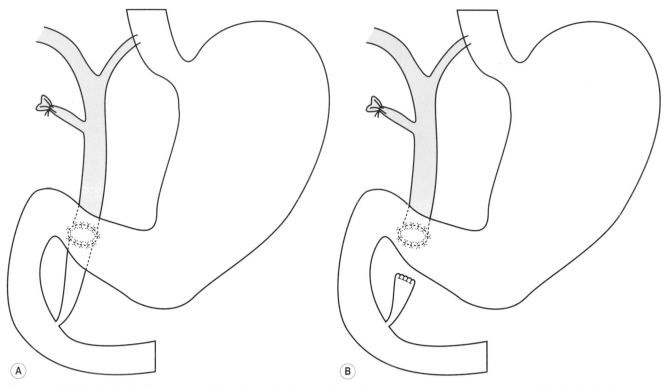

Figure 15 Choledochoduodenal anastomosis. (A) A side-to-side choledochoduodenal anastomosis. (B) An end-to-side choledochoduodenal anastomosis.

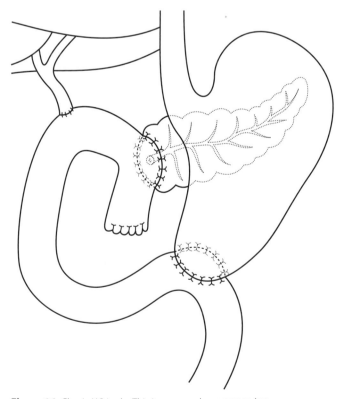

Figure 16 Classic Whipple. This is a non-pylorus preserving pancreaticoduodenectomy. The head of the pancreas has been resected. There is a gastrojejunostomy, with an afferent and efferent limb. The afferent limb leads to the hepatico- and pancreaticojejunostomies. Note that the pancreaticojejunostomy is past the hepaticojejunostomy and is often found almost at the end of the afferent limb.

Box 3 The afferent loop

How to identify and enter the afferent loop
- The afferent loop is almost always more difficult to access than the efferent loop.
- The afferent loop is usually adjacent to the lesser curve.
- If it is not possible to intubate the afferent loop, place the patient to prone or supine position.
- A wire can be advanced into the correct loop, and the endoscope guided over the wire into the loop.
- If this fails, a CRE wire-guided balloon is sometimes useful. It can be inflated in the loop, and the endoscope then guided into the loop. These procedures should be performed under fluoroscopic guidance to avoid complications.

How do I know if I am in the afferent loop?
There are several tools you can use to determine if the endoscope is in the correct limb:
- Use fluoroscope to confirm that the endoscope is moving towards the right hypochondrium.
- The presence of bile.

---

partial gastrectomy with end-to-side gastrojejunostomy (Fig. 17). The operation may also be known as a Polya and Hoffmeister, depending on how the gastrojejunostomy is performed. A duodenoscope should be used initially. If this is unsuccessful, it can be exchanged for a forward viewing endoscope. There is a native papilla, but the pancreatico-biliary anatomy is reversed as described in the pancreaticoduodenectomy.

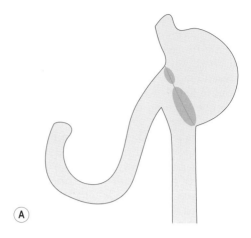

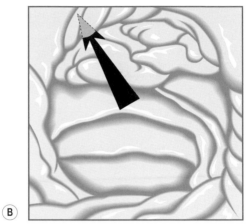

Figure 17 Gastrojejunal anastomosis. (A) Demonstrates the relationship of the afferent and efferent limbs in a gastrojejunal anastomosis (Finisterer type procedure). (B) Note the location of the afferent loop – it is at the top left under the fold and is the more difficult limb to enter.

8.9. Gastric bypass surgery

There are two types of gastric bypass surgery performed. In patients with gastric outlet obstruction, a side-to-side loop gastrojejunostomy is performed. Patients undergoing gastric bypass surgery as a treatment of obesity often have a gastric pouch which is separated from the rest of the stomach. The pouch empties into an end-to-side gastrojejunostomy. A jejunojejunostomy connects the other part of the stomach, duodenum and jejunum in a Roux-en-Y configuration. Although it is occasionally possible to reach the anastomosis with a duodenoscope, a forward viewing endoscope is usually required. There is a native papilla, but as with a Billroth II or pancreaticoduodenectomy, the anatomy is reversed with the bile duct between 5 and 6 o'clock.

Box 4 Jejunojejunal anastomoses

- Enteric anastomoses can either be in the 'Y' configuration, which presents the endoscopist with two lumens to choose from, or in a side-to-side anastomosis, which appears as three lumens.
- The afferent loop is usually the most difficult loop to enter.

Box 5 How to reach the papilla in a patient with an afferent limb

- The afferent limb should be approached in a similar manner to a colonoscopy, with repeated shortening of the endoscope and removal of loops.
- Contrast can be injected either through a catheter or a CRE balloon (if reflux of contrast is a problem). This is useful where there are sharp angulations to determine the direction of the afferent loop.
- External manual compression can be useful.
- Take care not to stretch the anastomosis, as perforation can occur.

8.10. Cannulating the bile duct and pancreatic duct in patients with Billroth II or Whipple's procedure

In Billroth II the ampulla will be intact, while in a Whipple's or other reconstructive surgery there will be a surgical anastomosis (i.e. choledochoenteric anastomosis), and the pancreatic and bile duct anastomoses are usually found separately in the jejunum. The pancreatic duct is often located just proximal to the end of the loop, while the biliary orifice is located proximal to the pancreatic orifice, on the anti-mesenteric wall. As the papilla has been reached retrograde through the afferent loop, the anatomy is reversed by 180° with the biliary orifice found between 5 and 6 o'clock rather than the normal 11 o'clock position (Fig. 18). A

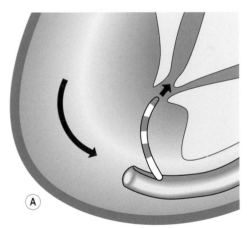

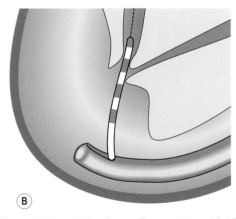

Figure 18 Cannulating the papilla in a patient with a Billroth II. As the papilla has been reached retrograde through the afferent loop, the anatomy is reversed by 180° with the biliary orifice found between 5 and 6 o'clock rather than the normal 11 o'clock position.

straight catheter can be used to cannulate the bile duct or pancreatic duct. It is helpful to maintain an *en-face* position and exaggerated distance away from the ampulla. A standard cannula is sometimes useful, as a standard sphincterotome may make biliary cannulation difficult in this situation due to its pre-curve. In our experience, guidewire cannulation is particularly useful in these circumstances.

8.11. Rendezvous procedure

A percutaneous transhepatic catheter (PTC) is inserted by an interventional radiologist prior to or at the same time as the ERCP.

Technique

- Identify the percutaneous catheter (Fig. 19)
- Insert a sphincterotome into the catheter
- The percutaneous catheter containing the sphincterotome is retracted into the bile duct
- The sphincterotome is placed in the papilla and a standard sphincterotomy performed.

Alternative techniques

- Use the PTC catheter as a guide, and cannulate alongside the catheter using a sphincterotome with a wire.
- A guidewire is inserted percutaneously (Fig. 20). The guidewire is retrieved using a snare and gently pulled into the instrument channel. A sphincterotome is then inserted over the guidewire and a standard sphincterotomy is performed.
- A variation of this is where a catheter has been placed by radiology. Insert a guidewire through the catheter (Fig. 21). The percutaneous guidewire is retrieved using a snare and pulled out of the instrument channel. The guide catheter is mounted on the guide wire in the bile duct. The stent is pushed through the stenosis.

> **! Warning!!**
>
> It is very important to work closely with radiology. Large catheters should not be removed without prior discussion with radiology, as these can cause bile to leak into the peritoneum.

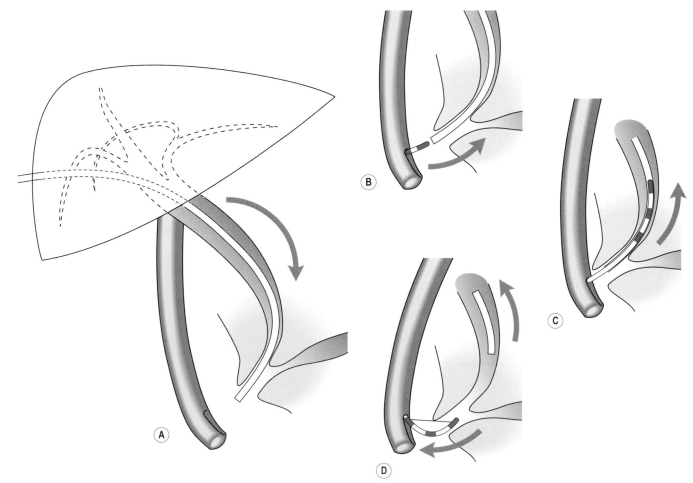

Figure 19 Rendezvous procedure. (A) A PTC catheter is inserted by an interventional radiologist. (B) The catheter is identified. (C) The sphincterotome is advanced in the catheter. Once percutaneous catheter containing the sphincterotome is retracted into the bile duct, the PTC catheter is withdrawn. (D) Biliary sphincterotomy is performed.

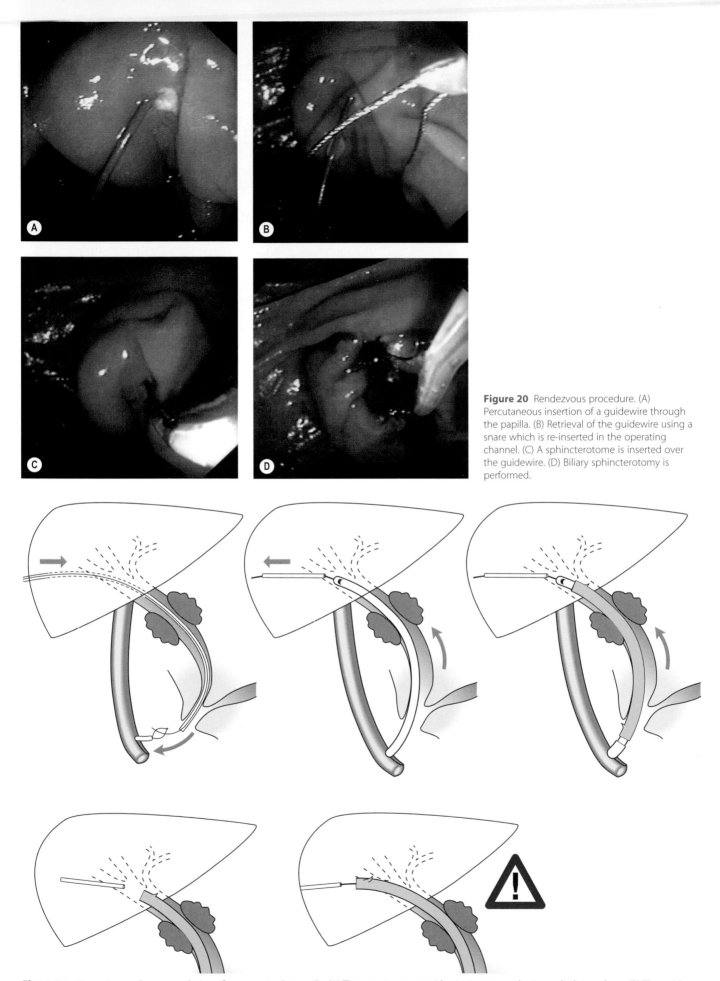

Figure 20 Rendezvous procedure. (A) Percutaneous insertion of a guidewire through the papilla. (B) Retrieval of the guidewire using a snare which is re-inserted in the operating channel. (C) A sphincterotome is inserted over the guidewire. (D) Biliary sphincterotomy is performed.

Figure 21 Alternative rendezvous technique for access to the papilla. (A) The percutaneous guidewire is recovered using a diathermy loop. (B) The guide catheter is mounted on the guidewire in the bile duct. (C) The stent is pushed through the stenosis. (D) Withdrawal of the guidewire before withdrawal of the catheters. (E) Stent in the hepatic parenchyma to be repositioned.

- If the sphincterotome is being advanced over the wire, a long wire (>450 cm) is required as it will need to pass from the liver, through the duodenoscope.
- Always manipulate the catheter/wire gently as liver laceration can occur.
- Some of the PTC catheters have a fixed pigtail to maintain their position in the duodenum. This must be either released or cut prior to removing the catheter or liver laceration can occur.
- It is advisable to insert a regular guidewire through the PTC catheter prior to manipulating it to minimize the risk of laceration

PTC, percutaneous transhepatic cholangiogram.

9. Successful cannulation rate

Cannulation of the papilla is successful in 95–98% of cases when performed by an experienced endoscopist. The pancreatic ducts are opacified on average in 90–95% of cases and the bile ducts in 85–90%. Failures are due to duodenal stenosis, a papillary lesion, or the intradiverticular location of the papilla.

In patients with altered anatomy, success rates depend on the type of surgery. Patients with a pyloroplasty, Billroth I, or choledochoduodenal anastomosis, have a similar success rate to normal ERCP. Patients with a Roux-en-Y have lower success rates of between 60% and 75%, provided the afferent loop is not too long or located transmesocolically.

10. ERCP in children

ERCP in children should be undertaken under general anesthesia. A diagnostic side-viewing duodenoscope may be used from the age of 1 year upwards. A therapeutic duodenoscope can be used in children over 5 foot. A 7.5 mm diameter duodenoscope with a 2.0 mm operating channel is available for use in children under the age of 1. There are few indications: bile duct stones, jaundice due to bile duct malformation, recurrent pancreatitis, pancreatic trauma, bile stones.

10.7 **Cytology, biopsies, and biochemical analysis**

Key Points

- Cytological analysis of bile and pancreatic juice have a sensitivity of between 35% and 70% and specificity of >90% for the diagnosis of cancer.
- Biopsies of the major papilla should be taken in all patients suspected of having autoimmune pancreatitis.
- Transpapillary biopsies can be performed following biliary sphincterotomy and have a similar sensitivity and specificity as cytology.
- The type of tumor and the number of passes made with a brush affect the sensitivity. Multiple passes should be made in a patient with a suspicious lesion.

1. Cytology

The cytological study of the bile or pancreatic juice can help to diagnose cancer of the bile ducts or pancreas and has a sensitivity of between 35% and 70%, with a specificity of >90%. Fluid can be collected by selective catheterization, or by collection of duodenal aspiration either after irrigation with saline or following stimulation with either CCK or secretin. Stents inserted into potentially neoplastic stricture should also be sent for cytological analysis.

2. Biopsies

Endoscopic transpapillary biopsies of a localized lesion or stenosis of the biliary or pancreatic ducts are more difficult, with a sensitivity of between 43% and 88% and a specificity of >90%. It is particularly difficult to introduce biopsy forceps through an intact papilla and to position them correctly within the lesion. Biopsies of the major papilla should

be taken in patients who are suspected of having auto-immune pancreatitis.

3. Brushing

The sensitivity of endoscopic transpapillary brush cytology is dependent on the type of tumor, as well as the number of passes made with the brush. Thus, it is important to brush multiple times, and to repeat brushing if the patient returns for repeat ERCP. Tumors which compress the bile duct (i.e. pancreatic) have a lower sensitivity than primary biliary cancer. If a pancreatic neoplasm is suspected, endoscopic ultrasound should be considered as the initial procedure of choice to obtain tissue.

A new technique, inserting a guidewire through a stricture and collecting juice above the stricture, has a high sensitivity (93%) and specificity (100%) in a single study. Further studies are required to confirm these promising results.

4. Biochemical examination of bile and pancreatic juice

4.1. Collection of bile juice

The biochemical study of bile should be carried out before contrast is injected. Optimal collection requires deep biliary cannulation with a catheter with three lateral holes in its tip. The collection of pure bile samples is indicated in three circumstances:

- Severe cholangitis: Samples should be sent for culture and antibiotic sensitivity test
- Testing for lithogenic bile: Calcium bilirubinate crystals, bile pigments and cholesterol (Fig. 1) can be seen. This

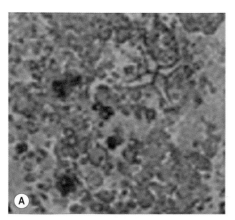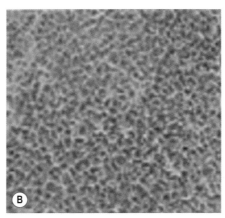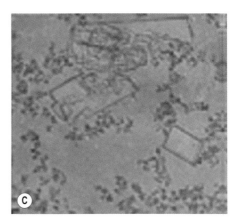

Figure 1 Crystallography of bile. (A) Calcium bilirubinate crystals. (B) Bile pigments. (C) Cholesterol crystals (translucent, larger) and calcium bilirubinate crystals (yellow and brown) obtained by bile sampling.

is used if microlithiasis is suspected in patients who have pancreatic or biliary clinical symptoms, and can be treated with ursodeoxycholic acid

• Pharmacokinetic study of drugs eliminated via the bile in relation to hepatobiliary disease.

4.2. Collection of pancreatic juice

Pure pancreatic juice can be collected for analysis of molecular markers as part of a research study. Pancreatic juice can also be collected after stimulation with secretin.

10.8 Pancreaticobiliary anatomy

Summary

1. **Normal and variant biliary anatomy** 393
2. **Post-surgical anatomy** 398

Key Points

- Understanding normal, variant and post-surgical pancreaticobiliary anatomy is essential.
- The Couinaud classification divides the liver into eight functionally independent segments.
- The most common variation of biliary anatomy is where the right posterior hepatic duct drains into the left hepatic duct, prior to its confluence with the right anterior hepatic duct.
- In patients undergoing laparoscopic cholecystectomy, surgeons should be informed of altered cystic duct anatomy.
- Pancreas divisum is the embryonic anomaly most commonly found in adults (5% of ERCP), characterized by the failure of the ventral and dorsal pancreatic ducts to fuse.

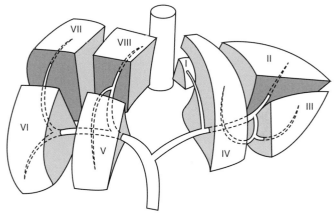

Figure 1 Normal segmental anatomy of the liver. This drawing shows normal biliary segmental anatomy, which is observed in 56% of individuals.

1. Normal and variant biliary anatomy

The Couinaud classification gives eight functionally independent segments, numbered I through VIII (Fig. 1). The segments are numbered in a clockwise manner starting with the caudate lobe (segment I). Each segment has its own vascular inflow, outflow, and biliary drainage. In the center of each segment there is a branch of the portal vein, hepatic artery, and bile duct. In the periphery of each segment, there is vascular outflow through the hepatic veins. The liver is divided by vascular structures. The right hepatic vein divides the right lobe into anterior and posterior segments. The middle hepatic vein divides the liver into right and left lobes, while the left hepatic vein divides the left lobe into medial and lateral parts. The portal vein divides the liver into upper and lower segments.

The biliary drainage runs in parallel to the portal venous supply. The right hepatic duct drains the segments of the right liver (V–VIII), with the right posterior duct draining the posterior segment (VI and VII), and the right anterior duct draining the anterior segments (V, VIII). The right posterior duct has an almost horizontal course, while the right anterior duct tends to have a more vertical course. The left hepatic duct is formed from tributaries draining segments II–IV. The common hepatic duct is formed by fusion of the right and left hepatic ducts. The duct draining the caudate lobe (I) usually joins the origin of the right or left hepatic duct. The cyst duct usually joins the common hepatic duct below the confluence of the right and left hepatic ducts (Fig. 2).

There are variations of this classic anatomy. The most common variant, which is present in up to 19% of the population, is where the right posterior duct drains into the left hepatic duct before its confluence with the right anterior duct (Fig. 3D). Another common variant, occurring in 12%

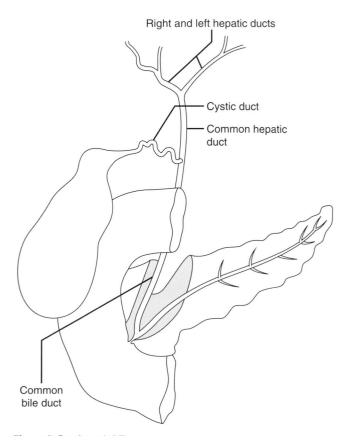

Right and left hepatic ducts

Cystic duct

Common hepatic duct

Common bile duct

Figure 2 Extrahepatic biliary tree.

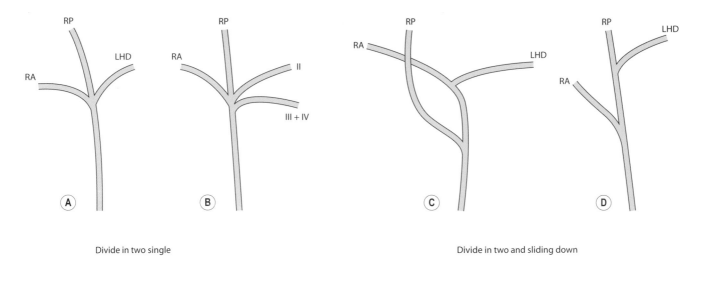

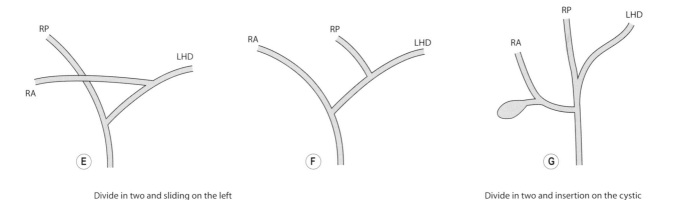

Figure 3 Hepatic duct variation. Variant anatomy most commonly affects the **right hepatic duct.** (A) The right posterior (RP), right anterior (RA) and left hepatic duct (LHD) insert together. This occurs in 12% of individuals. (B) Segments II, III and IV join the right anterior and posterior ducts in 3% of people. (C) This is the most common anatomical variation, occurring in 16% of individuals, where the right anterior hepatic duct (RA) drains into the left hepatic duct (LHD), prior to its confluence with the right posterior hepatic duct (RP). Other variations include insertion of the left hepatic duct into the right posterior hepatic duct, prior to insertion of the right anterior hepatic duct (4%) (D); insertion of the right anterior hepatic duct into the left hepatic duct followed by a confluence with the right posterior hepatic duct (5%) (E); insertion of the right posterior hepatic duct into the left hepatic duct which then joins the right anterior hepatic duct (1%) (F); and (G) confluence of the left hepatic duct with the right posterior hepatic duct which then join the right anterior hepatic duct (1–2%).

of individuals, is where the right posterior duct empties into the right aspect of the right anterior duct. Another common variant is where the right anterior, posterior, and left hepatic ducts drain simultaneously into the common hepatic duct (Fig. 3A). In these individuals, the right hepatic duct is virtually non-existent.

> ✏️ **Note**
>
> ERCP images can only be interpreted with the patient in dorsal decubitus position.

The cystic duct termination exhibits a number of variants. A common variation is where there is a low insertion of the cystic duct into the distal third of the common bile duct (9%) (Fig. 4). Another variation is where the cystic duct drains into the left side of the common hepatic duct.

The common bile duct terminates at the ampulla of Vater, where it joins the main pancreatic duct (Wirsung's duct)

(Fig. 5). There are a number of variations in the communication between the common bile duct and Wirsung's duct. It is important to be familiar with these variations when cannulating the papilla (Fig. 6). In the majority of cases (98%), the papilla has a single orifice (type I). The biliary duct and

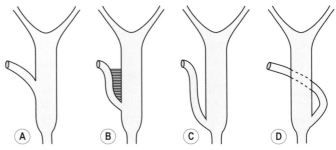

Figure 4 Variations in cystic ductal anatomy. The cystic duct termination exhibits a number of variants. A common variation is where there is a low insertion of the cystic duct into the distal third of the common bile duct (9%) (C). Another variation is where the cystic duct drains into the left side of the common hepatic duct (D).

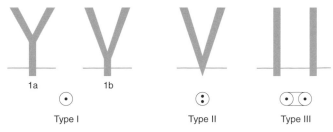

1a   1b

Type I   Type II   Type III

Figure 6 Variations in the communication between the common bile duct and Wirsung's duct. Type 1a has a long common bile duct (>1 cm) with one orifice. Type 1b has a short common bile duct with one orifice. Type 2 has a separate orifice for the bile and pancreatic ducts. Type 3 has separate orifices for the bile and pancreatic ducts at different points in the duodenum.

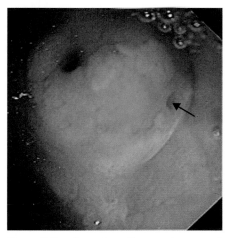

Figure 7 Type II opening with separate pancreatic (black arrow) and bile ducts.

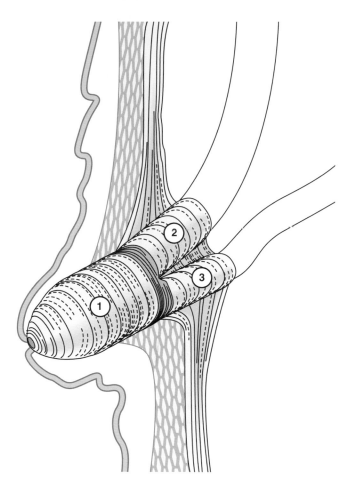

Figure 5 Ampulla of Vater with junction of the common bile duct and Wirsung's duct. (1) Common sphincter. (2) Choledochic sphincter. (3) Wirsung's duct sphincter.

the pancreatic duct may have separate openings in the papilla (type II) (Fig. 7) or openings at different points in the duodenum (type III). There are two types of common opening (or common channel):

- Type 1a corresponds to a long common channel with extraduodenal confluence of the two channels (Fig. 8).

- Type 1b corresponds to a common channel confined to the mucosa and to the duodenal submucosa.

When the common channel is >15 mm long, the frequency of congenital anomalies of the bile ducts (choledochal cyst, Caroli disease) and cholangiocarcinoma is believed to be higher.

The arterial supply of the papilla exhibits numerous anatomical variations, which are determined by the retroduodenal artery and the branch of the upper pancreaticoduodenal

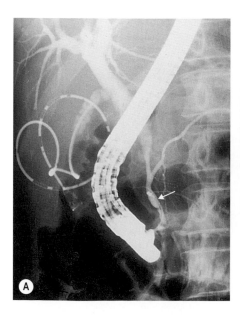

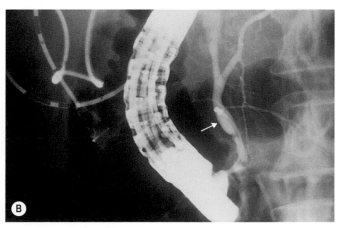

Figure 8 Type 1a common channel. These images illustrate a type 1a, with a long common channel (arrow).

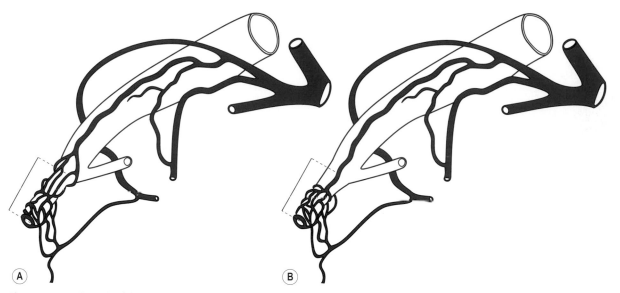

Figure 9 Arterial supply of the papilla. (A) This configuration is associated with a low hemorrhagic risk with sphincterotomy. (B) This configuration is associated with increased risk of bleeding due to a low arterial trunk which can be cut during sphincterotomy.

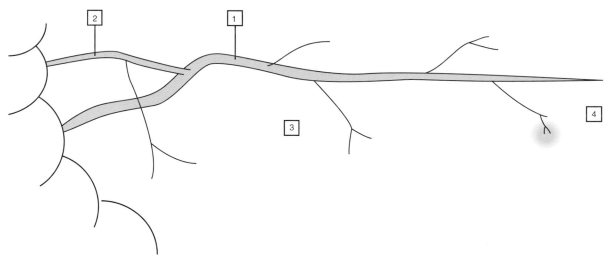

Figure 10 Normal pancreatic ductal anatomy. (1) Duct of Wirsung or pancreatic duct. (2) Duct of Santorini. (3) Secondary ducts. (4) Parenchyma.

artery. Significant bleeding can occur depending on the configuration of the blood vessels at the papilla (Fig. 9).

1.1. Normal pancreas and its variants

The main pancreatic duct rises steeply in the head, then crosses the upper abdomen horizontally or in a slightly ascending manner (Fig. 10). In healthy individuals, the shape of the pancreatic duct is variable, and diagnostic conclusions cannot be based on shape alone. Loops (ansa loops) may be observed, particularly in the isthmus (Fig. 11). The diameter of the pancreatic duct is on average 4 mm in the head of the pancreas, 3 mm in the body and 2 mm in the tail. The duct of Santorini usually connects the pancreatic duct to the accessory papilla. Collateral branches open perpendicular to the axis of the pancreatic duct. Their normal diameter should not exceed 1 mm. The diameter of the pancreatic duct increases with age. The aging of the pancreas is accompanied by irregularities in ductal diameter and may make differential diagnosis with incipient chronic calcifying pancreatitis difficult.

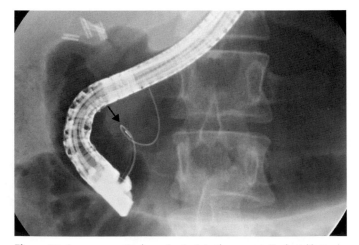

Figure 11 Ansa pancreatica loop. A wire is in the pancreatic duct. Note where the tip of the sphincterotome is (arrow) there is an alfa loop consistent with ansa pancreatica but the wire is in the direction of the common bile duct. Ensure careful injection.

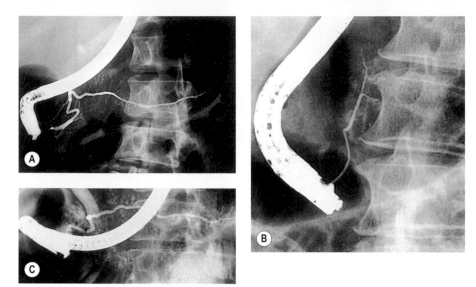

Figure 12 Normal pancreatogram and pancreas divisum. (A) Normal pancreatogram. (B) Ventral duct (pancreas divisum). (C) Dorsal duct (pancreas divisum).

1.2. Congenital anomalies of the pancreatic ducts

Annular pancreas is characterized by a ring of pancreatic tissue surrounding the descending portion of the duodenum. It is thought to be due to incomplete rotation of the pancreatic ventral bud. It is a rare anomaly in adults (0.1% of ERCP).

Pancreas divisum (Fig. 12) is the embryonic anomaly most commonly found in adults (5% of ERCP), characterized by the failure of the ventral and dorsal pancreatic ducts to fuse. A definite diagnosis can be obtained only by cannulation of the major papilla and the accessory (minor) papilla.

Cannulation of the major papilla opacifies the ventral pancreas (Fig. 12B). The ventral duct is short with a small diameter. The length varies from a few millimetres to 5 or 7 cm. If the duct is very short, injection of contrast medium results very quickly in acinarization, which must not be confused with a

submucosal injection. If the duct measures 3 or 4 cm, complete occlusion of the head of the pancreas by cancer must be excluded. Opacification of the dorsal pancreas (Fig. 12C) should be performed to confirm the diagnosis of pancreas divisum if the ventral pancreas is completely atrophic and invisible after catheterization of the major papilla. Opacification also allows visualization of lesions in the dorsal pancreas. Incomplete forms of pancreas divisum exist (Fig. 13).

Box 1 Problematic surgical anatomy

- Partial gastrectomy with Billroth II gastrojejunostomy.
- Whipple resection with Roux-en-Y limb of jejunum anastomosed to the biliary and pancreatic ducts.
- Pylorus preserving Whipple resection with Roux limb of jejunum anastomosed to the duodenal cap.
- Gastrojejunal bypass for obesity with a Roux limb of jejunum anastomosed to a small gastric pouch.
- Resection of the bile duct with anastomosis of the common hepatic duct (choledochojejunostomy) or hilum (hepatico-jejunostomy) to a Roux-en-Y limb of jejunum.
- Biliary diversion procedure with a Roux limb of jejunum draining the gastric remnant after partial gastrectomy.
- Total gastrectomy with anastomosis of the esophagus to a Roux limb of jejunum.

From Haber GB. Double balloon endoscopy for pancreatic and biliary access in altered anatomy (with videos). Gastrointest Endosc 66(3 Suppl):S47–S50, 2007.

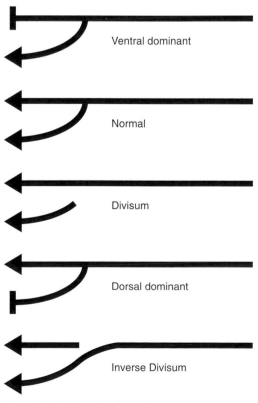

Ventral dominant

Normal

Divisum

Dorsal dominant

Inverse Divisum

Figure 13 Variations in pancreatic anatomy.

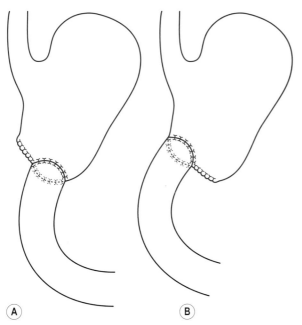

Figure 14 Gastroduodenal anastomoses. (A,B) represent two different types of gastroduodenal anastomoses. A Pean (A) anastomosis is commonly found in Europe, while a Billroth I is seen more frequently in the USA (B). These types of surgery were often performed for treatment of peptic ulcer disease and are seen less frequently now due to eradication of *H. pylori* and use of proton pump inhibitors.

2. Post-surgical anatomy

It is important to understand post surgical anatomy (see also Ch. 10.6), as it is encountered frequently due to the increase in obesity and gastric bypass surgery. Gastroduodenal anastomoses (Fig. 14) and certain types of choledochoduodenal anastomoses (Fig. 15) can usually be reached with a duodenoscope. The papilla is more difficult to reach in patients with Roux-en-Y anatomy (Fig. 16). A pediatric colonoscope, enteroscope or double/single balloon or spiral enteroscopy may be required to reach the papilla. The main problem in these patients is the length of small bowel that has to be

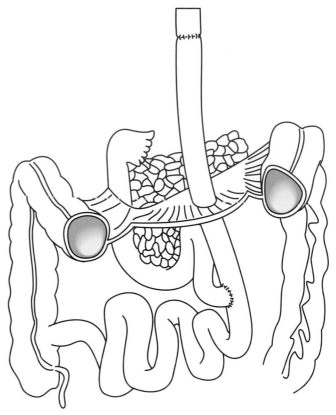

Figure 16 Roux-en-Y. This is the classic Roux-en-Y configuration found in patients with Billroth II, Finsterer and Polya anatomy. Note that the Roux limb can be either antero- or retrocolic (as found in this figure). Retrocolic Roux limbs have greater angulation and can be more difficult to traverse.

traversed. The shortest distance is encountered with a Billroth II (Fig. 17), with the longest distance typically associated with Roux-en-Y, associated with gastric bypass. Whether the limb has been placed antero- or retrocolic can also affect the ability to reach the papilla (Fig. 18). Retrocolic is associated with acute turns which can be difficult to negotiate but it's a short way to find papilla. Anterocolic is a long way to reach papilla.

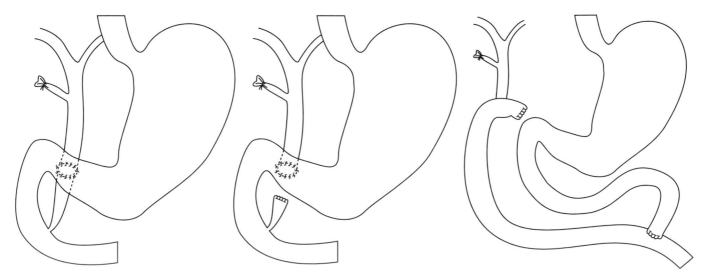

Figure 15 Choledochoduodenal anastomoses. (A) Side-to-side choledochoduodenal anastomosis. (B) End to side choledochoduodenal anastomosis. (C) Choledochojejunal anastomosis with Roux-en-Y anastomosis.

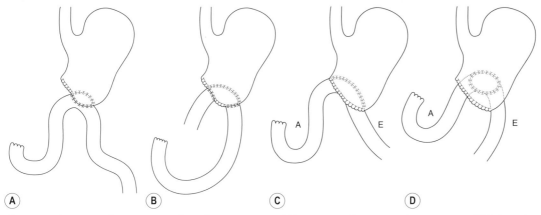

Figure 17 Gastrojejunal anastomoses. These figures represent different types of gastrojejunal anastomoses. (A) Polya is found more commonly in Europe, while a Billroth II (B) is performed commonly in the UK and USA for patients with pancreatic cancer in the head. (C,D) represent a classic and an isoperistaltic Finsterer gastrojejunostomy. Note that the Roux limbs are labelled A and E. A represents the afferent limb, which contains the papilla or choledochoenterostomy. E is the efferent limb which leads to the remaining small bowel. It is very important to check what limb you are in. This is usually done by looking for bile (afferent limb) and by using fluoroscopy to check your position. The endoscope should be going in the direction of the right upper quadrant. If you are not, you may be in the efferent limb.

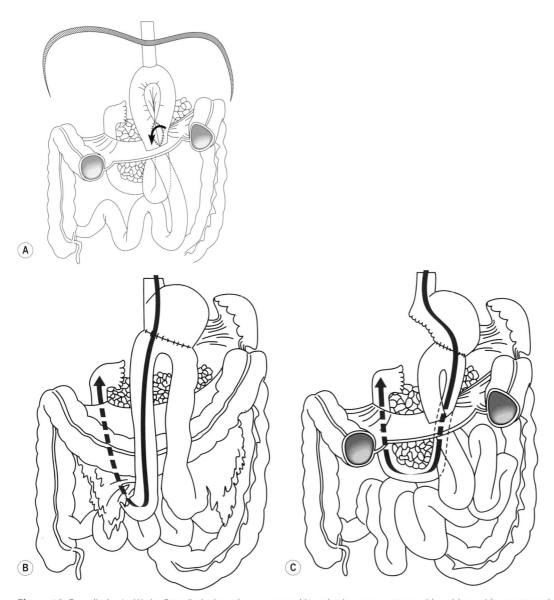

Figure 18 Roux limbs. In (A) the Roux limbs have been arranged in a classic omega pattern with a side-to-side anastomosis. The omega loop and retrocolic position make it difficult to reach the papilla. The configuration in (B) is better, as there is a relatively straight path to the papilla. (C) Demonstrates enterocolic Roux limb. Patients with this type of anatomy have less angulation of the bowel, compared with retro-colic Roux-limbs; however, the distance to the papilla is greater, which can make accessing the papilla challenging.

10.9 ERCP imaging technique

Summary

Introduction   400

1. Dilute or full strength contrast media?   400

2. How much contrast should be injected?   400

3. When and how many X-ray images should be taken?   400

4. Diagnostic problems and interpretation errors   400

Key Points

- It is essential that the highest quality radiographic images are obtained during ERCP.
- Full strength contrast is usually used, unless pancreatic or biliary stones are suspected.
- Images should be taken from different views to clearly define any abnormal area.
- Bubbles can be distinguished from stones by placing the patient in the reverse Trendelenburg position.

Introduction

It is very important that high quality radiographic images are obtained. The type of contrast used, the amount injected, and how to obtain good radiographic views are discussed below.

1. Dilute or full strength contrast media?

Contrast media can be used undiluted (300 mg iodine/mL), or diluted to 50%. In most cases, undiluted contrast is usually used. This provides excellent visualization of neoplastic stenoses or diseases of the small bile or pancreatic ducts. Diluted contrast is often used where biliary or pancreatic stones are suspected, as stones are often not seen if full strength contrast is used.

2. How much contrast should be injected?

Continue injecting until the intrahepatic bile ducts or the small pancreatic ducts are visible. Do not overfill the gallbladder (due to the risk of cholecystitis) or secondary pancreatic ducts (due to the risk of pancreatitis). Usually 3–5 mL of contrast medium is sufficient to opacify the pancreatic ducts, while 15–20 mL is required for the bile ducts. In patients who have a sphincterotomy, a balloon catheter may be required to allow adequate opacification of the ducts.

3. When and how many X-ray images should be taken?

X-rays should be taken at different stages. An image should be taken before injection and passing the endoscope, as well as in different stages of opacification (as you start injecting, once injection is completed and while contrast is emptying from the ducts). Images taken from different views (left lateral decubitus, dorsal decubitus with slight rotation to the right) can be used to clearly define abnormal areas, and to identify normal structures such as the cystic duct take off. An image of contrast emptying from the bile duct is taken after the duodenoscope has been removed. An image is often taken in the supine position after removing the duodenoscope to exclude perforation for medicolegal reasons. The pancreatic duct, however, empties quickly and images must be taken during the injection of the contrast medium.

4. Diagnostic problems and interpretation errors

Interpreting cholangiographic and pancreatographic images sometimes raises difficult problems, which should be borne in mind.

4.1. Stones or bubbles?

A filling defect corresponds in the majority of cases to a stone; however, occasionally it may be due to parasites (gallbladder with hydatid cyst, *Ascaris*, flukes), benign or malignant tumor fragments, hemobilia, or even air bubbles. To differentiate air bubbles from stones, tilt the table in such a way that the patient's head is elevated (reverse Trendelenburg position). This will cause air bubbles to rise and stones to fall (Fig. 1).

Errors of interpretation can be reduced by some simple principles:

- Use contrast medium diluted to 75% if stones are suspected.
- Use undiluted contrast medium if a tumor is suspected (dense bile due to stasis prevents accurate assessment of the limit of the tumor).
- Catheterization of the bile and pancreatic ducts must be selective and deep to achieve correct opacification which is the key to the correct interpretation of the images.
- In the left lateral decubitus and ventral position, air bubbles remain in the lower common bile duct, while stones rise to the hilum. In the dorsal decubitus position, the opposite occurs.
- A close examination of all the images, including those taken in the dorsal decubitus position, is essential. This allows the following to be confirmed:
  - Correct drainage of the bile and pancreatic ducts
  - Opacification of the left intrahepatic bile ducts

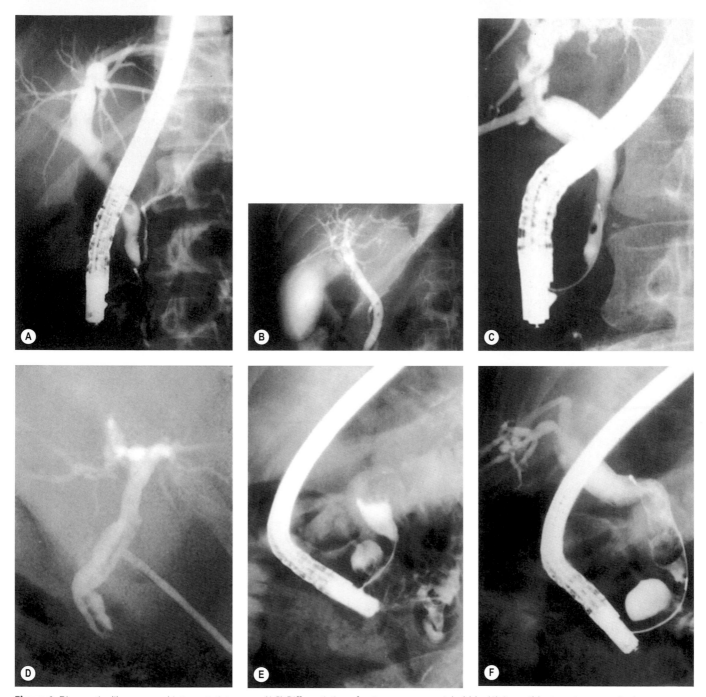

Figure 1 Diagnostic dilemmas and interpretation errors. (A,B) Differentiation of a stone versus an air bubble. (A) A possible stone is present in the common bile duct. A stone generally rises towards the intrahepatic bile ducts with a patient prone. (B) Air bubbles do not usually rise. (C) Adenoma arising in the common bile duct appears as a fixed, non-moving object. (D) Hemobilia. (E,F) False underfilling: stone occluding the lower common bile duct (complete filling necessary before drawing conclusions).

- A stone pushed by the injection into the intrahepatic bile ducts which has re-descended with the patient in dorsal decubitus.
- The catheter can be connected to a pump which injects contrast. This should be purged correctly with a constant drop-wise injection system to reduce the risk of injecting bubbles. A stone located in the papilla or in the bile duct may simulate the image of a tumor, by its immobility.
- A stone located in the papilla may not be identified and present a misleading tapered aspect. Images taken during

emptying show the normal lower common bile duct with a tapered appearance varying over time, related to the alternate contraction and relaxation of the sphincter of Oddi. A stone or a tumor yields a fixed image.
- A normal dilated bile duct, without visible stones, does not automatically rule out the possibility of stones. Microlithiasis may be present, the stone may be hidden in contrast medium, or the stone may have migrated since the clinical event.
- An image in which contrast does not appear to fill beyond the bile duct may correspond to obstruction

by a tumor or a false image due to incomplete opacification. This is also true for the left intrahepatic bile ducts, which fill only in excess pressure or in images taken with the patient in dorsal decubitus.

- The benign or malignant nature of a biliary stenosis is sometimes difficult to determine from the radiological appearance alone.
- Obstruction of the intrapancreatic bile duct may correspond to cancer of the pancreas or of the common bile duct.
- Dilation of the bile duct does not always correspond to sphincter of Oddi stenosis, particularly in elderly or cholecystectomized individuals.
- Cancer in the region of the ampulla of Vater infiltrating the ampulla is not endoscopically visible and may appear as irregular stricture of the lower common bile duct during opacification.
- Minor anomalies during pancreatography are difficult to interpret. They may correspond to incipient chronic pancreatitis or to a normal pancreas, particularly in the elderly.

- Compression of bile duct by the gallbladder may be secondary to cholecystitis, a stone impacted in the cystic duct or a tumor lesion (gallbladder cancer).
- Incomplete stenosis of the pancreatic duct may correspond to cancer or to pancreatitis.
- Complete stenosis of the pancreatic duct may be due to cancer, pancreatitis or to a technical fault (injection of air bubbles or incomplete opacification which must not be confused with pancreas divisum).
- Normal pancreatography does not rule out incipient chronic pancreatitis or cancer of the peripheral pancreas.
- Incorrectly filled intrahepatic bile ducts should be distinguished from sclerosing cholangitis.

Most of these diagnostic problems can be resolved by correct catheterization technique, rigorous analysis of the radiological images and precise knowledge of the limits of ERCP.

10.10 Abnormal imaging: classification and etiology

Summary

1. Cystic dilation of the bile duct   403
2. Cholangiocarcinoma   403
3. Gallbladder cancer   406
4. Primary sclerosing cholangitis   406
5. Other causes of biliary dilation   406
6. Intrahepatic cholestasis   406
7. Chronic pancreatitis   407
8. Pancreatic tumors   408

Key Points

- A knowledge of abnormal imaging is essential for anyone undertaking ERCP.
- Hilar cholangiocarcinoma is classified into four types depending on its extent into the intrahepatic biliary tree.
- Gallbladder cancer can present with Mirizzi's syndrome.
- Alternating stricturing and dilation is classic for primary sclerosing cholangitis.

1. Cystic dilation of the bile duct

Congenital cysts of the bile duct are rare. They are classified depending on their location in the biliary tree (Table 1, Figs 1–4). They can be associated with jaundice, abdominal discomfort, cholelithiasis, cholangitis, hepatic abscesses, recurrent pancreatitis, cirrhosis, portal hypertension, portal vein thrombosis, and are associated with an increased risk of cholangiocarcinoma.

2. Cholangiocarcinoma

Cholangiocarcinoma can be classified into three types based on its radiographic appearance (Fig. 5):

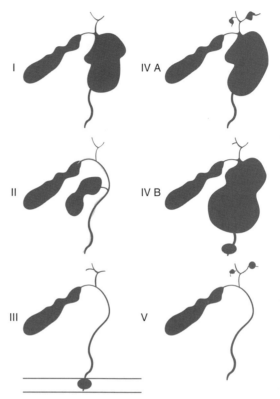

Figure 1 Classification of congenital bile duct cysts (Todani classification). Type I: Dilation of the entire common hepatic or common bile duct or segments of each. Type II: CBD diverticulum. Type III: Dilation of the intraduodenal portion of the CBD. Type IV: Dilation of the intra and extrahepatic biliary tree (Type IVa). Type IVb demonstrates dilation of the extrahepatic biliary tree alone. Type V: Single or multiple intrahepatic cysts.

Table 1 Classification of congenital bile duct cysts (Todani classification)

Type of cyst	Definition	Comment
I	Dilatation of the entire common hepatic or common bile duct or segments of each	Account for 80–90% of cysts. Treatment of choice is excision of the cyst and Roux-en-Y biliary-enteric anastomosis.
II	Diverticulum in the CBD	Surgical excision and primary closure over a T-tube.
III (choledochocele)	There is a dilatation of the intraduodenal portion of the CBD (Figs 2, 3)	<3 cm in diameter treat with sphincterotomy. ≥3 cm requires surgery.
IVa	Multiple dilatations of the intra- and extrahepatic biliary tree (Fig. 4)	Excision of the cyst and Roux-en-Y biliary-enteric anastomosis. No specific treatment of intrahepatic cysts. If disease is limited to specific intrahepatic segment these can be considered for surgical resection.
IVb	Multiple dilatations of the extrahepatic biliary tree	
V (Caroli disease)	Single or multiple intrahepatic cysts	If disease is limited to a single hepatic lobe, surgical resection can be considered. Transplantation can be considered in patients with decompensated cirrhosis.

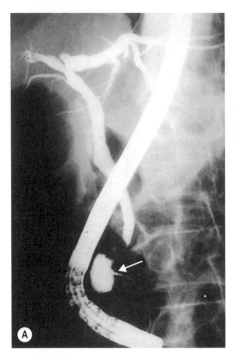

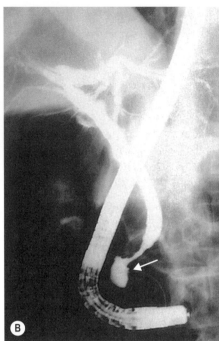

Figure 2 (A,B) Type III cyst (choledochocele). Note the dilatation of the intraduodenal portion of the CBD (arrow).

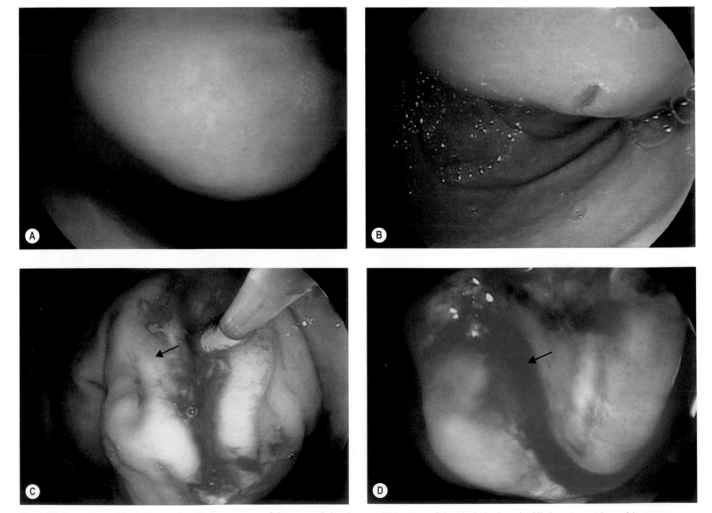

Figure 3 Type III cyst (choledochocele). (A) Appearance of the second duodenum. (B) Incision of the choledochocele. (C) Opening with a sphincterotome. (D) Appearance after opening with a sphincterotome.

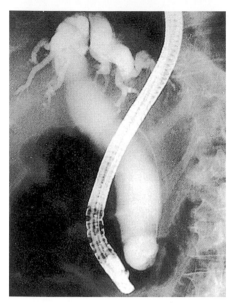

Figure 4 Type IVa cyst. This image demonstrates cystic dilation of the common bile duct and intrahepatic bile ducts

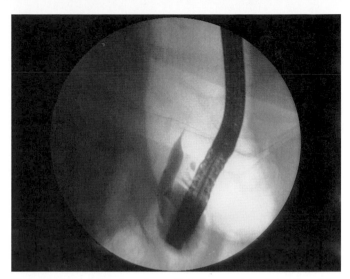

Figure 6 Type I cholangiocarcinoma. Note the complete obstruction of the bile duct.

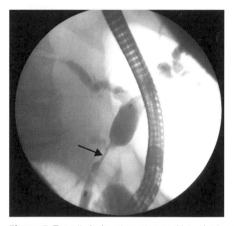

Figure 7 Type II cholangiocarcinoma. Note the irregular stenosis (arrow) with upstream dilation of the biliary tree.

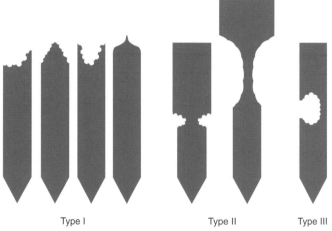

Type I   Type II   Type III

Figure 5 Cholangiocarcinoma. Cholangiocarcinoma can be classified based on its radiographic appearance: Type I, complete stenosis of the bile duct; Type II, incomplete stenosis and Type III, filling defect is present.

- Type I: complete stenosis (Fig. 6)
- Type II: incomplete stenosis (Fig. 7)
- Type III: filling defect.

In Type I, there is complete obstruction of the bile duct. In Type II, there is a stenosis of variable length with smooth or irregular contours with upstream dilation of the biliary tree. This is the most common type. Type III presents as a filling defect or as a fixed sessile or pedunculated lesion arising from the wall. This appearance may be confused with a stone; however, unlike a stone the tumor is immobile.

2.1. Hilar cholangiocarcinoma

Hilar cholangiocarcinoma is classified into four types, using the Klatskin classification (Fig. 8):

- Type I: involvement of the common hepatic duct
- Type II: invasion of the bifurcation without involvement of the secondary intrahepatic ducts

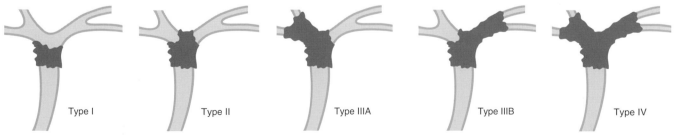

Type I   Type II   Type IIIA   Type IIIB   Type IV

Figure 8 Klatskin classification of hilar cholangiocarcinoma.

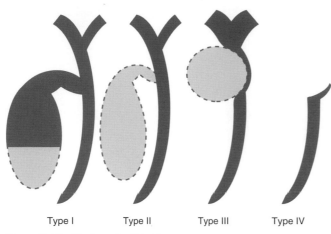

Figure 9 Classification of gallbladder cancers.

- Type III:
  - A: invasion of the bifurcation which extends into the right secondary intrahepatic duct
  - B: extends into the left secondary intrahepatic duct
- Type IV: invasion of the bifurcation, and involvement of secondary intrahepatic ducts on both sides.

3. Gallbladder cancer

Gallbladder cancer can also be classified based on its radiographic appearance into types I–IV (Fig. 9). It is rare to find an irregular filling defect in the gallbladder without alteration of the common bile duct (Types I and II). Gallbladder cancer can present with Mirizzi's syndrome (Type III). This radiographic appearance can also be due to cholecystitis, a stone impacted in the cystic duct or hepatic metastasis.

4. Primary sclerosing cholangitis

Primary sclerosing cholangitis (PSC) causes diffuse strictures of the common bile duct and intrahepatic bile ducts. Alternating stenosis and dilation is characteristic. It is important to emphasize the difficulty of diagnosing diffuse bile duct cancer in this group of patients, thus, the importance of histological and cytological samples. Strictures of the pancreatic duct are rarer in PSC, occurring in 8% of patients, while cystic duct involvement occurs in 18%. PSC can be classified into four intrahepatic and four extrahepatic types depending on the radiographic features (Fig. 10).

4.1. Intrahepatic radiographic changes in PSC

- *Type 1*: There is slight irregularity of ductal contour, localized stricture, no post-stenotic dilation. These features are often found at the bifurcation.
- *Type 2*: There is diffuse filiform stricture, alternating with moderate interstenotic dilations or with a normal ductal diameter. The strictures are predominant at the bifurcation, with reduced arborization.
- *Type 3*: There is complete occlusion of the peripheral ducts with multiple cystic, fusiform, sac-like dilations of the central ducts; there are strictures between dilations giving a string-of-pearls appearance.

- *Type 4*: There is diffuse ductal occlusion with stenoses of the remaining ducts; only the central ducts are filled with contrast medium. Large spaces are empty of any ducts.

4.2. Extrahepatic radiographic changes in PSC

- *Type 1*: There are moderate irregularities of the contours with no segmental or total stenosis without distinct strictures.
- *Type 2*: There is segmental stenosis of the common bile duct with irregular or regular edges, sparing part of the duct.
- *Type 3*: There is diffuse stricture with a string-of-pearls appearance along its length.
- *Type 4*: This has very irregular edges with alternating strictures and dilations, giving the appearance of a pseudodiverticulum.

5. Other causes of biliary dilation

- Sphincter of Oddi (see also Ch. 10.18) dysfunction (SOD) can be associated with a stricture of the sphincter, with diffuse dilation of the bile duct and pancreatic duct
- Postoperative stenoses (following cholecystectomy, liver transplantation, sphincterotomy) yield images of complete or incomplete stenosis which are short, and may be associated with stones. The bile duct are not diluted upstream of the obstacle (at an early stage).
- AIDS-related cholangiopathy.

6. Intrahepatic cholestasis

A diagnosis of intrahepatic cholestasis is made by demonstrating normal opacification of the whole bile duct with no

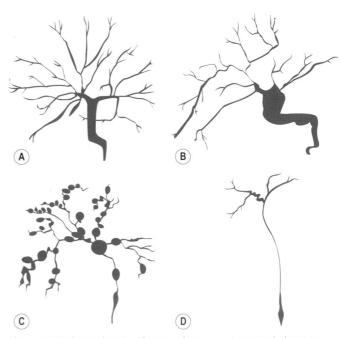

Figure 10 Radiographic classification of primary sclerosing cholangitis.

Table 2 Cambridge criteria for grading chronic pancreatitis

Grade	Main pancreatic duct	Side branches
Normal	Normal	Normal
Equivocal	Normal	>3 abnormal
Mild	Normal	>3 abnormal
Moderate	Abnormal	>3 abnormal
Severe	Abnormal with at least one of the following:	>3 abnormal
	Large cavity (>10 mm)	
	Duct obstruction	
	Intraductal filling defects	
	Severe dilation or irregularity	

filling defects, in particular by good filling of the intrahepatic bile ducts. Only deep, selective catheterization can yield complete images of the intrahepatic bile ducts.

7. Chronic pancreatitis

7.1. Pancreatographic alterations

The main duct is often normal initially, with a few collateral branches demonstrating localized dilation. CT, functional and pancreatic tests are usually normal at this stage.

Box 1 Kasugai's classification of chronic pancreatitis

Kasugai's classification distinguishes between three forms of the disease:
- Minor forms: a few collateral branches are abnormal and the pancreatic duct is normal
- Moderate forms: in addition to the above lesions, there are images of pancreatic duct irregularities
- Major forms: stenosis of the pancreatic duct, with pancreatic stones, pseudocysts, and common bile duct stenosis.

Endoscopic ultrasound may show changes within the parenchyma before any ductal changes appear. The diagnosis of chronic pancreatitis in the advanced form is rarely difficult: the main duct is dilated, tortuous and with defects (stones and protein deposits), stenosis and areas where the duct is disrupted. ERCP is useful in managing the complications of chronic pancreatitis. Chronic pancreatitis is usually graded using the Cambridge criteria (Table 2). Other classification systems used include the Kasugai classification (Box 1), and Crémer's classification (Fig. 11).

7.1.1 Crémer's classification

- *Type 0*: The pancreatic duct is normal and a few secondary ducts are abnormal. This form is difficult to distinguish from age-related changes in the ducts
- *Type I or minor pancreatitis*: This is divided into two subtypes. Type IA where the pancreatic duct has irregular contours and a few secondary ducts are altered

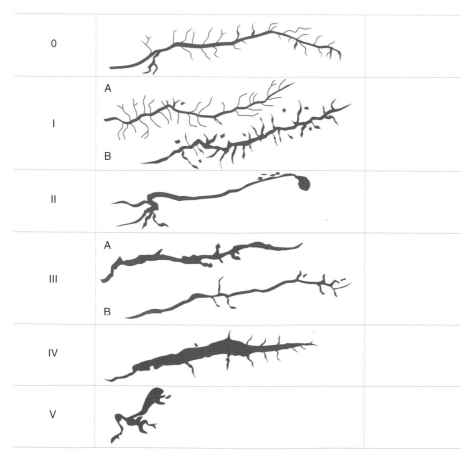

Figure 11 Crémer's classification of chronic calcifying pancreatitis.

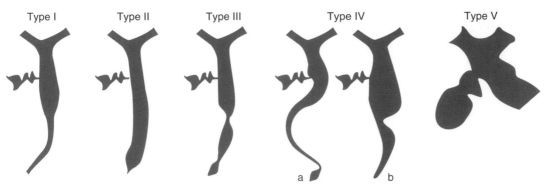

Figure 12 The cholangiographic appearance of the pancreatic pathology can be classified into Types I–V (Caroli–Sarles classification).

or dilated; type IB where all the secondary ducts are abnormal

- *Type II or focal pancreatitis*: This predominantly affects the head or the tail with macrocystic dilation of one or more secondary ducts. The morphology of the ducts in unaffected segments is normal
- *Type III or diffuse pancreatitis*: The pancreatic duct shows one or more stenoses (IIIB or IIIA) without marked dilation upstream. The secondary ducts are always abnormal
- *Type IV or cephalic pancreatitis*: The pancreatic head shows segmental stenosis with dilation upstream of all the ducts. *This type can be seen in cancers*
- *Type V or pancreatitis with cephalic filling limit*: The contrast medium does not fill the cephalic segment of the pancreatic duct. *This image suggests cancer of the head of the pancreas.*

Chronic pancreatitis can also affect the bile duct (Figs 12, 13). This can be classified into types I–IV depending on the radiographic appearance.

- *Type I* is the commonest alteration of the bile duct. There is an elongated, regular stenosis of the retropancreatic path of the common bile duct with or without dilation upstream and a gaping papilla.
- *Type II* corresponds to a stricture at the sphincter of Oddi with dilation upstream.
- *Type III* corresponds to an hourglass-shaped stenosis at the upper edge of the pancreas.
- *Type IV*, which may also be seen in pancreatic cancer, corresponds to localized lateral or anteroposterior compression of the intrapancreatic common bile duct (Type IVb).

8. Pancreatic tumors

The image of both biliary and pancreatic stenosis is characteristic of pancreatic cancer. In typical cases, stenosis is present in the upper part of the intrapancreatic common bile duct with the same image shown in the cephalic pancreatic

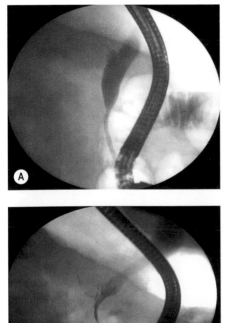

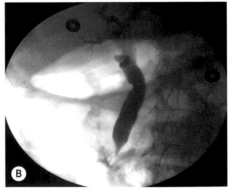

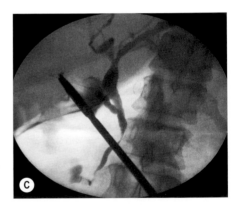

Figure 13 Changes in the bile duct and chronic pancreatitis. (A) Type I has an elongated stenosis. (B) Type II presents as a stricture at the sphincter of Oddi. (C) Type III has a stricture with an hour-glass appearance. (D) Type IVa there is compression by a pancreatic pseudocyst.

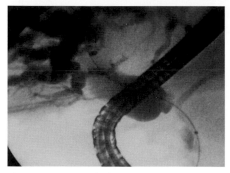

Figure 14 Type V, cholangiographic appearance of pancreatic cancer.

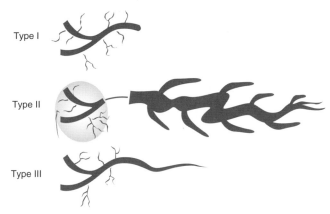

Type I

Type II

Type III

Figure 15 Radiographic changes of the pancreatic duct associated with pancreatic cancer.

duct. The pancreatic ductal changes are shown in Figure 15 and can be classified as shown below. Types I and II are the most frequent. The other forms of pancreatic cancer are far less common.

- *Type I*: There is complete stenosis of the pancreatic duct, with irregular, tapering stricture, or cystic dilation indicative of tumor necrosis.
- *Type II*: There is localized stenosis of the pancreatic duct with dilation of the ducts upstream.
- *Type III*: Infiltrating form. There is diffuse infiltration form, with a narrow, irregular pancreatic duct.
- *Type IV*: There are changes in the secondary ducts which show amputation, stenosis and dilation. The pancreatic duct is normal.
- *Type V*: There is dilation of the pancreatic duct and one or more branches, which contain radiotransparent filling defects which correspond to mucoid masses. This type is characteristic of adenomatous tumors of the pancreatic duct.

The bile duct can also be affected by pancreatic cancer. The radiographic appearances are discussed below, with stenotic and obstructive types being the commonest seen.

- *Stenotic type*: There is incomplete stenosis in the upper part of the head of the pancreas, away from the papilla, with marked dilation and horizontalization of the common bile duct, which is engulfed by the tumor. This appearance is characteristic of cancer of the head

of the pancreas (Type V of the Caroli–Sarles classification) (Figs 12, 14).
- *Obstructive type*: This involves complete stenosis of the common bile duct in the upper part of the head of the pancreas.
- *Angular type*: The bile duct is engulfed in the upper edge of the pancreas and shows angulation with rigid walls without proximal dilation (Type IVb of the Caroli–Sarles classification) (Fig. 12).

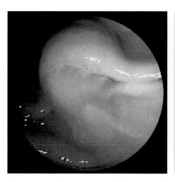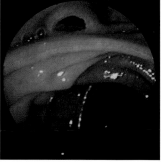

Figure 16 Appearance of the papilla in a patient with IPMN. The presence of mucin in the papilla is classic for IPMN.

Further Reading

Cremer M, Toussain J, Hermanu A, Deltenre M, de Toeuf J, Engelholm L: Les pancréatites chroniques primitives, *Classification sur base de la pancreatographie endoscopique Acta, Gastroenterol Belg* 39:522-546, 1976.

Liguory CI, Canard JM: Tumors of the biliary system, *Clinics in Gastroenteroly* 12(1):265-291, 1983.

Sarles H, Sarles JC, Guien C: Study of pancreatic and bile ducts in chronic pancreatitis, *Arch Mal App Dig* 47:664-683, 1958.

Ohto M, Ono T, Tsuchiya Y, Saisho H: *Cholangiography and pancreatography*, Tokyo New York, 1978, Ed. Igaku-Shoïn, pp 155-159.

10.11 **Endoscopic sphincterotomy**

Key Points

- The biliary orifice should be cut between the 11 o'clock and 12 o'clock position.
- The pancreatic orifice should be cut between the 1 o'clock and 3 o'clock position.
- The minor papilla is cut in from the 5 o'clock to 11 o'clock direction.
- Pre-cut sphincterotomy and fistulotomy should only be performed by an experienced endoscopist.
- Complications of sphincterotomy include perforation, bleeding, and pancreatitis.

Introduction

Endoscopic sphincterotomy is commonly performed as part of the treatment of biliary and pancreatic diseases. The success and complication rate depend not only on having appropriate equipment, but also on the experience and frequency with which the endoscopist performs sphincterotomies.

1. Indications

- To allow a diagnostic or therapeutic procedure to be performed
- To allow dilation of the biliary tree or pancreatic duct
- To allow the removal of stones from the biliary or pancreatic duct
- To allow cholangioscopy or pancreatoscopy
- As part of the treatment for:
  - Bile duct leak
  - Pancreatic fistula
  - Pseudocyst
  - Pancreatic duct rupture
- To treat sphincter of Oddi dysfunction or papillary stenosis
- Minor papilla sphincterotomy is performed in patients with recurrent acute pancreatitis in whom no other cause can be identified.

2. Biliary sphincterotomy technique

2.1. Standard technique

The standard technique was developed by Classen and Demling and consists of five steps:

1. The bile duct is cannulated deeply (Figs 1A, 2A)
2. Confirm that the sphincterotome is in the correct duct:
   - Contrast is injected to confirm that the correct duct has been cannulated and to confirm the diagnosis. It is important to look for and confirm the presence of stones, even if they have been demonstrated on recent imaging, as they may have passed spontaneously.
3. Place the sphincterotome in the cutting position:
   - This is achieved by withdrawing the sphincterotome until approximately half of the metal wire appears outside the papilla (Figs 1B, 2A). The wire should be positioned in the direction of the bile duct between 11 and 12 o'clock (Figs 1C, 2B).
4. Sphincterotomy
   - The sphincterotome is connected to the electrocautery unit. This should be done just before the endoscopist is ready to perform the sphincterotomy to avoid accidentally cutting the bile duct with the sphincterotome.
   - The papilla is cut using endo-cut mode. Cutting is carried out in a stepwise fashion.
5. Radiographic images
   - Images should be taken in the ventral and dorsal decubitus position. If sphincterotomy has been performed correctly, the bile duct drains completely into the duodenum on the images in dorsal decubitus. Images taken in dorsal decubitus should always be checked to confirm the absence of retropneumoperitoneum, which would indicate a perforation.

3. Pancreatic sphincterotomy technique

- If both biliary and pancreatic sphincterotomies are required, commence with the pancreatic sphincterotomy (Figs 3, 4). If the pancreatic orifice cannot be located, biliary sphincterotomy may be performed initially. This may then help to locate the pancreatic orifice.
- The pancreatic duct is cannulated with a sphincterotome and a 0.035 inch guidewire. Some practitioners use a smaller calibre wire to cannulate the pancreatic duct (0.025 inch wire), as theoretically this may decrease trauma to the pancreatic duct.

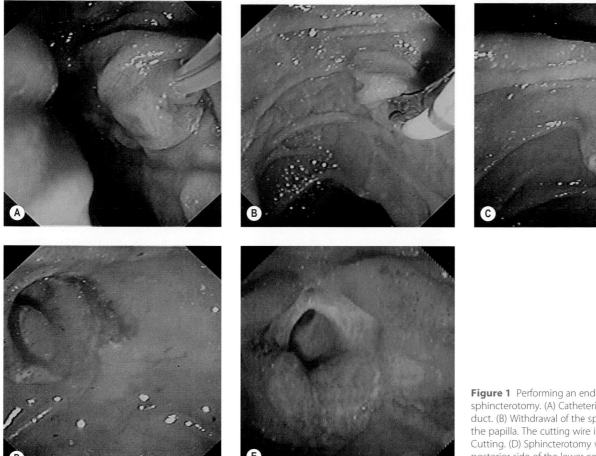

Figure 1 Performing an endoscopic sphincterotomy. (A) Catheterization of the bile duct. (B) Withdrawal of the sphincterotome from the papilla. The cutting wire is tensioned. (C) Cutting. (D) Sphincterotomy with a view of the posterior side of the lower common bile duct. (E) Sphincterotomy on day 15.

 Clinical Tip

Electrocautery settings for biliary and pancreatic sphincterotomy

40 pure-cut or

ERBE blended current.
- With ERBOTOM ICC 200:

Endo-cut on 120 W with hemostase 2
- With ERBE VIO 200 D (Chapter 1.4, Table 1):

Endo-cut I
- ■ effect 1 no coagulation
- ■ effect 2 with coagulation

- A pancreatogram should be obtained. Inject contrast gently to avoid acinarization, which increases the risk of pancreatitis.
- A 3–4 mm cut is made directing the sphincterotome towards the 1 o'clock position. An alternative technique is to place a stent and perform needle-knife sphincterotomy cutting down onto the stent. One study has shown that this decreases the rate of pancreatitis in patients with sphincter of Oddi dysfunction; however, it is technically demanding and should only be performed by experienced endoscopists.

- Minor papilla sphincterotomy can be performed using a sphincterotome, cutting in the 5 to 11 o'clock direction.

3.1. Problems with sphincterotomy

- The sphincterotome is not cutting properly:
  - ■ Check that you do not have too much of the sphincterotome within the infundibulum. The ideal cutting position is with the proximal one-third of the sphincterotome.
  - ■ Withdraw the sphincterotome a few millimeters to reduce the cutting wire surface area in contact with tissues (Fig. 5).
- I cannot orientate the sphincterotome in the 11–12 o'clock position. Try the following:
  - ■ Adjust your position using right/left wheel.
  - ■ Unbow the sphincterotome and advance it into the bile duct and withdraw it.
  - ■ Go to a long scope position.
  - ■ Alter your body position, by rotating your shoulders left or right. This will alter the position of the sphincterotome and will often allow you to perform a sphincterotomy using the edge of the wire.
- How far can I cut and how big should I make a biliary sphincterotomy?
  - ■ The average size of a sphincterotomy is between 10 and 15 mm. The papilla and the whole infundibulum (Figs 1D, 1E) should be cut until the

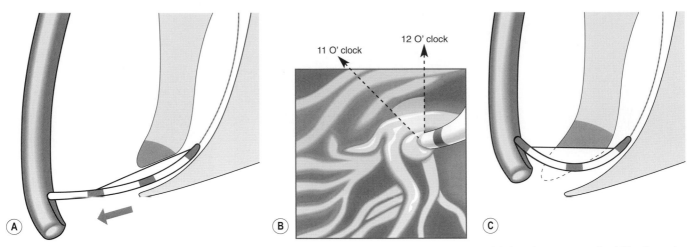

Figure 2 Biliary sphincterotomy. (A) Correct position of the sphincterotome before tensioning the cutting wire. (B) The sphincterotome should be directed between the 11 and 12 o'clock position (shaded area). (C) Sphincterotomy.

lumen of the lower common bile duct is visible and/or air appears in the bile.

- The length of the incision depends on the endoscopic anatomy, the diameter of the bile duct, the length of the infundibulum (Figs 6) and if you are removing stones, their size.
- How do I know if the biliary sphincterotomy is adequate?
  - There are several methods to assess the adequacy of a biliary sphincterotomy. There should be rapid emptying of contrast from the bile duct into the second portion of the duodenum on imaging.

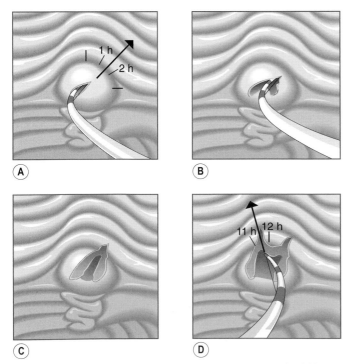

Figure 3 Pancreatic sphincterotomy. (A) The sphincterotome should be angled towards the 1 to 2 o'clock position. (B,C) Sphincterotomy performed. (D) Following pancreatic sphincterotomy, look for the biliary orifice between the 11 and 12 o'clock position.

- The biliary sphincter can sometimes be seen on imaging as a smooth tapering just above the papilla. This disappears as the sphincter is cut.
- Another method of assessing the size of the sphincterotomy is to insert the sphincterotome into the bile duct. Fully bow the sphincterotome and withdraw it. If it is easy to withdraw a fully bowed sphincterotome through the papilla this suggests that a generous sphincterotomy has been performed.
- How far can I cut and how big should a pancreatic sphincterotomy be?
  - As with a biliary sphincterotomy, the length of the incision depends on the endoscopic anatomy, the diameter of the pancreatic duct, the length of the infundibulum and if you are removing stones, their size.
- How do I know if the pancreatic sphincterotomy is adequate?
  - The adequacy of the sphincterotomy depends on why it is being performed (i.e. to remove stones, etc.). Some general tips are:
    - The length of the incision depends on the diameter of the bile duct, the length of the infundibulum and the size of the stones (if you are removing stones). When the size of the stones is bigger than the maximum potential diameter of the sphincterotomy, you can dilate the sphincterotomy to 15 mm (see section 7 below).
    - After performing a sphincterotomy, check fluoroscopy to see if contrast is draining from the duct or if there is a rapid drainage of bile. If it is not, you may need to extend the sphincterotomy.
    - Look for the loss of the sphincter on fluoroscopy. The sphincter is seen as a smooth tapering of the distal CBD, and is lost following sphincterotomy.
    - Check the size of the sphincterotomy by seeing if it will allow a fully bowed sphincterotome through.

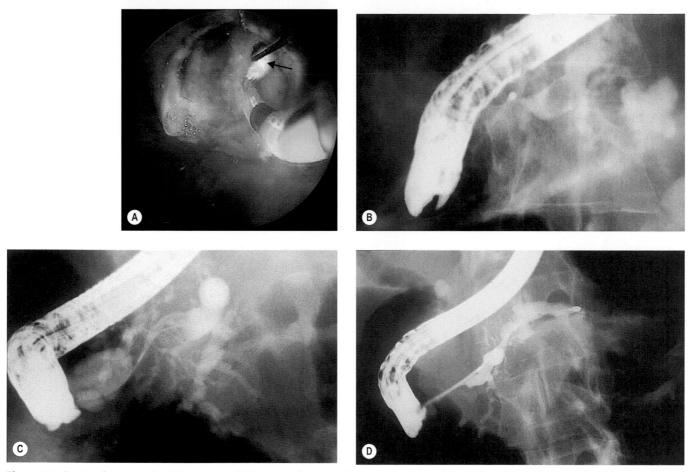

Figure 4 Indications for pancreatic sphincterotomy. (A) Removal of a pancreatic stone (arrow). Note the position of the prior pancreatic sphincterotomy towards 1 o'clock. (B) Stenosis of the main pancreatic duct in the head, with an upstream stone which caused a fistula following distal pancreatectomy. (C) Incomplete retrieval of the pancreatic stone. (D) Follow-up after complete removal of the stone: the fistula resolved 72 h later.

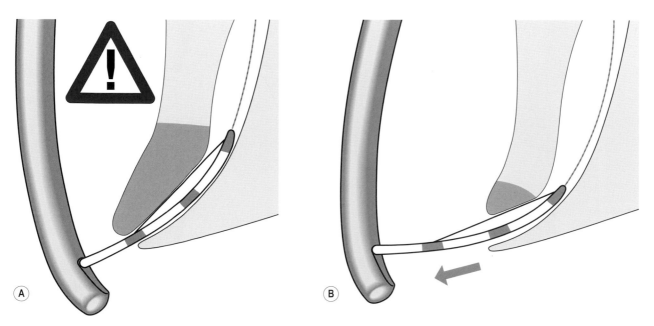

Figure 5 Wire position is critical to successful sphincterotomy. (A) Sphincterotome introduced too deeply into the bile duct; the current leaks away without cutting, with the resulting risk of rough cutting with hemorrhage and perforation. (B) Sphincterotome in the correct position.

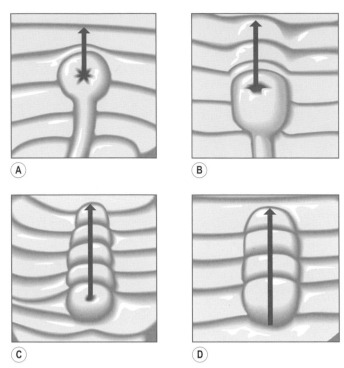

Figure 6 The size of the sphincterotomy can be affected by the type of infundibulum.

4. Special situations

4.1. Sphincterotomy in patients with a gastroenteric anastomosis (Billroth II/Whipple)

In patients with a gastroenteric anastomosis, the papilla is accessed through the afferent loop. As the papilla is approached through the afferent loop, the anatomy is reversed with the bile duct between 5 and 6 o'clock. Sphincterotomy is difficult to perform but extraction of stones is, by contrast, easier because it is done along the axis of the bile duct.

Techniques

- The standard technique described above can be used (Fig. 7), however caution must be used as the sphincterotome tends to cut in the direction of the pancreas (Fig. 8). Sphincterotomy should be performed towards the 5–6 o'clock position (Fig. 9), i.e. THE OPPOSITE OF NORMAL.

Equipment

Equipment is determined by which endoscope is used.

- Duodenoscope: Standard or specialized equipment. Special sphincterotomes can be used where the cutting wire is directed towards the bile duct.
- 160 cm enteroscope: Standard or specialized equipment
- >160 cm enteroscope: Standard ERCP equipment (sphincterotome, balloon, etc.) are not long enough to be used with these enteroscopes. A bespoke special length sphincterotome can be made.
- In difficult cases, a biliary stent can be placed. A pre-cut sphincterotomy can then be performed cutting down onto the stent.

4.2. Sphincterotomy in children

Sphincterotomy should not be performed in children unless there is a definite indication. If a sphincterotomy is performed, it should be generous to decrease the risk of subsequent stricture formation.

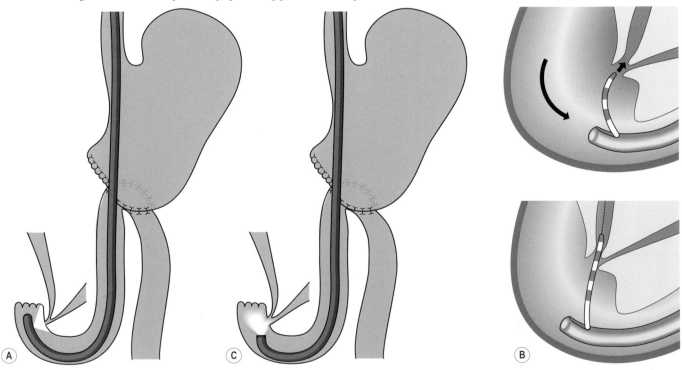

Figure 7 Altered anatomy. This is a diagram of a Finsterer operation, which is a variation of a Roux-en-Y. (A) Demonstrates centering the papilla. (B) After centering the papilla, the endoscope is withdrawn to allow cannulation in the direction of the bile duct, with the aid of a guidewire. (C) The same procedure performed using of a forward-viewing endoscope.

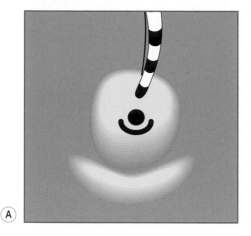

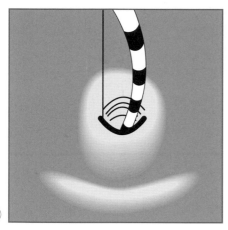

Figure 8 Incorrect orientation of the sphincterotome in a patient with a Roux-en-Y anastomosis (B). The sphincterotome tends to align in the direction of the pancreatic, rather than bile duct in patients with gastrojejunal anastomosis. Sphincterotomy should be performed towards the 5 or 6 o'clock position.

5. Sphincterotomy in difficult cases

In about 10% of cases, deep biliary cannulation is impossible and sphincterotomy cannot be performed. In these cases, the following techniques may be used in order of preference, depending on the anatomical conditions.

5.1. Sphincterotomy over a guidewire

Where cannulation is difficult, a triple lumen sphincterotome is used to cannulate the bile duct with a guidewire (Fig. 10). Once the guidewire is deeply inserted into the duct, contrast is injected to confirm the correct duct. The sphincterotome is then advanced over the guidewire into the duct and sphincterotomy performed as described above.

5.2. Pre-cut

In a pre-cut sphincterotomy the bile duct is identified by opening it from the papillary orifice. This can be performed using a regular sphincterotome; however, a short tip sphincterotome may be useful in these cases. This technique is used in the absence of an infundibulum or when a neoplastic lesion causes bile duct obstruction.

Technique

- Insert the sphincterotome into the papillary orifice. The sphincterotome rapidly comes up against the papillary orifice after a few millimeters (Fig. 11).
- Ensure that the electrocautery unit is set to use of pure cutting current.
- Tense the cutting wire.
- Using stepwise cuts, the sphincterotome is advanced in the direction of the bile duct.
- Try to locate the bile duct after each cut.
- When the bile duct has been located, cannulate the bile duct, and perform a standard sphincterotomy.

 Warning!

BEWARE! Pancreatitis and perforation are more common with pre-cut sphincterotomy due to cutting in the wrong direction.

5.3. Needle knife infundibulotomy

This involves cutting through the infundibulum to the bile duct. This technique should be used with a Type II or III infundibulum and should not be performed in a Type I or 0 infundibulum (Fig. 12). The ideal indication is a stone impacted in the papilla of Vater, where the stone serves as a block on which to open the infundibulum.

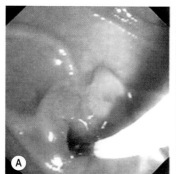
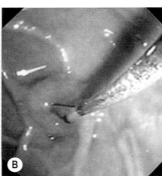
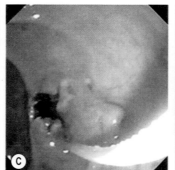
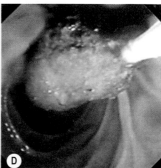

Figure 9 Endoscopic sphincterotomy in a patient with Billroth II gastrectomy. (A) Sphincterotome in position through a papilla open due to the passage of a stone. (B) Sphincterotome cutting wire tensioned. (C) Sphincterotomy completed. (D) Extraction of the stone.

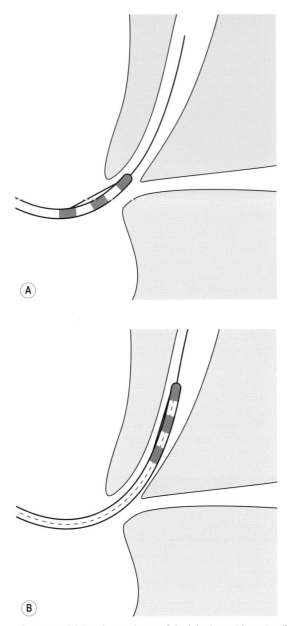

Figure 10 (A) Initial cannulation of the bile duct with a wire. (B) Successful deep cannulation achieved by guiding the sphincterotome over the guidewire.

Technique (Figs 13, 14)

- Optimize conditions by ensuring complete duodenal hypotonia.
- Ensure that the electrocautery unit is set to pure cutting current.
- The needle is advanced 3–5 mm and the guard fixed. The needle is then withdrawn into the catheter and the catheter inserted into the instrument channel.
- Take time to locate the optimal site. Practice the maneuver you are going to use once or twice. Use the elevator to control the needle. The aim of the technique is to gently cut down into the bile duct as if it were an onion where you are peeling back the layers.
- Advance the needle and cut down into the infundibulum in a stepwise manner. The cut can be made starting at the top and cutting down towards the os or from the os cutting up. The dissection is performed in a stepwise fashion, layer by layer. Wash generously to ensure adequate visualization. After each cut, try to locate the bile duct which has a white pearly appearance, before continuing.
- A flow of bile is proof that the bile duct has been cut. Do not cut any further, wash the area and try to identify and cannulate the biliary orifice. Once the bile duct has been cannulated, the sphincterotomy is extended with the aid of a standard sphincterotome.
- Do not proceed if you cannot see the bile duct after deep dissection, as it has probably been cut.

There is a high risk of perforation associated with this procedure. In this situation is better to stop and repeat the ERCP 24 hours later after the edema has receded.

> ### ✓ Clinical Tip
>
> - Pre-cut sphincterotomy or *infundibulotomy* should only be attempted when there is a definite therapeutic indication based on other imaging and never during diagnostic ERCP.
> - This procedure is associated with an increased risk of perforation, bleeding, and pancreatitis, and should only be performed by an experienced endoscopist.
> - It is often better to stop and repeat the ERCP 24 h later after the edema has resolved.

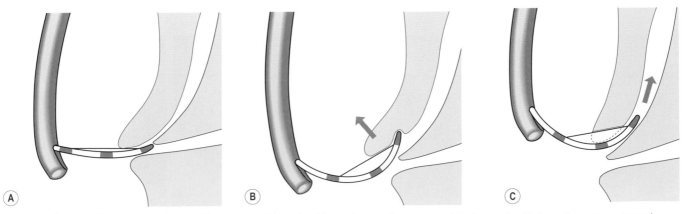

Figure 11 Pre-cut sphincterotomy using a sphincterotome. (A) Insert sphincterotomy as far as you can into the papilla. (B) Tense the cutting wire and perform a sphincterotomy on the section you can visualize. (C) Repeat the procedure until deep cannulation of the bile duct is achieved.

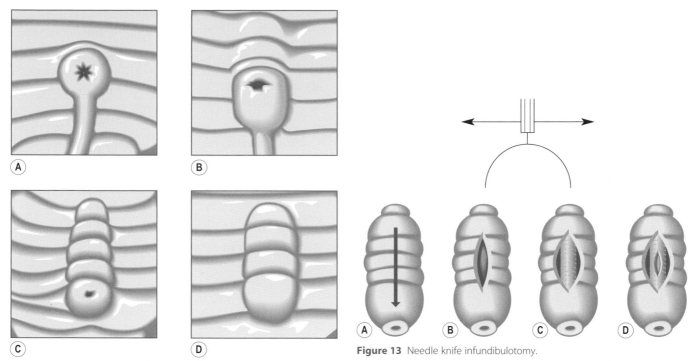

Figure 12 Classification of different types of infundibulae. Type 0: No infundibulum; Type 1: Infundibulum at the limit of visibility; Type 2: Projecting infundibulum; Type 3: Large infundibulum covering the papilla.

Figure 13 Needle knife infundibulotomy.

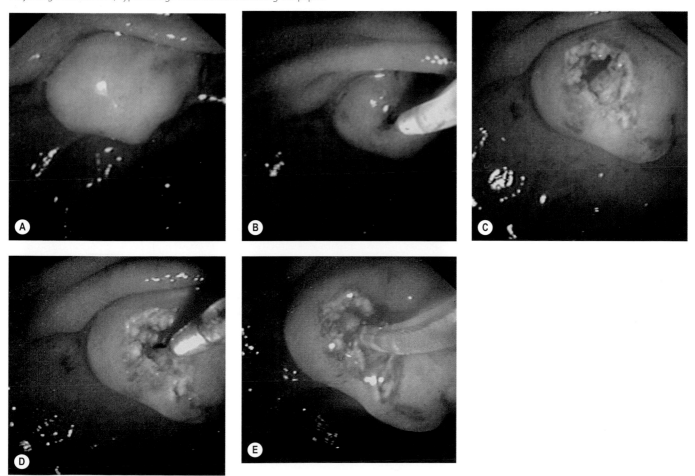

Figure 14 Needle knife infundibulotomy. (A) Examine the infundibulum to locate the optimal site. (B) Using the tip of the needle knife catheter, palpate the infundibulum to locate the optimum site. (C,D) Cut down into the infundibulum in a stepwise manner. Start slightly above the optimal site cutting from the top down. The dissection is performed in a stepwise fashion, layer by layer. (E) Cannulate the bile duct.

In cases where deep cannulation of the bile duct is difficult, a rendezvous procedure can be performed followed by biliary sphincterotomy.

6. Endoscopic balloon dilation of the Sphincter of Oddi

Endoscopic balloon dilation (EBD) of the biliary sphincter is an alternative to biliary sphincterotomy. The potential advantages of EBD over sphincterotomy are that it preserves the biliary sphincter, and also reduces the risk of bleeding compared with a biliary sphincterotomy. However, a single multi-center study in 237 patients randomized to either endoscopic sphincterotomy or balloon dilation was stopped early due to increased rates of pancreatitis (15.4% vs 0.8%), with two deaths due to pancreatitis in the dilation group. EBD can be considered as an alternative to endoscopic sphincterotomy in patients at high risk for endoscopic sphincterotomy such as those with a bleeding disorder, altered anatomy (i.e. Billroth II), or difficult anatomy such as a periampullary diverticulum. In patients with large CBD stones with a prior sphincterotomy, EBD can also be used as an alternative to extending the sphincterotomy. EBD is performed as follows:

- Cannulate the bile duct
- Confirm that the correct duct has been cannulated
- Insert an 8 mm biliary balloon over a guidewire
- Position the balloon so that the waist of the balloon is within the sphincter
- Inflate the balloon until the waist is no longer present under fluoroscopy and then deflate the balloon
- A guidewire should be maintained in the bile duct as access can occasionally be difficult following EBD

Further Reading

Disario JA, Freeman ML, Bjorkman DJ, et al: Endoscopic balloon dilation compared with sphincterotomy for extraction of bile duct stones, *Gastroenterology* 127(5):1291–1299, 2004.

Kethu SR, Adler DG, Conway JD, et al: ERCP cannulation and sphincterotomy devices, *Gastrointestinal Endoscopy* 71:435–445, 2010.

http://daveproject.org – This is an excellent site which provides videos on how to perform a sphincterotomy in normal, as well as altered, anatomy.

10.12 Biliary and pancreatic stone extraction techniques

Key Points

- The choice of which method to use is determined by the experience of the endoscopist and the size of the stones.
- Very small stones (<5 mm) often pass spontaneously or can be removed with a balloon.
- Stones measuring 5–15 mm can be removed either with a balloon or a basket.
- Giant stones (>1.5 cm) usually require mechanical lithotripsy to break them into smaller pieces before they can be removed.
- It is important to correctly align the duodenoscope for successful stone removal.
- When multiple stones are encountered, commence by removing the most distal stone.
- Once stones have been captured in a basket, the basket is withdrawn without closing it.
- A Dormia basket is usually used first to extract stones which are <1.5 cm. A basket with lithotripsy capability should always be used.
- Ensure that all the equipment required (Dormia basket, balloon, mechanical lithotripter, nasobiliary drain, etc.) is available prior to commencing an ERCP.

Introduction

Gallstones affect 10–20% of the Caucasian population while 10–15% of patients with symptomatic cholelithiasis will also have bile duct stones.

Transabdominal ultrasound is the least sensitive method for detecting bile duct stones. Helical contrast-enhanced CT has a sensitivity of between 71% and 73% and specificity of 98–97% for intrahepatic and extrahepatic gallstones, respectively. A systematic review comparing EUS and magnetic resonance cholangiogram (MRC) for the diagnosis of bile duct stones found that EUS had a sensitivity of 93%, specificity of 96%, compared with a sensitivity of 85%, specificity 93% for MRC. ERCP has a sensitivity of 79–90% and specificity of 92–100%. Intraoperative cholangiogram has a false positive rate of up to 5%. The sensitivity of MRC decreases when the bile duct is dilated (>10 mm) or when the stone measures <6 mm. False negative results occur in ERCP with small stones located within a dilated biliary duct, while false negative results for EUS occur in stones located in the upper portion of the common hepatic duct or within the intrahepatic ducts.

1. Bile duct stones

 Clinical Tip

Gallstones

- *Cholesterol gallstones*
  - Round and golden in color.
- *Calcium bilirubinate (pigment) gallstones*
  - Black, round and hard, contain calcium bilirubinate.
- *Primary bile duct stones*
  - Brown and shapeless stones. Consist of a mixture of calcium salts, unconjugated bilirubin, protein, bacteria and cholesterol.
- Risk factors for gallstone development:
  - Age, female sex, pregnancy, multiparous, genetic (Native Americans, Chileans)
  - Obesity, diabetes, weight loss
  - Drugs (exogenous estrogens, clofibrate, long-term octreotide), TPN
  - Diseases: Terminal ileal resection/disease (impaired enterohepatic circulation), gallbladder stasis, cirrhosis, hemolytic disease (pigment stones), hypertriglyceridemia (cholesterol stones), gallbladder stasis (diabetes mellitus, TPN, post-vagotomy, octreotide, somatostatinoma, spinal cord injury)
  - Biliary bacterial colonization (brown pigment stones)
  - Reduced exercise (men).

ERCP is the most common method for treating bile duct stones. Several methods can be used to remove stones; the choice of which method to use is determined by the experience of the endoscopist and the size of the stones. Very small stones (<5 mm) often pass spontaneously or can be removed with a balloon. Stones measuring between 5 and 15 mm can be removed either with a balloon or a basket. Giant stones (>1.5 cm) usually require mechanical lithotripsy to break them into smaller pieces before they can be removed. When stones are large, or where the patient's anatomy makes stone extraction difficult, electrohydraulic or laser lithotripsy may be required. Laparoscopic bile duct exploration is an alternative to ERCP (Fig. 1). Prophylactic cholecystectomy should be offered to all patients following clearance of their bile duct, unless they are poor operative candidates.

Box 1 Extraction of bile duct stones is successful in almost all cases

- 65–0% in a single session.
- 85% with multiple sessions.
- 95–99% with lithotripsy.

2. Pancreatic duct stones

Approximately one-third of patients with chronic pancreatitis have pancreatic duct stones. It is unclear whether pancreatic stones worsen the clinical course of chronic pancreatitis and glandular destruction. There is, however, evidence that they may contribute to pain associated with chronic pancreatitis due to increased intrapancreatic pressures.

Indications for pancreatic duct stone removal include:

- Patients with symptomatic chronic pancreatitis. The most suitable patients are those with ≤3 stones measuring <10 mm, located in the head or body with no downstream strictures or impacted stones.
- Patients with pancreatic pseudocyst.

3. Equipment

- Guidewire
- Sphincterotome
- Dormia basket with lithotripsy capability
- Biliary balloon
- Biliary and pancreatic stents

Specific equipment is required for lithotripsy, which is discussed later in this chapter.

4. Technique

A balloon or Dormia basket can be used to extract most stones. The decision of which to use is based on personal preference and experience; however, many experienced ERCPists use a Dormia basket first, with a balloon used where residual stones remain following a pull through with

Box 2 Definitions

Cholelithiasis
- Stones in the gallbladder.
- 5–10% will have choledocholithiasis.

Choledocholithiasis
- Stones in the biliary tree.
- 90% will have cholelithiasis.
- Primary choledocholithiasis are stones that arise within the biliary tree.
- Secondary choledocholithiasis are stones that arise in the gallbladder and then migrate into the biliary tree.

Microlithiasis
- Stones or particles only visible under a microscope.

Sludge
- A suspension of crystals and/or calcium salts.

Box 3 Predictors of choledocholithiasis

Very strong
- Common bile duct stone on transabdominal US.
- Clinical ascending cholangitis.
- Bilirubin >4 mg/dL.

Strong
- Dilated common bile duct on US (>6 mm with gallbladder *in situ*).
- Bilirubin level 1.8–4 mg/dL.

Moderate
- Abnormal liver biochemical test other than bilirubin.
- Age older than 55 years.
- Clinical gallstone pancreatitis.

Assigning a likelihood of choledocholithiasis based on clinical predictors
- Presence of any very strong predictor: High.
- Presence of both strong predictors: High.
- No predictors present: Low.
- All other patients: Intermediate.

(Reproduced with permission from Maple JT, Ben-Menachem T, Anderson MA et al. The role of endoscopy in the evaluation of suspected choledocholithiasis. *Gastrointestinal Endoscopy* 2010.)

a Dormia basket, for the extraction of small stones, or small fragment following lithotripsy.

4.1. Balloons

Balloons are used exclusively for small stones, or after a Dormia basket has been used. A selection of balloons are available in different sizes. A balloon is ideal for small (<5 mm) stones, or to remove small fragments after mechanical lithotripsy, but can be difficult to use in a large, dilated bile duct as the stone can slide past the balloon.

4.1.1. Balloon technique

- The balloon is inserted above the stone. If there are several stones, the stones are removed one at a time, starting with the stone closest to the papilla.
- Modern balloons can be inflated to several different sizes using the same balloon. The size of the bile duct should be estimated and a balloon should be chosen that is the same size or slightly larger than the width of the duct.
- A balloon can be used to remove intrahepatic stones. Place a guidewire above the stones and then insert the balloon over the guidewire. The size of the duct is assessed and the balloon inflated to a similar diameter. Take care to ensure that the diameter of the balloon is

Box 4 Indications for stone removal: ERCP in acute pancreatitis

- There are four randomized trials of ERC compared with conservative management in patient's acute pancreatitis.
- ERC is indicated in patients with severe pancreatitis and evidence of biliary obstruction within 24–72 h of admission.

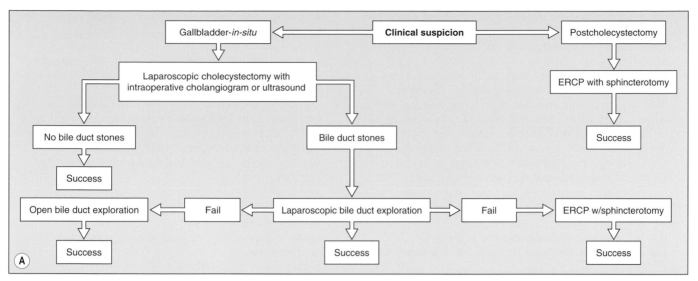

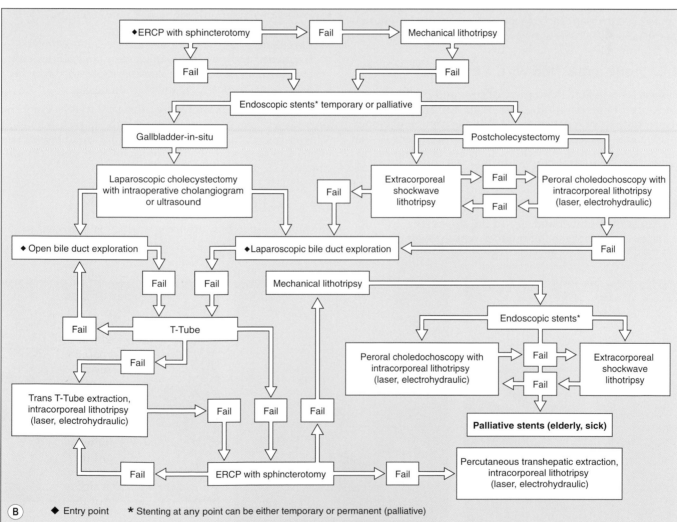

Figure 1 (A) Standard treatment of choledocholithiasis. (B) Specialized treatment of difficult bile duct stones. (With permission from Ginsberg G, Kochman ML, Norton I, et al, editors. Clinical gastrointestinal endoscopy, Saunders, 2005, London, p 677.)

not too large as there is a risk of perforation of the bile duct.

- The balloon is inflated above the stone and is gently pulled as far as the papilla.
- It is important to ensure that the duodenoscope is correctly aligned to successfully remove the stone through the sphincterotomy. Check the position of the scope – the balloon/bile duct should be aligned at 90° to the scope. The tip of the duodenoscope should be positioned directly below the papillary orifice abutting the opening. Often the scope will need to be inserted slightly, the tip deflected downwards and right. If this is not successful, gently turn the shaft of the scope clockwise while keeping constant pressure on the balloon.
- If this fails, the balloon may need to be deflated slightly to allow it to pass through the sphincterotomy.

In cases where there is a large stone but it is not possible to extend the sphincterotomy, a balloon sphincteroplasty can be used to dilate the os to allow the stones to be removed (see Chapter 10.11, Section 11.6).

4.2. Stone extraction with a basket

Baskets are available in a variety of sizes and configurations. 'Memory' or non-deforming baskets are also available which return to their original shape, facilitating capture of stones. Wire-guided baskets also exist. It is important to ensure that the basket is compatible with a mechanical lithotripter so that stones can be crushed if required.

4.2.1. Basket technique

- Assess the number and size of the stones. The stones must be small enough to pass through the

distal duct and sphincterotomy to prevent stone impaction.

- The closed basket covered by its plastic sheath is inserted over the stones. If this is difficult, a guidewire can be placed above the stones and the basket inserted over the guidewire.
- The basket is opened and the stone snared by opening and closing the basket. Sometimes vigorous shaking of the fully open basket inside the bile duct may help to bring the stones into the basket. Take care when opening the basket not to displace stones into the intrahepatic ducts.
- The basket is gently withdrawn as far as the papilla *without closing it* (Figs 2, 3). It is important to ensure that the duodenoscope is correctly aligned as described above to successfully remove the stone through the sphincterotomy.
- If the stone continually slips out of the basket, then the basket can be closed gently around the stone.
- Where there are multiple stones, commence by removing the most distal stone.
- Abundant lavage will help to remove small stones or fragments, and even to mobilize very large stones and remove them. If the stones are very large, they may be broken mechanically by the Dormia basket.

Common bile duct stones are often very friable. Once the large stones have been removed with the basket, a balloon catheter is sometimes required to remove small stone fragments and to obtain an occlusion cholangiogram demonstrating a clear biliary tree.

4.2.2. Problems with the Dormia basket

The stone is snared in the basket, which is impacted in the sphincterotomy opening.

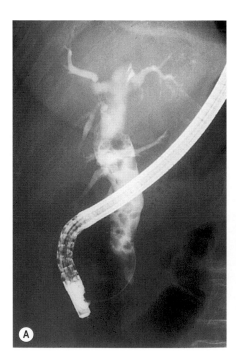
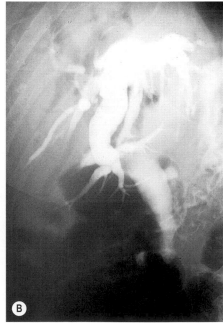
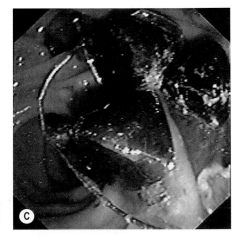

Figure 2 Removal of stones using a Dormia basket. (A) Stones in the common bile duct. (B) Extraction of stones using a Dormia basket. (C) Clear bile duct at the end of the procedure.

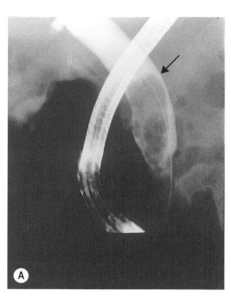
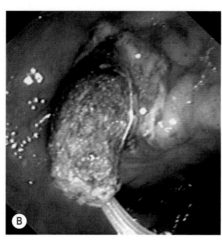
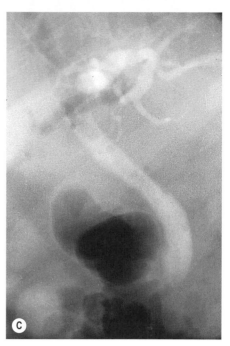

Figure 3 Removal of distal CBD stones. (A) Large stone (arrow) in the lower common bile duct. (B) A large sphincterotomy was performed, followed by retrieval of the stone with a Dormia basket. (C) Bile duct with no evidence of stones at end of the procedure.

There are several solutions.

- Withdraw the endoscope gradually and firmly, maintaining firm traction on the basket so that the endoscope and basket are integral. This may allow the stone to pass through the sphincterotomy orifice.
- Advance the endoscope so that the tip of the endoscope is against the papilla. Force the basket into the operating channel. The basket will close as it is withdrawn into the operating channel, crushing the stones (Fig. 4).
- The basket should be attached to a lithotripter and the stones crushed (see *Lithotripsy technique without withdrawal of the endoscope*, below).

Other options include extending the sphincterotomy, intra- or extracorporeal lithotripsy.

In cases where this fails, which is extremely rare, a nasobiliary drain can be inserted (see Chapter 10.19). The Dormia catheter is exteriorized like the nasobiliary drain. By pulling on it slightly every day, the stone and the Dormia become disimpacted within 48–72 h when the edema around the sphincterotomy subsides.

4.3. Reasons for failure to clear the bile duct of stones

In 65–70% of cases, the bile duct will be cleared of stones at the first attempt. Reasons for failure to extract the stone at the first attempt include:

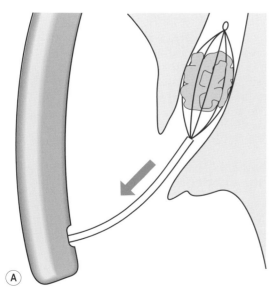
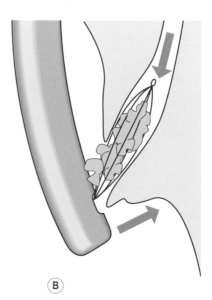

Figure 4 Wedged Dormia basket with stone. The endoscope is advanced so that the tip of the endoscope is against the papilla. The basket is forced into the operating channel. The stones are crushed as the basket closes as it is withdrawn into the operating channel.

Clinical Tip

Etiology of intrahepatic bile duct stones

- Primary stones
  - Parasitic infestations (*Clonorchis sinensis*).
  - Biliary infections.
  - Congenital factors/ductal abnormalities.
  - Intrahepatic cholangiocarcinoma.
  - Previous hepatobiliary surgery/strictures.
  - Cystic fibrosis.
  - Caroli's disease.
- Secondary stones
  - Stones which have refluxed into the intrahepatic system.

- Stone moulded to the bile duct or stones which are larger than the endoscopic sphincterotomy. These stones are often 'giant' stones measuring >1.5 cm
- Clot around the edges of the endoscopic sphincterotomy impeding maneuvers
- Stones in the intrahepatic bile ducts (see Clinical Tip, below)
- Bile duct stenosis
- Missed stones, noticed on follow-up images.

If there were multiple stones or if there is any doubt about a possible residual stone, follow-up ERCP should preferably be performed a few days later to make sure that the bile duct is clear.

Clinical Tip

Management of intrahepatic stones

- Primary stones
  - Avoid sphincterotomy unless definitive therapy is planned due to increased risk of recurrent cholangitis.
  - Patients with residual stones are at increased risk of cholangitis and cholangiocarcinoma.
  - Stone removal can be difficult due to the anatomy, strictures and peripheral location of stones; however, it has been shown to be successful in 64% of patients in one study, with 22% developing recurrent stones.
  - Alternatives to ERC include PTC with intracorporeal lithotripsy, ESWL with intracorporeal lithotripsy, hepatic resection or hepaticojejunostomy.
- Secondary stones
  - Sometimes a small, light stone may be pushed into the intrahepatic bile ducts during injection. It is difficult to snare the stone in this situation. The fluoroscopy table can be raised or the patient placed in the decubitus position, which causes the stone to descend with gravity into the common bile duct, making it more accessible for extraction.
  - Alternatively, insert a guidewire above the stone, followed by the balloon.
  - If this fails, a balloon can be placed just below the stone, inflated to fully fill the duct, and then rapidly retracted. This creates suction, which can pull the stone down.

Box 5 Mirizzi's syndrome

- Type I consists of external compression of the common hepatic duct by a stone in the cystic duct or gallbladder neck.
- Type II involves erosion of the stone into the common hepatic duct with subsequent fistula formation. Surgery is more difficult in this group due to increased risk of bile duct trauma.
- ERCP findings are of a smooth narrowing of the bile duct.
- Bile duct stenting or intracorporeal lithotripsy are sometimes successful.
- Mirizzi's syndrome is rare. Gallbladder cancer is a differential diagnosis and should always be considered.

5. Lithotripsy

Lithotripsy is used for large stones which are too big to fit through the sphincterotomy, stones located above a stenosis, or stones which cannot be snared with the basket catheter.

5.1. Mechanical lithotripsy

Mechanical lithotripsy is the most commonly used technique to extract bile duct stones when standard techniques fail. Mechanical lithotripsy can be performed with the endoscope in place, or after the endoscope has been removed (Soehendra lithotripter). The overall success rate for bile duct clearance with mechanical lithotripsy is 80–90% although 20–30% of patients require more than one session.

5.1.1. Lithotripsy technique without withdrawal of the endoscope

The lithotripter consists of a metal sheath covering a polyethylene catheter which contains the basket. The end of the catheter is attached to a lithotripter handle. The basket should be connected to the handle and tested to ensure that it is working prior to inserting it. The catheter is quite rigid and can be difficult to introduce and manipulate. In these cases, a wire-guided lithotripsy basket can be used.

5.1.2. Mechanical lithotripsy technique with duodenoscope in place

- The bile duct is cannulated with the catheter (Fig. 5).
- The catheter is advanced above the most distal stone. The basket is then opened.
- When the stone has been snared, the catheter is withdrawn until the basket with the stone touches the metal sheath.
- The stone is then fragmented by forcing the stone against the metal sheath by closing the basket wires.

5.1.3. Mechanical lithotripsy technique with removal of the duodenoscope

The technique uses the Soehendra lithotripter, and is used infrequently. Stones that are located more proximally in the bile duct must be captured and brought to the papilla before using the Soehendra lithotripter.

- Make sure that the stone has been snared correctly by the Dormia basket and that it is not caught on one side.
- Withdraw the endoscope while continuing to apply traction to the Dormia basket (Fig. 6).

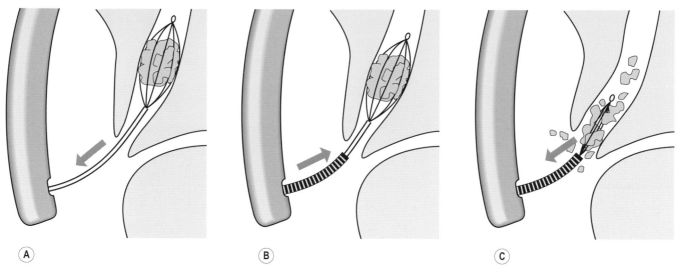

Figure 5 Lithotripsy technique without withdrawal of the endoscope. (A) The stone is snared in a Dormia basket. (B) The basket with withdrawn. (C) The stones are crushed against the metal sheath.

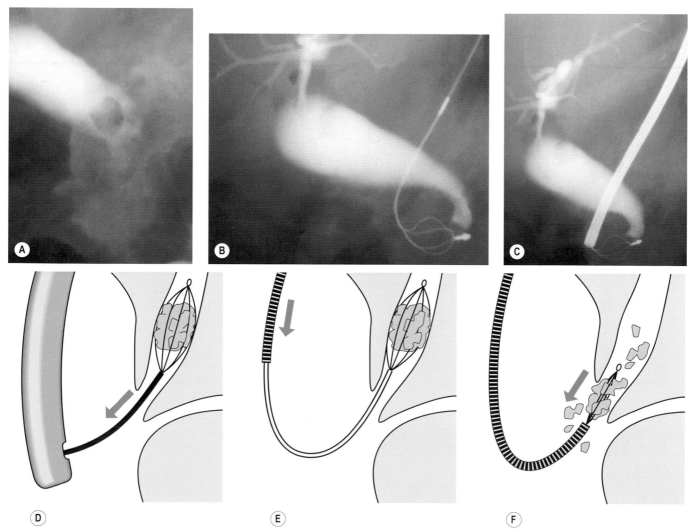

Figure 6 Soehendra mechanical lithotripter. (A) Stone that cannot be removed. (B) The endoscope is retracted. The Dormia wire is in position. (C) The endoscope is replaced by a metal sheath. (D) Insertion of the Soehendra lithotripter. (E) Removal of the endoscope and insertion of the metal sheath. (F) Basket withdrawn into the metal sheath.

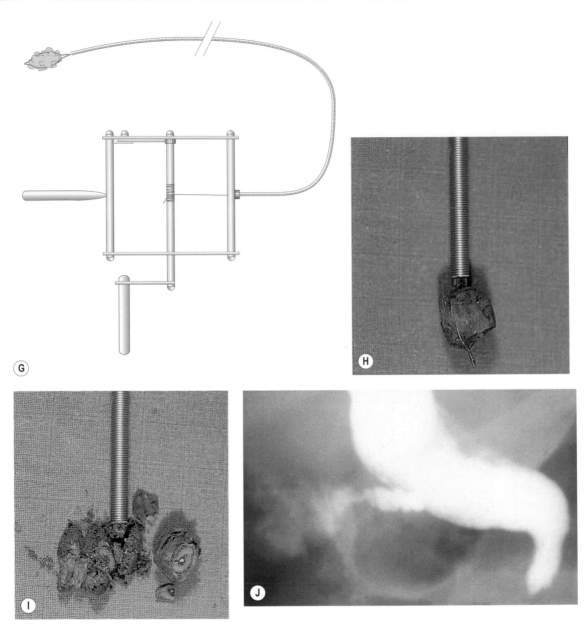

Figure 6, Continued (G) Soehendra mechanical lithotripter assembled and ready for use. (H) Stone snared in the Dormia in contact with the metal sheath. (I) The Dormia basket withdraws into the metal sheath, crushing the stone. (J) The bile duct is clear of stones after extraction of the fragments.

- Slide the metal sheath under fluoroscopic control onto the Dormia until it makes contact with the stone.
- Attach the end of the Dormia basket to the lithotripter handle.
- Apply steady traction to the handle (a winch, crank or rack system can be used).

- The Dormia basket is withdrawn into the metal sheath crushing the stone.
- The stone fragments are then removed by lavage, with the Dormia basket or a balloon.

5.2. Electrohydraulic lithotripsy

Electrohydraulic lithotripsy (EHL) is normally performed in combination with pancreatoscopy or cholangioscopy (Fig. 7). Cholangioscopy can be performed anterograde (via a percutaneous route) or retrograde (through a duodeno-scope). EHL fragments stones by means of a shock wave. This shock wave is generated by the creation of an electric high voltage spark between two electrodes located at the tip of the fibre. These sparks generate an expansion in the surrounding liquid, causing a shock wave.

Application of EHL is best achieved under direct visualization since shock waves can damage the biliary epithelium, or cause perforation or bleeding (<1% risk).

✓ Clinical Tip

Stenting for refractory CBD stones

Stenting can be used in high-risk surgical patients to provide temporary drainage. Stone size has been reported to decrease after stenting. However, long-term stenting should be avoided as a treatment for large stones, as this is associated with significantly more long-term complications compared with patients who have complete clearance of stones.

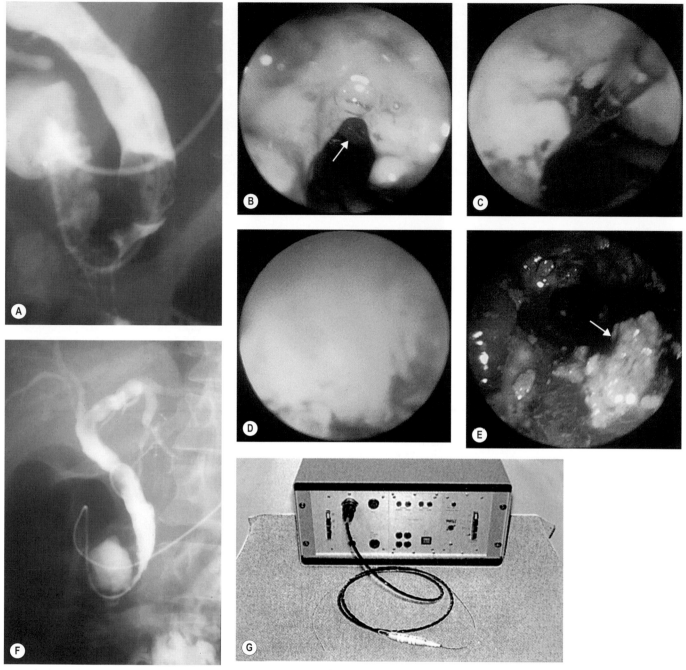

Figure 7 Electrohydraulic lithotripsy performed via per oral cholangioscopy. Radiographic images: (A) Large stone which cannot be removed via a sphincterotomy. (B) Stone visible through the sphincterotomy orifice (arrow) which should not be enlarged. (C) Lithotripsy probe facing the stone in the submerged second part of the duodenum. (D) Stone debris during firing. (E) Fragmented stone (arrow). (F) Bile duct with no evidence of residual stones at the end of the procedure. (G) LithoTron lithotripsy box.

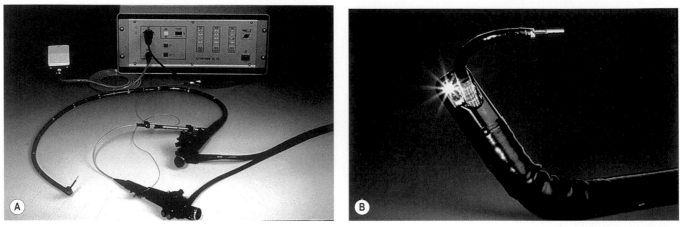

Figure 8 Equipment for per oral lithotripsy. (A) Therapeutic duodenoscope with lithotripsy box. (B) Choledoscope with EHL probe in position.

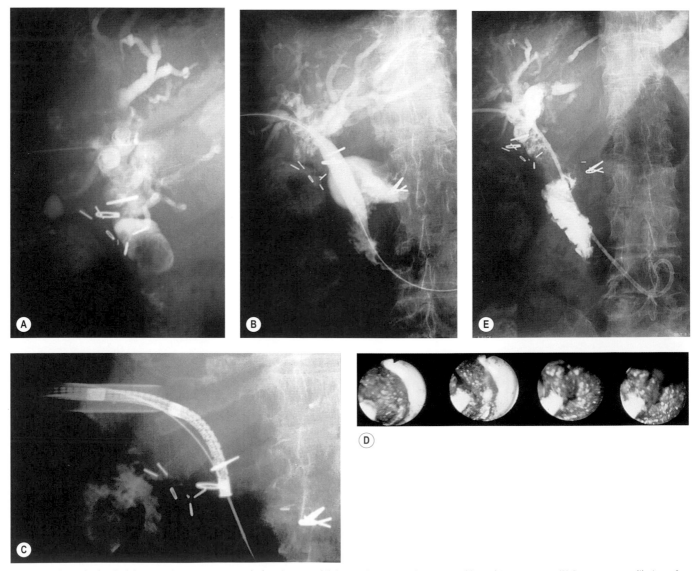

Figure 9 Electrohydraulic lithotripsy by percutaneous cholangioscopy. (A) Stone that cannot be removed by sphincterotomy. (B) Percutaneous dilation of the tract. (C) Percutaneous choledoscopy. (D) Lithotripsy of the stone under visual control. (E) A percutaneous cholangiogram revealing no residual stones.

5.2.1. Retrograde EHL technique

- The cholangioscope is inserted into the bile duct. The bile duct is irrigated with saline to allow visualization of the stone and also to generate a medium for the EHL.
- The EHL probe is advanced through the working channel with care taken to avoid bending (Fig. 8).
- The EHL probe is then positioned both endoscopically and fluoroscopically so that it abuts or is very close to the center of the stone.
- Take care to ensure that the probe is not abutting the bile duct wall.
- The EHL is fired. Commonly used setting is 70 W for 1–2 s, increasing by 10 W to a maximum of 100 W.
- The stone fragments are then removed using either a basket or a balloon.

Cholangioscopy with EHL can also be performed via a percutaneous route (Fig. 9) or directly thought an anstomosis (Fig. 10).

5.3. Laser lithotripsy

Laser lithotripsy is an alternative to EHL. It permits precise targeting of the stone, reducing the risk of bile duct injury.

There are three endoscopic laser lithotripsy systems for bile duct stones, the neodymium:yttrium-aluminum-garnet (Nd:YAG), the flashlamp pulsed dye, and flashlamp pulsed dye with an automatic stone recognition system. Laser lithotripsy is expensive compared with EHL, and not readably available.

5.4. Extracorporeal lithotripsy

Extracorporeal shock wave lithotripsy (ESWL) is an alternative for patients who have bile duct stones which are not amenable to endoscopic removal. Shock waves are applied externally to target large stones under fluoroscopic control. A pancreatic stent is often sufficient for targeting. For very small stones, contrast may need to be instilled via the nasopancreatic drain. The fragments are then removed by endoscopy. ESWL has several drawbacks. Only a small portion of bile duct stones are calcified, necessitating instillation of contrast via a nasobiliary catheter before targeting radiolucent stones. Several treatment sessions are usually required. Despite these limitations, success rates of up to 90% have been reported. ESWL can be considered in patients in whom mechanical or contact electrohydraulic lithotripsy has been unsuccessful before attempting percutaneous access to the bile duct.

Further Reading

Chopra KB, Peters RA, O'Toole PA, et al: Randomised study of endoscopic biliary endoprosthesis versus duct clearance for bileduct stones in high-risk patients, *Lancet* 348:791–793, 1996.

Fan ST, Lai EC, Mok FP, et al: Early treatment of acute biliary pancreatitis by endoscopic papillotomy, *N Engl J Med* 28:228–232, 1993.

Folsch UR, Nitsche R, Ludke R, et al: Early ERCP and papillotomy compared with conservative treatment for acute biliary pancreatitis. The German Study Group on Acute Biliary Pancreatitis, *N Engl J Med* 336:237–242, 1997.

Maple JT, Ben-Menachem T, Anderson MA, et al: The role of endoscopy in the evaluation of suspected choledocholithiasis, *Gastrointest Endosc* 71:1–9, 2010.

Neoptolemos JP, Bailey IS, Carr-Locke DL, et al: Sphincter of Oddi dysfunction: results of treatment by endoscopic sphincterotomy, *Br J Surg* 75:454–459, 1988.

10.13 Biliary and pancreatic stents: insertion techniques

Key Points

- 10 Fr diameter is optimum for plastic stent patency.
- Plastic stents are cheaper than self-expanding metal stents (SEMS); however, they occlude more quickly, requiring repeat intervention.
- SEMS are associated with decreased incidence of cholangitis, decreased risk of occlusion and reintervention, and rapid resolution of jaundice compared with plastic stents.
- SEMS should be placed in patients with a life expectancy of more than 6 months, with malignant disease.
- Placement of a pancreatic stent should be considered in patients at high risk of pancreatitis.
- Placement of multiple stents over a 6–12 month period is effective for management of benign biliary or pancreatic strictures.

Introduction

Endoscopic treatment of biliary stenoses uses plastic stents and self-expanding metal stents (SEMS) which, apart from their miniaturization, are no different in terms of materials or design from stents used in other parts of the digestive tract. Stents are very effective and have come to dominate the palliative treatment of biliary and pancreatic cancers. Pancreatic stents have a slightly different design to bile duct stents with the aim of minimizing trauma to the pancreatic duct. Thus, they are a smaller caliber, more flexible, with an increased number of side holes to facilitate drainage from pancreatic side branches, and have no internal flap to prevent inward migration.

1. Indications

1.1. Biliary stent insertion

- Treatment of benign strictures (PSC, postoperative/transplant)
- Treatment of malignant biliary strictures (ampullary, biliary, pancreatic or metastases) (Fig. 1)
- Treatment for a bile duct leak/perforation/fistula (Figs 2, 3)
- Temporary management to bypass obstructing bile duct stone.

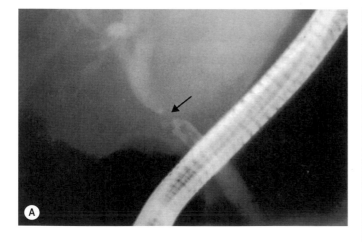

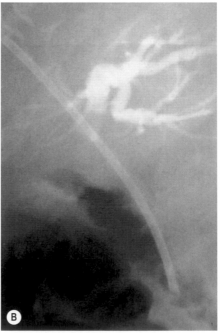

Figure 1 Postoperative stenosis. (A) Postoperative stenosis of the common hepatic duct (arrow). (B) Insertion of a 10 Fr stent to calibrate the stenosis after dilation of the stricture.

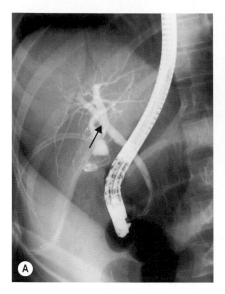

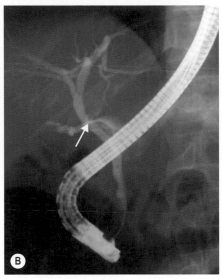

Figure 2 (A) Fistula (arrow) after laparoscopic cholecystectomy treated by external drainage and endoscopic sphincterotomy. (B) Biliary leak due to loosening of the surgical clip on the cystic duct (arrow) after laparoscopic cholecystectomy treated by endoscopic sphincterotomy.

Box 1 Indication for stent placement: ascending cholangitis

- 10% of patients will fail to respond to supportive care and antibiotics and require urgent ERCP.
- In patients with severe cholangitis who are hemodynamically unstable (septic shock, multi-organ failure, coagulopathy), biliary sphincterotomy and stent insertion should be performed providing biliary drainage. Stone removal can be delayed until the patient is more stable.
- In patients who are stable, biliary sphincterotomy and stone removal should be performed at the initial ERCP.

Biliary stent insertion is indicated for patients with inoperable pancreatic cancer. In patients who are surgical candidates, some studies have found that preoperative ERCP increases the risk of cholangitis because of contamination and hence increases postoperative morbidity. However, other studies have shown that in patients with severe jaundice, preoperative drainage reduces operative mortality. ERCP with stent insertion should be performed if there is evidence of cholangitis, whenever the obstructed bile duct has been filled with contrast medium, or if early surgery is not feasible.

1.2. Indications for pancreatic duct stent insertion (Fig. 4)

- Treatment of benign pancreatic duct stricture.
  Stent insertion is indicated in patients with symptomatic stricture (pain), with or without upstream ductal dilation. Technical success rates of 72–100%, with a reduction in pain in 75–94% and long-term relief in 52–74% of patients are reported
- Bypass obstructing pancreatic duct stone
- Pancreatic fistula or ductal disruption

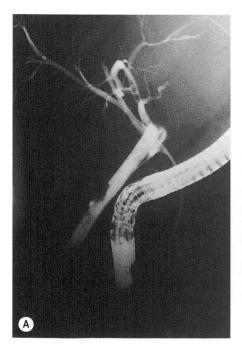

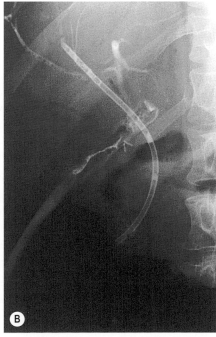

Figure 3 Treatment of a biliary fistula. (A) A drain has been placed and contrast can be seen passing from the biliary tree through the fistula and into the drain. (B) A bile duct stent was inserted.

431

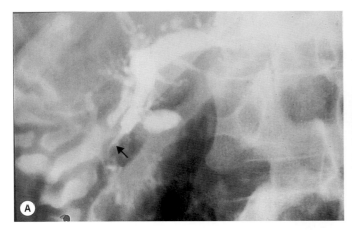

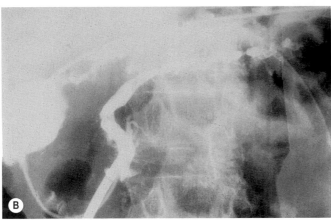

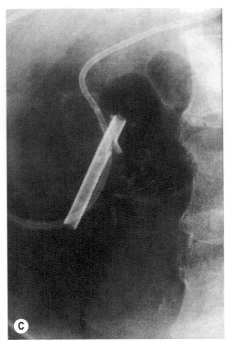

Figure 4 Pancreatic stent insertion for stenosis. This patient had symptomatic stenosis of the main pancreatic duct in the head. (A) Initial pancreatogram. Note the dilated main pancreatic duct in the body and tail with visible side branches consistent with chronic pancreatitis. There is a stricture in main pancreatic duct in the head (arrow). (B) A pancreatic stent and nasopancreatic drain were inserted with resolution of her symptoms. (C) Complete drainage of contrast from the pancreatic duct confirms that the stent and drain are working correctly.

- Pseudocyst drainage
- Serve as a guide for sphincterotomy
- Malignant pancreatic duct obstruction.

  This is a rare indication for pancreatic duct stenting, but has been shown in two studies, with small patient numbers, to reduce pain in patients with malignant obstruction of the pancreatic duct and severe pain
- Prevent procedure-related pancreatitis.

  The published literature on the benefits of prophylactic pancreatic stenting is conflicting. Four randomized controlled trials have shown a significant decrease in the risk of post-ERCP pancreatitis, while two studies have demonstrated no benefit. A meta-analysis concluded that stenting decreased the risk of post-ERCP pancreatitis by two-thirds (15.5% vs 5.8%) in selected patients. Consider placing 2–5 cm long 3 Fr or 5 Fr stent in the following patients:
  - Suspected or documented sphincter of Oddi dysfunction
  - Post-ampullectomy
  - Pancreatic endotherapy/sphincterotomy/ following aggressive instrumentation of the pancreatic duct
  - Balloon dilation of an intact sphincter
  - Difficult biliary cannulation with repeated cannulation of the pancreatic duct
  - Following pre-cut sphincterotomy.

1.3. Indications for the insertion of self-expanding metal biliary stents

1.3.1. Treatment of malignant stenosis

- Pancreatic cancer.

  The role of SEMS vs plastic stent for treatment of pancreatic cancer is discussed below (see Clinical Tips box).
- Cholangiocarcinoma.

  Treating very long stenoses or patients with a life expectancy of only a few days should be avoided. Type I, II, and III hilar invasion (see Fig. 13 for classification of cholangiocarcinoma) may benefit from plastic stents initially, replaced by two metal stents if secondary obstruction occurs and expected survival is acceptable.

1.3.2. Treatment of benign stenosis

Fully covered SEMS have been used to manage benign biliary stenosis; however, the number of studies is small. We currently treat benign strictures with multiple plastic stents, reserving SEMS for refractory strictures.

2. Equipment

2.1. Plastic biliary stents

Plastic stents vary in caliber, length, material and configuration (See Biliary and Pancreatic stents by Somogyi L et al in

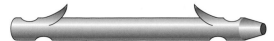

Figure 5 Plastic biliary stent.

the further reading section for detailed description of available stents). Plastic stents come in straight (angled, curved) or pigtail shapes. Pigtail stents are useful when there is a risk of stent migration (i.e. pseudocyst) and can have a single pigtail or one at each end (double pigtail). One of the most commonly placed stents is an Amsterdam-type straight plastic stent (Fig. 5). These are made with holes at the extremity of the stent to facilitate the flow of bile. The distal end is tapered to aid insertion, with a flap at both ends to prevent migration. New stents with novel designs continue to be developed. An example of this is the wing stent, which dispenses with the central lumen in favor of a plastic tube with a ribbed surface in a star shape. This maintains the duct caliber and acts as a wick for flow of juice along its surface, thus avoiding occlusion of side branch openings.

Biliary stents come in a range of diameters from 5 to 12 Fr and in a range in lengths from 1 cm to >15 cm. A 10 Fr (3.3 mm) diameter has been shown to be optimum for stent patency, with no additional benefit in patency using larger diameter stents. Smaller diameter stents can be used for tight strictures which will not permit insertion of a 10 Fr stent, while 3 Fr or 5 Fr stents are usually used in the pancreas. A therapeutic duodenoscope with a 4.2 mm operating channel can insert any diameter stent.

 Clinical Tips

Plastic or metal stent for inoperable cancer?

- Endoscopic stent placement has been shown to improve quality-of-life in patients with malignant biliary obstruction.
- Compared with surgical bypass, patients with endoscopically placed stents have no difference in survival, with more frequent readmissions for stent occlusion, recurrent jaundice and cholangitis but have lower morbidity and procedure-related mortality.
- The decision of which stent to place is based on the patient's life expectancy and cost-effectiveness.
- A plastic stent should be placed in patients with pancreatic adenocarcinoma and liver metastases (average life expectancy of 2.7 months).
- A partially covered SEMS is indicated in patients with distal stricture and an estimated survival of longer than 6 months.
- Uncovered SEMS should be used in patients with a malignant hilar stricture.

2.2. Self-expanding metal biliary stents

SEMS were developed to overcome the problem of early stent occlusion, to which plastic stents are prone. The internal

diameter of self-expanding metal biliary stents, when expanded, is 30 Fr, four times that of plastic stents. They therefore have advantages as regards speed of regression of jaundice, duration of hospitalization and fewer instances of secondary occlusion and repeat ERCP.

The majority of SEMS are made of nitinol, a super elastic nickel-titanium alloy with thermal shape memory. Elgiloy, a cobalt based alloy, is used in some stents. SEMS are available in a variety of designs and sizes with different delivery systems. Membrane coated SEMS, covered with silicone, polyurethane, or Teflon, are available which decreased tumor ingrowth through the metal latticework. Fully covered removable SEMS have also been developed for treatment of benign strictures.

All SEMS systems consist of a stent constrained in a plastic outer sheath over a small-caliber catheter with a tapered tip (Fig. 7). An uncovered SEMS has an outer diameter of between 7 and 8.5 Fr, while a covered stent measures 10 Fr. The stent is compressed onto a catheter and held in place with a sheath. The SEMS is deployed by withdrawing the sheath, allowing the stent to expand. *Some stents shorten by up to 30% while others maintain their length, a characteristic which must be taken into consideration when choosing the length of the stent and during deployment.*

2.3. Equipment for the insertion of stents

- Guidewire with radio-opaque and visual markers on distal end.
  A 0.035 inch guidewire can usually be used to cannulate the bile duct and major or minor papilla, but a range of sizes (0.018–0.025 inch) and types of wires (mixed hydrophilic and pure hydrophilic) should be available.
- Guide and pusher catheters (Figs 6, 7).
  (Guiding catheters are only required for stent ≥10 Fr).
- Stents of various lengths and diameter.

3. Technique

Pre-ERCP imaging is important, and is *essential* in patients with suspected cholangiocarcinoma (see Hilar stenosis below). An MRI provides information about the site and length of the stricture which can facilitate targeted cannulation and stenting, while minimizing the risk of cholangitis.

3.1. Biliary plastic stent insertion technique

- Cannulate the bile duct and obtain a cholangiogram. If a stricture is present, assess the location, type and extent of the stricture.
- A 10 Fr stent is usually inserted unless there is a very tight stricture. In these cases, the stricture should be dilated prior to inserting a stent or a smaller stent inserted. The shortest possible stent should be chosen

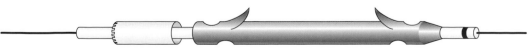

Figure 6 Stent insertion equipment. This figure shows the guidewire, with the white guide catheter (with black marking), the stent (blue) and the pusher catheter.

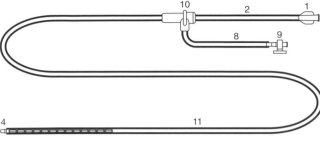

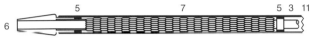

Figure 7 Wallflex metal stent. (1) Stainless steel end of the tube. (2) Stainless steel tube. (3) Stent delivery catheter. (4) Stent delivery catheter tip. (5) Radio-opaque markers. (6) Catheter lumen. (7) Undeployed stent. (8) T-connector. (9) T-connector tap. (10) T-connector connection. (11) Sheath.

that will extend just above the stricture without the end of the stent impacting on the opposing duodenal wall.

- A short sphincterotomy is often performed to facilitate insertion of the stent. However, a sphincterotomy is not essential prior to stent placement and should be avoided if a patient has abnormal coagulation.
- Insert a guidewire into the intrahepatic biliary tree and remove the catheter or sphincterotome over the wire. Avoid inserting excessive wire as this can made stent insertion difficult.
- For 10 Fr stents, a guide catheter is inserted. There are two markers on the distal end of the guide catheter which are 7 cm apart, which are visible both endoscopically and fluoroscopically (Fig. 6). The catheter should be advanced until the distal end is past the stricture and both markers are in the bile duct. Avoid inserting excessive catheter as this can make stent insertion difficult.

Box 2 Covered or uncovered SEMS?

- Successful deployment is identical.
- Studies evaluating the risk of tumor ingrowth in covered versus uncovered SEMS, including randomized controlled trials (see below), have produced mixed results. A recent randomized study of almost 400 patients showed no difference in mortality, stent occlusion or complication rates between covered or uncovered metal biliary stents inserted for malignant biliary strictures.

  Some, but not all, studies have reported increased risk of cholecystitis and pancreatitis with covered stents. One large prospective, randomized trial showed no difference in complication rates between the two groups. There was an increased risk of migration in the covered stent group, but no difference between the groups with respect to pancreatitis or cholecystitis.
- Migration is slightly commoner with covered stents (0–4.5% of cases) compared with 0–1% of cases with non-coated stents.
- Biliary hemorrhage is more frequent with non-covered SEMS than covered SEMS (3.6% versus 0%).
- We use partially covered SEMS in patients with malignant disease.
- Fully covered SEMS can be used in patients with benign strictures which have failed to respond to plastic stenting; however, large clinical experience in these cases is not currently available.

Box 3 How to determine the length of a stricture

There are several different methods for assessing stricture length.
- Place the catheter/sphincterotome above the stricture. Keep your fingers on the same spot on the catheter as you withdraw it. Stop once it reaches the duodenum. The distance between your fingers and the biopsy cap is the length of stent required to reach above the stricture.
- The guide catheter has two markings 7 cm apart which can be used to measure the length of a stricture.
- Therapeutic duodenoscopes measure approximately 12 mm in diameter. The length of the stricture can be estimated using this.

- The stent is inserted into the biopsy channel taking care not to catch the back flap, and advanced with a pusher catheter.
- The endoscope should be kept as close as possible to the papilla to prevent the stent looping in the duodenum. The stent is advanced pushing the stent forward with the pusher catheter, as well as using the elevator and the 'up/down' wheel which is used to assist forward movement of the stent into the biliary tree. This combination of movements is repeated until the stent is in the correct position (Figs 8, 9).
- Check that the stent is in the correct position above the stenosis with fluoroscopy, then withdraw the guidewire, and catheters. Keep constant pressure on the pusher catheter while withdrawing the guide catheter to prevent the stent from moving back into the duodenum.
- Bile should be seen flowing from the stent. A dorsal decubitus image can be obtained to confirm the passage of contrast medium from the bile duct into the second duodenum. Late images should be obtained if there is any doubt that the stent is not working properly.

3.2. Biliary SEMS insertion technique

SEMS insertion is similar to plastic biliary stent insertion.

- Cannulate the bile duct and obtain a cholangiogram. Avoid filling segments that will not be drained. Assess the stricture as described above, and insert a guidewire across it. A stiff guidewire often aids insertion.
- Choose the stent length. Remember that for many SEMS, the initial length of the closed stent shortens by 30% when it is deployed.
- Insert the stent over the guidewire.
- Insertion into the papilla can be difficult. Optimize the angle of the duodenoscope to the bile duct. Use the elevator to help elevation. The duodenoscope position should be altered so that the angle with the bile duct is optimized.
- Most stents have two markers identifying the proximal and distal end of the stent. The stent should be manipulated so that the stricture is in the middle of the stent, with approximately 1 cm of the stent remaining outside the duodenum.

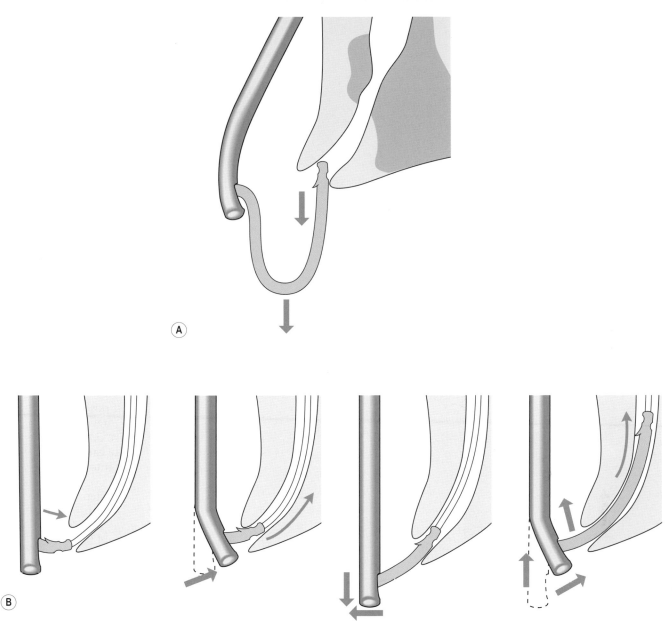

Figure 8 Correct technique for plastic stent insertion. (A) The endoscope should be as close as possible to the papilla to prevent the stent looping in the duodenum, which may cause the procedure to fail. (B) The stent progresses up the bile duct as a result of movements combining upwards deflection, withdrawal of the endoscope and forward pressure on the stent.

- During deployment of the stent, the position of the stent should be monitored both fluoroscopically and endoscopically. The sheath covering the stent is withdrawn gradually holding the tip in one hand without retraction. Constant backwards pressure by the endoscopist is usually required to prevent the stent advancing up the duct. The distal end of the stent opens first (Fig. 10). When the stent is deployed, it shortens from its distal to proximal end. Careful attention must be paid to ensure that the stent remains correctly positioned, watching the distal end under fluoroscopy and the proximal end endoscopically. The stent is deployed when the sheath covering it is fully withdrawn.
- The bile duct can be opacified to check that drainage is occurring correctly and that the stent is working

properly. The stent will achieve its maximum diameter after 1 week (Fig. 11).

3.3. Pancreatic stent insertion technique

3.3.1. Plastic stent insertion

Pancreatic stents are inserted using the same technique described in the biliary stent section through the major papilla or minor papilla.

- Cannulate the pancreatic duct with a sphincterotome and a wire. Obtain a pancreatogram. If a stricture is present, note its location, type and extent.
- A pancreatic sphincterotomy is performed if multiple stent changes are likely (i.e. treatment of a chronic pancreatitis stricture) or for certain pathologies.

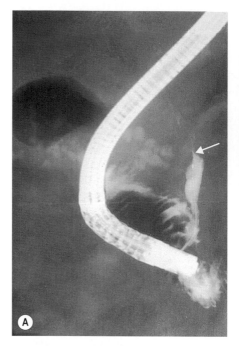

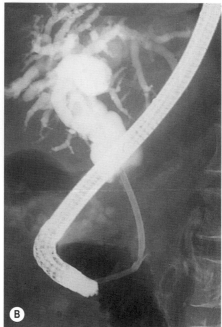

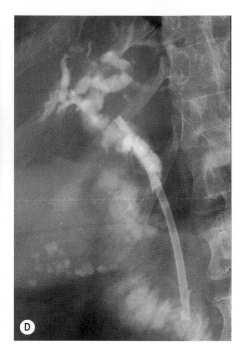

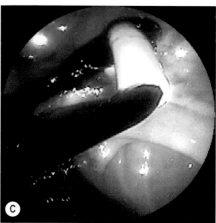

Figure 9 Insertion of a plastic biliary stent. (A) Neoplastic stenosis of the lower common bile duct (arrow). (B) Insertion of the stent across the stricture. (C) Flow of black stasis bile from a plastic biliary stent. (D) Drainage of contrast from the biliary system confirming correct placement of stent across the stricture.

- Gently advance the guidewire. The depth of insertion of the guidewire depends on the length of the stent being inserted. In general, the guidewire is advanced across the neck of the pancreas and into the body. If a stricture is present, the guidewire should be advanced until it is several centimetres beyond the stricture.
- Remove the catheter or sphincterotome over the wire.
- Unlike a bile duct stent, pancreatic stents do not need a guide catheter and are inserted directly over a wire. The stents usually come with a pusher catheter; however, a regular catheter or sphincterotome can also be used.
- Pancreatic stents are smaller and shorter than bile ducts stents and insertion is usually easier. It is therefore important to insert the stent slowly, taking care not to insert the distal end of the stent into the duct. The tip of the endoscope should be kept at a distance to the papilla using the up/down wheel, to allow good visualization of the stent as it is inserted. If necessary, the distal third of the stent can be marked with a black marker before inserting it into the endoscope.

- Check that the stent is in the correct position above the stenosis with fluoroscopy, then withdraw the guidewire and catheter.

✓ Clinical Tips

What size pancreatic stent to insert?

- The stent should be sufficiently long to remain outside the papilla and go a few centimetres past the stenosis. Very short stents are used for stenosis of the papilla.
- Stent length is calculated by pancreatography. The fluoroscopic magnification which increases anatomical distances by a factor of 30% on average should be taken into account.
- Smaller diameter and unflanged stents have been shown in some, but not all studies, to be associated with less ductal changes and are more effective in preventing post ERCP pancreatitis. The diameter of the stent should not exceed the size of a normal downstream duct. We usually use a 5 Fr stent with an external flange if a stent is being inserted for pancreatitis prophylaxis.

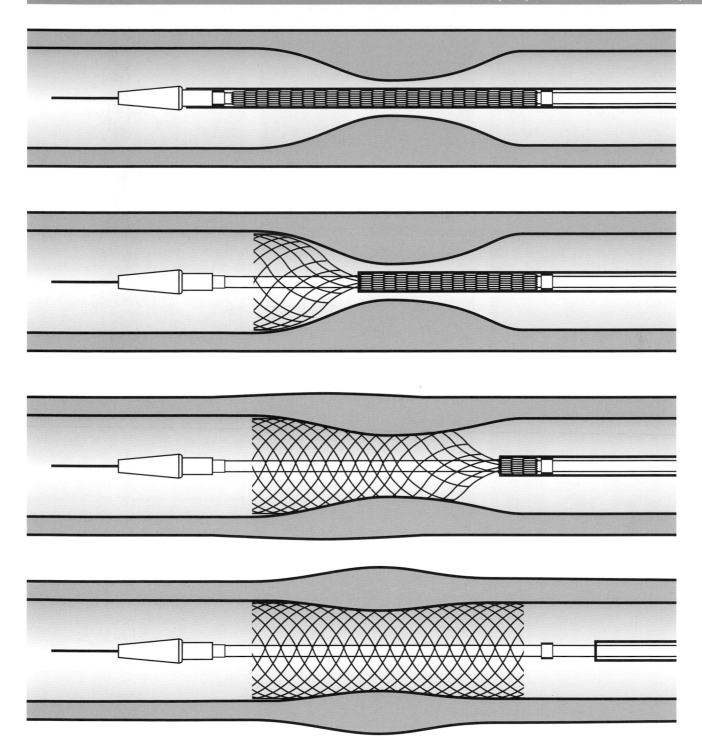

Figure 10 Expansion of a metal stent (uncoated Wallflex). The stent starts to deploy distally. The stent should be deployed under constant endoscopic and fluoroscopic guidance.

3.3.2. Pancreatic stent removal

- Pancreatic stents inserted for pancreatitis prophylaxis should be removed between after 24 h and within 2 weeks.
- Pancreatic stents inserted for treatment of pancreatic stricture are usually changed every 3–6 months, with repeat stenting, with sequential stent insertion should be performed until the stricture has resolved. If the patient has found no improvement in their symptoms surgical options should be considered.

4. Problems with stent insertion

4.1. Problems with plastic stent insertion

Difficulty advancing the stent:

- Ask the endoscopy assistant to keep a steady pressure on the guide catheter. Use intermittent fluoroscopy to ensure that the guide catheter does not move and to aid manipulation of the stent past the stricture (Fig. 12).

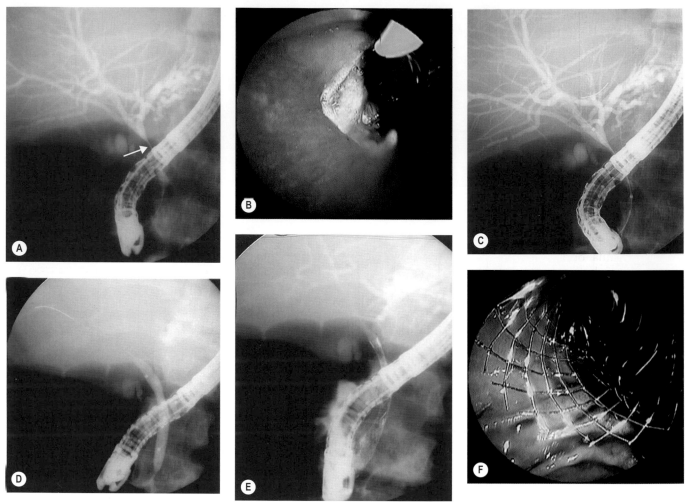

Figure 11 Insertion of a SEM biliary stent. (A) A stenosis is present just below the hilum (arrow) due to breast cancer metastasis. (B) Sphincterotomy with flow of black bile due to stasis is seen. (C,D) Dilation of the stricture with a balloon. (E) Fluoroscopic view of SEMS deployment. (F) Endoscopic view of SEMS with flow of black bile indicating effective drainage.

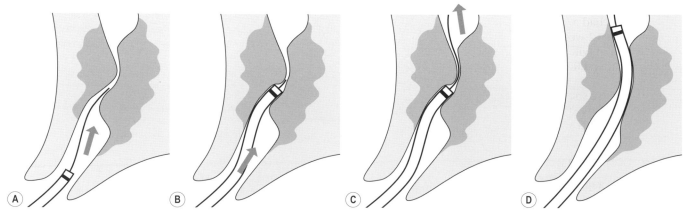

Figure 12 Manipulation of the wire and stent through a stricture with multiple angulations. (A) Insert the wire as far as the stricture. (B) Gently advance the catheter over the wire. (C) Advance the wire through the next section of the stricture. (D) Advance the catheter over the wire and through the stricture.

- Check the amount of wire/guide catheter in the bile duct. If this is excessive, it can make insertion of the stent difficult.
- Keep the duodenoscope close to the papilla. A loop will dissipate the force exerted on the stent.
- Take the locks off the big and small wheels.

In cases where there is an impassable stricture, a rendezvous procedure, where radiology insert a percutaneous wire or stent, may be required (see Ch. 10, Sec. 8.11 for further details).

5. Stent insertion in specific situations

5.1. Bile duct leak

- A bile leak can present with choleperitoneum, external biliary fistula, or obstructive jaundice with or without features of cholangitis.
- ERCP is the gold standard for diagnosing bile duct leak.
- A careful cholangiogram is essential, with early films used to identify stones (present in 20% of patients with bile leaks). A complete intrahepatic cholangiogram must be obtained to exclude a leak from an intrahepatic branch (a balloon may be required if a sphincterotomy has been performed).
- Bile leaks are classified by the Bergman classification:
  - Type A: Leak from the cystic duct, aberrant or peripheral hepatic radicles
  - Type B: Major bile duct leaks with or without concomitant biliary strictures
  - Type C: Bile duct strictures without bile leaks
  - Type D: Complete transaction of the duct with or without excision of some portion of the biliary tree.
- The aim of ERCP is to remove any stones, and eliminate the transpapillary pressure gradient either by a sphincterotomy, stent insertion or both.
- Type A: Sphincterotomy and/or stent insertion is successful in 95% of cases. Bile leak should close within 1 week. Remove stent 6 weeks later unless the patient has had a liver transplant, in which case remove the stent at 12 weeks
- Type B: Stent will need to be inserted and left in place for 3 months. ERCP success rate of between 71% and 79%
- Type C: These should be treated in the same manner as a benign biliary stricture (see below)
- Type D: ERCP is sometimes successful.

5.2. Benign biliary strictures

Endoscopic therapy has very good results for the treatment of benign strictures, with success rates of between 80% and 89% and fewer complications compared with surgical management. Up to 20% of patients will develop recurrent strictures, the majority recurring during the first 6 months follow-up; 18% have stent occlusion requiring early exchange. The results of stenting of distal CBD stricture due to chronic pancreatitis are less impressive due to their fibrotic nature. Early endoscopic stenting is important, with improved results in strictures diagnosed early.

The optimum number of stents and timing of their exchange has not been determined. A reasonable approach is to:

- Perform a sphincterotomy to facilitate stent placement
- Dilate the stricture if required. Remove any sludge or stones
- Insert as many stents as the stricture will allow. This is normally two 10 Fr stents initially, with sequential stents inserted at 2–3 month intervals. Usually a total of 3–5 stents are inserted and left for up to 12 months.

5.3. Benign pancreatic strictures

Successful stenting with decompression of the ductal obstruction in patients with chronic pancreatitis has proved successful in relieving pain in approximately 75% of patients. Multiple sequential stents should be placed in a similar manner to that used for treating benign biliary strictures. If pancreatic duct stones are present, extracorporeal shock-wave lithotripsy (ESWL) should be performed prior to stenting.

5.4. Pancreatic duct fistula

ERCP with stent insertion is indicated for patients with pseudocyst or pancreatic ductal disruption.

5.5. Malignant duodenal infiltration

Duodenal obstruction occurs in 10–20% of patients with pancreaticobiliary malignancies. Surgical bypass is associated with up to 10% procedure-related mortality and prolonged hospital stay. When duodenal and biliary obstruction occur simultaneously, a metal SEMS should be inserted first, followed by a metal enteral stent. This is because access to the bile duct is technically difficult following enteral metal stenting unless the metal stent is placed proximal to the ampulla.

Where it is not possible to pass the duodenal stricture with the duodenoscope, pass a guidewire through the stricture under fluoroscopic guidance. Dilate the stricture, and without withdrawing the TTS balloon, deflate it slightly and use it to guide the endoscope through the stricture. If this fails, a short enteric stent can be placed, with the aim of placing the distal end of the stent proximal to the ampulla. Alternatively, combined percutaneous and endoscopic management (rendezvous procedure) or surgical bypass can be considered.

If a duodenal stent has been placed across the papilla, the bile duct can sometimes be successfully accessed through the wire mesh. There are also reports of using APC to disrupt the wire mesh, allowing access to the bile duct.

5.6. Hilar stenosis

ERCP should not be undertaken in a patient with suspected cholangiocarcinoma until adequate radiographic imaging has been performed. An MRI provides information about resectability, and provides information for the endoscopist about the site and length of the stricture which facilitated targeted cannulation and stenting, minimizing the risk of cholangitis (see Ch. 10.6).

- Several studies have shown that draining one side of the liver is equally effective as draining both sides.

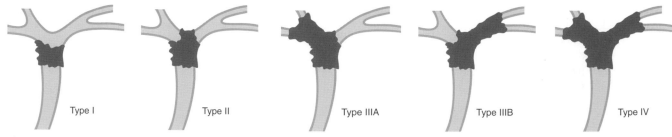

Figure 13 Klatskin classification of hilar tumors. Klatskin I: involvement of the common hepatic duct. Klatskin II: invasion of the bifurcation without involvement of the secondary intrahepatic ducts. Klatskin IIIa: invasion of the bifurcation which extends into the right secondary intrahepatic duct. Klatskin IIIb: extends into the left secondary intrahepatic duct. Klatskin IV: invasion of the bifurcation, and involvement of secondary intrahepatic ducts on both sides.

- Type I, II, and III hilar invasion (Fig. 13) may benefit from plastic stents initially, replaced by two metal stents if secondary obstruction occurs and expected survival is acceptable.
- Any segment which has been accessed must be drained in these patients to avoid cholangitis.
- Insertion of stents into Bismuth Type IV cholangiocarcinomas is very difficult and percutaneous drainage should be considered in these patients.
- Plastic, SEMS or a combination of plastic and SEMS can be used.

Hilar cholangiocarcinoma is classified using the Klatskin classification:

- Type I: involvement of the common hepatic duct
- Type II: invasion of the bifurcation without involvement of the secondary intrahepatic ducts
- Type III:
  - A – invasion of the bifurcation which extends into the right secondary intrahepatic duct
  - B – extends into the left secondary intrahepatic duct
- Type IV: invasion of the bifurcation, and involvement of secondary intrahepatic ducts on both sides.

5.6.1. Technique

The stents are inserted as described above in plastic and SEMS stent insertion.

- Examine the MRI beforehand and use it as a roadmap. Minimize the use of contrast, and use the guidewire to guide you, as any segment which has contrast in it will need to be drained to decrease the risk of cholangitis.

- Aspirate bile before injecting. Contrast should not be injected until a guidewire has been introduced into a dilated duct.

The left hepatic duct is usually the more difficult to cannulate and should be cannulated first.

Bilateral placement of SEMS can be performed a number of ways:

- A short sphincterotomy is often performed to facilitate insertion of the stent. However, a sphincterotomy is not essential prior to stent placement and should be avoided if a patient has abnormal coagulation.
- Insert a guidewire into the intrahepatic duct (Fig. 14). If both sides are to be drained, insert a second wire into the opposite intrahepatic duct. There should now be one wire in the right and one wire in the left hepatic duct.
- For bilateral plastic stent insertion, insert a 10 Fr stent into the duct which was more difficult to access (Fig. 15). After successful placement of the first stent the second stent can be placed.

 Clinical Tips

- Always insert the first stent into the side that was more difficult to cannulate.
- Be careful not to displace the second wire when inserting or deploying the first stent!

5.6.2. Techniques for SEMS insertion

For SEMS, stents can be inserted side-by-side, or one stent can be placed through the other stent.

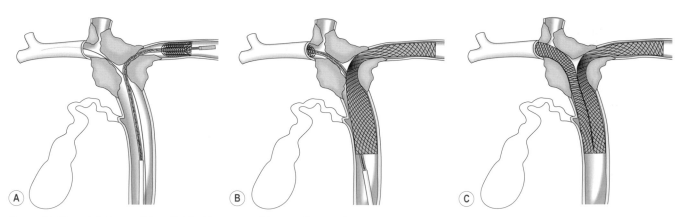

Figure 14 Bilateral drainage of Type IIIa Klatskin tumour with two self-expanding metal stents.

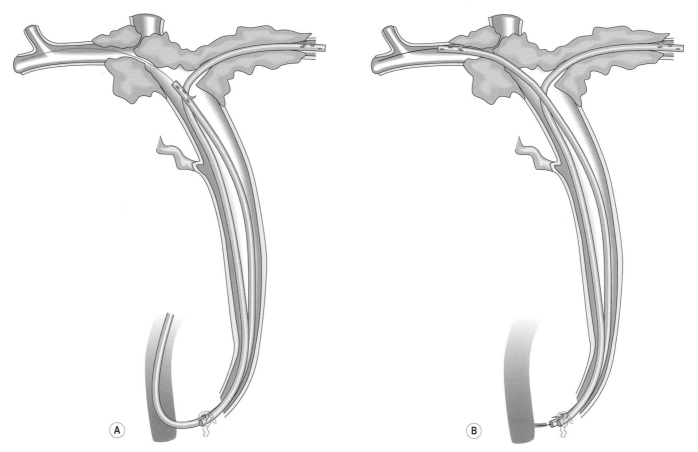

Figure 15 (A) Insertion of two stents to drain both hepatic lobes effectively. Note that the more difficult side to cannulate (left hepatic duct) is stented first (sketch). (B) Plastic stent in the right liver.

Technique 1

- Insert the SEMS into the duct which was more difficult to access and deploy this under fluoroscopic and endoscopic monitoring.
- Insert the second SEMS along the second wire (Fig. 14). It can sometimes be difficult to advance a second SEMS after the first SEMS has been deployed. Some manufacturers (TaeWoong Medical, Kimpo, Korea) have developed SEMS which have wider mesh holes in the middle portion of the stent, facilitating cannulation and stenting through the original stent.

Technique 2

- Insert a plastic stent into whichever intrahepatic duct was most difficult to cannulate.
- Then insert a SEMS into the opposite duct. The plastic stent prevents the first SEMS fully deploying.
- A wire can then be placed alongside the plastic stent and a second SEMS inserted.

Technique 3

One company now produces two 7 Fr SEMS (Cook Medical).

- Insert the first SEMS into the side which was more difficult to cannulate.
- Then insert the second SEMS into the opposite side. The two stents are then deployed one after the other.

6. Outcome of stenting

- 80% of subhilar stenoses and 60% of stenoses at or above the hilum can be successfully stented.
- 95% of biliary and pancreatic neoplastic lesions can be drained using a combination of radiology and endoscopy.
- Failures are due to the usual causes of catheterization problems (diverticulum, Billroth II, etc.), in addition to obstacles created by tumor (duodenal stenosis, failure of sphincterotomy due to neoplastic duodenal invasion, failure of the guidewire to pass through, or failure of the stent to pass through the stenosis).
- The average time to plastic stent occlusion is 3 months (range 1 week to 2 years). The bilirubin level should normalize by 1 month. SEMS have longer patency with an average of 8 months.
- Patients with neoplastic strictures who have persistent cholestasis, despite stenting, have a poor short-term prognosis. Survival is longer in cases where there is a stricture in the lower common bile duct rather than the upper section of the biliary tree. Hilar tumors result in shorter survival, due mainly to the difficulties of performing the technique in this area and to inadequate drainage regardless of the method used.
- PDT can be used to prolong patency in patients with inoperable cholangiocarcinoma (see Ch. 10.16).

Further Reading

Bergman JJ, Burgemeister L, Bruno MJ, et al: Long-term follow-up after biliary stent placement for postoperative bile duct stenosis, *Gastrointest Endosc* 54(2):154–161, 2001.

Fazel A, Quadri A, Catalano MF, et al: Does a pancreatic duct stent prevent post-ERCP pancreatitis? A prospective randomized study, *Gastrointest Endosc* 57(3):291–294, 2003.

Fumex F, Coumaros D, Napoleon B, et al: Similar performance but higher cholecystitis rate with covered biliary stents: results from a prospective multicenter evaluation, *Endoscopy* 38(8):787–792, 2006.

Harewood GC, Pochron NL, Gostout CJ: Prospective, randomized, controlled trial of prophylactic pancreatic stent placement for endoscopic snare excision of the duodenal ampulla, *Gastrointest Endosc* 62(3):367–370, 2005.

Isayama H, Komatsu Y, Tsujino T, et al: A prospective randomised study of 'covered' versus 'uncovered' diamond stents for the management of distal malignant biliary obstruction, *Gut 2004* 53(5):729–734, 2004.

Kahaleh M, Brock A, Conaway M, et al: Covered self-expandable metal stents in pancreatic malignancy regardless of resectability: a new concept validated by a decision analysis, *Endoscopy* 39(4):319–324, 2007.

Singh P, Das A, Isenberg G, et al: Does prophylactic pancreatic stent placement reduce the risk of post-ERCP acute pancreatitis? A meta-analysis of controlled trials, *Gastrointest Endosc* 60(4):544–550, 2004.

Soderlund C, Linder S: Covered metal versus plastic stents for malignant common bile duct stenosis: a prospective, randomized, controlled trial, *Gastrointest Endosc* 63(7):986–995, 2006.

Sofuni A, Maguchi H, Itoi T, et al: Prophylaxis of post-endoscopic retrograde cholangiopancreatography pancreatitis by an endoscopic pancreatic spontaneous dislodgement stent, *Clin Gastroenterol Hepatol* 5(11):1339–1346, 2007.

Somogyi L, Chuttani R, Croffie J, et al: Biliary and pancreatic stents, *Gastrointest Endosc* 63(7): 910–919, 2006.

Tarnasky PR, Palesch YY, Cunningham JT, et al: Pancreatic stenting prevents pancreatitis after biliary sphincterotomy in patients with sphincter of Oddi dysfunction, *Gastroenterology* 115(6):1518–1524, 1998.

Website: http://daveproject.org – This is an excellent resource with multiple videos demonstrating ERCP techniques.

10.14   Biliary and pancreatic balloon dilation

Key Points

- Balloon or Soehendra dilators can be used.
- Efficacy of dilation can be assessed by post-dilation cholangiogram or pancreatogram.
- Dilation is often combined with multiple stent insertion to allow remodeling of benign strictures.

1. Equipment

- Catheter/sphincterotome
- Guidewire (ensure that hydrophilic wires, in various sizes, are available)
- Balloons in a variety of sizes (4–10 mm for bile duct and pancreatic duct) and 10–15 mm for sphincterotomy and lengths (2–6 cm)
- Soehendra dilators in a variety of tip sizes (3 Fr to 11.5 Fr).

 Clinical Tips

Balloon or Soehendra dilator

- The choice of which to use is based mainly on availability and personal experience.
- A Soehendra dilator is useful for proximal stricture at the papilla or in the head of the pancreas, while balloon dilatation is often effective for common bile duct or pancreatic duct strictures.
- Great care must be taken when dilating a sphincterotomy. The choice of which CRE balloon size to use (8–10, 10–12, 12–15) is dependent on the size of the stone, the sphincterotomy and the common bile duct.

2. Technique

2.1. Dilation of a bile duct stricture

- The bile duct is cannulated and a cholangiogram obtained to assess the location, length and features of the stricture.

- A biliary sphincterotomy is often performed to aid insertion of the balloon or dilator.
- A guidewire is advanced across the stricture.
- If a balloon is being used, it is advanced until the center of the balloon is in the middle of the stricture (confirmed with fluoroscopy).
- The balloon is then inflated for 1 min with intermittent fluoroscopy. The 'waist' of the stricture should be seen to disappear.
- If a Soehendra dilator is used, the stricture is assessed in terms of diameter and an appropriate size dilator chosen. The dilator is advanced over the guidewire and through the stricture and then withdrawn.
- Following dilation, a repeat cholangiogram is obtained to assess whether a residual stricture is present.
- A stent is often inserted after dilation to assist with stricture remodeling.

2.2. Dilation of a pancreatic duct stricture

- The technique is very similar to that described for bile duct strictures.
- The pancreatic duct is cannulated and a pancreatogram obtained. The stenosis is assessed in terms of its location and length.
- A pancreatic sphincterotomy is usually performed.
- The guidewire is advanced across the stricture and either a balloon or Soehendra dilator advanced over the guidewire as described previously. Always check the guidewire position prior to inserting the dilator or balloon into the pancreatic duct.
- A post-dilation pancreatogram is obtained.
- A stent is usually inserted after dilation to decrease the risk of pancreatitis and to assist with stricture remodeling.

10.15 Endoscopic ampullectomy

Key Points

- Endoscopic ampullectomy is an alternative to pancreaticoduodenectomy.
- The ampulla should always be carefully inspected to detect small adenomas or adenocarcinomas.
- Ampullary lesions can be polypoid, ulcerated, infiltrating or mixed.
- The majority can be identified endoscopically and diagnosis confirmed with biopsy.
- CT and EUS should be performed to exclude advanced disease.
- Placement of pancreatic duct stent should be considered to decrease the risk of acute pancreatitis.
- Acute complications include acute pancreatitis, retroperitoneal perforation and bleeding.
- 10–25% will have local recurrence.

Introduction

A range of ampullary lesions can occur including villous and tubulovillous adenomas, hemangiomas, leiomyomas, leiomyofibromas, lipomas, neurogenetic tumors, and invasive adenocarcinoma. These tumors can be sporadic or arise in the setting of familial adenomatous polyposis (FAP). They can arise from biliary, pancreatic or duodenal mucosal origin and present with cholestasis, jaundice, dilation of the biliary or pancreatic duct and, in some cases, anemia due to bleeding.

The diagnosis is made by duodenoscopy, which allows visualization of the lesion and biopsies. They are usually easy to diagnose. They often have a polypoid or ulcerated surface and are rarely infiltrating (Fig. 1). Occasionally, these lesions can be more subtle, associated with an abnormal pit pattern or irregular contour. Biopsies should always be taken if the ampulla is abnormal, and are positive in 65% and 90% of polypoid or ulcerative lesions respectively. In practice, a papilla with ulceration always corresponds to cancer, even if endoscopic biopsies are negative. Polypoid lesions are suitable for macrobiopsies using a diathermy loop which give an accurate diagnosis in 90% of cases. Infiltrating cancer is rarer and more difficult to recognize endoscopically, but biopsies obtained with forceps generally allow confirmation of cancer. An endoscopically normal papilla does not rule out diagnosis of a tumor of the ampulla of Vater region, particularly if intrapapillary spread has occurred. In these cases, biliary and pancreatic opacification is required. Findings of a dilated bile duct above an irregular stenosis is indicative of bile duct involvement. Ideally, preoperative histological diagnosis should be made, and if necessary, a sphincterotomy may be made to allow intrapapillary biopsies to be taken. EUS is used to assess the T and N stage and to confirm that there is no invasion of common bile duct or pancreatic duct, while CT is used to exclude distant spread in patients with adenocarcinoma.

⚠ Warning!

Biopsying the ampulla

Biopsies should be taken AWAY from the pancreatic orifice to avoid pancreatitis. A safe place to biopsy is the upper left quadrant.

The standard curative treatment for ampullary tumors has until recently been exclusively surgical with a pancreaticoduodenectomy. This is associated with significant morbidity of 20–40%, with mortality of 2–10%. An alternative is surgical ampullectomy with lymph node sampling. However, morbidity is still significant and recurrence-free and disease-free survival appears to be inferior to pancreaticoduodenectomy. Endoscopic mucosal resection is an alternative for adenomas or microinvasive carcinoma.

1. Indications

1.1. What patients are suitable for ampullectomy?

1.1.1. Endoscopic ampullectomy

- Ampullary adenomas:
  - All patients
- Ampullary adenocarcinoma:
  - Well-differentiated
  - <6 mm tumors
  - No infiltration of the submucosa (T1 has a <4% risk of lymph node metastases)
  - No intraductal involvement beyond the papillary cavity.

1.1.2. Pancreaticoduodenectomy

- Ampullectomy with positive margins
- ≥T2 disease or tumor involving the pancreatic or bile duct.

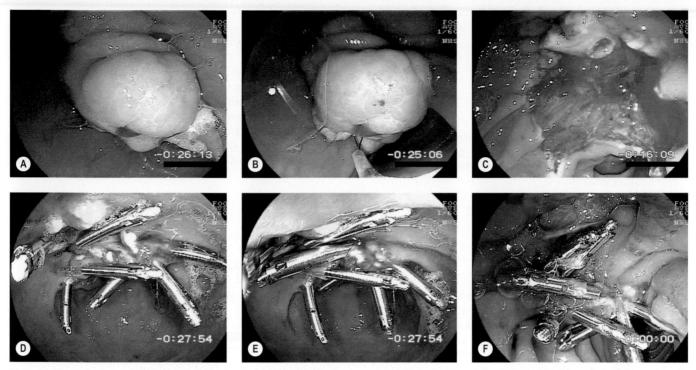

Figure 1 Papillary adenoma. (A) Endoscopic image of a large ampullary adenoma. (B) A snare is placed completely around the adenoma and then resected with snare cautery. (C) The endoscopic appearance of the papilla following ampullectomy. (D) Six Clips. (E) Eight Clips. (F) Control 3 days later.

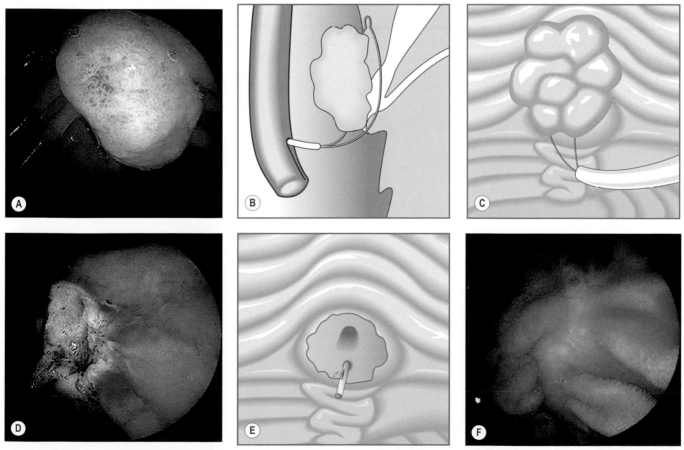

Figure 2 Endoscopic ampullectomy. (A) The papilla is examined. (B,C) A snare is placed over the polypoid lesion. (D) Following polypectomy. (E) A plastic stent is inserted into the pancreatic duct. (F) Follow-up 2 months after papillectomy. Note the clean scar without recurrence with the biliary sphincterotomy orifice in the upper part of the scar.

2. Equipment

- Duodenoscope
- Catheter/sphincterotome
- Guidewire
- Pancreatic stent
- ERBE
- Snare
  - A variety of snares can be used. We use a hexagonal snare as it can be used to remove large adenoma when fully open, or can be used half closed for smaller lesions.
- Roth basket or equivalent
- Clips/adrenaline (epinephrine)/APC.

3. Technique

- The papilla is inspected (Fig. 2A).
- Submucosal injection may be performed beforehand. It demonstrates a line of demarcation allowing the endoscopist more latitude to remove the entire ampulla. The disadvantage is that it can induce edema, which can obscure the pancreatic orifice.
- Ampullectomy without submucosal injection may allow removal of the ampulla along with the sphincter of Oddi allowing easier recognition of the pancreatic orifice following resection.
- A snare is placed over the polyp (Fig. 2B,C). The tumor is then removed, ideally *en bloc*, using pure cutting current (40 W) or endo-cut mode (pure cutting current has a theoretical decreased risk of pancreatitis but increased risk of acute bleeding, endo-cut is associated with decreased risk of acute bleeding). Pure cutting current is used as this may decrease the risk of acute pancreatitis (See Ch. 1.4, Table 1).

- The specimen is then retrieved with a Roth basket or equivalent. Make sure that this is open and ready for use prior to commencing polypectomy.
- The polypectomy site should be inspected (Fig. 2D). Minor bleeding can be treated with injection of epinephrine (adrenaline). More significant bleeding should be treated with clip placement, or coagulation with a Coagrasper.
- The pancreatic duct is then identified and cannulated, and a pancreatic duct stent inserted. (Fig. 2E).

4. Follow-up

- Remove the pancreatic duct stent between 1–7 days post-ERCP
- Repeat endoscopy with a side viewing scope at 2 , 6, 12, 18, 24, and 36 months with or without EUS at 6, 18, and 24 months.

5. Complications

- Acute pancreatitis (6–18% of cases)
- Retroperitoneal perforation (0.9–3%)
- Hemorrhage (12%)
- Cholangitis (3.3%)
- Stenosis of the bile or pancreatic ducts is an uncommon complication. This can be avoided by systematic biliary sphincterotomy
- Recurrence:
  - 10–25% have local recurrence
  - 75% of these can be treated endoscopically
  - A pancreaticoduodenectomy is required in 10% of cases.

10.16   Photodynamic therapy

Key Points

- Photodynamic therapy has been used to treat unresectable cholangiocarcinoma.
- Histologic diagnostic of cholangiocarcinoma is necessary before phototherapy by brushing vigorously (multiple times).
- It induces local tumour necrosis.
- Several studies have shown increased survival times, improvement in quality-of-life and decreased bilirubin levels.

Introduction

> **Box 1** Clinical criteria for the diagnosis of cholangiocarcinoma
>
> The presence of these six clinical criteria have a predictive positive value of 95%:
> - Isolated jaundice
> - Age over 60 years old
> - No biliary tract surgery
> - No gallstones
> - Normal common bile duct
> - Stenosis limited to the hilum.

Cholangiocarcinoma is an intraductal malignancy of the extra or intrabiliary ducts, accounting for 1% of digestive cancers. The diagnosis of cholangiocarcinoma is based on clinical (Box 1) imaging (EUS, MRI, ERCP), as well as cytology obtained at ERCP or EUS. Classic appearances of a cholangiocarcinoma arising in the bile duct are shown in Figure 1. Cholangiocarcinomas arising at the hilum are classified, based on the Klatskin classification (see p440, Fig. 8). All patients should be assessed by a multidisciplinary team to determine resectability (Box 2).

CBD cancers are classified as having complete stenosis (type I), incomplete stenosis (type II) and filling defect (type III) (see Ch. 10.10, Fig. 5).

Recent studies, have examined the role of photofrin photodynamic therapy (PDT) and biliary stent placement in patients with non-resectable hilar cholangiocarcinoma. A study by Harewood et al involving 8 patients, demonstrated an increased median survival time compared with the use of a prosthesis alone (276 days vs 47–127). Ortner (2003) performed a study in 39 patients who were randomized to double plastic stent insertion or double plastic stent insertion plus Photofrin-PDT. The latter group had a significant increase in survival median (493 days vs 98), an increase in the Karnofsky index, quality-of-life and a significant decrease in bilirubin levels. A second randomized trial of biliary stent

> **Box 2** Criteria for unresectability of cholangiocarcinoma
>
> **General criteria**
> - Presence of adjacent organ invasion.
> - Presence of disseminated disease.
> - Presence of retropancreatic or paraceliac metastatic lymph nodes.
> - Presence of distant liver metastases.
> - Presence of invasion of the portal vein or hepatic artery.
>   - Some centers will consider an *en bloc* resection with vascular reconstruction.
>
> **Hilar tumors**
> - Presence of hepatic duct involvement of the second radicals bilaterally.
> - Presence of atrophy of one lobe of the liver with encasement of the contralateral portal vein branch.
> - Presence of atrophy of one liver lobe with contralateral secondary biliary radical involvement.
> - Involvement of bilateral hepatic arteries.
> - Encasement or occlusion of the main portal vein proximal to its bifurcation.

versus biliary stent and PDT in 32 patients, demonstrated that 4 weeks after treatment, most patients in the PDT group had almost complete elimination of bile duct stenosis in the treated area. The PDT group had longer median survival times (21 months) compared with the stent alone group (7 months).

PDT involves injection of an intravenous porphyrin photosensitizer, followed by endoscopic application of light to the tumour bed, inducing local tumoral necrosis.

Potential benefits of PDT (with stent insertion) include:

- Extension of median time survival
- Improve quality of life
- Improve Karnofsky index
- Decreased bilirubin level.

1. Indications

PDT can be considered in a patient with unresectable cholangiocarcinoma.

2. Technique

- Patients received Photofrin intravenously at a dose of 2 mg/kg 48 h before the ERCP.
- ERCP is performed to define the proximal and distal extent of intraductal tumor. It is essential to insert a

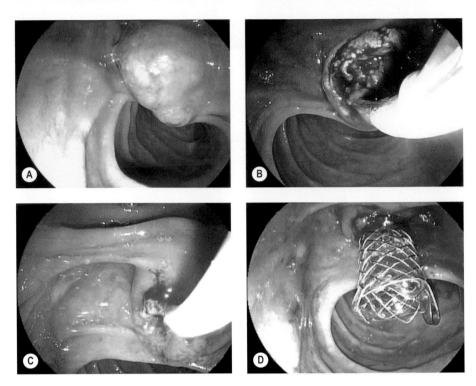

Figure 1 (A) Adenocarcinoma arising within a choledochal cyst. (B) Sphincterotomy was performed with multiple biopsies confirming adenocarcinoma. (C) PDT is performed. (D) A self-expanding metal stent was inserted post-PDT.

stent at the time of PDT. A SEMS can be inserted prior to PDT or a plastic stent and reinserted immediately after PDT. The following technique described PDT after insertion of a SEMS. If a plastic stent or SEMS is present it should be removed before PDT and reinserted immediately after PDT.

- A 6 Fr guiding catheter is inserted. The laser diffuser fiber is advanced through the catheter and positioned at the level of the biliary stricture.
- Radiomarkers on the diffuser tip are used to assist accurate positioning. The catheter should be placed so that there is a 5 mm proximal and distal overlap with normal tissue.
- Laser light is applied at a wavelength of 630 nm with a diode laser.
- The dose applied depends on the site of the cancer:
  - A fluence of 150 J/cm diffuser length is applied with an illumination time of 6 min. If a second illumination is required, the fluence is reduced to 130 J/cm. This dose is associated with 3–10 mm of tissue destruction around the diffuser.
  - At the hilum, laser light is applied at a wavelength of 630 nm with a fluence of 180 J/cm fiber diffuser length and an illumination time of 720 s. If a

second session is required, the fluence is reduced to 130 J/cm fiber diffuser length, and an illumination time of 520 seconds.
- Tumor segments can be treated sequentially, progressing from proximal to distal.

> **⚠ Warning!**
>
> PDT should only be used after the biliary tree has been drained with a stent and any infection (cholangitis) treated. At the hilum, laser light is applied at a wavelength of 630 nm with a fluence of 180 J/cm fiber diffuser length and an illumination time of 720 seconds. If a second illumination is required, the dose is reduced to 130 J/cm fiber diffuser length and an illumination time of 520 seconds.

3. Complications

- Cholangitis
- Cholecystitis
- Stenosis
- Skin photosensitization.

Further Reading

Harewood GC, Baron TH, Rumalla A, et al: Pilot study to assess patient outcomes following endoscopic application of photodynamic therapy for advanced cholangiocarcinoma, *J Gastroenterol* 20:415–420, 2005.

Kahaleh M, Mishra R, Shami VM, et al: Unresectable cholangiocarcinoma: comparison of survival in biliary stenting alone versus stenting with photodynamic therapy, *Clin Gastroenterol Hepatol* 6(3):290–297, 2008.

Ortner ME, Caca K, Berr F, et al: Successful photodynamic therapy for nonresectable cholangiocarcinoma: a randomized prospective study, *Gastroenterology* 125:1355–1363, 2003.

Zoepf T, Jakobs R, Arnold JC, et al: Palliation of nonresectable bile duct cancer: improved survival after photodynamic therapy, *Am J Gastroenterol* 100:2426–2430, 2005.

10.17 **Cholangioscopy**

Key Points

- It can be performed via percutaneous or per-oral route.
- It is time consuming and may require two endoscopists depending on the technique used.
- Cholangioscopy and pancreatoscopy can be performed.
- It is useful for stones which are refractory to routine treatment.
- It is also useful for direct visualization of stricture, particularly if cancer is suspected.
- Cholangioscopes are fragile and great care is needed to avoid damaging them.

Introduction

Cholangioscopy can be performed by the per-oral transpapillary or percutaneous transhepatic route. It allows direct visual assessment of the biliary tree, tissue sampling, and therapeutic interventions.

Percutaneous cholangioscopy (Fig. 1) is performed through a previously created stable cutaneobiliary fistula that has been sequentially dilated to 14–18 Fr. It requires an endoscopist and two assistants. Percutaneous cholangioscopes are used which are shorter and wider than per-oral cholangioscopes (external diameter 4.1–4.9 mm) and have biopsy channels of between 1.7 and 2.2 mm in diameter.

Per-oral cholangioscopy and pancreatoscopy can be performed using a 'mother–baby' system (Fig. 2). This requires two experienced endoscopists. The cholangioscope has an outer diameter of 2–3.5 mm and a biopsy channel, which allows insertion of biopsy forceps or lithotripsy probes. The cholangioscope is introduced into the bile duct using a standard duodenoscope with a (4, 2 mm) operating channel.

Per-oral cholangioscopy can also be performed with an axial endoscope in patients with a sufficiently wide choledochoduodenal anastomosis (Fig. 3) or following an endoscopic sphincterotomy in a patient with a Billroth II gastrectomy. Recent developments include the introduction of a videocholangioscope with narrow-band imaging, ultraslim scopes (external diameter 2.09 mm) which can be inserted without a prior sphincterotomy, and can be performed with only one operator. Ultrathin pancreatoscopes have also been developed with external diameters of between 0.5 and 0.8 mm.

'Spyglass' is a relatively new system, which has the advantage of requiring only one operator to perform cholangioscopy. It can be performed either percutaneously or per-oral.

It has four-way directional steering, and therapeutic procedures, including optically directed biopsies, EHL and laser lithotripsy, can be performed through the accessory channel. Similar to cholangioscopes, spyglass is fragile, but it is reusable and can be reused approximately 12 times if treated with care. Its image is generated by a 6000 pixel fiberoptic probe, whose image quality is inferior to that obtained with modern cholangioscopes. Spyglass is still in its infancy, and its exact role has yet to be determined.

1. Indications

- Lithotripsy
  - Although lithotripsy can be performed under fluoroscopic control using an inflatable balloon to center the probe within the lumen, direct visualization of the target intuitively enhances the success of stone fragmentation and minimizes complication, particularly if the duct is tortuous or angulated.
  - Treatment of CBD or pancreatic duct stones.
  - Treatment of Mirizzi syndrome (particularly Type II; see Ch. 10.12).
  - Treatment of intrahepatic bile duct stones.
- Laser photocoagulation of bile duct tumours
  - Photocoagulation may be used curatively to destroy an adenoma or palliatively to reduce the tumour mass of an unresectable cholangiocarcinoma. Reduction in tumour mass may facilitate biliary drainage. This technique may be useful after failure to pass through the stenosis radiologically after failure by the transpapillary route. An Nd: YAG laser is used.
  - A follow-up examination to determine whether adenomas have been destroyed should be carried out a few months later.
- Assessment and biopsy of indeterminate biliary or pancreatic strictures (Fig. 4). One study found that per-oral cholangioscopy was significantly superior to ERCP in diagnosing malignancy in PSC patients with dominant stenoses.
- Assessment of indeterminate filling defects.
- To guide cannulation of a stricture where ERCP has failed.
- To facilitate placement of gallbladder stents.
- Preoperative assessment to document the proximal and distal spread of cholangiocarcinomas of the hilum.
- To assess main duct IPMN.

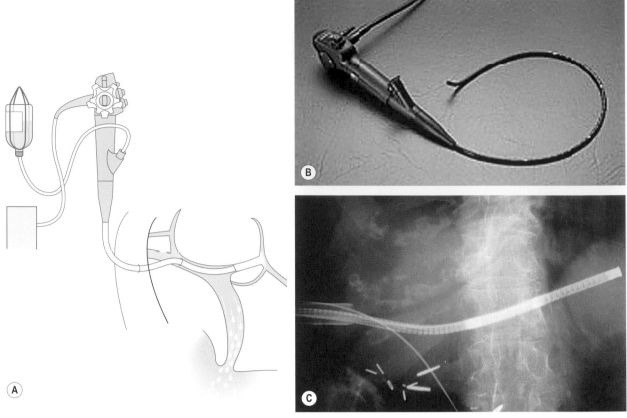

Figure 1 Percutaneous cholangioscopy of the left hepatic duct. (A) Demonstrates insertion of the cholangioscope through the cutaneobiliary fistula, with saline, from irrigation, passing into the duodenum. (B) Fujinon videoendoscope. (C) Percutaneous insertion of the endoscope through the skin into the left hepatic ductal system.

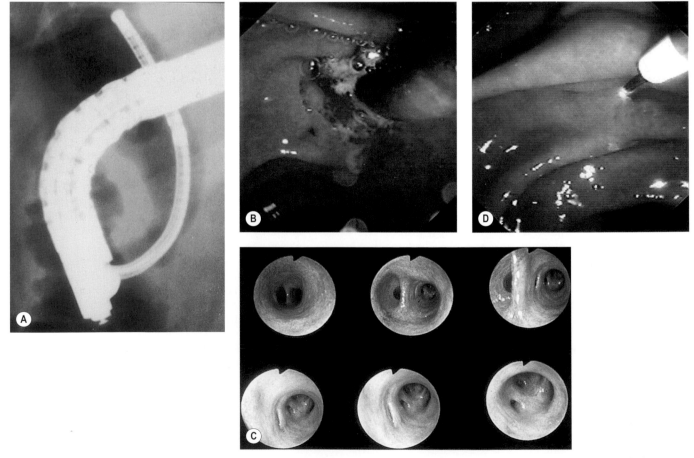

Figure 2 Olympus per-oral cholangioscopy fiberscope. (A) A fine endoscope is mounted in the bile duct by means of a duodenoscope with standard duodenoscope with a 3.2 mm operating channel. (B) A cholangioscope is inserted into the bile duct after a biliary sphincterotomy has been performed. (C) Close up of the small optical fiber mounted in a catheter prior to insertion through an intact papilla. (C) Endoscopic appearance of the intrahepatic bile ducts with cholangioscope. (D) Close up of the small optical fiber mounted in a catheter prior to insertion through an intact papilla, the ancestor of the spyglass in 1989.

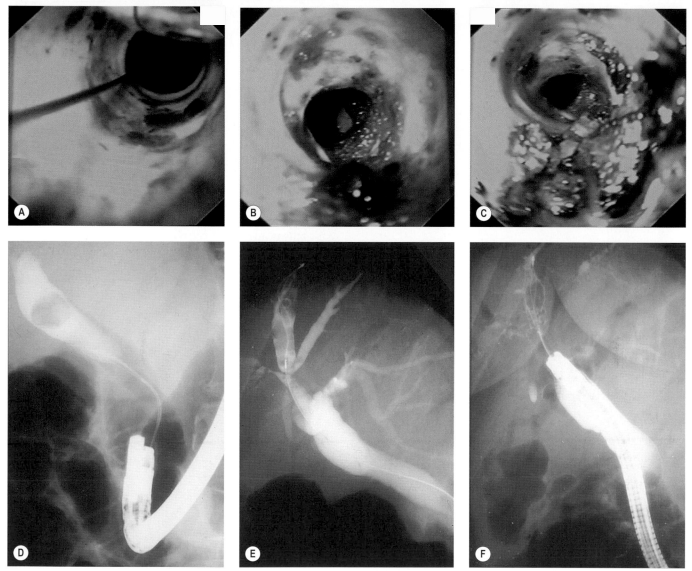

Figure 3 Extraction of intrahepatic stones with cholangioscopy in a patient with a gastrojejunal anastomosis (Billroth II). (A) Dilation of stenosis under visual control (the endoscope against the balloon reveals the stenosis). (B,C) The stenosis after dilation. (A) Extraction of intrahepatic stones by cholangioscopy after dilation of bile duct stenosis. (D) Extraction of a stone from the common bile duct below the stenosis. (E) Stones above a stenosis of the intrahepatic bile duct draining segment VIII. (F) Clear intrahepatic bile duct (an endoscope with axial vision has been inserted into the bile duct via the sphincterotomy orifice).

2. Equipment

2.1. General equipment

- Endoscope:
  - Percutaneous cholangioscopes
  - Per-oral cholangioscope
  - Per-oral pancreatoscope
  - Spyscope
- Guidewire
- Sterile balloon and Dormia catheters
- Biopsy forceps or 'SpyBite' biopsy forceps
- EHL or laser lithotripsy. The equipment should be ready and primed for firing before the examination
- A three-way tap which is fitted in the operating channel to allow for constant lavage and the introduction of instruments

- Irrigation pump and footswitch. A constant irrigation system is prepared, comprising a 3 L bag of physiological saline and an irrigation pump.

2.2. Percutaneous cholangioscopy

- A sterile fenestrated drape
- Two straight Amplatz guides
- Catheter
- Dilators of different diameters
- A flexible 18 Fr sheath
- Wells (sterile water, Telebrix and alcohol with iodine) and syringes, compresses, forceps, scalpel blades, suture thread, etc.
- Sterile gown, gloves.

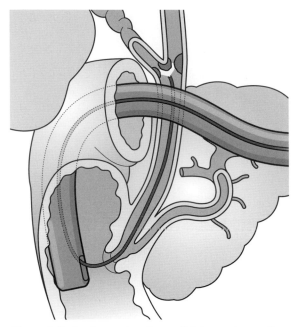

Figure 4 Cholangioscopy in strictures. This image shows a Spyscope inserted to the level of a stricture. Cholangioscopy with either a mother and baby scope or Spyscope is useful for the assessment of strictures. It allows direct visualization, tissue sampling and can also be used to guide selective cannulation. (Redrawn with permission from Boston Scientific Corporation.)

2.3. Spyglass system

- Optic probe.
  The optic probe contains a 6000 pixel fiberoptic bundle surrounded by light fibers. It has a 70° field of view.
- Delivery catheter.
  The delivery catheter has several functions. It protects the optic probe, and can also be used to direct the probe, as the tip of the catheter can be steered in four directions. It has four channels (Fig. 5); 1.0 mm channel for the fiberoptic probe, a second 1.2 mm accessory channel, and two further channels for irrigation. The delivery catheters are single use only.
- Spyglass camera
- Spyglass ocular.
  This is an optical coupler that interfaces with the Spyglass probe and video camera head
- Lightsource.
  300 W high intensity white light
- Isolation transformer
- Irrigation pump and footswitch.

2.4. Spyglass accessories

- 'SpyBite' biopsy forceps. SpyBite (Fig. 6) is a single use biopsy forceps designed specifically to be used with the Spyscope. It is inserted through the accessory channel

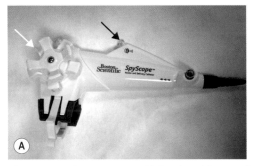
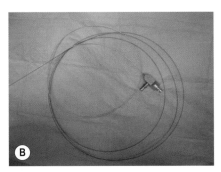
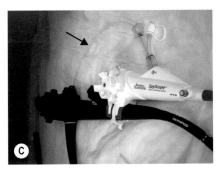

Figure 5 Spyglass equipment. (A) Spyglass delivery catheter. A guidewire or SpyBite can be inserted (black arrow), while the tip of the catheter can be moved in four directions (white arrow). (B) The Spyglass catheter (yellow) through which the optic probe has been placed. (C) The spyglass delivery catheter attached to the duodenoscope, with the delivery catheter and optic probe (arrow) inserted.

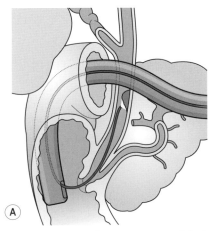
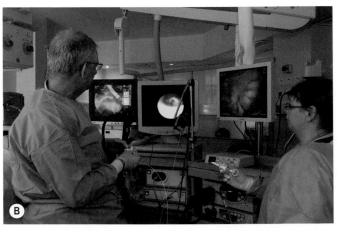

Figure 6 (A) Biopsy forceps in common bile duct used with Spyglass (SpyBite) (Redrawn with permission from Boston Scientific Corporation). (B) Pancreaticoscopy in pancreatic stricture with stone. Biopsy forceps (SpyBite) to do tissue sampling of the stricture before dilatation and extraction the pancreatic stone.

in the delivery catheter and allows targeted biopsies to be taken from within the pancreaticobiliary tree. It requires a minimum working channel of 1.2 mm. It is 286 cm in length with a jaw diameter of 1 mm closed and 4 mm open.

- EHL and laser lithotripsy. Spyglass is compatible with Northgate 1.9 Fr biliary probe and EHL generator, as well as with Lumenis slimline 365 μm laser probe and Lumenis VersaPulse Power Suite 20 W Holmium Laser Generator.
- A short wire system cannot be used with Spyglass. A 450 cm guidewire is required.

3. Technique

3.1. General

- The fluoroscopy table should be protected from moisture (the examination requires constant irrigation)
- The patient is positioned in the dorsal decubitus position for per-oral cholangioscopy
- Antibiotic prophylaxis is usually given for percutaneous cholangioscopy.

3.2. Percutaneous cholangioscopy

- This requires an interventional radiologist and endoscopist.
- The procedure is performed under sterile conditions.
- The patient is positioned in dorsal decubitus, leaning slightly to one side:
    ■ To access the left bile ducts, the head rests on the left part of the table. The patient is leaning slightly to the left (Fig. 1). The left bile ducts are accessed from the right bile ducts.

    ■ To access the right bile ducts, the head rests on the right part of the table. The patient is leaning to the right. The right bile ducts are accessed from the left bile ducts (Fig. 7).
- A percutaneous transhepatic drain is inserted under fluoroscopic control. The radiologist inserts drains with a diameter of approximately 10 Fr. 3 to 4 days later the transhepatic channel is dilated. A guidewire is inserted into the hepatic segment to be examined. A second safety guidewire is left in the duodenum through the papilla, which is then fixed to the drapes. The drain is removed. Dilators of increasing sizes are slid onto the guidewire until a channel of sufficient diameter to admit a flexible 18 Fr sheath is obtained.
- The cholangioscope is inserted through the sheath. Constant irrigation is used to distend the hepatic ducts and allow visualisation of the bile ducts.
- On completion of the procedure a biliary drain is reinserted to prevent the fistulous tract from closing.

3.3. Per-oral cholangioscopy

- An endoscopic sphincterotomy is usually required.
- The bile duct is cannulated and a guidewire inserted.
- The cholangioscope is inserted through the operating channel of the duodenoscope.
- The cholangioscope is guided into the bile duct over the wire using a combination of manipulation of the duodenoscope and tip angulation of the cholangioscope. It is important to avoid aggressive use of the elevator as this can damage the cholangioscope.

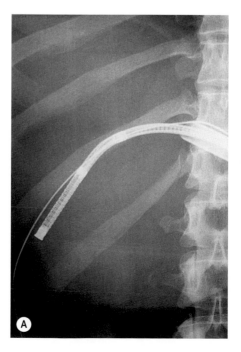
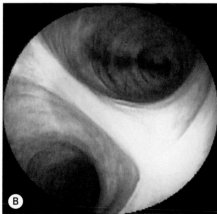
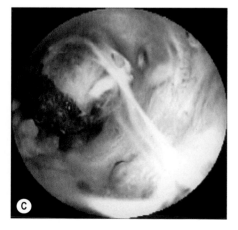

Figure 7 Percutaneous cholangioscopy. (A) Percutaneous cholangioscope inserted into the right intrahepatic bile duct. (B) Cholangioscopic images of normal intrahepatic bile ducts. (C) Stone within the intrahepatic bile ducts.

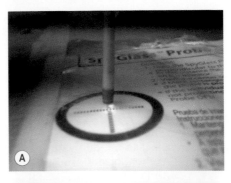

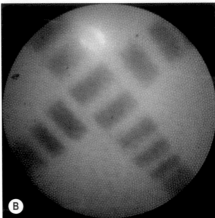

Figure 8 Spyglass – Focusing. The Spyprobe is focused by placing it approximately 1 cm above an X marked on a sheet (A). Initially focus using the ring on the ocular. The ideal focus gives a slightly grainy image (B).

- The bile duct is lavaged with normal saline via a three way tap on the instrument channel. It is important to ensure adequate drainage of the saline from the biliary tree following removal of the cholangioscope to avoid cholangitis.

A working channel of 1.2 mm is required for biopsies or lithotripsy.

3.4. Spyglass

3.4.1. Focus

- Always focus and white balance before starting the procedure.
- Focus it with the Spyprobe approximately 1 cm above an X marked on a sheet. Initially focus using the ring on the ocular. The ideal focus is where it is slightly grainy (Fig. 8).
- Usually, if this is done correctly it does not need to be refocused in the duct. Occasionally, it will need fine tuning using the ring on the ocular.

3.4.2. Technique

- Set up and test the Spyglass before commencing.
  - Focus the optical probe.
  - Insert the probe to the distal end of delivery catheter, then withdraw it 2 cm. This ensures that the probe is not damaged if the elevator is used to assist entry into the bile duct.

> **Box 1** Problem shooting with Spyglass

Blurred
- 'Speck of black'
  - Wipe the tip of the spyprobe with alcohol or a dry 4 × 4.
  - Wipe the end of the spyprobe, which plugs into the ocular, with alcohol or a dry 4 × 4.
  - Take a Q-tip and wipe down the end of the ocular where the spyprobe connects to the ocular.

Poor visualization
- Excessive contrast can give a 'fuzzy' view. Try to avoid excessive contrast and if this occurs, use water irrigation to dilute the contrast.
- Is the optical probe outside the delivery catheter? If it is blue, it is still within the delivery catheter. Gently push the optical probe forward until it is just outside the delivery catheter with a rim of blue on the outside.
- The optical probe is outside the delivery catheter but visualization is poor. Withdraw the optical probe until it is just inside the delivery catheter and then push it forward a fraction until a rim of blue is still just visible. The optimum position is to have it just outside the blue protective tubing, where you can still see the blue rim on the outside of the image.
- Still cannot see?
  - Use gentle, controlled left arm movements to reposition the optical probe within the duct
  - Flush with water
  - Check the position of the probe within the Spyscope
  - Check that the optical probe is properly focused.

Cannot advance accessory instruments?
- Pull the Spyglass fiber approximately 2 cm back into the delivery catheter.
- Withdraw the delivery catheter toward the duodenum without removing it from the bile duct. It is often possible to advance the biopsy forceps or other instruments once this maneuver has been performed.
- If this fails, check the position of the duodenoscope and try to minimize the angle at the tip by either inserting or withdrawing the duodenoscope slightly.
- Keep the forceps closed gently. If they are tightly held, it makes the tip very rigid. Occasionally opening and closing the forceps within the Spyscope is sufficient to allow them to advance.

- Cannulate the common bile duct and obtain a cholangiogram.
- Although a sphincterotomy is not absolutely necessary, it facilitates cannulation of the bile duct with the delivery catheter. Insert a guidewire.
- Insert the delivery catheter with optical probe (Fig. 5). Ensure the elevator is down to avoid damaging the optical probe. Try to cannulate the bile duct using none or minimal elevator.
- Insert the delivery catheter to the area of interest. Then gently push the optical probe forward until the probe is just outside the blue delivery catheter. In the ideal position, the blue delivery catheter can still just be seen.
- The water jet should be used to aid visualization of the bile duct. Avoid using excessive amounts of water, especially if there is a stricture distal to where the spyglass has been inserted.

- The optical probe can be maneuvered through rotation of duodenoscope, while small adjustments are made using the four-way directional wheels.
- Withdraw the delivery catheter until the area of interest is identified.
- To reinsert the Spyglass, withdraw the optical probe inside the delivery catheter and reinsert the delivery catheter.
- Biopsies:
  - Check that the forceps are closed and then insert the Spybite forceps into the device port of the Spyscope catheter. If a guidewire is not being used, the Spybite forceps can be preloaded into the delivery catheter before commencing the procedure.
  - Ensure that the elevator is down as the forceps are advanced.

4. Complications

Complications include:

- Cholangitis (1%).
  Prophylactic antibiotics are required with percutaneous cholangioscopy. Some endoscopists also use them with per-oral cholangioscopy.
- Pancreatitis.
  This can be associated with sphincterotomy. If pancreatoscopy is being performed, care should be taken to avoid infusing excessive amounts of saline during lavage.
- Trauma to the bile duct with ulceration is usually associated with lithotripsy.
- Bile duct perforation (rare).

Further Reading

Chathadi KV, Chen YK: New kid on the block: development of a partially disposable system for cholangioscopy, *Gastrointest Endosc Clin N Am* 19(4):545–555, 2009.

Iqbal S, Stevens PD: Cholangiopancreatoscopy for targeted biopsies of the bile and pancreatic ducts, *Gastrointest Endosc Clin N Am* 19(4):567–577, 2009.

Itoi T, Neuhaus H, Chen YK: Diagnostic value of image-enhanced video cholangiopancreatoscopy, *Gastrointest Endosc Clin N Am* 19(4):557–566, 2009.

Petersen BT: Cholangioscopy for special applications: primary sclerosing cholangitis, liver transplant, and selective duct access, *Gastrointest Endosc Clin N Am* 19(4):579–586, 2009.

Website: http://daveproject.org This is an excellent site, which provides videos featuring different techniques used in cholangioscopy.

Summary

Key Points

- Sphincter of Oddi (SOD) is a benign, non-calculous obstruction to the flow of bile or pancreatic juice through the papilla.
- Patients are classified as SOD Type I, II or III.
- SOD is associated with abdominal pain post-cholecystectomy, elevated LFTs associated with pain which resolve, dilated bile or pancreatic duct and acute recurrent pancreatitis.
- Patients are at increased risk of acute pancreatitis and pancreatic stent insertion should be considered.

Introduction

Sphincter of Oddi dysfunction (SOD) is a benign, non-calculous obstruction to the flow of bile or pancreatic juice through the pancreaticobiliary junction (i.e. the sphincter of Oddi). SOD can be due to either abnormal contraction of the sphincter, most commonly a hypertonic sphincter or due to stenosis of the sphincter, which can occur after inflammation. As it is impossible to differentiate a hypertonic sphincter from stenosis, SOD is used to incorporate both groups.

Patients with SOD are classified as biliary type I, II or III based on the presence or absence of abnormal LFTS and CBD dilatation (Table 1). A pancreatic classification (Table 2) has also been developed but is less commonly used. Delayed biliary drainage was used in the original SOD classification; however, it has been removed from the modified classification, as it is rarely performed and is found in 60% of patients without SOD.

SOD classically presents as paroxysmal epigastric or right upper quadrant pain radiating to the back or scapulae, associated with elevated liver function tests, in patients in whom all other causes have been excluded. Both the pain and the liver function tests resolve completely between episodes. The pain may occur several years after a cholecystectomy was performed and should be the same character to the pain leading to the cholecystectomy. Alternatively, patients may have continued pain that was not relieved by the cholecystectomy. The Rome III criteria (Box 1) are used to diagnose SOD. All the criteria are required, with patients subdivided into functional gallbladder, functional SOD or functional pancreatic SOD disorder, depending on whether they have a gallbladder or abnormal amylase, lipase or liver function tests.

Alternatives methods of diagnosing SOD have been developed. These include provocation test with cholecystokinin (bile duct diameter increases by ≥2 mm), secretin (increase in pancreatic duct diameter by ≥1.5 mm), and hepatobiliary scintigraphy.

1. Indications

- Patients in whom ERCP with SOD manometry should be considered are those who:
  - Fulfill Rome III criteria.
  - SOD Type II.
  - Patients with Type I should have sphincterotomy without manometry. International societies do not currently recommend SOM in patients with Type III SOD outside of a clinical trial.
- Pancreatic SOM should be performed in patients fulfilling the Rome III criteria, in whom there is unexplained recurrent acute pancreatitis, after ruling out biliary microlithiasis.

Box 1 Rome III criteria for the diagnosis of SOD

Patients must have epigastric and/or right upper quadrant pain and ALL of the following:
- Symptoms recur at different intervals (not daily)
- The pain is not relieved by bowel movements, postural change or antacids
- The pain builds up to a steady level
- The pain is moderate to severe enough to interrupt the patient's daily activities
- Episodes last 30 min or longer
- Other structural diseases have been excluded.

Functional gallbladder

- Above symptoms plus normal LFTs[a], bilirubin, amylase, lipase and gallbladder.

Functional bile duct

- Above plus normal amylase and lipase in patients with cholecystectomy.

Functional pancreatic duct

- Above plus elevated amylase or lipase.

[a]LFTs, liver function tests.

Table 1 Modified Hogan–Geenen classification of biliary SOD (also known as the Milwaukee classification)

Group	Findings	Comment
Biliary Type I	Typical biliary pain and history of cholecystectomy	Biliary sphincterotomy can be performed without the need for SOM. 90–95% symptomatic improvement with biliary sphincterotomy.
	>LFTs[a] with pain on at least two occasions followed by normalization of LFTs	
	CBD >12 mm[b]	
Biliary Type II	Typical biliary pain and history of cholecystectomy	SOM strongly recommended. Patients with abnormal manometry have 85% chance of improvement with biliary sphincterotomy. Patients with normal manometry have a 30% chance of improvement in their symptoms.
	Plus one of the following:	
	>LFTs with pain on at least two occasions followed by normalization of LFTs	
	Dilated CBD >12 mm	
Biliary Type III	Typical biliary pain and history of cholecystectomy	SOD is rare. 30–40% improvement if SOM is positive. <10% if SOM negative.
	No other abnormalities	

SOM, sphincter of Oddi manometry.
[a]Twice upper level of normal of SGOT and alkaline phosphatase.
[b]12 mm is taken as the upper limit of normal *post-cholecystectomy*.

Sphincter of Oddi manometry is technically difficult and is associated with significant side-effects and should only be performed in tertiary referral centres with pancreaticobiliary experience. Anticholinergics, cholinergics, nitrates, calcium channel blockers and narcotics should be discontinued at least 12 h pre-ERCP as these affect sphincter pressures. It is important to consider sedation issues prior to commencing manometry. Many patients are on large doses of narcotics and are difficult to sedate. Benzodiazepines and propofol can be used as these do not affect sphincter pressures. Pethidine (meperidine) affects phasic wave contractions but not the basal sphincter pressures but can be used as the diagnosis of SOD is made on the basal sphincter pressures. Glucagon should be avoided during manometry.

2. Technique

A perfusion catheter consists of three separate ports 2 mm from each other. The catheter is attached to a pump which perfuses the catheter 0.25 mL of water per min. As the catheter is pulled through the sphincter, a continuous reading is generated of any pressure changes. A solid-state pressure transducer has been developed; however, most units continue to use the water perfused catheter. Both biliary and pancreatic manometry should be performed as manometry can be normal in one duct but abnormal in the other. There are several types of catheters available including wire-guided.

Table 2 Hogan-Geenen classification of pancreatic SOD

Group	Findings	Comment
Pancreatic Type I	Unexplained recurrent acute pancreatitis	Consider pancreatic sphincterotomy. No need for SOM[b].
	>Amylase or lipase[a] on at least two occasions	
	Homogeneous dilation of the main and secondary pancreatic ducts	
	Delayed drainage of contrast from the pancreatic duct >9 min	
Pancreatic Type II	Unexplained recurrent acute pancreatitis	Perform SOM.
	Plus at least one of the following:	
	>Amylase or lipase[a] on at least two occasions	
	Homogeneous dilation of the main and secondary pancreatic ducts	
	Delayed drainage of contrast from the pancreatic duct >9 min	
Pancreatic Type III	Pancreatic type pain	Do not perform SOM unless within a clinical trial.
	No other abnormalities	

SOM, sphincter of Oddi manometry.
[a]Amylase or lipase 1.5× times the upper limit of normal.
[b]>6 mm diameter in the head; >5 mm diameter in the body.

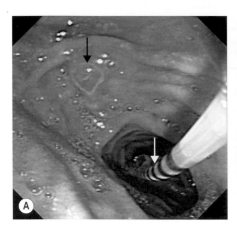
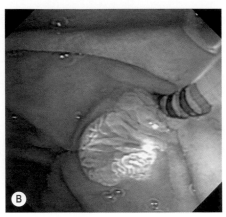

Figure 1 (A) The manometry catheter is zeroed in the duodenum. Note the position of the catheter in the middle of the lumen and not touching the mucosa (white arrow). The ampulla is marked with a black arrow. (B) The bile duct is cannulated with the manometry catheter.

2.1. Biliary sphincter of Oddi manometry

- Check that the manometry equipment is set up and working. The catheter should be perfused at 0.25 mL/min using distilled water through a low-compliance pump.
- A separate intraduodenal catheter is attached to the end of the duodenoscope. This provides a continuous reading of the intraduodenal pressure. If not using a separate intraduodenal catheter, zero the catheter in the duodenum before the pull through.
- Patients must be placed completely supine or prone to allow accurate pressure measurement.
- Insert the duodenoscope into the second part of the duodenum and inspect the papilla to exclude an ampullary tumour.
- Insert the perfusion catheter into the duodenum until all the rings are outside the endoscope. Zero the catheter in the duodenum (Fig. 1).
- Cannulate the CBD, obtain a cholangiogram to exclude other causes for pain, and determine the diameter of the CBD.
- Achieve deep cannulation with the catheter. Ensure that it is not impacted against the wall. Withdraw the catheter unit – the first ring is visible outside the papilla. Maintain this position for 30 seconds while obtaining manometric readings. Repeat this maneuver at each ring.
- A minimum of two catheter withdrawals (pull throughs) are made.

- Contrast present in the biliary tree after 45 min is considered delayed drainage; however, this is rarely performed.

Pancreatic sphincter of Oddi manometry is performed in the same manner as biliary manometry.

2.2. Interpretation of sphincter of Oddi manometry results

> A diagnosis of SOD is made on a basal SO pressure elevation of >40 mm in multiple leads which is sustained for at least 30 seconds.

2.3. Complications of SOD

Patients with SOD have a higher risk of acute pancreatitis of up to 31% compared with patients undergoing ERCP for other indications. A large, multicentre study of 2347 patients, found the pancreatitis rate was highest (21.7%) in patients with sphincter of Oddi dysfunction, and lowest in patients whose indication was bile-duct stone removal (4.9%). Given the increased risk of pancreatitis, it is important ensure that the catheter is correctly positioned and avoid prolonged perfusion of the pancreatic duct. A pancreatic duct stent should also be inserted following completion of the procedure as this has been shown to decrease the risk of pancreatitis in some studies.

Further Reading

Behar J, Corazziari E, Guelrud M, et al: Functional gallbladder and sphincter of Oddi disorders, *Gastroenterology* 130(5):1498–1509, 2006.

Chen YK, Foliente RL, Santoro MJ, et al: Endoscopic sphincterotomy-induced pancreatitis: increased risk associated with nondilated bile ducts and sphincter of Oddi dysfunction, *Am J Gastroenterol* 89:327–333, 1994.

Fogel EL, Eversman D, Jamidar P, et al: Sphincter of Oddi dysfunction: pancreaticobiliary sphincterotomy with pancreatic stent placement has a lower rate of pancreatitis than biliary sphincterotomy alone, *Endoscopy* 34:280–285, 2002.

Freeman ML, Nelson DB, Sherman S, et al: Complications of endoscopic biliary sphincterotomy, *N Engl J Med* 335:909–918, 1996.

Sherman S, Ruffolo TA, Hawes RH, et al: Complications of endoscopic sphincterotomy: a prospective series with emphasis on the increased risk associated with sphincter of Oddi dysfunction and nondilated bile ducts, *Gastroenterology* 101:1068–1075, 1991.

Tarnasky P, Cunningham J, Cotton P, et al: Pancreatic sphincter hypertension increases the risk of post-ERCP pancreatitis, *Endoscopy* 29:252–257, 1997.

10.19 **Nasobiliary drain insertion**

Summary

Introduction   459

1. Indications   459

2. Equipment   459

3. Technique   459

4. Complications   460

Key Points

- Nasobiliary drain (NBD) is an important technique to be aware of.
- It is most commonly used in cases of cholangitis, when there is incomplete clearance of bile duct stones.
- Nasobiliary drains are contraindicated in patients who are uncooperative or confused.
- Fluoroscopy is required to ensure that the drain remains in place while the duodenoscope is withdrawn.

Introduction

The use of a nasobiliary drain (NBD) has become rare and has been replaced by stent insertion. Two indications remain for nasobiliary drain: the presence of an intrahepatic abscess and extracorporeal lithotripsy.

1. Indications

The indications for insertion of a nasobiliary drain include:

- Cholangitis.
   A common indication is obstructive jaundice secondary to a stricture with cholangitis.
- CBD stones
   - With cholangitis: in critically ill patients, a NBD is sometimes initially inserted, with stone removal later
   - Incomplete clearance of CBD stones to prevent cholangitis
   - If it is unclear if duct has been cleared (i.e. stones), a repeat cholangiogram can be obtained
- Papillary edema. After papillary dilatation for stone extraction.
- Drainage
   - Intrahepatic abscess
   - Bile leak
   - Hemobilia
- Lavage of the bile duct to facilitate the removal of stones
- To facilitate cholangiography for extracorporeal lithotripsy with fluoroscopic guidance for targeting
- Infusion if necessary of substances to dissolve stones
- Alternative to stent insertion.

2. Equipment

- Nasobiliary drain: Nasobiliary drains are made of polyethylene. They are 250 cm in length, and have an external diameter ranging from 5 Fr to 10 Fr. They have a preformed duodenal loop for anchoring it in the bile duct. 5–6 Fr are used if the drain is being inserted into the intrahepatic ducts. Nasobiliary drains come with a straight or pigtail distal end which can be an alfa or contra-alfa loop. The drain has several lateral orifices at the distal end for the effective drainage of the bile duct, and is radio-opaque so that its position can be monitored. Sometimes cutting the distal end of the drain can make it easier to insert.
- Guidewire: Manipulation of the drain is facilitated by a guidewire, which must be at least 400 cm long due to the length of the drain. The guidewire is used to straighten the curves and facilitate insertion in the bile duct.

3. Technique

- The nasobiliary drain should be inserted deep in the bile duct as far as the hilum. If there are problems inserting the nasobiliary drain directly in the bile duct, a guidewire can be placed and the nasobiliary drain inserted over the guidewire.
- The nasobiliary drain is usually inserted following a sphincterotomy, however, it can be inserted without a prior sphincterotomy.
- The guidewire is then withdrawn, allowing the drain to regain its initial shape in the duodenum and bile duct.
- The duodenoscope is removed under fluoroscopic control, leaving the drain in position (Fig. 1).
- The nasobiliary drain now needs to be moved from the mouth to the nose (Fig. 2).
   - Insert a tube through the nose in the same manner that you would insert a nasogastric tube. The tube is designed to curve from the nose into the oral cavity where it is retrieved. When this does not happen, use a laryngoscope and McGill forceps to visualize and retrieve the tube. The tube is now brought out through the mouth (Fig. 2A).
   - The nasobiliary drain is inserted into the tube (Fig. 2B).
   - The tube, with the nasobiliary drain attached, is then gently pulled out of the nose (Fig. 2C).
- The drain is stitched to the bridge of the nose. This is the most effective means of preventing the drain being moved either voluntarily or involuntarily.

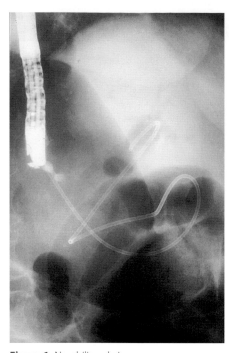

Figure 1 Nasobiliary drain.

A drain may be left in position for several days to weeks. It is well tolerated and allows the patient to eat normally.

4. Complications

Unsuccessful attempts to insert a drain are rare but may be due to severe post-sphincterotomy hemorrhage preventing the biliary orifice being located, or to large, numerous stones preventing the drain reaching the hilum. Spontaneous or accidental migration used to occur when simple Teflon catheters were used. Migration is rare with modern drains owing to the duodenal pre-curve.

Complications are rare but include pharyngeal and abdominal discomfort, diarrhea, vomiting, particularly after infusion of solution to dissolve stones, and aspiration pneumonia. A nasobiliary drain should not be inserted in a patient with altered consciousness. Ensure that the patient is alert and cooperative before using the nasogastric tube for lavage.

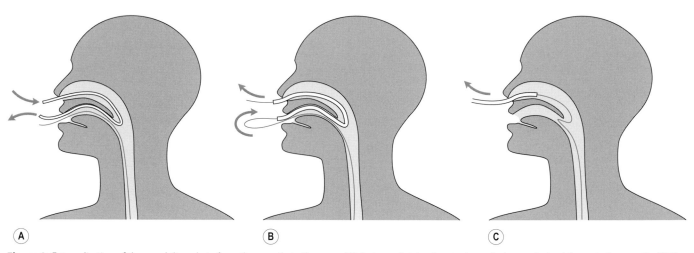

(A) (B) (C)

Figure 2 Externalization of the nasobiliary drain from the mouth to the nose. (A) A stomach tube, inserted nasally, is exteriorized through the mouth. (B) The nasobiliary drain is inserted into the stomach tube. (C) The stomach tube is retrieved with the nasobiliary drain through the nose.

Further Reading

Itoi T, Sofuni A, Itokawa F, et al: Role of endoscopic nasobiliary drainage indication and basic technique, *Dig Endosc* 18:S105–S109, 2006.

10.20 Complications of ERCP

Key Points

- The commonest cause of post-ERCP complications is cardiopulmonary.
- Always ensure that the ERCP is indicated.
- Endoscopist experience, as well as patient and procedure factors, are related to the risk of complications.
- Complications are graded as mild, moderate or severe, based on consensus guidelines.

Introduction

It is essential for any ERCPist to be aware of potential complications and methods to decrease their risk. The commonest complication following endoscopic retrograde cholangiopancreatography (ERCP) is cardiopulmonary. ERCP-related complications include pancreatitis, bleeding, perforation, sepsis, and death (Table 1). Complications are graded as mild, moderate or severe (Table 2) based on consensus guidelines.

Clinical Tips

- Retroperitoneal is seen in up to 30% of patients post sphincterotomy.
- Elevated amylase levels occur in up to 75% of patient post ERCP. Clinical correlation is important.

1. Pancreatitis

Post-ERCP pancreatitis complicates between 1.9 and 5.4% of ERCP procedures. The majority of cases are mild or moderate with a 0.4% of severe pancreatitis, with an 0.04% risk of death. Elevated amylase levels (up to 600 IU/L) are common, occurring in up to 75% of patients, and are not indicative of pancreatitis. A commonly used definition of post-ERCP pancreatitis is a three-fold rise in the serum amylase 24 h post-procedure, associated with abdominal pain requiring hospitalization.

Risk factors for pancreatitis can be divided into endoscopist, patient, and procedure-related factors (Table 3). It is important to realize that risk factors are additive. There are several potential methods of decreasing the risk of pancreatitis, including:

- Adequate training of the endoscopist is a very important factor in decreasing the risk of pancreatitis
- Adequate case volume to acquire and maintain experience
- Avoidance of diagnostic ERCP when an alternative and less invasive method is available (i.e. MRCP)
- Avoidance of pancreatic duct cannulation if not indicated
- Limited cannulation time to avoid trauma to the papilla
- Limited injection number and volume of contrast to avoid pancreatic overfilling
- Use of endocut I effect 1 (Table 1 in Chapter 1.4) or pure cutting current, especially when performing pancreatic sphincterotomy
- Insertion of plastic stent in high-risk patients (sphincter of Oddi, post-pancreatic sphincterotomy).

2. Bleeding

Sphincterotomy is the major cause of ERCP-related bleeding. The risk of bleeding post-sphincterotomy is 2% with 0.1% mortality. Bleeding can occur up to 10 days post-ERCP, with 50% occurring immediately post-sphincterotomy. Bleeding is graded as mild, moderate or severe (Table 2). Anatomical, patient, and technical risk factors have been identified (Table 4). In contrary, arterial supply of the papilla cannot be identified. (See Ch. 10.8, Fig. 9).

Most acute bleeding following sphincterotomy stops spontaneously. In cases where bleeding continues, initial management includes spraying with adrenaline (epinephrine) (1/10 000), followed by injection of adrenaline (epinephrine) into the papilla between 10 and 12 o'clock. Hemoclips can be used for more significant bleeding. Electrocautery

Box 1 Three types of perforation occur in ERCP

- Retroperitoneal duodenal perforation.
- Perforation of the bile ducts.
- Free bowel wall perforation of the duodenum.

Table 1 Risk of complications associated with ERCP

Complication	Risk (%)
Pancreatitis	1.9–5.4
Bleeding	2–3
Sepsis	1.4–1.7
Perforation	0.3–1
Other	0.3–1.1
Death	0.4–1.3

Data from Cotton, PB et al 1991; 37:383. Freeman et al 1996, Rabenstein et al 1998.

Warning!

- Always ensure that an obstructed biliary system is adequately drained.
- 87% of patients with incomplete drainage develop cholangitis.

can also be used. A biliary balloon can be used to tamponade the bleeding site. This is done by inserting the balloon into the common bile duct, inflating the balloon, and then withdrawing it to the papilla. Deflate the balloon after a few minutes if the bleeding has ceased. In cases of refractor bleeding angiography with embolization can be attempted, while surgery is undertaken if all other measures have failed. Of note, some authors recommend completing a sphincterotomy, despite bleeding, as this may have a beneficial effect on allowing full retraction of a partially severed vessel.

The risk of bleeding can be decreased by proper assessment of patients prior to ERCP. Discontinuation of anticoagulation (warfarin 3–5 days, clopidogrel 7 days, low molecular weight heparin/heparin) prior to the procedure as well as ensuring that clotting (INR <1.3) and platelet count (>50 000) are sufficient prior to sphincterotomy (see Ch. 2.1).

3. Sepsis

Sepsis-related complications include ascending cholangitis, acute cholecystitis, liver abscess, infected pancreatic pseudocyst, and peritonitis. Endocarditis can occur, but is uncommon. Ascending cholangitis is the most common septic complication, with a particularly high risk in patients with an obstructed biliary tree, which is inadequately drained. Patients with an undrained obstructed biliary tree should receive prophylactic antibiotics, as should patients with a pancreatic pseudocyst (see Ch. 2.2).

4. Perforation

ERCP-related perforation can be retroperitoneal duodenal perforation, perforation of the bile duct or free bowel wall perforation of the duodenum (Fig. 1). Retroperitoneal duodenal perforation is the most common, often occurring after a sphincterotomy extends past the intramural portion of the bile duct. Perforation of the bile duct is rarer, and can occur following dilation, particularly when performed in the setting of malignancy. Guidewire perforation can also occur. Free bowel wall perforation is rare and is associated with ERCP undertaken in patients with altered anatomy, such as Billroth II. It can also occur in the presence of a peri-ampullary diverticulum. Esophageal, gastric and jejuna perforation have also been reported.

It is important to think about possible perforation in a post-ERCP patient who is unwell as swift identification and appropriate management is important. An AXR and erect CXR should be performed, followed by a CT abdomen, which is the most sensitive method of detecting perforation,

Table 2 Consensus guidelines for grading severity of post-ERCP complications

	Mild	Moderate	Severe
Bleeding	Clinical evidence of bleeding (i.e. not just endoscopic) Hb drop <3 g No need for transfusion	≤4 units transfused No angiographic intervention or surgery	≥5 units transfused Medical treatment >10 days or Surgical or percutaneous intervention
Perforation	Very slight leak of contrast Resolved ≤3 days with medical management	Definite perforation Resolved with medical treatment between 4 and 10 days	Medical treatment >10 days or Percutaneous or surgical intervention
Pancreatitis	Amylase ×3 normal at >24 h post-procedure Requires hospital admission ≤3 days	Hospitalization 4–10 days	Hospitalization >10 days or Hemorrhagic pancreatitis, phlegmon, or pseudocyst or Intervention (drainage or surgery)
Cholangitis	Temp >38°C for 24–48 h	Hospitalization >3 days due to septic illness or intervention (endoscopic or percutaneous)	Septic shock or surgery
Basket impaction	Basket released spontaneously or by repeat endoscopy	Percutaneous intervention	Surgery

From PB Cotton et al. Endosocpic sphincterotomy complications & their management: an attempt at consensus. GIE 1991; 37: 383–93.

Table 3 Risk factors associated with post-ERCP pancreatitis

Patient related factors	Non-dilated duct
	Younger age
	Normal bilirubin
	Pre-existing pancreatitis or history of post-ERCP pancreatitis
	Sphincter of Oddi dysfunction
Procedure related factors	Sphincterotomy
	Pre-cut sphincterotomy
	Pancreatic sphincterotomy
	Biliary sphincteroplasty (dilation of sphincter of Oddi)
	Difficult cannulation (prolonged or repeated)
	Acinarization due to overfilling of the pancreatic duct with contrast
	Repeated injection of contrast into the pancreatic duct
	Sphincter of Oddi manometry

From Roger Williams, BSG 2006 Complications of Endoscopy (available on the BSG website).

if doubt exists. Management is determined by the type of perforation and clinical picture. Retroperitoneal air is a common finding (up to 75%) in patients post-sphincterotomy. In patients who are clinically asymptomatic, conservative management (nil PO, IV fluids, IV antibiotics) and observation are usually successful. Retroperitoneal perforation is also usually successfully managed with conservative treatment (nil PO, IV fluids, IV antibiotics, nasogastric or duodenal suction). In contrast, patients with free bowel wall perforation, or perforation of the esophagus, stomach or jejunum, usually require surgery.

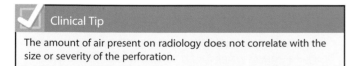

Clinical Tip

The amount of air present on radiology does not correlate with the size or severity of the perforation.

5. Impacted basket

Impacted basket occurs less frequently due to lithotripsy; however, it is important to be aware of their management should it occur. The first step is to withdraw the endoscope gradually and firmly, maintaining firm traction on the basket so that the endoscope and basket are integral. This may allow the stone to pass through the sphincterotomy orifice. If this fails, advance the endoscope so that the tip of the endoscope is against the papilla. Force the basket into the operating channel. The basket will close as it is withdrawn into the operating channel, crushing the stones

(See Ch. 10.12, Fig. 4). If this is unsuccessful, the basket should be attached to a lithotripter and the stones crushed (see Ch. 10.17). Other options include extending the sphincterotomy, intra- or extracorporeal lithotripsy. If a Dormia basket remains impacted in the sphincterotomy, and lithotripsy equipment is not available, a nasobiliary drain should be inserted (see Ch. 10.19). The Dormia catheter is exteriorized like the nasobiliary drain. By pulling on it slightly every day, the stone and the Dormia become disimpacted within 48–72 h, when the edema around the sphincterotomy subsides.

6. Stent-related complications

Complications occur with both plastic and SEMS stents which are summarized below.

6.1. Plastic biliary stent complications

- Pancreatitis.
  This is reported to occur more frequently in patients undergoing biliary stent placement for proximal biliary strictures. Sphincterotomy may reduce this risk by relieving stent-related compression of the pancreatic orifice.
- Stent migration.
  This occurs in between 1.7% and 10% of stents, with proximal migration more common in malignant strictures, and distal migration in benign stricture.

Table 4 Risk factors associated with bleeding

Anatomical factors	Billroth II partial gastrectomy
	Peri-ampullary diverticulum
	Stenosis of the ampulla of Vater
	Impacted common bile duct stone
Patient related factors	Coagulopathic
	Anti-coagulation within 3 days of the procedure
	Child's grade C cirrhosis
	Renal failure with hemodialysis
	Bleeding during the procedure
	Bleeding as an indication for the procedure (i.e. attempted hemostasis)
	Preceding cholangitis
Procedure related factors	Length of the sphincterotomy made
	Extension of a prior sphincterotomy
	Uncontrolled sphincterotomy (zipper cut)
	Needle knife sphincterotomy
	Low case volume

From Roger Williams, BSG 2006 Complications of Endoscopy (available on the BSG website).

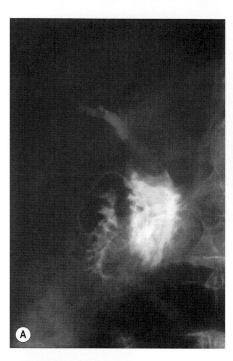
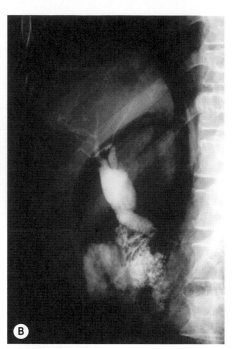
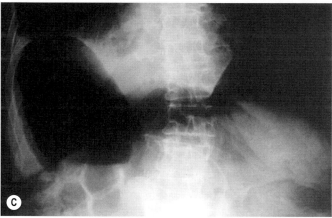

Figure 1 Perforation. (A) Leak of contrast medium around the lower common bile duct. (B) Retropneumoperitoneum: triangular area of radiolucency surrounding the right kidney. (C) Pneumoperitoneum.

- Rare complications include perforation secondary to the passage of the stent in the portal vein or perforation of the duodenal wall by the lower end of the stent. This is possible if the stent is too long and too rigid.
- Cholecystitis is rare. It occurs as a result of secondary obstruction of the cystic duct by the stent or by tumor growth.
- Late stent occlusion (defined as occurring >30 days post-ERCP). This is due to bacterial infection and biofilm/sludge adhesion or due to tumor ingrowth in patients with cancer.
- Cholangitis associated with failed or inadequate stent position or stent occlusion. Cholangitis is far commoner in cases of hilar stenosis because it is difficult to insert two stents endoscopically to drain both lobes effectively with a Bismuth Type II or III stricture. Any segment which has been accessed must be drained in these patients. Percutaneous stenting can complete or replace failure of endoscopic stenting.

Box 2 Retrieving migrated plastic stents

- Some 80–90% of migrated bile duct stents can be successfully retrieved endoscopically.
- If the stent is still visible, gently grasp the end of the stent with either a snare or a large (i.e. rat-tooth) forceps. Take care when grasping the stent, not to push it further up the duct.
- Insert a guidewire above the stent. Then insert a balloon over the wire. Inflate the balloon beside the distal end of the stent. If the stent has migrated within a stricture or in a non-dilated bile duct, the balloon can be inflated above the stent and then gently retracted towards the duodenum.
- If this fails, a snare or a basket can be placed around the distal end of the stent, and then gently withdrawn into the duodenum.
- A closed biopsy forceps can be passed through the stent and then opened once it is outside the proximal end of the stent and gently withdrawn into the duodenum.
- If it is not possible to retrieve the stent, a second stent can be placed and a repeat attempt made at a later date.

6.2. Complications of biliary SEMS

- Early cholangitis is rare due to the quality of drainage achieved (as with other drainage methods, some cases of existing cholangitis persist despite correct drainage)
- Stent migration
- Hemorrhage due to erosion of the duodenal wall over the stent
- Secondary obstruction.

SEMS can obstruct due to tumor infiltration through or outside the stent. SEMS become blocked less often and more slowly than plastic stents. In cases of benign stenosis, obstruction is possible due to the appearance of inflammatory granuloma. These tissue obstructions can be treated by inserting a metal stent or a plastic stent in the metal stent or by various local techniques such as APC.

6.3. Plastic pancreatic stent complications

Immediate complications include pancreatitis, bleeding and ductal rupture. Late complications include stent occlusion, which will occur in 50% of stents at 6 weeks, and 100% at 9 weeks. Stent migration, pancreatitis, duct disruption, injury or structuring. Changes can occur in the pancreatic duct including dilation of side branches, duct narrowing and ductal irregularity due to stent placement. These have been reported to occur in between 36% and 80% of patients and persist after stent removal in 30%. Using smaller diameter stent and those without side flanges may decrease the risk.

7. Papillary stenosis

There is a 1–4% risk of papillary stenosis following endoscopic sphincterotomy. This occurs when the initial sphincterotomy is small, with subsequent fibrosis and stenosis. Stenting or balloon dilation is often successful.

8. Contrast allergy

Contrast allergy is rare; however, patients with a known sensitivity should be premedicated with oral steroids the day before ERCP or IV steroids the day of the procedure and non-ionic or low osmolarity contrast media should be used.

9. Other complications

Many other complications have been reported, including injection of contrast into the portal vein, hepatic or superior mesenteric artery, duodenal pneumatosis following sphincterotomy, pneumothorax, pneumomediastinum, and pneumoperitoneum, all of which can occur following perforation, while pneumothorax has been reported following ERCP without perforation. Other rare complications include portal vein gas or air embolism; hemorrhage from trauma to the spleen or liver or vascular trauma; acute angle glaucoma can occur in patients given anticholinergics.

Further Reading

Chapman RW: Complications of ERCP. BSG Guidelines in gastroenterology. www.bsg.org.uk/clinical-guidelines/endoscopy/index.html.

Cotton PB, Garrow DA, Gallagher J, et al: Risk factors for complications after ERCP: a multivariate analysis of 11,497 procedures over 12 years, *Gastrointest Endosc* 70:80–88, 2009.

Cotton PB, Lehman G, Vennes J, et al: Endoscopic sphincterotomy complications and their management: an attempt at consensus, *Gastrointest Endosc* 37:383–393, 1991.

Freeman ML, Nelson DB, Sherman S, et al: Complications of endoscopic biliary sphincterotomy, *N Engl J Med* 335:909, 1996.

Okabe Y, Tsuruta O, Kaji R, et al: Endoscopic retrieval of migrated plastic stent into bile duct or pancreatic pseudocyst, *Dig Endosc* 21:1–7, 2009.

Singh P, Das A, Isenberg G, et al: Does prophylactic pancreatic stent placement reduce the risk of post-ERCP acute pancreatitis? A meta-analysis of controlled trials, *Gastrointest Endosc* 60(4):544–550, 2004.

Index

Page numbers followed by 'f' indicate figures, 't' indicate tables and 'b' indicate boxes.